Anna L Macdonald.

D1422431

Anna L Macdonald.

ORAL HISTOLOGY
Development, Structure, and Function

ORAL HISTOLOGY
Development, Structure, and Function

A.R. Ten Cate, B.D.S., B.Sc., Ph.D.
Vice-Provost, Health Sciences
Professor of Dentistry
Faculty of Dentistry
University of Toronto
Toronto, Canada

FOURTH EDITION

with 812 illustrations

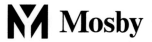 Mosby

St. Louis Baltimore Boston Chicago London Madrid Philadelphia Sydney Toronto

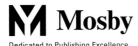
Mosby
Dedicated to Publishing Excellence

Editor-in-Chief: Don Ladig
Executive Editor: Linda L. Duncan
Developmental Editor: Melba Steube
Project Manager: John Rogers
Production Editor: George B. Stericker, Jr.
Production: Graphic World Publishing Services
Manufacturing Supervisor: Karen Lewis
Designer: Julie Taugner
Cover Design: Elizabeth Rohne Rudder

FOURTH EDITION

Printed in the United States of America
Composition by Graphic World, Inc.
Printing/binding by Maple-Vail Book Mfg Group, Binghamton

Mosby–Year Book, Inc.
11830 Westline Industrial Drive
St. Louis, Missouri 63146

Library of Congress Cataloging in Publication Data
Ten Cate, A. R. (Arnold Richard)
  Oral histology : development, structure, and function / A.R. Ten
Cate. —4th ed.
    p.   cm.
  Includes bibliographical references and index.
  ISBN 0-8016-7966-4
  1. Teeth—Histology. 2. Mouth—Histology.   I. Title.
  [DNLM: 1. Mouth—anatomy & histology. 2. Dentition. 3. Mouth—
physiology.   WU 101 T289o 1994]
  RK280.T46 1994
  611′.31—dc20
  DNLM/DLC
  for Library of Congress   93-33602
                                                  CIP

94 95 96 97 98 / 9 8 7 6 5 4 3 2 1

Contributors

Anne Carlyle Dale, B.A., D.D.S.

Associate Professor, Faculty of Dentistry
University of Toronto
Toronto, Canada

Jack G. Dale, D.D.S.

Associate Professor, Faculty of Dentistry
University of Toronto
Toronto, Canada

Dale R. Eisenmann, D.D.S., Ph.D.

Professor, Department of Oral Biology
University of Illinois at Chicago
College of Dentistry
Chicago, Illinois

Richard P. Ellen, D.D.S.

Professor, Faculty of Dentistry
University of Toronto
Toronto, Canada

Donald H. Enlow, M.S., Ph.D.

Thomas Hill Distinguished Professor Emeritus
Department of Orthodontics
Case Western Reserve University
Cleveland, Ohio

Eric Freeman, D.D.S., M.Sc.D.

Professor, Faculty of Dentistry
University of Toronto
Toronto, Canada

Murray W. Hill, Ph.D.

Professor, Faculty of Dentistry
University of Western Australia
Perth, Australia

Christopher A. Squier, M.A., Ph.D., D.Sc., F.R.C.Path.

Professor, Assistant Dean for Research and Director
Dows Institute for Dental Research
College of Dentistry
University of Iowa
Iowa City, Iowa

A. R. Ten Cate, B.D.S., B.Sc., Ph.D.

Professor, Faculty of Dentistry
University of Toronto
Toronto, Canada

Calvin D. Torneck, D.D.S., M.S., F.R.C.D.(C)

Professor, Faculty of Dentistry
University of Toronto
Toronto, Canada

S. William Whitson, Ph.D.

Professor, Department of Biomedical Sciences
Southern Illinois University School of Dental
  Medicine
Alton, Illinois

Preface

THE interval between editions of this book is approximately four years, and the student using the text may question whether the advances in the subject are of a pace sufficient to warrant continued new editions, especially as the book is designed for use by undergraduate students learning the subject matter for the first time.

I believe it is essential that the undergraduate student be exposed to current data in a straightforward manner. To do otherwise denies recognition that dentistry is a profession rooted in a university setting that demands the advancement of knowledge.

Each year at the annual meeting of the International Association for Dental Research some 2500 papers are presented, which totals 10,000 papers between editions of this book. Many papers, of course, are not concerned with the structure and function of the dental tissue, but sufficient are, and therefore justify the four-year cycle in publication. New illustrative material has been added, but it is the text that has changed the most to reflect new knowledge and ideas. I am hopeful that the delicate balance between maintaining currency, the ex-position of controversy, and the provision of basic data has been presented in this edition in such a way as to benefit the undergraduate student.

A.R. Ten Cate

ACKNOWLEDGMENTS

In the 16 years since this book was first conceived, I have never had a denial from colleagues to publish their material. They have always been most cooperative and their assistance is acknowledged by referencing the source material. However, for this edition, I would like to acknowledge the special assistance of Professor Irma Thesleff, University of Helsinki, who helped me explain the rapidly developing field of cytokines as they relate to dental development, and to Drs. Antonio Nanci and Marc McKee, University of Montreal, for constructive comments on the subject of amelogenesis.

Contents

1 **General Embryology,** 1
A.R. Ten Cate

2 **Embryology of the Head, Face, and Oral Cavity,** 15
A.R. Ten Cate

3 **Structure of the Oral Tissues,** 45
A.R. Ten Cate

4 **Development of the Tooth and Its Supporting Tissues,** 58
A.R. Ten Cate

5 **Fibroblasts and Their Products,** 81
A.R. Ten Cate

6 **Epithelial-Mesenchymal Relations,** 100
A.R. Ten Cate

7 **Hard Tissue Formation and Destruction,** 111
A.R. Ten Cate

8 **Bone,** 120
S.W. Whitson

9 **Dentinogenesis,** 147
A.R. Ten Cate

10 **Dentin-Pulp Complex,** 169
C.D. Torneck

11 **Amelogenesis,** 218
D.R. Eisenmann

12 **Enamel Structure,** 239
D.R. Eisenmann

13 **Development of the Periodontium,** 257
A.R. Ten Cate

14 **Periodontium,** 276
E. Freeman

15 **Physiological Tooth Movement: Eruption and Shedding,** 313
A.R. Ten Cate

16 **Surface Coatings of the Teeth,** 342
R. Ellen

17 **Salivary Glands,** 356
A.C. Dale

18 **Oral Mucosa,** 389
C.A. Squier, M.W. Hill

19 **Temporomandibular Joint,** 432
A.R. Ten Cate

20 **Repair and Regeneration of Dental Tissue,** 456
A.R. Ten Cate

21 **Childhood Facial Growth and Development,** 469
D.H. Enlow, J.G. Dale

ORAL HISTOLOGY
Development, Structure, and Function

CHAPTER 1

General Embryology

THIS first chapter covers enough general embryology to explain the development of the head, particularly the structures in and around the mouth. It provides a background for understanding the origins of the tissues associated with facial and dental development and helps clarify the etiology of many of the congenital defects that manifest themselves in these tissues.

GERM CELL FORMATION AND FERTILIZATION

The human somatic (body) cell contains 46 chromosomes, 46 being the diploid number for the cell. Two of these are sex chromosomes; the remainder are autosomes. Each chromosome is paired so that every cell has 22 homologous sets of paired autosomes, with one chromosome derived from the mother and one from the father. The sex chromosomes, designated X and Y, are paired XX in the female and XY in the male. Interestingly, the X and Y chromosomes contain the genes for enamel formation and the X-linked gene controls tooth size and tooth form.

Fertilization involves the fusion of male and female germ cells (the spermatozoa and ova, collectively called gametes) to form a zygote, which commences the formation of a new individual. Obviously, the fusion of two cells with 46 chromosomes each is not possible; if it were, a cell with 92 chromosomes would result, and in the next generation a cell with 184, and so on! Thus germ cells are required that have half as many chromosomes (the haploid number), so that on fertilization the original complement of 46 chromosomes will be reestablished in the new somatic cell. The process by which germ cells are produced with half the number of chromosomes of the somatic cell is called *meiosis*, as distinct from *mitosis* (which describes the division of somatic cells).

Before mitotic cell division begins, DNA is first replicated during the "S" (synthetic) phase of the cell cycle so that the amount of DNA is doubled to a value known as tetraploid (which is 4 times the amount of DNA found in the germ cell). During mitosis the chromosomes containing this tetraploid amount of DNA are split and distributed equally between the two resulting cells; thus they both have a diploid DNA quantity and chromosome number, which duplicates the parent cell exactly.

Meiosis, on the other hand, involves two sets of cell divisions occurring in quick succession. Before the first division, DNA is replicated to the tetraploid value as in mitosis. In the first division the number of chromosomes is halved so each daughter cell contains a diploid amount of DNA distributed in a haploid number of chromosomes. The second division involves the splitting and separation of the chromosomes; thus the final composition of each cell is haploid with respect to both its DNA value and its chromosome number.

Meiosis is introduced in this textbook because the process occasionally malfunctions, producing zygotes with an abnormal number of chromosomes and resulting in individuals with congenital defects that sometimes affect the mouth and teeth. An abnormal number of chromosomes can, for example, be brought about by the failure of a homologous chromosome pair to separate during meiosis, so that the daughter cells contain either 24 or 22 chromosomes. If, on fertilization, the gamete containing 24 chromosomes fuses with a normal gamete (containing 23), the resulting zygote will possess 47 chromosomes, with one homologous pair having a third component. Thus the cells are trisomic for a given pair of chromosomes. If, on the other hand, one member of the homologous chromosome pair is missing, a condition known as monosomy prevails. This condition is very rare. The best known example of trisomy is Down's syndrome, or trisomy 21 (formerly known as mongolism). Among features of Down's syndrome are facial clefts, a shortened palate, a protruding and fissured tongue, and delayed eruption of teeth. Other types of trisomy usually result in early death of the infant and are beyond the scope of this book. Trisomy and monosomy can also occur in relation to the sex chromosomes, but in such cases they rarely manifest themselves as dental defects.

About 10% of all human malformations are caused by an alteration in a single gene. Such alterations are transmitted in several ways, two of which are of special importance. First, if the malformation results from autosomal dominant inheritance, the affected gene is generally inherited from only one parent. The trait usually appears in every generation and can be transmitted by the affected parent to statistically half of the children. Examples of autosomal dominant conditions include achondroplasia, cleidocranial dysostosis, osteogenesis imperfecta, and some forms of amelogenesis imperfecta, with the latter two conditions resulting in abnormal formation of the dental hard tissues (Fig. 1-1). Second, when the malformation is due to autosomal recessive inheritance, the abnormal gene can express itself only when it is received from both parents. Examples of this condition include chondroectodermal dysplasia, some cases of microcephaly, and cystic fibrosis. Many other congenital malformations with a genetic basis exist but are beyond the scope of this book.

All the above conditions are examples of abnormalities in the genetic makeup or *genotype* of the individual and are classified as genetic defects. The expression of the genotype is affected by the environment in which the embryo develops, and the final outcome of development is termed the *phenotype*. Adverse factors in the environment can result in excessive deviation from a functional and accepted norm; and when this occurs, the outcome is described as a congenital defect. Teratology is the study of such developmental defects.

SOME GENERAL CONCEPTS

Before the events that follow fertilization are described in detail, it is important to state and grasp some important concepts associated with development.

Prenatal development occupies 10 lunar months. Precise timing of developmental events in humans is problematic because of the difficulty in determining the exact time of fertilization and because of variations in the rate of early development. Early development has been divided into 23 stages or horizons based on a combination of external features and the development of internal systems. Another, and perhaps more common, way of comparing embryos for descriptive purposes is to use a measurement known as the crown-rump (CR) length. This measurement, however, can be made only after the embryo assumes shape, at about 3 weeks of gestation.

Prenatal development is divided into three successive phases. The first two when combined constitute

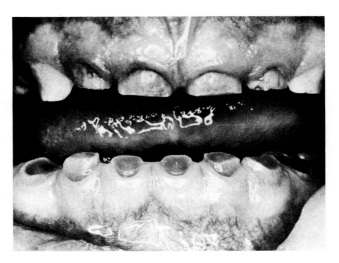

FIG. 1-1 Dentition of a child with dentinogenesis imperfecta, an autosomal dominant genetic defect. The dental tissues are poorly formed and rapidly lost to function. (Courtesy Dr. N. Levine.)

the *embryonic* stage, and the third is the *fetal* stage. The forming individual is described as an embryo or fetus depending on its developmental stage.

The first phase begins at fertilization and spans the first 4 weeks or so of development. It involves largely cellular proliferation and migration, with some differentiation of cell populations. Few congenital defects result from this period of development because, if the perturbation is severe, the embryo is lost. If less severe, the proliferative response can compensate by a process of cell renewal.

The second phase spans the next 4 weeks of development and is characterized largely by the differentiation of all major external and internal structures (morphogenesis). This is a particularly vulnerable period for the embryo because it involves many intricate embryologic processes; it is during this period that many recognized congenital defects develop.

From the end of the second phase to term, further development is largely a matter of growth and maturation, and the embryo is now called a fetus (Fig. 1-2).

INDUCTION, COMPETENCE, AND DIFFERENTIATION

Induction, competence, and differentiation are important concepts in embryology. All the cells of an individual stem from the zygote. Clearly, they have differentiated somehow into populations that have assumed particular functions, shapes, and rates of turnover. Such a population of cells is said to be compart-

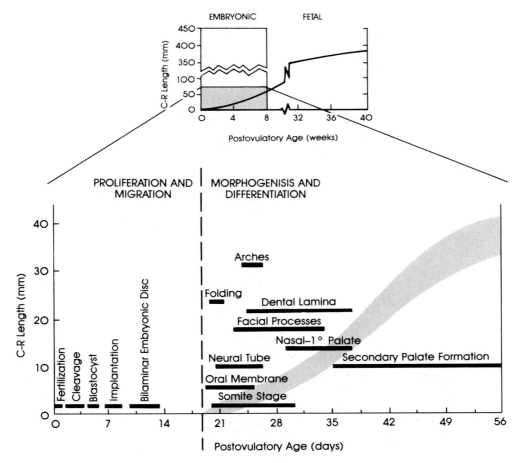

FIG. 1-2 Sequences of development. In the upper small diagram the distinction between embryonic and fetal stages is shown. The *shaded area* is expanded in the lower diagram, which distinguishes the stages of proliferation and migration and morphogenesis and differentiation. The timing of key events is also indicated. (Redrawn and modified from Waterman RE, and Meller SM: In Shaw J H, et al [eds]: *Textbook of oral biology,* Philadelphia, 1978, WB Saunders.)

mentalized; successive generations of cells in a given compartment may either remain constant or differentiate—that is, change their characteristics and establish a new population of cells. The process that initiates differentiation is termed induction; an inducer is the agent that "persuades" cells to be induced. Furthermore, each compartment of cells must be competent to respond to the induction process. There is evidence that over time populations of embryonic cells vary their competence, from no response to maximum response and then back to no response. In other words, there is a window of competence of varying duration for different populations of cells. The concepts of induction, competence, and differentiation apply in the development of the tooth and its supporting tissues and will be referred to often in later chapters. The whole question

of induction, competence, and differentiation revolves very much around cells' expressing their surface receptors at particular times. These receptors are able to capture and respond to a variety of influences (e.g., hormones) and locally produced molecules (e.g., transforming growth factor and other extracellular matrix substances), and their effects will be discussed further in Chapters 5 and 6.

FORMATION OF THE THREE-LAYERED EMBRYO

After fertilization, mammalian development involves a phase of rapid proliferation and migration of cells, with little or no differentiation. This proliferative phase lasts until three germ layers have formed. In summary:

The fertilized egg initially undergoes a series of rapid divisions leading to the formation of a ball of cells called the *morula*. Fluid seeps into the morula, and its cells realign themselves to form a fluid-filled hollow ball, the *blastocyst*. Within the blastocyst two cell populations can now be distinguished: those lining the cavity (the primary yolk sac), called *trophoblast* cells, and a small cluster within the cavity, called the inner cell mass or *embryoblast* (Fig. 1-3). The embryoblast cells form the embryo proper whereas the trophoblast cells are associated with implantation of the embryo and forma-tion of the placenta; they will not be considered fur-ther here.

The embryoblast rapidly differentiates so that at about 8 days a two-layered germ disk can be distin-guished. The upper or *ectodermal* layer forms the floor of a cavity (the amniotic cavity) that has developed within the embryoblast, and the lower or *endodermal* layer forms the roof of a second cavity (the secondary yolk sac) that develops from the migration of peripheral cells of the endodermal layer. This configuration, de-picted in Figure 1-4, is completed after 2 weeks of

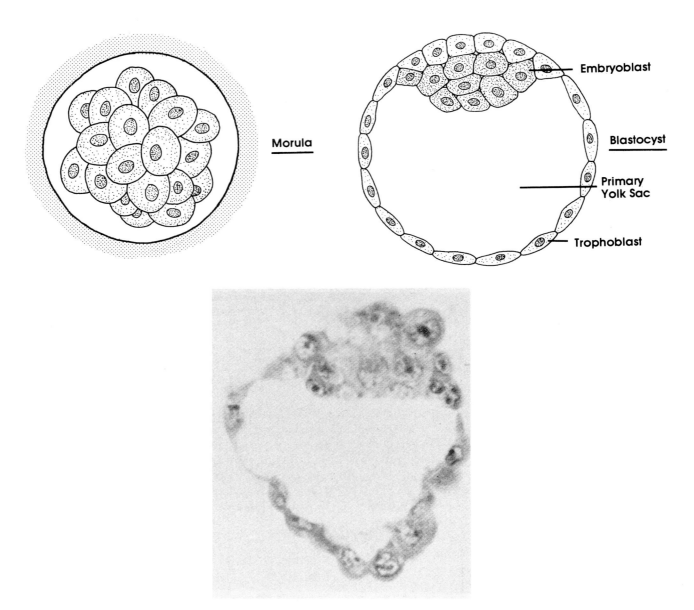

FIG. 1-3   Differentiation of the morula into a blastocyst. At this time cells differentiate into embryoblasts (involved in development of the embryo) and trophoblasts (involved in maintenance). (From Hertig AT, et al: *Contrib Embryol* 35:199, 1954.)

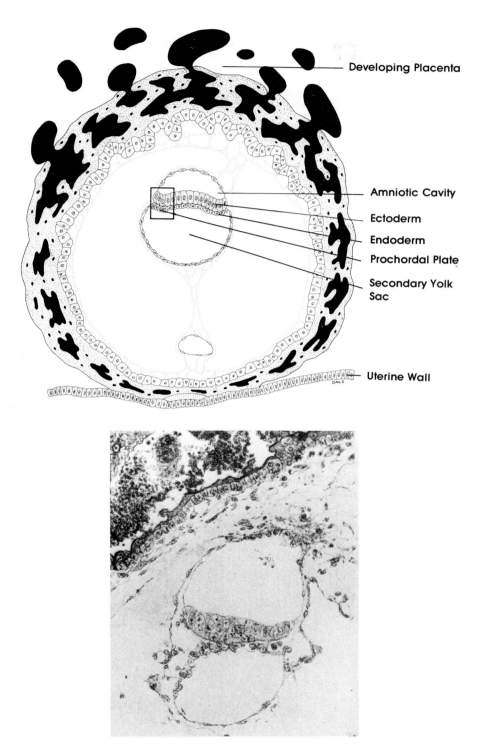

Developing Placenta

Amniotic Cavity

Ectoderm

Endoderm

Prochordal Plate

Secondary Yolk Sac

Uterine Wall

FIG. 1-4   Thirteen-day human blastocyst. An amniotic cavity has formed within the ectodermal layer. Proliferation of endodermal cells forms a secondary yolk sac. The bilaminar embryo is well established, and formation of the prochordal plate has given rise to the craniocaudal axis of the embryo. (From Brewer JI: *Contrib Embryol* 27:85, 1938.)

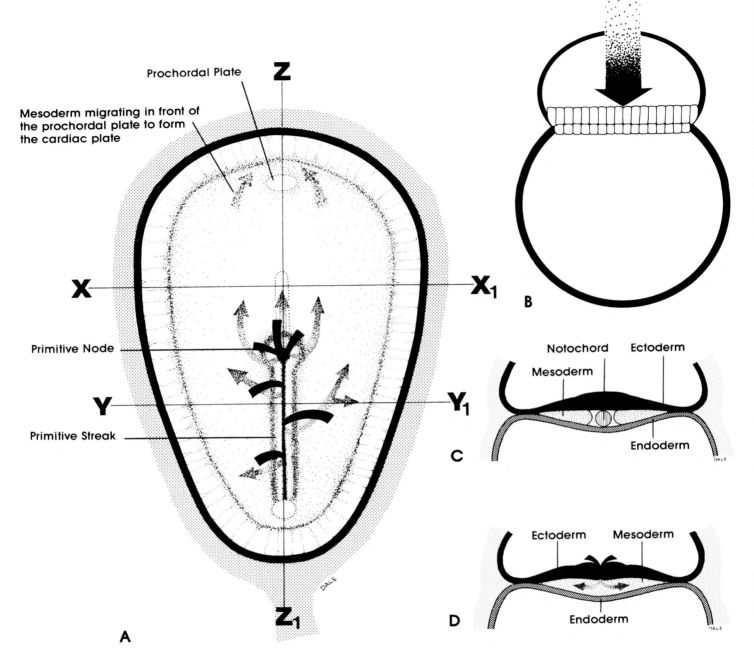

FIG. 1-5 Conversion of the bilaminar embryo into a tri-laminar embryo. **A** depicts the floor of the amniotic cavity, formed by ectodermal layer of the bilaminar embryo. **B** provides the orientation. The primitive streak is a narrow groove *(solid line along the Z-Z₁ axis)* terminating in a circular depression called the primitive node. Surface ectodermal cells migrate to the streak *(solid lines),* and mesodermal cells migrate from the streak *(shaded lines)* between the ectodermal and endodermal layers. A notochordal process extends forward from the primitive node. **C** is a transverse section through X-X₁ showing the notochord flanked by mesoderm. **D** is a section through Y-Y₁ is shown, and **E** a section through Z-Z₁.

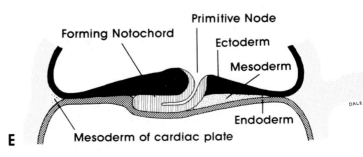

development. During that time the axis of the embryo is established and is represented by a slight enlargement of the ectodermal and endodermal cells at the head (or rostral) end of the embryo in a region known as the *prochordal plate*. At the prochordal plate there is firm union between the ectodermal and endodermal cells.

During the third week of development the bilaminar embryonic disk is converted to a trilaminar disk. As already described, the floor of the amniotic cavity is formed by ectoderm and within it, along the midline, a structure called the *primitive streak* develops (Fig. 1-5, *A*). This structure is a narrow groove with slightly bulging areas on each side. The rostral end of the streak finishes in a small depression called the primitive node, or pit. At the node, cells of the ectodermal layer divide and migrate between the ectoderm and endoderm to form a solid column that pushes forward in the midline as far as the prochordal plate. Through canalization of this cord of cells, the *notochord* is formed to support the primitive embryo (Fig. 1-5, *A*, *C*, and *E*). Elsewhere alongside the primitive streak, cells of the ectodermal layer divide and migrate toward the streak, where they invaginate and spread laterally between the ectodermal and endodermal layers to form a third layer of cells, the *mesoderm* (Fig. 1-5, *A* and *D*). As well as spreading laterally, cells spread progressively forward, passing on each side of the notochord and prochordal plate. The cells that accumulate anterior to the prochordal plate as a result of this migration give rise to the *cardiac plate*, the structure in which the heart forms (Fig. 1-5, *E*). As a result of these cell migrations, the notochord and mesoderm now completely separate the ectoderm from the endoderm (Fig. 1-5, *C*), except in

the region of the prochordal plate and in a similar area of fusion at the tail (caudal) end of the embryo, the cecal plate.

FORMATION OF THE NEURAL CREST AND FATE OF THE GERM LAYERS

The series of events leading to the formation of the three-layered, or triploblastic, embryo during the first 3 weeks of development has now been sketched. These initial events involve cell proliferation and migration. During the next 3 to 4 weeks of development, major tissues and organs differentiate from the triploblastic embryo. Included are the head and face and the tissues contributing to development of the teeth. Key events involve the differentiation of nervous system and neural crest tissues from the ectoderm, the differentiation of mesoderm, and the folding of the embryo in two planes along the rostrocaudal (head-tail) and lateral axes.

The nervous system develops as a thickening within the ectodermal layer at the rostral end of the embryo. This thickening constitutes the neural plate, which rapidly forms raised margins (the neural folds). These, in turn, encompass and delineate a deepening midline depression, the neural groove (Fig. 1-6). The neural folds eventually fuse so that a neural tube separates from the ectoderm forming the floor of the amniotic cavity, with mesoderm intervening. From the neural tube the brain and spinal cord develop. In avian embryos, which have been most extensively studied, a group of cells can be distinguished differentiating at the crest of the neural folds. These are the neural crest cells (Figs. 1-7 and 1-8). In mammalian embryos this same group of cells separate from the lateral aspect of the

Neural Groove
Neural Fold

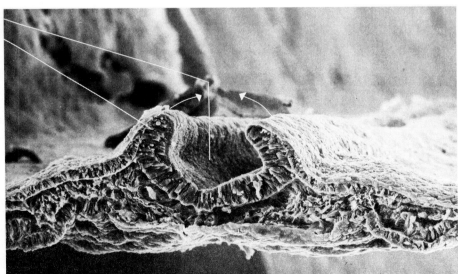

FIG. 1-6 Scanning electron micrograph of neural fold elevation. (From Tosney KW: *Dev Biol* 89:13, 1982.)

Neural Crest Cells

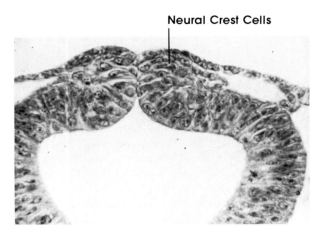

FIG. 1-7 Photomicrograph illustrating the origin and development of neural crest cells in the embryo. (From Noden DM: In Garrod DR [ed]: *Receptors and recognition: specificity of embryological interactions,* London, 1978, Chapman & Hall.)

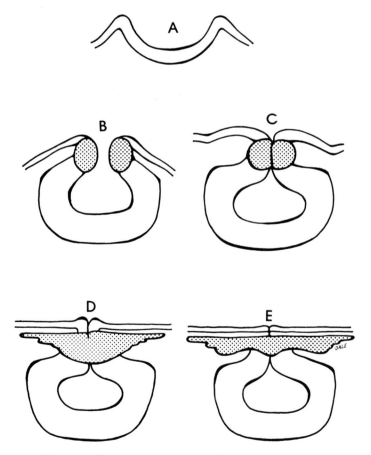

FIG. 1-8 Successive stages of development of the neural crest *(dotted area),* based on reconstructions from chick embryos. (From Tosney KW: *Dev Biol* 89:13, 1982.)

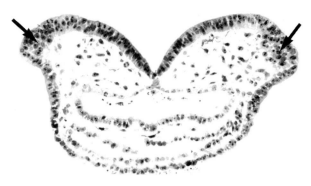

FIG. 1-9 Mouse embryo. Differentiation of neural crest cells *(arrows)* from the lateral aspect of the neural plate. (Courtesy Dr. AG Lumsden.)

neural plate (Fig. 1-9) rather than from its crest. Even so, the term *neural crest* has become entrenched and is retained here; however, this species difference does preclude a mixing of neural crest cells across the midline, as happens in avian embryos. These cells have the capacity to differentiate extensively within the developing embryo (Fig. 1-10), giving rise to a number of structures—the sensory ganglia, sympathetic neurons, Schwann cells, pigment cells, meninges, and cartilage of the branchial arches. They also form most of the embryonic connective tissue in the facial region. The contribution of neural crest cells is so extensive, and their contribution so significant, that they have been considered as a fourth germ layer. It is known that the migratory pattern of neural crest tissue is not intrinsic but rather is determined by the host tissues, which express factors that delineate the migratory pathway (Chapter 6).

In a dental context the proper migration of neural crest cells is essential for development of the face and teeth. In the Treacher-Collins syndrome (Fig. 1-11), for example, full facial development is prevented by an interference with the migration of neural crest cells to the facial region. All the tissues of the tooth (except enamel) and its supporting apparatus are derived directly from the neural crest, and their depletion will prevent proper dental development.

FOLDING OF THE EMBRYO

A crucial developmental event is the folding of the embryo in two planes, along the rostrocaudal axis and along the lateral axis (Fig. 1-12). The head fold is critical to the formation of a primitive *stomatodeum* or oral cavity, for it is through this fold that ectoderm comes to line the stomatodeum, with the stomatodeum being

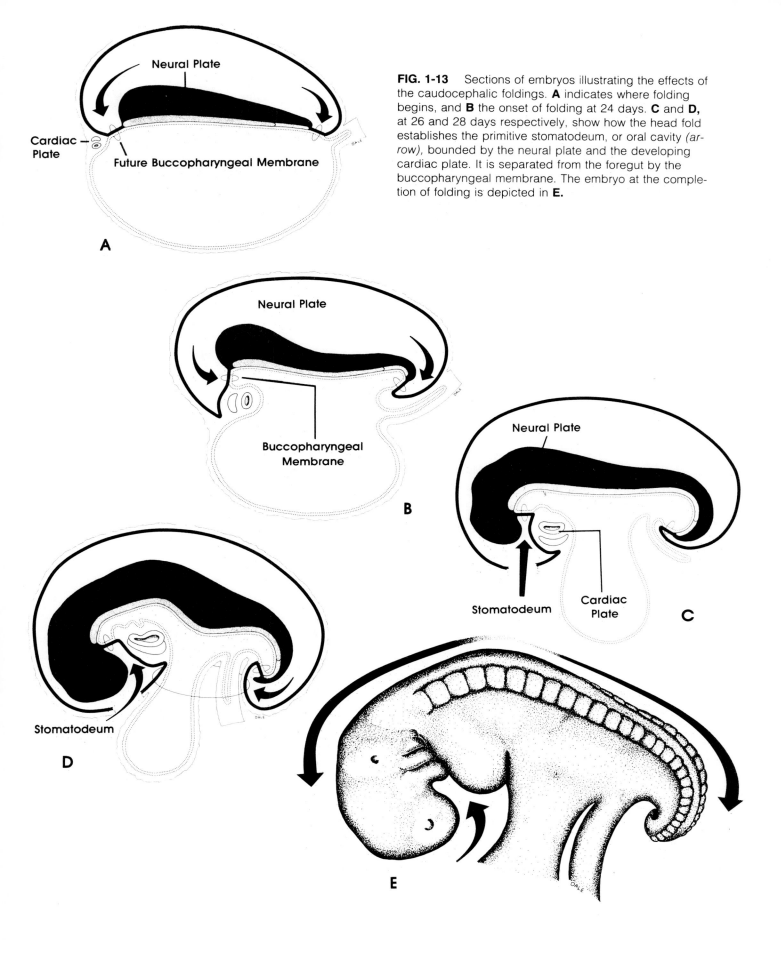

FIG. 1-13 Sections of embryos illustrating the effects of the caudocephalic foldings. **A** indicates where folding begins, and **B** the onset of folding at 24 days. **C** and **D,** at 26 and 28 days respectively, show how the head fold establishes the primitive stomatodeum, or oral cavity *(arrow),* bounded by the neural plate and the developing cardiac plate. It is separated from the foregut by the buccopharyngeal membrane. The embryo at the completion of folding is depicted in **E.**

Neural Plate

Cardiac Plate

Future Buccopharyngeal Membrane

A

Neural Plate

Buccopharyngeal Membrane

B

Neural Plate

Stomatodeum

Cardiac Plate

C

Stomatodeum

D

E

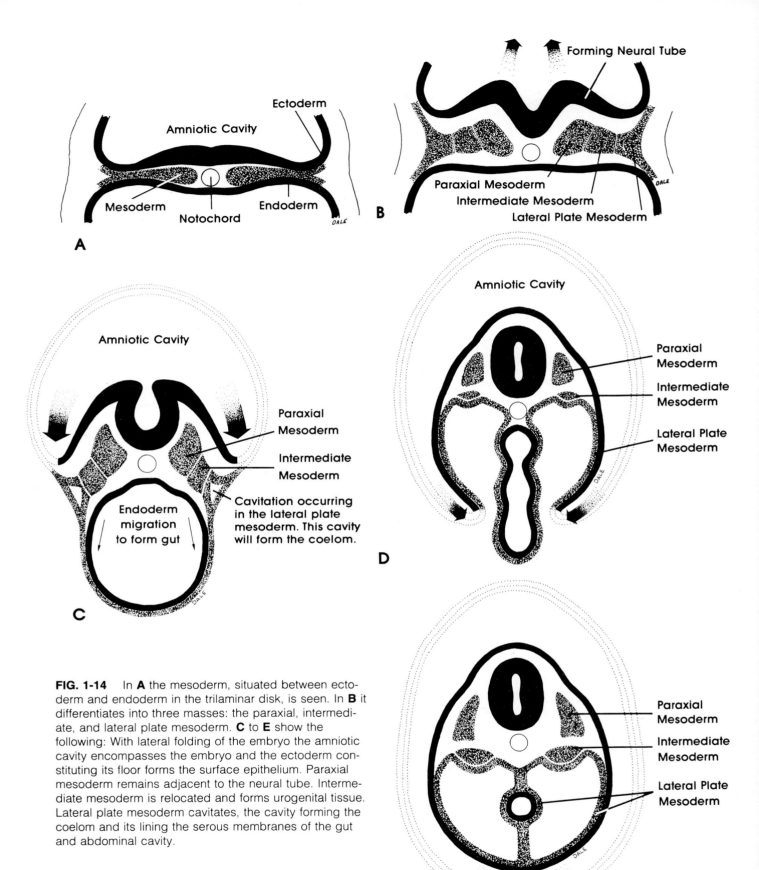

FIG. 1-14   In **A** the mesoderm, situated between ecto-derm and endoderm in the trilaminar disk, is seen. In **B** it differentiates into three masses: the paraxial, intermedi-ate, and lateral plate mesoderm. **C** to **E** show the following: With lateral folding of the embryo the amniotic cavity encompasses the embryo and the ectoderm con-stituting its floor forms the surface epithelium. Paraxial mesoderm remains adjacent to the neural tube. Interme-diate mesoderm is relocated and forms urogenital tissue. Lateral plate mesoderm cavitates, the cavity forming the coelom and its lining the serous membranes of the gut and abdominal cavity.

endoderm forms the gut. The final disposition of the mesoderm is shown in Figure 1-15, as are the derivatives of the ectoderm, endoderm, and neural crest. It is worth explaining here that one of the derivatives of mesoderm is *mesenchyme*, or embryonic connective tissue. Neural crest cells also give rise to mesenchyme. Such mesenchyme is termed *ectomesenchyme*, in recognition of its derivation.

This chapter has described the early stages of embryonic development, which mainly involve rapid cell proliferation and some histodifferentiation, leading quickly to the formation of a trilaminar disk consisting of three layers—ectoderm, mesoderm, and endoderm—with a head-tail axis established. The nervous system arises from the ectoderm of this disk through the development of folds; these folds also spin off neural

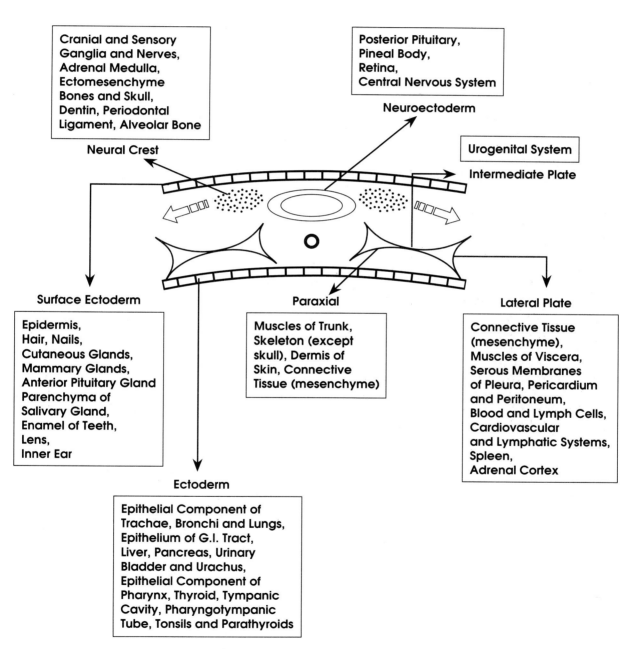

FIG. 1-15   Derivatives of the germ layers and neural crest.

crest cells, which contribute extensively to many tissues of the embryo, including most of the dental tissues. All the tissues of the embryo arise from these four cell populations. The shape of the embryo is determined by the folding of the disk in two planes, along the rostrocaudal and lateral axes, with the rostral fold being crucial to the establishment of a primitive mouth. The origin of some genetic defects has been explained; the effect of environmental factors on embryogenesis will be discussed in the next chapter. Environmental factors have relatively little impact on the production of congenital defects during the early stages of development, because their effects are masked. If damage is slight, proliferative activity can easily compensate for it by replacement with new cells. If the damage is severe, the embryo dies. Environmental effects are significant, however, in the later stages of embryonic development.

BIBLIOGRAPHY

Arey LB: The history of the first somite in human embryos, *Contrib Embryol* 27:233, 1938.

Brewer JI: A human embryo in the bilaminar blastodisc stage, *Contrib Embryol* 27:85, 1938.

Hamilton WJ, Mossman HW: *Human embryology,* ed 4, Cambridge, 1972, Heffer.

Hertig AT, Rock J, Adams EC, Mulligan WJ: On the preimplantation stages of the human ovum: a description of four normal and four abnormal specimens ranging from the second to the fifth day of development, *Contrib Embryol* 35:199, 1954.

Innes PB: The ultrastructure of early cephalic normal crest cell migration in the mouse, *Anat Embryol* 172:33, 1985.

Johnston MC: A radioautographic study of the migration and fate of the cranial neural crest cells in the chick embryo, *Anat Rec* 156:143, 1966.

Langman J: *Medical embryology, human development: normal and abnormal,* ed 5, Baltimore, 1985, Williams & Wilkins.

Moore KL: *The developing human: clinically orientated embryology,* ed 4, Philadelphia, 1989, WB Saunders.

Noden DM: The role of the neural crest in patterning of avian cranial, skeletal, connective, and muscle tissues, *Develop Biol* 96:144, 1983.

Noden DM: Craniofacial development: new views on an old problem, *Anat Rec* 208:1, 1984.

Noden DM: Origins and patterning of craniofacial mesenchymal tissues, *J Craniofac Genet Develop Biol Suppl* 2:15, 1986.

Sperber GH: *Craniofacial embryology,* Bristol UK, 1989, John Wright & Sons.

Tan SS, Morriss-Kay G: The development and distribution of the cranial neural crest in the rat embryo, *Cell Tissue Res* 240:403, 1985.

Tosney KW: The segregation and early migration of cranial neural crest cells in the avian embryo, *Develop Biol* 89:13, 1982.

CHAPTER 2

Embryology of the Head, Face, and Oral Cavity

IN the previous chapter the folding of the three-layered embryo was described; of course, the rostral or head fold is of importance here. Recall that the neural tube results from the formation and fusion of neural folds, which sink beneath the surface ectoderm. The anterior portion of this neural tube shows massive expansion as the brain forms; but there is always some mesenchyme (embryonic connective tissue) between the developing brain and the surface epithelium, except where the olfactory and orbital placodes form, and here there is direct fusion of neuroectoderm with the surface epithelium. Neural crest cells contribute to and intermingle with this mesenchyme, except anterior to the expanding forebrain. This configuration explains why neural crest cells, once they have differentiated into ectomesenchyme, provide much of the connective tissue associated with the face (Fig. 2-1).

BRANCHIAL (PHARYNGEAL) ARCHES AND THE PRIMITIVE MOUTH

When the stomatodeum first forms, it is delimited rostrally by the neural plate and caudally by the developing cardiac plate. The buccopharyngeal membrane separates it from the foregut (Fig. 2-2), but this soon breaks down so that the stomatodeum communicates directly with the foregut. Laterally the stomatodeum becomes limited by the first pair of *pharyngeal* or *branchial* arches. The branchial arches form in the pharyngeal wall (which first consists of a sheet of lateral plate mesoderm sandwiched between ectoderm externally and endoderm internally) as a result of proliferating lateral plate mesoderm and subsequent reinforcement by migrating neural crest cells. Six cylindrical thickenings thus form (the fifth is a transient structure in humans) that expand from the lateral wall of the

pharynx, pass beneath the floor of the pharynx, and approach their anatomic counterparts expanding from the opposite side. In doing so, the arches progressively separate the primitive stomatodeum from the developing heart (Fig. 2-3). The arches are clearly seen as bulges on the lateral aspect of the embryo and are externally separated by small clefts called *branchial grooves*. On the inner aspect of the pharyngeal wall are corresponding small depressions called *pharyngeal pouches* that separate each of the branchial arches internally. In aquatic vertebrates the pharyngeal pouches and branchial grooves fuse and eventually break down to form the gill clefts. In humans the grooves and pouches have other functions (Figs. 2-4 and 2-5).

Fate of Grooves and Pouches

The first groove and pouch are involved in the formation of the external auditory meatus, tympanic membrane, tympanic antrum, mastoid antrum, and pharyngotympanic or eustachian tube. The second, third, and fourth grooves are normally obliterated by overgrowth of the second arch, but sometimes they persist as a cervical sinus that may or may not open into the side of the neck. The second pouch is also largely obliterated by the development of the palatine tonsil; a part persists as the tonsillar fossa. The third pouch expands dorsally and ventrally into two compartments, and its connection with the pharynx is obliterated. The dorsal component gives origin to the inferior parathyroid gland whereas the ventral component, with its anatomic counterpart from the opposite side, forms the thymus gland. The fourth pouch also expands into dorsal and ventral components. The dorsal component gives origin to the superior parathyroid gland, and the ventral portion gives rise to the ultimobranchial body, which in turn gives rise to the parafollicular cells of the thyroid

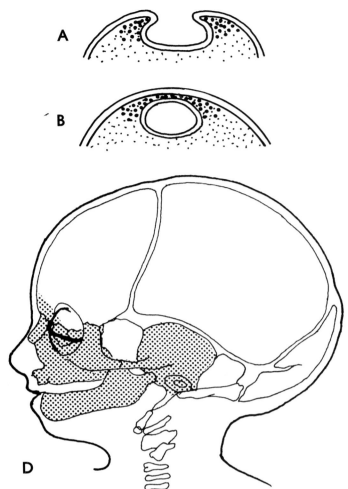

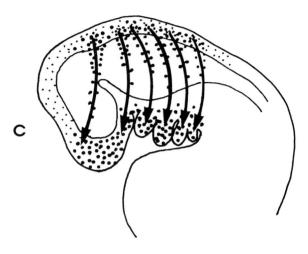

FIG. 2-1 Contribution of mesodermal mesenchyme and ectomesenchyme in the development of skeletal structures of the head. **A,** Separation of neural crest cells as the neural tube forms. **B,** With separation of the neural tube from the surface ectoderm, an intervening layer of mesenchymal-ectomesenchymal tissue is established. **C,** Migration of neural crest tissue into the developing facial and branchial arch region. Note that neural crest tissue does not intermingle with the mesenchyme anteriorly in front of the developing forebrain. **D,** Bones of the skull and face *(stippled)* derived from the neural crest.

FIG. 2-2 Sagittal section through a 25-day embryo showing the stomatodeum delimited by the neural plate above and the developing cardiac plate below. The buccopharyngeal membrane separates the stomatodeum from the foregut.

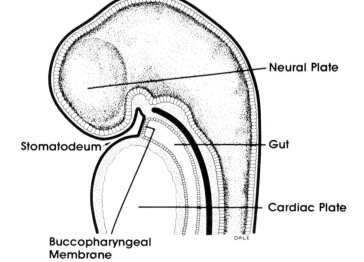

Neural Plate

Stomatodeum

Gut

Cardiac Plate

Buccopharyngeal Membrane

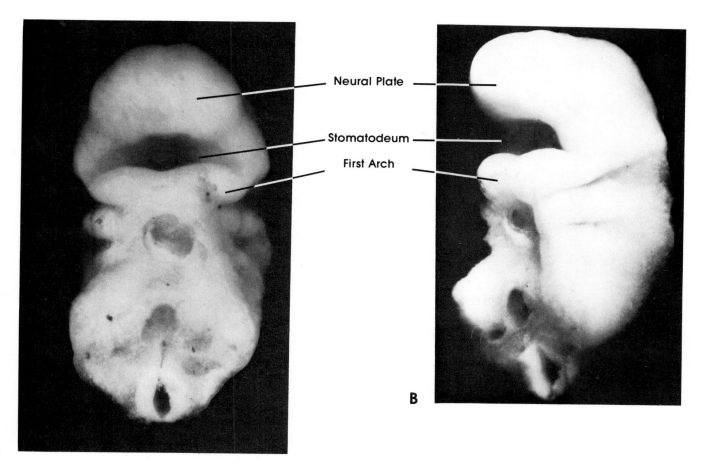

FIG. 2-3   A 26-day embryo. **A,** Viewed from the front. **B,** Viewed from the side. The structures limiting the stomatodeum are clearly recognizable. (Courtesy Dr. Hideo Nishimura.)

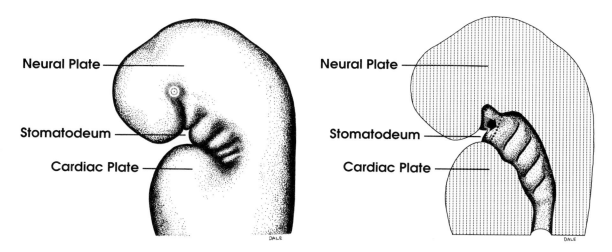

FIG. 2-4   A, Development of pharyngeal arches and the clefts between them in a 35-day embryo. **B,** Midline section showing reflection of the arches on the pharyngeal wall. The dotted line *(arrow)* represents the site of attachment of the buccopharyngeal membrane.

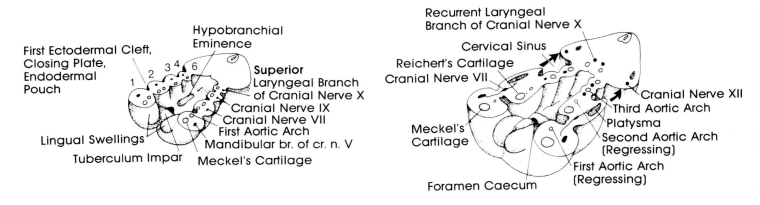

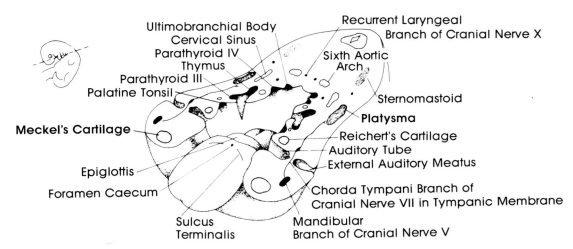

FIG. 2-5 Progressive stages in development of the pharyngeal arches and their derivatives during the second month in utero. (From Shaw JH, et al: *Textbook of oral biology,* Philadelphia, 1978, WB Saunders.)

gland. The fifth pouch in humans is rudimentary and thus either disappears or becomes incorporated into the fourth pouch (Fig. 2-5).

Anatomy of an Arch

Every branchial arch has the same basic plan. The inner aspect is covered by endoderm (ectoderm in the case of the first arch, since this forms in front of the buccopharyngeal membrane, which delineates the junction of the stomatodeum [lined by ectoderm] from the foregut [lined by endoderm]) and the outer surface by ectoderm. The central core consists of mesenchyme derived from lateral plate mesoderm, which is surrounded by mesenchyme derived from the neural crest. The neural crest mesenchyme (called ectomesenchyme) condenses to form a bar of cartilage, the arch cartilage. The cartilage of the first arch is called *Meckel's* cartilage, and that of the second *Reichert's*, after the

anatomists who first described them. The other arch cartilages are not named. Some of the mesenchyme surrounding this cartilaginous bar develops into striated muscle. The first arch musculature gives origin to the muscles of mastication, and the second arch musculature to the muscles of facial expression. Each arch also contains an artery and a nerve. The nerve consists of two components, one motor (supplying the muscle of the arch) and one sensory. The sensory nerve divides into two branches: a posttrematic branch, supplying the epithelium that covers the anterior half of the arch, and a pretrematic branch, passing forward to supply the epithelium that covers the posterior half of the preceding arch. The nerve of the first arch is the fifth cranial (or trigeminal) nerve; that of the second is the seventh cranial (or facial) nerve; and that of the third the ninth cranial (or glossopharyngeal) nerve. Structures derived from any arch carry with them the nerve supply of that

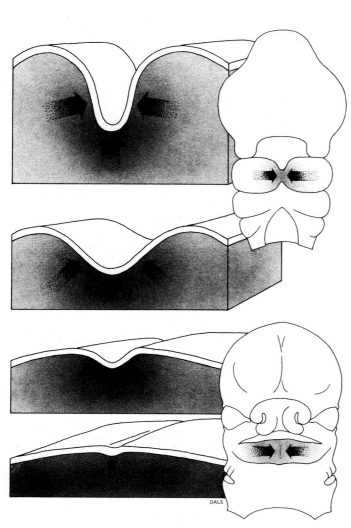

FIG. 2-6 Apparent fusion of facial processes by the elimination of a furrow between them. Compare with Fig. 2-7.

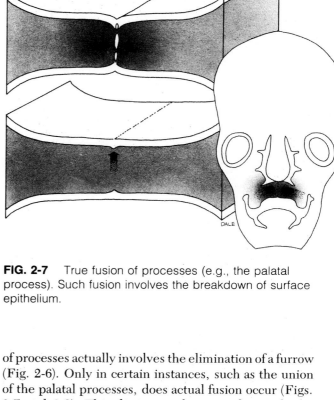

FIG. 2-7 True fusion of processes (e.g., the palatal process). Such fusion involves the breakdown of surface epithelium.

arch. Thus the muscles of mastication are innervated by the trigeminal nerve and the muscles of facial expression by the facial nerve.

Fusion of Processes

The first, second, and third branchial arches play an important role in the development of the face, mouth, and tongue. Classically, the formation of the face is described in terms of the formation and fusion of several processes or prominences. This terminology may be confusing, however. In some instances these processes are swellings of mesenchyme that cause furrows between apparent processes, so that the ostensible fusion of processes actually involves the elimination of a furrow (Fig. 2-6). Only in certain instances, such as the union of the palatal processes, does actual fusion occur (Figs. 2-7 and 2-8). This distinction being understood, the conventional term *process* rather than the more accurate terms swelling or prominence will be used to describe the further development of the face and oral cavity.

To recapitulate: The primitive stomatodeum is at first bounded above (rostrally) by the neural plate, below (caudally) by the developing heart, and laterally by the first branchial arch. With spread of the arches midventrally, the cardiac plate is eliminated from the stoma-

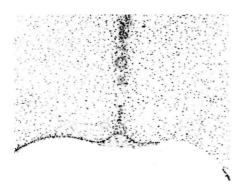

FIG. 2-8 Photomicrograph of the line of fusion between palatal processes. Remnants of the surface epithelium are visible along the line of fusion.

todeum and the floor of the mouth is formed by the epithelium covering the mesenchyme of the first, second, and third branchial arches.

At about 24 days the first branchial arch establishes another process, the *maxillary process,* so that the stomatodeum is now limited cranially by the frontal prominence covering the rapidly expanding forebrain, laterally by the newly formed maxillary process, and ventrally by the first arch (now called the *mandibular process*) (Fig. 2-9).

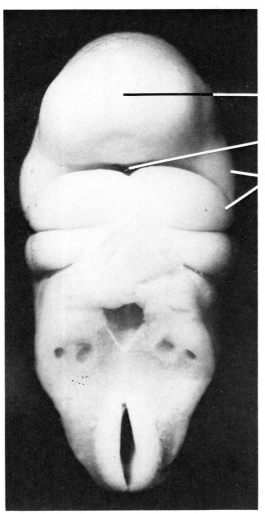

Frontal Prominence

Stomatodeum

First Arch — { Maxillary
              Mandibular

FIG. 2-9 A 27-day embryo viewed from the front. Note the beginning elements for facial development and the boundaries of the stomatodeum. (Courtesy Dr. Hideo Nishimura.)

FORMATION OF THE FACE

Early development of the face is dominated by the proliferation and migration of ectomesenchyme involved in the formation of the primitive nasal cavities. At about 28 days, localized thickenings develop within the ectoderm of the frontal prominence, just rostral to the opening of the stomatodeum. These thickenings are the olfatory placodes. Rapid proliferation of the underlying mesenchyme around the placodes bulges the frontal eminence forward and also produces a horseshoe-shaped ridge that converts the olfactory placode into the nasal pit. The lateral arm of the horseshoe is called the *lateral nasal process*, and the medial arm the *medial nasal process*. Between the two nasal processes is a now depressed area called the *frontonasal process*. The medial nasal processes of both sides, together with the frontonasal process, give rise to the middle portion of the nose, middle portion of the upper lip, anterior portion of the maxilla, and *primary palate* (Fig. 2-10).

The maxillary process grows medially and approaches both the lateral and the medial nasal processes but remains separated from them by distinct grooves. The medial growth of the maxillary process pushes the medial nasal process toward the midline, where it merges with its anatomic counterpart from the opposite side, eliminating the frontonasal process. In this way the upper lip is formed from the maxillary processes of each side and the medial nasal process, with fusion occurring between the forward extent of the maxillary process and the lateral face of the medial nasal process. The lower lip is formed, of course, by fusion of the two mandibular processes. The merging of the two medial nasal processes results in the formation of that part of the maxilla carrying the incisor teeth and the primary palate as well as part of the lip. These steps in facial development are shown in Figures 2-11 and 2-12.

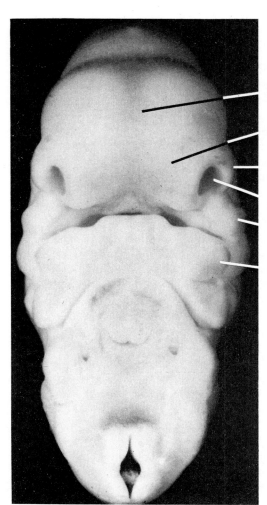

Frontal
Prominence

Medial Nasal
Process

Lateral Nasal
Process

Nasal Pit

Maxillary
Process

Mandibular
Process

FIG. 2-10 A 34-day embryo viewed from the front. The nasal pits have formed, thereby delineating the lateral and medial frontonasal processes. (Courtesy Dr. Hideo Nishimura.)

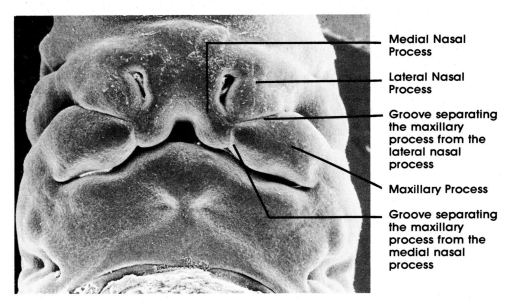

FIG. 2-11 Scanning electron micrograph of a human embryo at 7 weeks. (Courtesy Dr. K.K. Sulik.)

An unusual type of fusion occurs between the maxillary process and the lateral nasal process. As with most other processes associated with facial development, the maxillary and lateral nasal processes are initially separated by a deep furrow. The epithelium in the floor of the groove between them forms a solid core that separates from the surface and eventually canalizes to form the nasolacrimal duct. Once the duct has separated, the two processes merge by infilling of the mesenchyme.

The face develops between the twenty-fourth and thirty-eighth days of gestation. By this time some of the epithelium covering the facial processes can already be distinguished as odontogenic, or tooth forming (Fig. 2-12). On the inferior border of the maxillary process and the superior border of the mandibular arch, where the lateral margin of the stomatodeum is formed, the epithelium begins to proliferate and thicken. This thickened area is the odontogenic epithelium. Odontogenic epithelium also develops on the lateral aspect of the medial nasal process; but not until the thirty-seventh day of development, when the processes fuse, can a single plate of thickened epithelium, the *primary epithelial band*, be observed. Thus the primary epithelial band is an arch-shaped continuous plate of odontogenic epithelium that forms in the upper jaw from four separate zones of epithelial proliferation, the middle two associated with the medial nasal process. Two zones, one in each mandibular process, form the primary epithelial band of the lower jaw.

Formation of the Palate

Initially there is a common oronasal cavity bounded anteriorly by the primary palate and occupied mainly by the developing tongue. Only after the development of the *secondary palate* is distinction between oral and nasal cavities possible. The palate proper develops from both primary and secondary components.

The formation of the primary palate from the frontonasal and medial nasal processes has already been described. The formation of the secondary palate occurs between 7 and 8 weeks of development and results from the fusion of shelves formed from each maxillary process. These shelves, the *palatine shelves* or processes, are first directed downward on each side of the tongue. After the seventh week of development the tongue is withdrawn from between the shelves, which now elevate and fuse with each other above the tongue and with the primary palate (Figs. 2-13 to 2-15). The closure of the secondary palate involves an intrinsic force in the palatal shelves whose nature has not yet been determined. The high concentration of glycosaminoglycans, which attract water and make the shelves turgid, has been suggested, as has the presence of contractile fibroblasts in the palatal shelves. Another factor in the closure of the secondary palate is displacement of the tongue from between the palatal shelves by the growth pattern of the head.

In the embryo between 7 and 8 weeks, the tongue and mandible are small relative to the upper facial com-

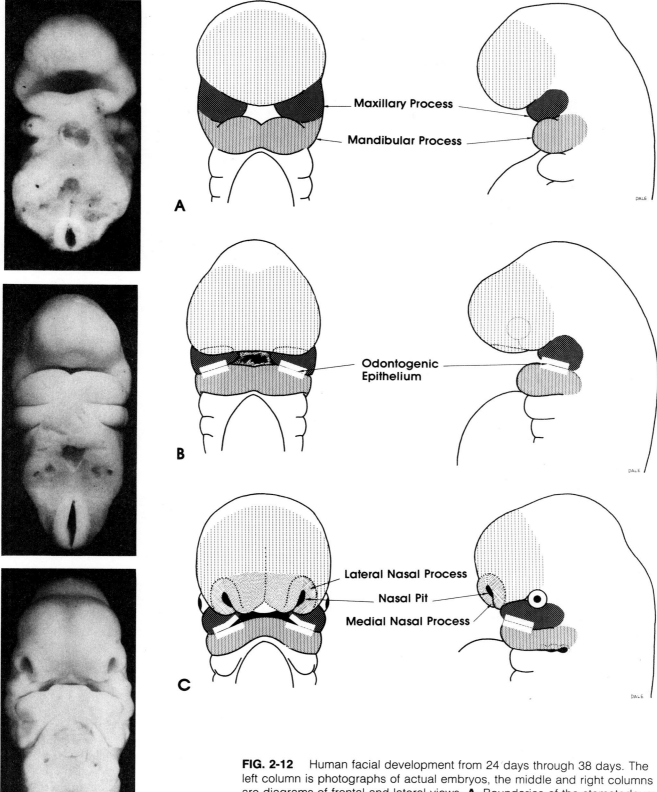

FIG. 2-12 Human facial development from 24 days through 38 days. The left column is photographs of actual embryos, the middle and right columns are diagrams of frontal and lateral views. **A,** Boundaries of the stomatodeum in a 26-day embryo. **B,** A 27-day embryo. The nasal placode is about to develop, and the odontogenic epithelium *(white bars in the diagram)* can be identified. **C,** A 34-day embryo. The nasal pit, surrounded by lateral and medial processes, is easily recognizable.

Continued.

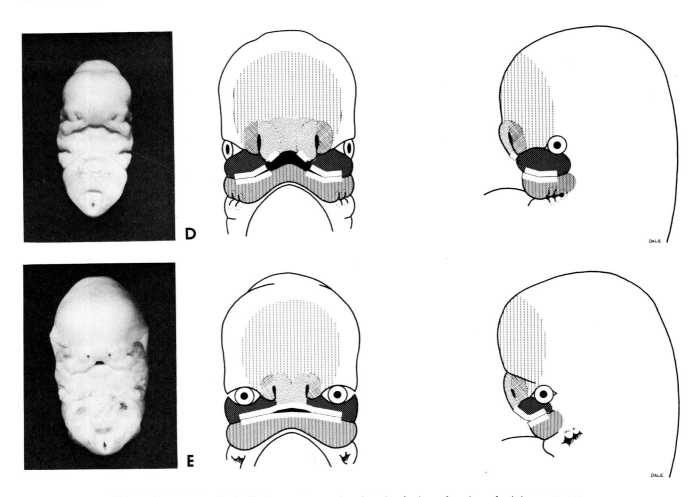

FIG. 2-12 *cont'd*   **D,** A 36-day embryo, showing the fusion of various facial processes that are completed by 38 days, **E. (A** to **E** courtesy Dr. H. Nishimura. Drawings adapted from Nery FB, et al: *Arch Oral Biol* 15: 1315, 1970.)

plex and the lower lip is positioned behind the upper one. The head is folded onto the developing thoracic region and the tongue occupies an elevated position between the palatal shelves (Fig. 2-16, *A* and *B*). By 9 weeks, the upper facial complex has lifted away from the thorax and thus permits the tongue and lower jaw to grow forward, so that the lower lip is now positioned in advance of the upper and the tongue is situated below the palatal shelves (Fig. 2-16, *C* and *D*).

For fusion of the palatal shelves to occur, and (for that matter) fusion of any other processes, it is necessary to eliminate their epithelial covering. As the two palatal shelves meet, there is adhesion of the epithelia so that the epithelium of one shelf becomes indistinguishable from that of the other and a midline epithelial seam forms. To achieve this fusion, there is cessation of DNA synthesis within the epithelium some 24 to 36 hours before epithelial contact. Surface epithelial cells are sloughed off as they undergo physiologic cell death to expose the basal epithelial cells. These cells have a carbohydrate-rich surface coat that permits ready adhesion and the formation of junctions to achieve fusion of the processes. A midline seam is thus formed that consists of two layers of basal epithelial cells. This midline seam must be removed to permit ectomesenchymal continuity between the fused processes. Even though the epithelial cells of the seam continue to divide, growth of the seam fails to keep pace with palatal growth so that the seam first thins to a single layer of cells and then breaks up into discrete islands of epithelial cells. The basal lamina surrounding these cells is then lost, and the epithelial cells lose their epithelial characteristics and assume fibroblastlike features. In other words, epithelial cells transform into mesenchymal cells.

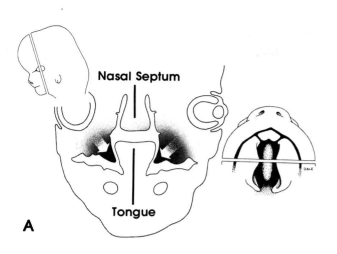

A

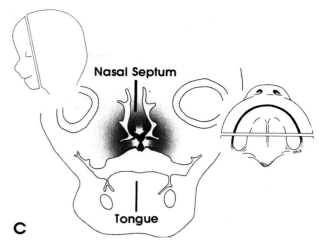

C

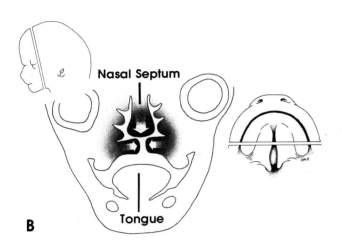

B

FIG. 2-13 Formation of the secondary palate. **A,** At 7 weeks the palatal shelves are forming from the maxillary processes and are directed downward on each side of the developing tongue. **B,** At 8 weeks the tongue has been depressed and the palatal shelves are elevated but not fused. **C,** Fusion of the shelves and the nasal septum is completed.

FORMATION OF THE TONGUE

The tongue begins to develop at about 4 weeks. Recall that the pharyngeal arches meet in the midline beneath the primitive mouth. Local proliferation of the mesenchyme then gives rise to a number of swellings in the floor of the mouth (Figs. 2-5 and 2-17). First, a swelling (the *tuberculum impar*) arises in the midline in the mandibular process and is flanked by two other bulges, the *lingual swellings.* Very quickly these lateral lingual swellings enlarge and merge with each other and the tuberculum impar to form a large mass from which the mucous membrane of the anterior two thirds of the tongue is formed. The root of the tongue arises from the *hypobranchial eminence,* a large midline swelling developed from the mesenchyme of the third arch. The mesenchyme of the third arch rapidly overgrows that of the second arch, which is thereby ex-

cluded from further involvement in the development of the tongue.

The hypobranchial eminence gives rise to the mucosa covering the root, or posterior third, of the tongue. Some authorities divide the hypobranchial eminence into an anterior copula (which gives origin to the mucosa covering the root of the tongue) and a hypobranchial eminence (which gives rise to the epiglottis). The tongue separates from the floor of the mouth by a downgrowth of ectoderm around its periphery, which subsequently degenerates to form the lingual sulcus and gives the tongue mobility. The muscles of the tongue have a different origin: they arise from the occipital somites, which have migrated forward into the tongue area, carrying with them their nerve supply, the twelfth cranial (hypoglossal) nerve (Fig. 2-18).

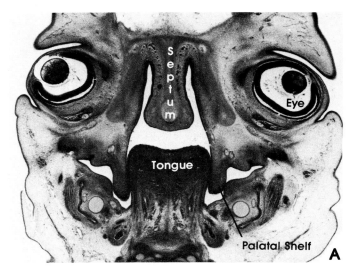

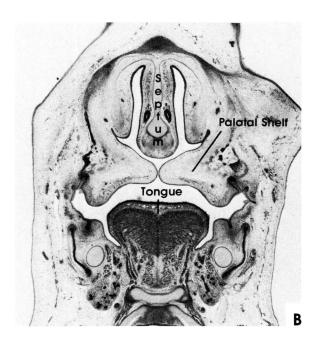

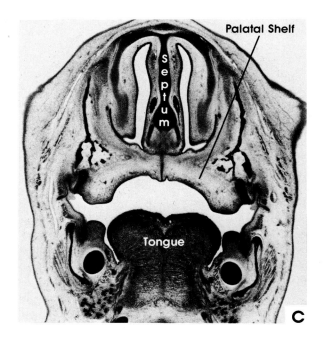

FIG. 2-14   Formation of the secondary palate. Coronal sections through human embryos at approximately 7 weeks, **A,** 8 weeks, **B,** and 9 weeks, **C.** The initial disposition of palatal shelves on each side of the tongue is shown in **A,** their elevation coincident with depression of the tongue in **B,** and their final fusion with each other and with the nasal septum in **C.** (**A** to **C** from Diewert VM: *Am J Anat* 167:495, 1983.)

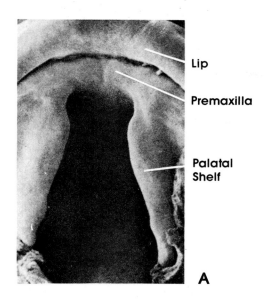

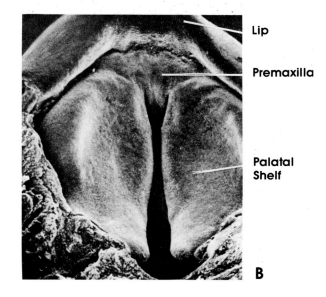

FIG. 2-15 Palatal shelves in the, **A,** 7-week and, **B,** 8-week human embryo corresponding approximately to Figs. 2-13, *A* and *B,* and 2-14, *B.* (**A** and **B** from Waterman RE, Miller SM: *Anat Rec* 180:111, 1974.)

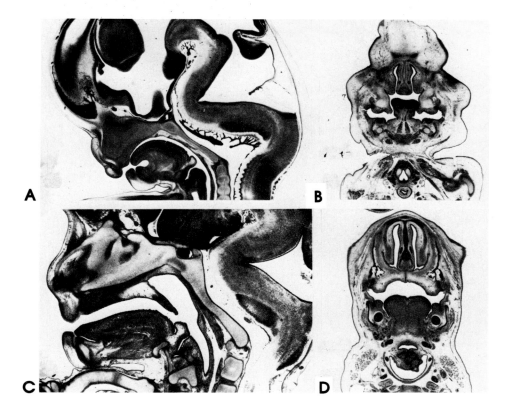

FIG. 2-16 Sagittal and coronal sections through human embryos between 7 and 9 weeks. **A,** The folded head has the upper lip in front of the lower with the tongue elevated. **B,** Palatal shelves are positioned on each side of the tongue. **C,** At 9 weeks the head is raised, so that the tongue is not only lowered but has also grown forward. The lower lip is now slightly in front of the upper. **D,** In this coronal section the palatal shelves have fused over the lowered tongue. (**A** to **D** from Diewert V: In Dixon AD, Sarnat BG, [eds]: *Factors and mechanisms influencing bone growth,* New York, 1982, Alan R Liss, pp 229 to 242.)

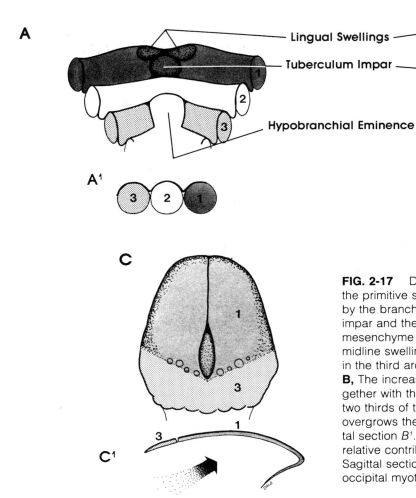

FIG. 2-17 Development of the tongue. **A,** The floor of the primitive stomatodeum, viewed from above, is formed by the branchial arches. Three swellings, the tuberculum impar and the paired lingual swellings, appear in the mesenchyme of the first arch beneath the epithelium. A midline swelling *(the hypobranchial eminence)* appears in the third arch. *A',* Sagittal section through the arches. **B,** The increased swelling of the lingual swellings, together with the tuberculum impar, will form the anterior two thirds of the tongue. The hypobranchial eminence overgrows the second arch. This is depicted in the sagittal section *B'.* **C,** Final disposition of the tongue and the relative contributions of the first and third arches. *C',* Sagittal section. The *arrow* depicts the route of incoming occipital myotomes that form the tongue muscle.

This unusual development of the tongue explains its innervation. Since the mucosa of the anterior two thirds of the tongue is derived from the first arch, it is supplied by the nerve of that arch, the fifth cranial (trigeminal) nerve, whereas the mucosa of the posterior third of the tongue, derived from the third arch, is supplied by the ninth cranial (glossopharyngeal) nerve. As already explained, the motor supply to the muscles of the tongue is the twelfth cranial nerve.

The development of the tongue and palate and the formation of the oral cavity are summarized diagrammatically in Figure 2-19, which illustrates midline sagittal sections through the developing embryo at progressively later stages of gestation.

FIG. 2-18 Occipital somites migrating forward into the floor of the mouth to form the musculature of the tongue.

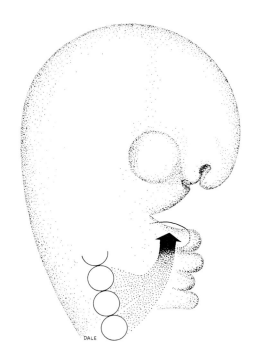

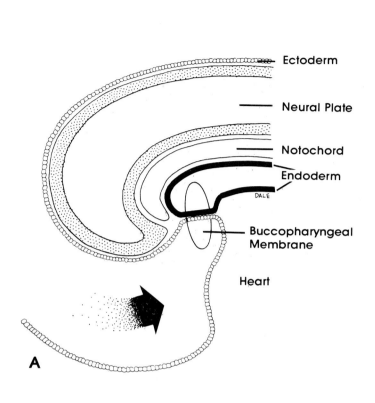

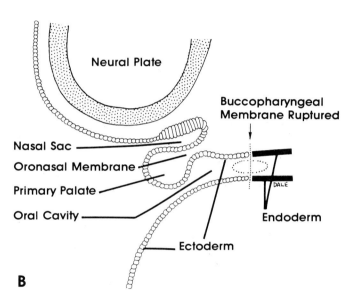

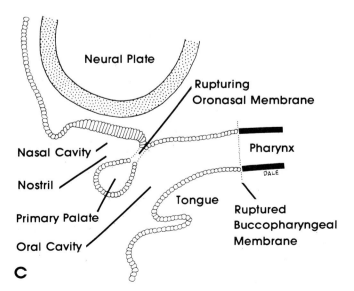

FIG. 2-19 Development of the oral cavity as seen in midsagittal section. **A,** Head fold and formation of the stomatodeum, or oral cavity. **B,** Formation of the nasal pit and primary palate. **C,** How continuity is established between the presumptive nasal and oral cavities.

Continued.

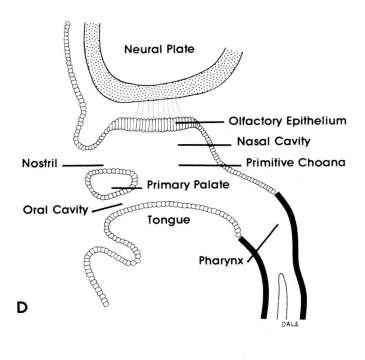

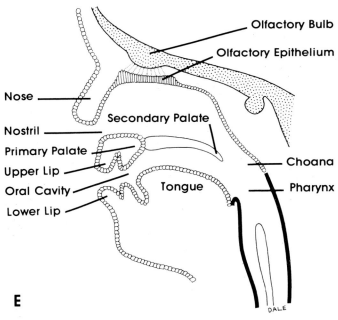

FIG. 2-19 *cont'd.*   **D** and **E,** Final anatomy of the nasal and oral cavities established by development of the secondary palate.

DEVELOPMENT OF THE SKULL

The skull can be divided into three components: (1) the cranial vault, (2) the cranial base, and (3) the face (Fig. 2-20). Its development is complex, and some understanding of skull evolution is required to provide a simple description. Early vertebrates possessed a series of cartilaginous boxes protecting the brain and sensory organs, which together formed the neurocranium, and a viscerocranium supporting the branchial arches around the beginning of the alimentary tract (Fig. 2-21).

This configuration can be seen in the approximately 12-week-old human fetus if only those bones of the skull that form in cartilage are depicted (Fig. 2-22). The cartilaginous cranial base is represented by the nasal and orbital cartilages (which once surrounded sense organs) and the petrosal and occipital bones from the original neurocranium. The petrosal bone has incorporated the otic capsule. The only parts of the viscerocranium contributing to the skull are the terminal parts of the first and second arch cartilages, which become ear ossicles. This cartilaginous base undergoes endochondral ossification. Membranous bone, formed directly in mesenchyme with no cartilaginous precursor, forms the cranial vault and face (Fig. 2-23). Some of these membrane-formed bones may develop secondary cartilages to provide rapid growth.

This is an extremely abbreviated account of skull development; for further details standard texts on embryology should be consulted. Here only the development of the jaws is considered in detail.

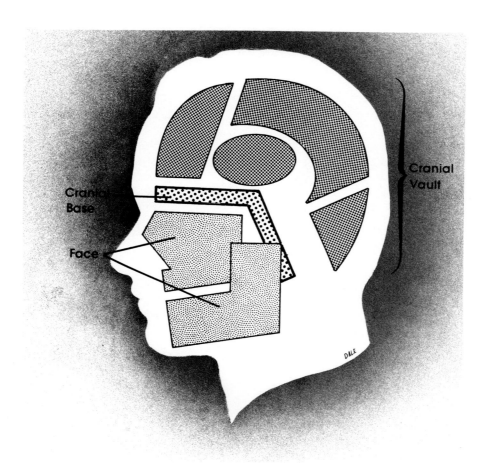

FIG. 2-20 Subdivisions of the skull.

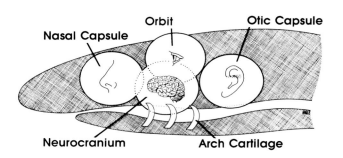

FIG. 2-21 Skull evolution. Cartilaginous boxes surrounding the sensory organs and brain form the neurocranium. Branchial arch cartilages constitute the viscerocranium.

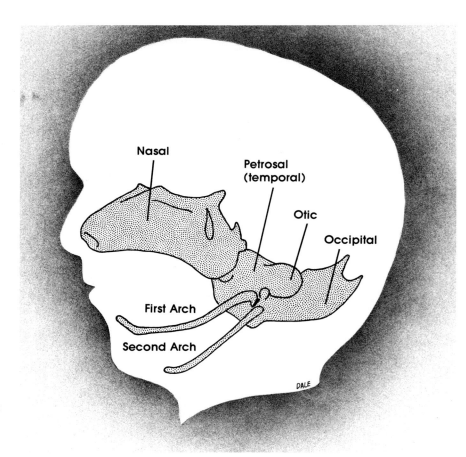

FIG. 2-22 Cartilaginous components in the developing head of a 3-month embryo. Membranous bones have been omitted. (Redrawn from Osborn JW [ed]: *Dental anatomy and embryology*, 1981, Blackwell Scientific Publications.)

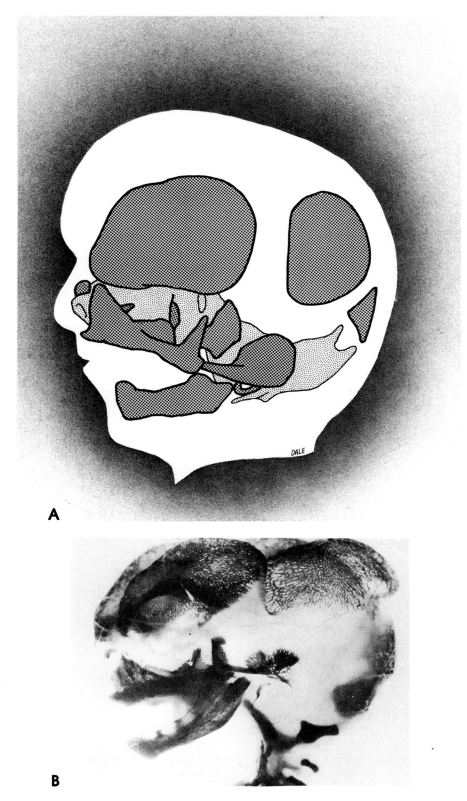

FIG. 2-23   **A,** Same diagram with the membrane-formed bones added. **B,** A 62-day cleared human embryo in which the mineralized bone has been stained with alizarin red.

DEVELOPMENT OF THE MANDIBLE AND MAXILLA

It is appropriate now to discuss the development of the bones of the jaw and the joint between them. Both the mandible and the maxilla form from the tissues of the first branchial arch, the mandible forming within the mandibular process and the maxilla within the maxillary process.

Development of the Mandible

The cartilage of the first arch (Meckel's cartilage) forms the lower jaw in primitive vertebrates. In humans it has a close positional relationship to the developing mandible but makes no contribution to it. At 6 weeks of development this cartilage extends as a solid hyaline cartilaginous rod, surrounded by a fibrocellular capsule, from the developing ear region (otic capsule) to the midline of the fused mandibular processes (Fig. 2-24). The two cartilages of each side do not meet at the midline but are separated by a thin band of mesenchyme. The mandibular branch of the trigeminal nerve (the nerve of the first arch) has a close relationship to Meckel's cartilage, beginning two thirds of the way along the length of the cartilage. At this point the mandibular nerve divides into lingual and inferior alveolar branches, which run along the medial and lateral aspects of the cartilage respectively. The inferior alveolar nerve further divides into incisive and mental branches more anteriorly.

On the lateral aspect of Meckel's cartilage, during the sixth week of embryonic development, a condensation of mesenchyme occurs in the angle formed by the division of the inferior alveolar nerve and its incisive and mental branches. At 7 weeks intramembranous ossification begins in this condensation, forming the first

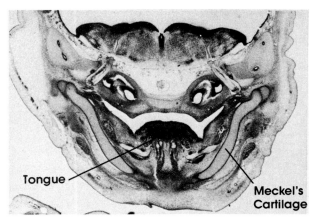

FIG. 2-24 Slightly oblique coronal section of an embryo demonstrating almost the entire extent of Meckel's cartilage. (From Diewert VM: *Am J Anat* 167: 495, 1983.)

bone of the mandible (Fig. 2-25). From this center of ossification, bone formation spreads rapidly anteriorly to the midline and posteriorly toward the point where the mandibular nerve divides into its lingual and inferior alveolar branches. This spread of new bone formation occurs anteriorly along the lateral aspect of Meckel's cartilage, forming a trough that consists of lateral and medial plates that unite beneath the incisive nerve. This trough of bone extends to the midline, where it comes into close approximation with a similar trough formed in the adjoining mandibular process. The two separate centers of ossification remain separated at the mandibular symphysis until shortly after birth. The trough is soon converted into a canal as bone forms over the nerve joining the lateral and medial plates.

Similarly, a backward extension of ossification along the lateral aspect of Meckel's cartilage forms a gutter, later converted into a canal, that contains the inferior alveolar nerve. This backward extension of ossification proceeds in the condensed mesenchyme to the point where the mandibular nerve divides into the inferior alveolar and lingual nerves. From this bony canal, extending from the division of the mandibular nerve to the midline, medial and lateral alveolar plates of bone develop in relation to the forming tooth germs, so that the tooth germs come to occupy a secondary trough of bone. This trough is partitioned; and thus the teeth come to occupy individual compartments, which finally are totally enclosed by growth of bone over the tooth germ. In this way the body of the mandible is essentially formed (Fig. 2-26).

The ramus of the mandible develops by a rapid spread of ossification posteriorly into the mesenchyme of the first arch, turning away from Meckel's cartilage (Fig. 2-27). This point of divergence is marked by the lingula in the adult mandible, the point at which the inferior alveolar nerve enters the body of the mandible.

Thus by 10 weeks the rudimentary mandible is formed almost entirely by membranous ossification—with (it must be stressed) little direct involvement of Meckel's cartilage (Figs. 2-28 and 2-29). Meckel's cartilage has the following fate: Its most posterior extremity forms the malleus of the inner ear and the sphenomalleolar ligament. From the sphenoid to the division of the mandibular nerve into its alveolar and lingual branches, the cartilage is totally lost but its fibrocellular capsule persists as the sphenomandibular ligament. From the lingula forward to the division of the alveolar nerve into its incisive and mental branches, Meckel cartilage is totally resorbed. Forward from this point to the midline there is some evidence that the cartilage makes a contribution to the mandible by means of endochondral ossification.

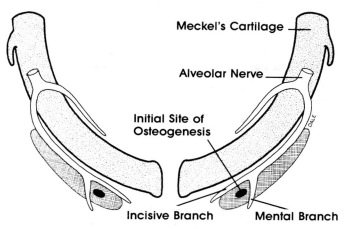

FIG. 2-25 Site of initial osteogenesis related to mandible formation.

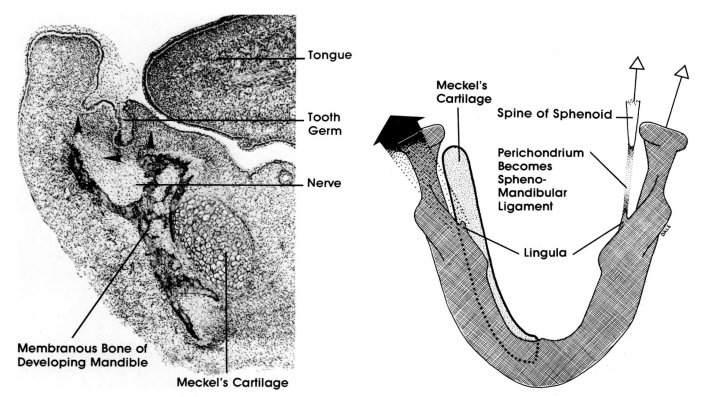

FIG. 2-26 Photomicrograph of a coronal section through an embryo showing the general pattern of membranous bone deposition associated with formation of the mandible. The relationship among nerve, cartilage, and tooth germ is evident. *Arrows* indicate the future directions of bone growth to form the neural canal and lateral and medial alveolar plates. Compare this with the development of the maxilla (Fig. 2-33).

FIG. 2-27 Spread of mandibular ossification away from Meckel's cartilage at the lingula.

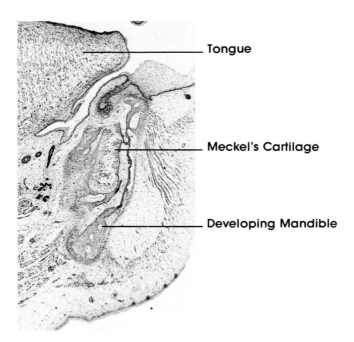

Tongue

Meckel's Cartilage

Developing Mandible

FIG. 2-28 Photomicrograph of a sagittal section through the developing jaw of an embryo showing how membrane bone forms around Meckel's cartilage as it forms the body of the mandible. Compare this with Fig. 2-29, which is at a higher magnification.

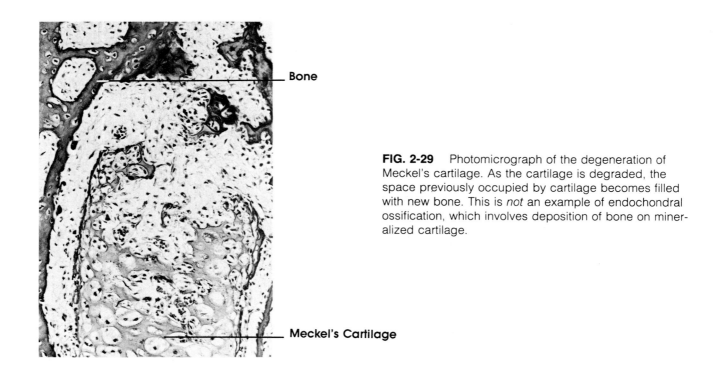

Bone

Meckel's Cartilage

FIG. 2-29 Photomicrograph of the degeneration of Meckel's cartilage. As the cartilage is degraded, the space previously occupied by cartilage becomes filled with new bone. This is *not* an example of endochondral ossification, which involves deposition of bone on mineralized cartilage.

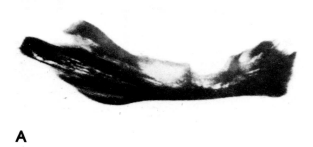

A

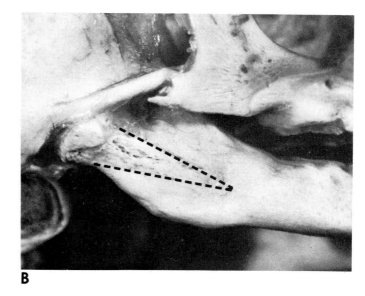

B

FIG. 2-30 Condylar cartilage. **A,** A radiograph of the mandible of a midterm fetus shows the carrot-shaped wedge of new bone that has formed from the condylar cartilage. This can also be seen in a dried fetal mandible, **B. C,** Histology of the same, showing the distinction between cartilaginous and intramembranous ossification. (**A** and **B** from Scott JH, Dixon AD: *Anatomy for students of dentistry,* London, 1979, Churchill Livingstone; **C** from Chif JG, et al: *Sequential atlas of human development,* Seoul Korea, 1992, Medical Publishing Co.)

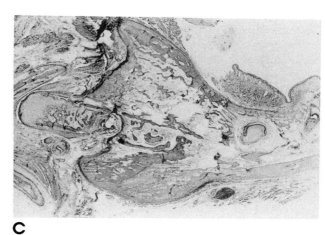

C

The further growth of the mandible until birth is strongly influenced by the appearance of three secondary (growth) cartilages and the development of muscular attachments: the condylar cartilage, which is most important, the coronoid cartilage, and the symphysial cartilage. These cartilages are called *secondary* cartilages, to distinguish them from the *primary* Meckel's cartilage; they have a different histologic structure from the primary cartilages in that their cells are larger and there is less intercellular matrix.

The *condylar* cartilage appears during the twelfth week of development and rapidly forms a cone or carrot-shaped mass that occupies most of the developing ramus (Fig. 2-30). This mass of cartilage is quickly con-

verted to bone by endochondral ossification (Chapter 8), so that at 20 weeks only a thin layer of cartilage remains in the condylar head. This remnant of cartilage persists until the end of the second decade of life, providing a mechanism for growth of the mandible, in the same way as the epiphyseal cartilage does (Chapter 21).

The *coronoid* cartilage appears at about 4 months of development, surmounting the anterior border and top of the coronoid process. It is a relatively transient growth cartilage and disappears long before birth.

The *symphysial* cartilages, two in number, appear in the connective tissue between the two ends of Meckel's cartilage but are entirely independent of it. They are obliterated within the first year after birth.

Small islands of cartilage may also appear as variable and transient structures in the developing alveolar processes.

Thus the mandible is a membrane bone, developed in relation to the nerve of the first arch and almost entirely independent of Meckel's cartilage. It has neural, alveolar, and muscular elements (Fig. 2-31) and its growth is assisted by the development of secondary cartilages. At birth the mandible is recognizable as such; its further growth is discussed in Chapter 21.

Development of the Maxilla

The maxilla also develops from a center of ossification in the mesenchyme of the maxillary process of the first arch. No arch cartilage or primary cartilage exists in the maxillary process, but the center of ossification is closely associated with the cartilage of the nasal capsule. As in the mandible, the center of ossification appears in the angle between the division of a nerve (that is, where the anterosuperior dental nerve is given off from the inferior orbital nerve). From this center, bone formation spreads posteriorly below the orbit toward the developing zygoma and anteriorly toward the future incisor region (Figs. 2-32 and 2-33). Ossification also spreads superiorly to form the frontal process. As a result of this pattern of bone deposition, a bony trough forms for the infraorbital nerve. From this trough a downward extension of bone forms the lateral alveolar plate for the maxillary tooth germs. Ossification also spreads into the palatine process to form the hard palate. The medial alveolar plate develops from the junction of the palatal process and the main body of the forming maxilla. This plate, together with its lateral counterpart, forms a trough of bone around the maxillary tooth germs, which eventually become enclosed in bony crypts in the same way as described for the mandible.

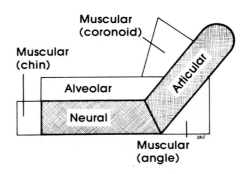

FIG. 2-31 Differing developmental blocks for the mandible.

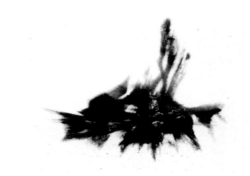

FIG. 2-32 Maxilla of a midterm fetus. The developing processes are apparent. (From Scott JH, Dixon AD: *Anatomy for students of dentistry,* London, 1979, Churchill Livingstone.)

FIG. 2-33 Coronal section through an embryo showing the general pattern of membranous bone deposition associated with formation of the maxilla. The relationship between cartilage, nerve, and tooth germ is evident. *Arrows* indicate the future directions of bone growth to form the lateral and medial alveolar plates. Compare this with the developing mandible in Fig. 2-25.

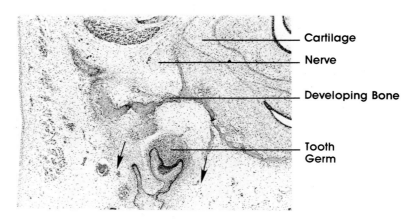

A secondary cartilage also contributes to the development of the maxilla. A *zygomatic*, or *malar*, cartilage appears in the developing zygomatic process and for a short time adds considerably to the development of the maxilla. At birth, the frontal process of the maxilla is well marked but the body of the bone consists of little more than the alveolar process containing the tooth germs and small though distinguishable zygomatic and palatal processes. The body of the maxilla is relatively small because the maxillary sinus has not developed. This sinus forms during the sixteenth week as a shallow groove on the nasal aspect of the developing maxilla. At birth it is still a rudimentary structure about the size of a small pea. The growth changes occurring in the maxilla after birth are described in Chapter 21.

Problem of the Premaxilla

The preceding has been a simplified account of the development of the maxilla. In the past, considerable discussion has focused on the number of ossification centers involved in the development of the maxilla and, possibly, that of the premaxilla. It has been suggested that two other centers of ossification exist in the premaxillary part of the bone, which is thought to reflect a separate identity for the premaxilla, a separate bone found in most mammalian jaws including those of primates. A separate premaxilla does not, however, occur in humans. It was formerly thought that in humans ossification from the main body of the maxilla spread anterior to, and overgrew, the premaxillary centers, thereby eliminating any premaxilla.

Because it is possible to distinguish an apparent suture line on the palatal surface of the maxilla diverging from the incisive fossa and running to the septa that separate the lateral incisors from the canines, a premaxilla was presumed to have existed sometime during maxillary development. However, recent study of serial sections through the developing human maxilla has established that what seems to be multiple centers is in fact a lamina of bone of complex shape that has developed from one ossification center. This new finding simplifies the explanation of maxillary development though it does not explain the suturelike grooves found delineating a possible premaxilla (Fig. 2-34).

Common Features of Jaw Development

From this account of jaw development it can be appreciated that in their development the mandible and maxilla have much in common. Both begin from a single center of membranous ossification related to a nerve and to a primary cartilage, both form a neural element related to the nerve, and both develop an alveolar element related to the developing teeth. Finally, both develop secondary cartilages to assist in their growth.

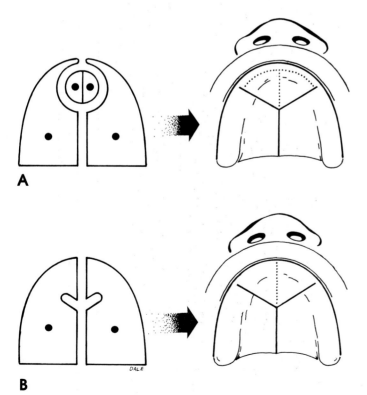

FIG. 2-34 Problem of the premaxilla. **A,** It is supposed that there are separate centers of ossification for the maxilla and the premaxilla and that bone from maxillary centers spreads and grows over the facial surface of the premaxilla. **B,** It is assumed that no separate center of ossification for the premaxilla exists and that the maxillary center is C shaped with the concavity filling in and leaving an incomplete suture.

DEVELOPMENT OF THE TEMPOROMANDIBULAR JOINT

The temporomandibular joint (TMJ) is an articulation between two bones initially formed from membranous centers of ossification. Before the condylar cartilage forms, there is a broad band of undifferentiated mesenchyme between the developing ramus of the mandible and the developing squamous tympanic bone. With formation of the condylar cartilage, this band is rapidly reduced in width and converted into a dense strip of mesenchyme. The mesenchyme immediately adjacent to this strip breaks down to form the joint cavity and the strip becomes the articular disk of the joint.

The complicated changes that occur during embryogenesis between the fourth and eighth weeks of development have now been described. They lead to, among other things, the formation of the face, mouth, and tongue and their associated structures. From 8 weeks onward, development is essentially a matter of growth.

CONGENITAL DEFECTS

It should be obvious that the development of an individual is a complicated and delicately balanced process; malfunctions will produce congenital defects. The genetic basis of some of these defects has already been discussed. Environmental factors, including teratogens (agents causing congenital defects), must also be considered. It is worth emphasizing that the time at which environmental factors exert their effect can be critical. If a teratogen exerts its effect during the first 4 weeks of life, when the embryo is developing rapidly, it usually damages so many cells that death of the embryo occurs. If only a few cells are damaged, however, normal proliferation is great enough that minor damage is readily eliminated. It is more than likely that many teratogenic agents acting in this first phase of development are not appreciated since the embryo dies and is miscarried. A possible exception is alcohol, whose effects are manifested in the so-called fetal alcohol syndrome, which does not necessarily kill the early embryo but stunts its repair potential. It is during the next stage of development, between 4 and 8 weeks, when histodifferentiation and organ differentiation are taking place, that teratogenic agents are most likely to produce malformation. The subsequent growth phase is not as susceptible to teratogenic agents.

Not surprisingly, therefore, most teratogenic agents leading to facial and dental malformations exert their effects during the period of histodifferentiation and morphogenesis within the embryo. It is estimated that one of every 700 live births in the United States has a cleft lip or palate or both. Orofacial clefts constitute approximately 13% of all reported anomalies and represent the second most common malformation. Some of the various types of cleft lip and palate that can be readily understood from a knowledge of embryology include microstomia (which is an excessive merging of the mandibular and maxillary processes), the converse or macrostomia (an oblique facial cleft resulting from failure of the maxillary and mandibular processes to fuse), and the rare mandibular cleft (Figs. 2-35 and 2-36).

Clefts have different etiologies. Those of the lip and anterior maxilla result from defective development of the embryonic primary palate. Often when such clefts occur, the distortion of facial development prevents the palatal shelves from making contact when they swing into the horizontal position; thus clefts of the primary palate are often accompanied by clefts of the secondary (hard and soft) palate. Facial clefts usually result from a deficiency of mesenchyme in the facial region, brought about by failure of neural crest to migrate or failure of the facial mesenchyme to proliferate.

When clefts of the palate occur with no corresponding facial cleft, the etiology is somewhat different. Such palatal clefts may result from (1) failure of the shelves to contact each other because of a lack of growth or because of a disturbance in the mechanism of shelf elevation, (2) failure of the shelves to fuse after contact has been made because the epithelium covering the shelves does not break down or is not resorbed, (3) rupture after fusion of the shelves has occurred, or (4) defective merging and consolidation of the mesenchyme of the shelves.

The types of environmental factors affecting the embryo can be classified into five groups: (1) infectious agents, (2) x-irradiation, (3) drugs, (4) hormones, and (5) nutritional deficiencies. The classic example of an *infectious agent* causing a congenital defect is the rubella virus, which induces German measles. Among the widespread malformations that result from this infection of the mother are cleft palate and deformities of the teeth. The teratogenic effect of *x-irradiation* is well understood, and it is recognized that many defects, including cleft palate, can result from the irradiation of pregnant women. It should also be remembered that as well as affecting the embryo directly, x-irradiation may also affect the germ cells of the fetus, causing genetic mutations that will lead to congenital malformations in succeeding generations. It has not been established whether *hormones* are capable of producing congenital abnormalities in humans, although they certainly can in experimental animals. When cortisone is injected into mice and rabbits, it causes a high percentage of cleft palates in the offspring. The same is also true for nutritional deficiencies, especially vitamin

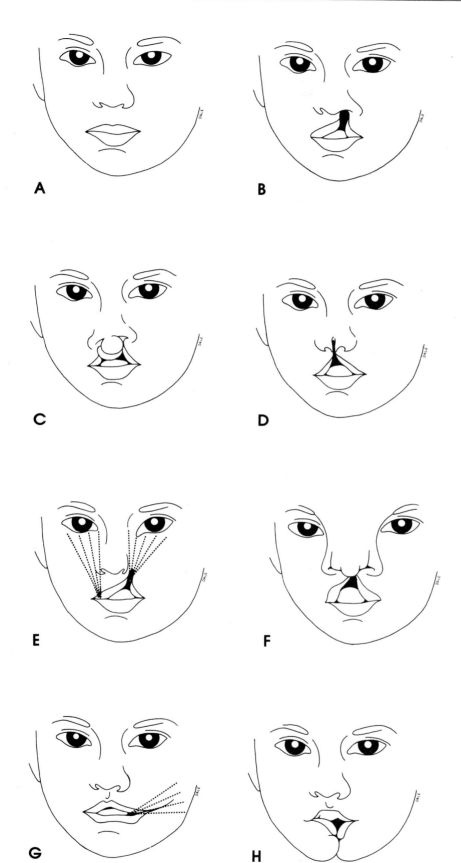

FIG. 2-35 Various types of facial clefts: **A,** normal; **B,** unilateral cleft lip; **C,** bilateral cleft lip; **D,** median cleft lip; **E,** oblique facial cleft; **F,** median cleft (frontonasal dysplasia); **G,** lateral facial cleft; **H,** mandibular cleft.

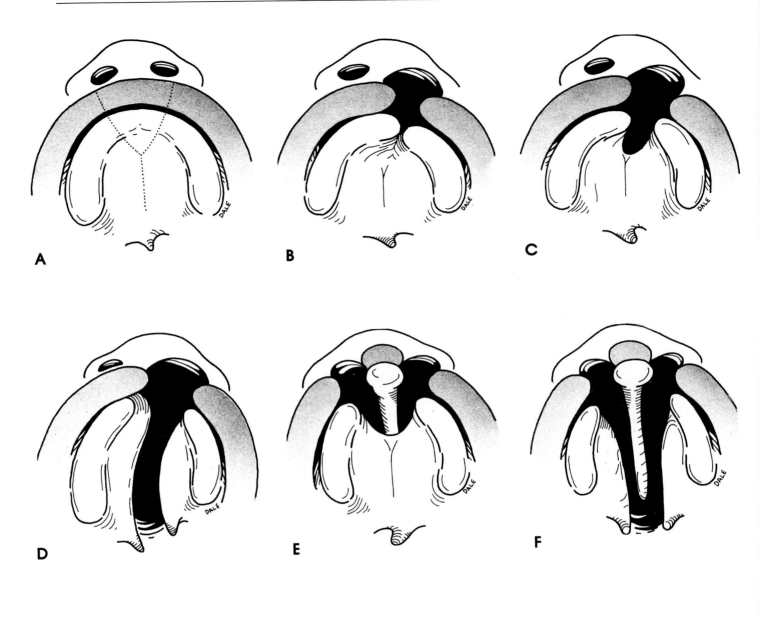

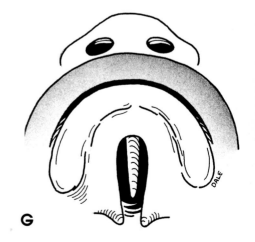

FIG. 2-36 Palatal clefts seen from a ventral view: **A,** normal; **B,** cleft of lip and alveolus; **C,** cleft of lip and primary palate; **D,** unilateral cleft lip and palate; **E,** bilateral cleft lip and primary palate; **F,** bilateral cleft lip and palate; **G,** cleft palate only.

deficiencies. Although vitamin deficiencies have been shown to be teratogenic in experimental animals, this effect has not been demonstrated in humans.

BIBLIOGRAPHY

Babiarz BS, Allenspach AL, Zimmerman EF: Ultrastructural evidence of contractile systems in mouse palates prior to rotation, *Develop Biol* 47:32, 1975.

Barry A: A development of the branchial region of human embryos with special reference to the fate of the epithelia. In Pruzansky S (ed): *Congenital anomalies of the face and associated structures*, Springfield Ill, 1961, Charles C Thomas.

Baume LJ: Ontogenesis of the temporomandibular joint, *J Dent Res* 41:1327, 1962.

Baume LJ, Holz J: Ontogenesis of the human temporomandibular joint: development of the temporal component, *J Dent Res* 49:864, 1970.

Burdi AR: Morphogenesis of mandibular dental arch shape in human embryos, *J Dent Res* 47:50, 1968.

De Beer GR: The differentiation of neural crest cells into odontoblasts in ambystoma and re-examination of the germ-layer theory, *Proc R Soc* 134B:377, 1947.

Dickson DR, Grant JC, Sicher H, et al: Status of research in cleft palate anatomy and physiology. I, *Cleft Palate J* 11:471;II, *Cleft Palate J* 12:131, 1973.

Diewert VM: Contributions of differential growth of cartilages to changes in craniofacial morphology. In Dixon AD, Sarnat BG, editors: *Factors and mechanisms influencing bone growth*, New York, 1982, Alan R Liss.

Diewert VM: A morphometric analysis of craniofacial growth and changes in spatial relations during secondary palatal development in human embryos and fetuses, *Am J Anat* 167:495, 1983.

Dixon AD: The development of the jaws, *Dent Pract Dent Rec* 9:10, September 1958.

Furstman L: The early development of the human temporomandibular joint, *Am J Orthod* 49:672, 1963.

Greene RM, Platt RM: Developmental aspects of secondary palate formation, *J Embryol Exp Morphol* 36:225, 1976.

Goss AN: Human palatal development in vitro, *Cleft Palate J* 12:210, 1975.

Hasell JR, Orkin RW: Synthesis and distribution of collagen in the rat palate during shelf elevation, *Develop Biol* 49:80, 1976.

Hazleton RD: Origin and migration of facial muscle primordia and their significance in the development of the cranial nervous system, *J Can Dent Assoc* 35:271, 1969.

Hudson CD, Shapiro BL: A radioautographic study of deoxyribonucleic acid synthesis in embryonic rat palatal shelf epithelium with reference to the concept of programmed cell death, *Arch Oral Biol* 18:77, 1973.

Humphrey T: The relation between human fetal mouth opening reflexes and closure of the palate, *Am J Anat* 125:317, 1969.

Jacobsen A: Embryological evidence for the nonexistence of the premaxilla in man, *J Dent Assoc South Africa* 10:189, 1955.

Johnston MC: Abnormal organogenesis of facial structures. In Wilson JG, Fraser FC (eds): *Handbook of teratology*, Philadephia, 1975, WB Saunders.

Johnston MC, Listgarten MA: The migration interaction and early differentiation of oro-facial tissues. In Slavkin HS, Bavetta LA (eds): *Developmental aspects of oral biology*, New York, 1972, Academic Press.

Johnston MC, Pratt RM: The neural crest in normal matrix influences of gene expression. In Slavkin HC, Greulich RC (eds): *Extracellular matrix influences of gene expression*, New York, 1975, Academic Press.

Krause BS, Decker JD: The prenatal interrelationships of the maxilla and premaxilla in the facial development of man, *Acta Anat* 40:278, 1960.

Krause BS, Kitamura H, Latham RA: *Atlas of the developmental anatomy of the face*, New York, 1966, Harper & Row.

Kvinnsland S: Observations on the early ossification process of the mandible as seen in plastic embedded human embryos, *Acta Odontol Scand* 27:643, 1969.

Kvinnsland S: Observations on the early ossification of the upper jaw, *Acta Ondontol Scand* 27:649, 1969.

Larsson KS: Closure of the secondary palate and its relation to sulphomucopolysaccharides, *Acta Odontol Scand* 20 (suppl 31):1, 1962.

Lessand JL, Wee AL, Zimmerman EF: Presence of contractile proteins in mouse fetal palate prior to shelf elevation, *Teratology* 9:113, 1974.

Levy BM: Embryological development of the temporomandibular joint. In Sarnar BG (ed): *The temporomandibular joint*, ed 2, Springfield Ill, 1964, Charles C Thomas.

Lockshin RA, Beaulaton J: Programmed cell death, *Life Sci* 15:1549, 1974.

Nishimura H: Incidence of malformations in abortions. In Fraser FC, McKusick VA (eds): *Congenital malformations*, New York, 1969, Exerpta Medica.

Pourtois M: Morphogenesis of the primary and secondary palate. In Slavkin HS, Bavetta LA (eds): *Developmental aspects of oral biology*, New York, 1972, Academic Press.

Perry HT, Xu Y, Forbes DP: The embryology of the temporomandibular joint, *J Craniomandib Pract* 3:126, 1985.

Pratt RM, Hassell JR: Appearance and distribution of carbohydrate-rich macromolecules on the epithelial surface of the developing rat palatal shelf, *Develop Biol* 45:192, 1975.

Ross RB, Johnston MC: *Cleft lip and palate*, Baltimore, 1972, Williams & Wilkins.

Saxen L: Association between oral clefts and drugs taken during pregnancy, *Int J Epidemiol* 4:37, 1975.

Shah RM: A cellular mechanism for the palatal shelf reorientation from a vertical to a horizontal plane in hamster: light and electron microscopic study, *J Embryol Exp Morphol* 53:1, 1979.

Shapiro BL, Sweney L: Electron microscopic and histochemical examination of oral epithelial mesenchymal interaction (programmed cell death), *J Dent Res* 48:652, 1969.

Slavkin HC: *Developmental craniofacial biology*, Philadelphia, 1979, Lea & Febiger.

Sperber GH: *Craniofacial embryology,* Bristol UK, 1973, John Wright & Sons.

Symons NBB: The development of the human mandibular joint, *J Anat* 86:326, 1952.

Walker BE: The association of mucopolysaccharides with morphogenesis of the palate and other structures in mouse embryos, *J Embryol* 9:22, 1961.

Waterman RE, Meller SM: A scanning electron microscope study of secondary palate formation in the human, *Anat Rec* 175:464, 1973.

Waterman RE, Meller SM: Alterations in the epithelial surface of human palatal shelves prior to and during fusion: a scanning electron microscopic study, *Anat Rec* 180:111, 1974.

Weston JA: The migration and differentiation of neural crest cells, *Adv Morphogr* 8:41, 1970.

Wood NK, Wragg LE, Stuteville OH, et al: Osteogenesis of the human upper jaw: proof of the nonexistence of a separate premaxillary centre, *Arch Oral Biol* 14:1331, 1969.

Wood PJ, Kraus BS: Prenatal development of the human palate, *Arch Oral Biol* 7:137, 1962.

Youdelis RA: The morphogenesis of the human temporomandibular joint and its associated structures, *J Dent Res* 45:182, 1966.

Youdelis RA: Ossification of the human temporomandibular joint, *J Dent Res* 45:192, 1966.

CHAPTER 3

Structure of the Oral Tissues

THIS chapter gives a brief account of the histology of the tooth and its supporting tissues (Fig. 3-1). The immediate environment of the tooth (oral mucosa, salivary glands, and plaque), the bones of the jaw, and the articulations between the jaws (temporomandibular joints) are also discussed. The intention here is to provide a simple description of the subject matter contained later within this book, setting the stage for more detailed consideration.

THE MOUTH

The mouth may be described in a number of ways to include its several structures. In functional terms, if an individual rinses orally with a harmless disclosing solution, the dye will be found to extend posteriorly to a line running across the roof of the mouth just beyond the junction of the hard and soft palates and to a line corresponding to this on the dorsum of the tongue. On the basis of this description the surface area of the visible structures within the mouth has been measured (Table 3-1).

THE TOOTH

Teeth constitute approximately 20% of the surface area of the mouth, the upper teeth significantly more than the lower teeth (24 cm² to 20 cm²). Teeth serve a number of functions. In humans the one most commonly associated with them is mastication; but teeth are also essential for proper speech and, in modern times, for esthetics. In the animal kingdom, teeth have important roles as weapons of attack and defense. To fulfill most of these functions, teeth need to be hard and firmly attached to the bones of the jaws. In most submammalian vertebrates the teeth are fused directly to the jawbone. Although this provides a firm attachment, it is a brittle arrangement and such teeth are frequently broken and lost during normal function. To compensate, many successional teeth form to ensure continued function of the dentition.

In mammals teeth are attached to the bones of the jaw by a fibrous ligament, the *periodontal ligament* (PDL). This arrangement provides an attachment with enough flexibility to withstand the forces of mastication. Accordingly, far fewer teeth are lost to normal function

| **TABLE 3-1** | Surface areas (cm²) of different regions of the mouth |

	Teeth	Palate	Upper and lower buccal and lower lingual gingival and alveolar mucosa	Buccal vestibular mucosa	Ventral surface of tongue and floor of mouth	Dorsum of tongue	Total area
Mean 10 males	46.1 ±4.6	20.7 ±1.8	47.0 ±7.0	50.0 ±3.4	26.6 ±5.0	26.3 ±1.5	217.3 ±11.7
Mean 10 females	44.5 ±5.3	19.5 ±1.9	46.2 ±7.9	50.5 ±2.3	26.3 ±3.2	25.1 ±2.0	212.1 ±14.0
Combined mean	45.3 ±5.0	20.1 ±1.9	46.6 ±7.4	50.2 ±2.9	26.5 ±4.2	25.7 ±1.8	214.7 ±12.9
Percent total area	21.1	9.4	21.7	23.4	12.3	12.0	100.0

From Collins LM, Dawes C: *J Dent Res* 66:1300, 1987.

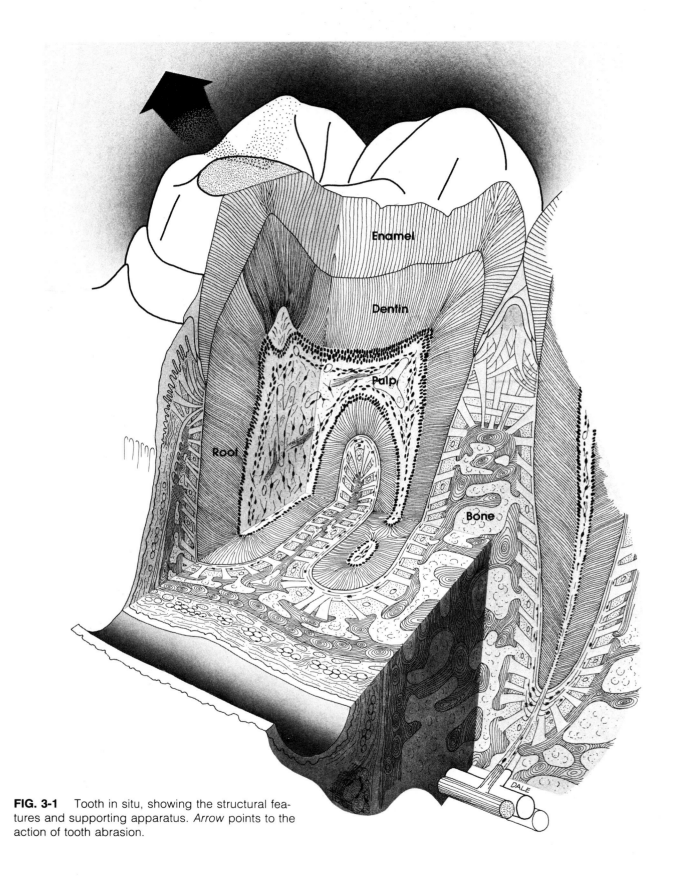

FIG. 3-1 Tooth in situ, showing the structural features and supporting apparatus. *Arrow* points to the action of tooth abrasion.

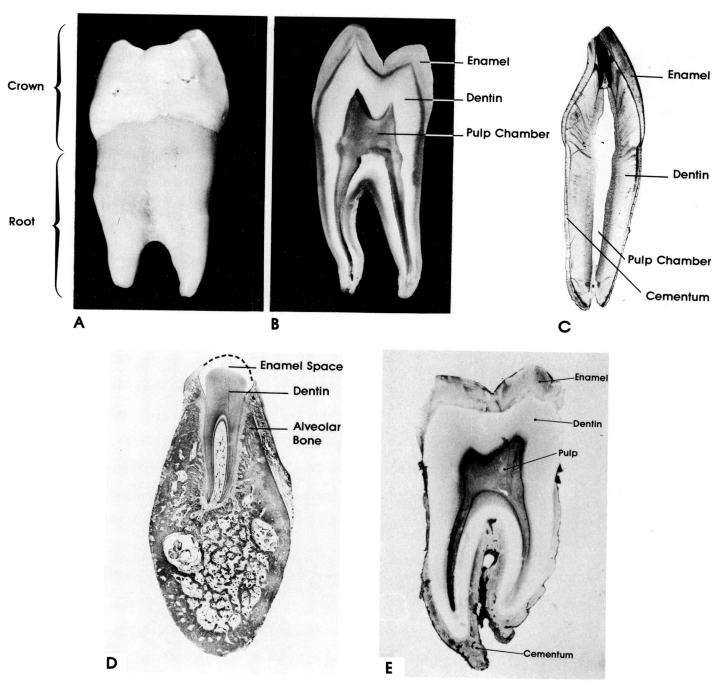

FIG. 3-2 Various ways of examining the tooth. **A,** Single tooth. **B,** Tooth cut longitudinally to show the disposition of enamel, cementum, dentin, and pulp chamber. **C,** Ground section. Note that it is relatively thick and contains no soft tissue. The enamel is retained for microscopic examination. **D,** Demineralized histologic section of an erupted tooth. It is much thinner, but the enamel is lost and cannot be studied. **E,** Specially prepared thick section (100 μm) in which all the dental tissues are retained.

and the need for continual replacement of teeth no longer exists. In humans and most mammals a limited succession of teeth still occurs, not to compensate for continual loss of teeth but to accommodate the growth of the face and jaws. The face and the jaws of a human child are small and consequently can carry only a few teeth of small size. These small teeth constitute the *deciduous* or *primary* dentition. With growth a large increase in the size of the jaws occurs, necessitating not only more teeth but larger ones. Because teeth cannot increase in size once they are formed, the deciduous dentition becomes inadequate and must be replaced by a *permanent* or *secondary* dentition consisting of more and larger teeth.

Anatomically the tooth consists of a crown and a root; the junction between the two is the cervical margin (Fig. 3-2). The term *clinical crown* denotes that part of the tooth visible in the oral cavity. Although teeth vary considerably in shape and size (compare an incisor to a molar), histologically they are similar.

Enamel

The anatomic crown is covered by a hard, acellular, inert tissue called *enamel*, the most highly mineralized tissue found in the body. Enamel consists of about 96% inorganic material made up mainly of hydroxyapatite crystallites with traces of organic material enveloping each crystallite. This very high inorganic content renders enamel particularly vulnerable to demineralization in the acid environment created by bacteria, leading to dental caries. The high mineral content of enamel also determines much of its microscopic structure. The hydroxyapatite crystallites within enamel are preferentially packed; it is this difference in crystallite orientation that is responsible for much of the histologic structure of enamel. The way the crystals are aligned creates a structure of enamel *rods* or *prisms*, separated by an interrod substance that also consists of apatite crystallites aligned in a different direction from those found in the rods (Fig. 3-3).

The cells responsible for the formation of enamel, the *ameloblasts*, cover the entire surface of the enamel as it formed but are rapidly lost as the tooth emerges into the oral cavity. The loss of these cells renders enamel a nonvital and insensitive tissue that, when destroyed by any means (usually wear or caries), cannot be replaced or regenerated. However, although enamel is a dead tissue in a strict biologic sense, it is permeable; and ionic exchange can occur between the enamel and the environment of the oral cavity, in particular the saliva. When topical fluoride is applied to the enamel surface, the tooth becomes more resistant to dissolution in acid as a result of the substitution (by ionic exchange) of the fluoride ion for the hydroxyl radical in the hydroxyapatite crystal.

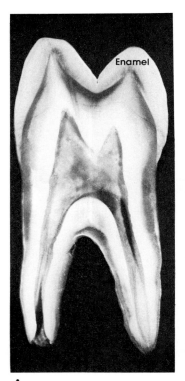

Enamel

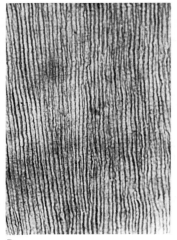

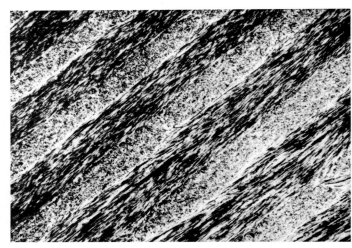

FIG. 3-3   Enamel. **A,** Its location. **B,** Its rod structure as seen in ground sections with the light microscope. **C,** Small fragment of enamel (electron micrograph). It consists of a mass of crystallites. The change in crystallite orientation creates an appearance of structure.

A   **B**   **C**

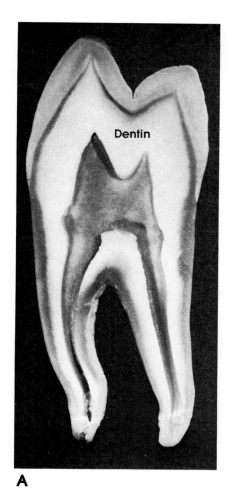

A

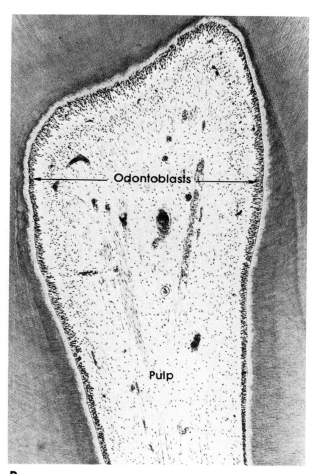

B

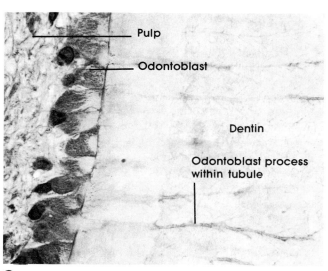

C

FIG. 3-4 Dentin and pulp. **A,** Dried tooth cut longitudinally. Dentin forms its bulk. Note the pulp chamber. **B,** In a demineralized section the pulp is retained and odontoblasts (cells that form dentin) outline the periphery. **C,** These cells at higher magnification with their processes extending into the tubular dentin.

Dentin

Because of its exceptionally high mineral content, enamel is a very brittle tissue, so brittle that it is unable to withstand the forces of mastication without fracture unless it has the support of a more resilient tissue. *Dentin* is this more resilient tissue, forming the bulk of the tooth, that supports the enamel and compensates for its brittleness.

Dentin is a hard, elastic yellowish white, avascular tissue enclosing the central pulp chamber (Fig. 3-4). By weight it is approximately 70% mineralized with hydroxyapatite crystals. Its organic component is mainly the fibrous protein collagen. A characteristic feature of dentin is its permeation by closely packed tubules traversing its entire thickness and containing the cytoplasmic extensions of the cells that once formed it and later maintain it. These cells are called *odontoblasts;* their cell bodies are aligned along the inner edge of the dentin, where they form the peripheral boundary of the dental pulp (Fig. 3-4, *B*). The very existence of odontoblasts makes dentin a vastly different tissue from enamel. Not only is dentin a sensitive tissue but, more important, it is capable of repair, since the odontoblasts can be stimulated to deposit more dentin as the occasion demands.

Pulp

The central pulp chamber, enclosed by dentin, is filled with a soft connective tissue called *pulp*. Anatomically, it is the practice to distinguish between dentin and pulp and it is easy to appreciate why this is the case. Dentin is a hard tissue whereas the pulp is soft (and is lost in dried teeth, leaving a clearly recognizable empty chamber). Embryologically, histologically, and functionally, however, dentin and pulp are the same and should be considered together. This unity is exemplified by the classic functions of the pulp: it is (1) formative, in that it produces the dentin that surrounds it, (2) nutritive, in that it nourishes the avascular dentin, (3) protective, in that it carries nerves that give dentin its sensitivity, and (4) reparative, in that it is capable of producing new dentin when required. All these functions of the dental pulp relate also to dentin.

In summary: The tooth proper consists of two hard tissues, the acellular enamel and the supporting dentin; the latter is a specialized connective tissue whose formative cells are in the pulp. These tissues bestow on teeth the properties of hardness and resilience. Also, because both tissues are mineralized, they give teeth a unique permanence; thus teeth have provided many important clues in tracing human evolution. For ex-

ample, the identification of Peking man *(Pithecanthropus erectus)* provides a fascinating story based on the discovery in 1921 by Zdansky of a single fossil molar tooth. Zdansky made no mention of his discovery until 1926, when Davidson Black, a Canadian professor of anatomy at Peking University, claimed from photographs and a written description, that the tooth was hominid and, with the discovery of two further teeth, that "the newly discovered specimen displays in the details of its morphology a number of interesting and unique characters, sufficient, it is believed, to justify the proposal of a new hominid genus." This bold conclusion was made from dental evidence alone but subsequently confirmed with the discovery of further fossilized skeletal remains.

Their indestructibility also gives teeth special importance in forensic science, for example, as a means of identification.

SUPPORTING TISSUES OF THE TOOTH

The tooth is attached to the jaw by a specialized supporting apparatus that consists of *alveolar bone*, the periodontal ligament and *cementum*, all protected by the *gingiva*.

Periodontal Ligament

The periodontal ligament (PDL) is a highly specialized connective tissue, about 0.2 mm in width, situated between the tooth and the alveolar bone (Fig. 3-5). Its principal function is to connect the tooth to the jaw, which it must do in such a way that the tooth will be able to withstand the considerable forces of mastication. This requirement is met by the masses of collagen fiber bundles that span the (theoretical) space between the bone and the tooth and by a gellike incompressible matrix. Each collagen fiber bundle is very much like a spliced rope in which individual strands can be continually remodeled without the overall fiber losing its architecture and function. In this way the collagen fiber bundles can adapt to the stresses placed on them. The PDL has another important function, a sensory one. Recall that tooth enamel is an inert tissue and therefore insensitive; yet the moment our teeth come into contact with each other, or when there is a grain of sand in a sandwich, we know it. Part of this sense of discrimination is provided by sensory receptors within the PDL.

At one extremity the fibers of the PDL are embedded in bone, and at the other the collagen fiber bundles are embedded in cementum.

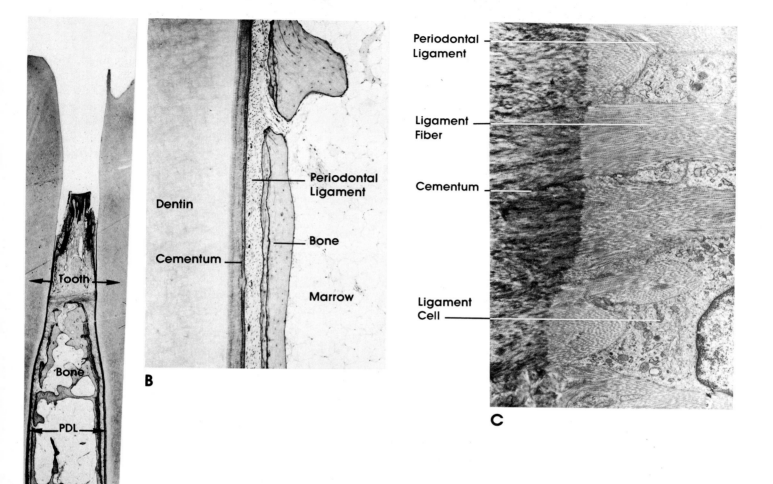

Dentin

Periodontal Ligament

Bone

Cementum

Marrow

B

Periodontal Ligament

Ligament Fiber

Cementum

Ligament Cell

C

Tooth

Bone

PDL

A

FIG. 3-5 Periodontal ligament. **A,** Supporting apparatus of the tooth at low magnification in longitudinal section. **B,** Light microscopic histology of the PDL. Note the fibrocellular nature of this structure. **C,** Fine structure of part of the PDL. In this electron micrograph the bundles of collagen fibers *(at right)* insert into acellular cementum *(at left)*. Between the fiber bundles are parts of ligament cells. (**C** courtesy Dr. M. Listgarten.)

Cementum

Cementum is hard and bonelike. It covers the roots of the teeth and is firmly "cemented" to the dentin of the root. It is a mineralized connective tissue very similar to bone except that it is avascular. It is about 50% mineralized, again with hydroxyapatite crystals, and its organic matrix is largely collagen.

There are two types of cementum. That attached to the root dentin and covering it from the cervical margin to the root apex is acellular and thus is called *acellular* cementum. This type is often covered, in turn, by *cellular* cementum, wherein the cells that formed it (the cementoblasts) have become trapped in lacunae within their own matrix very much as the osteocytes come to occupy lacunae in bone. Although there are variations in the distribution pattern of acellular and cellular cementum, both types function to anchor the PDL fiber bundles to the tooth.

It is worth stressing here that bone, the PDL, and cementum together form a functional unit of special importance when orthodontic tooth movement is undertaken.

ORAL MUCOSA

The oral cavity is lined by a mucous membrane that consists of two layers, an epithelial layer and a connective tissue layer (the lamina propria). This oral mucosa is particularly well adapted for the functions it has to perform (Fig. 3-6). Although its major functions are lining and protecting, it also is modified to serve as an exceptionally mobile tissue that permits free movement of the lip and cheek muscles. In other locations it serves as the organ of taste.

Histologically the oral mucosa can be classified as (1) masticatory, (2) lining, and (3) specialized. The *masti-*

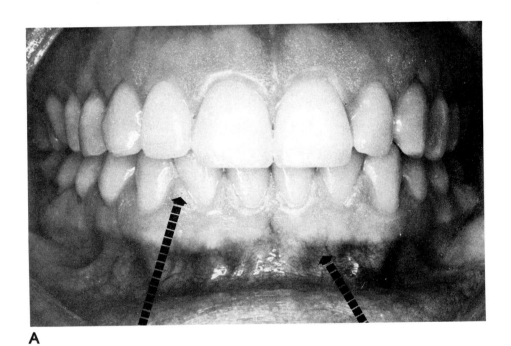

A

FIG. 3-6 Oral mucosa. **A,** Note the difference between tightly bound mucosa of the gingiva (gum) and mobile mucosa of the labial sulcus. This distinction can be seen in histologic section, **B,** where the gingival epithelium is tightly bound to bone by a dense fibrous connective tissue. In **C** the sulcular epithelium is supported by a much looser connective tissue.

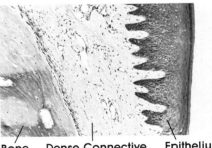

Bone Dense Connective   Epithelium
      Tissue

B

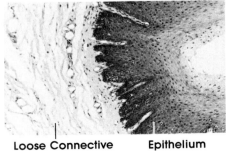

Loose Connective   Epithelium
Tissue

C

catory mucosa covers the gingiva and hard palate. It is tightly bound down by the lamina propria to the underlying bone (Fig. 3-6, *B*) and the covering epithelium is heavily keratinized to withstand the constant pounding of the food bolus during mastication. The *lining* mucosa, by contrast, must be as flexible as possible to perform its function of protection. Its epithelium is not keratinized; its lamina propria is structured for mobility (Fig. 3-6, *C*) and is not tightly bound down to underlying structures. The *specialized* mucosa is that tissue covering the surface of the tongue. Although functionally it is masticatory mucosa, it contains papillae and taste buds that serve special functions.

A unique feature of the oral mucosa is that it is perforated by the teeth. This anatomic feature has profound implications in the initiation of periodontal disease. The teeth are the only structures that perforate epithelium anywhere in the body. Epidermal appendages such as nails and hair are epithelial invaginations, but an epithelial continuity is always maintained. This perforation by teeth means that a junction must be established between the gum and the tooth.

Gingiva

The mucosa immediately surrounding an erupted tooth is known as the gingiva. In functional terms the gingiva consists of two parts, that facing the oral cavity (which is masticatory mucosa) and that facing the tooth (which is involved in attaching the gingiva to the tooth and also forms part of the periodontium). An arbitrary distinction between the two components can be made by drawing a line from the crest of the alveolar process to the crest of the gingiva. As it happens, the junction of the oral mucosa and the tooth is not very tight: antigens can easily pass through it and initiate inflammation in gum tissue (marginal gingivitis).

Saliva and Plaque

Saliva is a complex fluid that in health almost continually bathes those parts of the tooth exposed within the oral cavity. Consequently, it represents the immediate environment of the tooth. It is produced by three paired sets of major salivary glands—the parotid, submandibular, and sublingual glands—and by the many minor salivary glands scattered throughout the oral cavity. To give a precise account of the composition of saliva is very difficult because not only are the secretions of each of the major and minor salivary glands different but their volume may vary at any given time. In recognition of this variability, the term *mixed saliva* is used to describe the fluid of the oral cavity. Regardless of its precise composition, saliva has a variety of functions. It keeps the mouth moist, facilitates speech, lubricates food, and helps with taste by acting as a solvent for the food molecules. It also contains a digestive enzyme (amylase). Not only does it dilute noxious material mistakenly taken into the mouth, it cleanses the mouth; and it contains antibodies as well as acts like a buffer and therefore plays an important role in maintaining the pH of the oral cavity. Some idea of the importance of saliva to our well-being can be gained by recalling the morning "dry mouth" that accompanies a cold.

The basic histologic structure of the major salivary glands is very similar. A salivary gland may be likened to a bunch of grapes. Each "grape" is the *acinus* or *terminal secretory unit*, a mass of secretory cells surrounding a central space. The spaces of the acini open into ducts running through the gland that are called successively the intercalated, striated, and excretory ducts (Fig. 3-7), analogous to the stalks and stems of the bunch of grapes. These ducts are more than passive conduits, however; their lining cells have a function in determining the final composition of saliva.

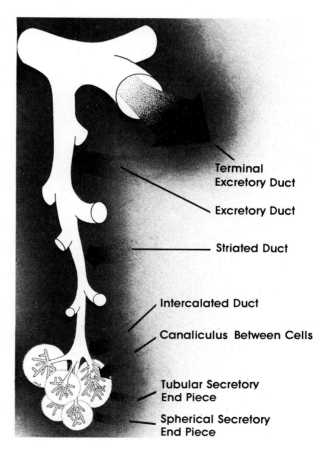

FIG. 3-7 Ductal system of a salivary gland.

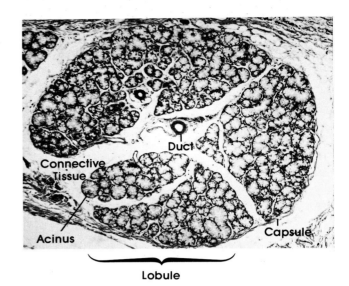

FIG. 3-8 Low-powered photomicrograph of a salivary gland showing its lobular organization.

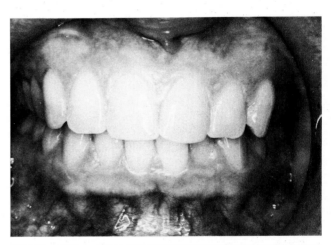

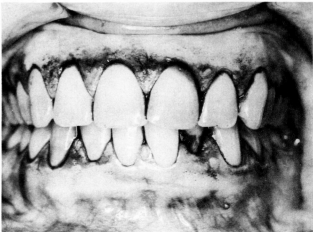

FIG. 3-9 Dental plaque. In the lower photograph a disclosing solution has been used to show the plaque that accumulates after 2 days. The plaque is especially prominent at the cervical margins and on the inset lower left incisor, which has escaped the beneficial action of previous brushing.

The ducts and acini constitute the *parenchyma* of the gland, the whole of which is invested by a connective tissue stroma carrying blood vessels and nerves. This connective tissue not only supports each individual acinus, it also divides the gland into a series of lobes or lobules and, finally, encapsulates it (Fig. 3-8).

A complex mixture of microorganisms—the normal flora of the mouth, salivary proteins, and desquamated epithelial cells—is attached to the surfaces of the teeth, especially when oral hygiene is poor, and forms a structure known as dental plaque (Fig. 3-9). Including a description of *dental plaque* in a textbook of normal dental histology might be questioned; however, plaque is practically a normal feature of the mouth, and its consideration here is justifiable. (Plaque and its activities will be discussed in greater detail in Chapter 16.)

BONES OF THE JAW

Mention has been made that teeth are attached to bone by the PDL. This bone, the alveolar bone, constitutes the alveolar process, which is firmly attached to the basal bone of the jaws (Fig. 3-10). As noted in the description of jaw development in Chapter 2, the alveolar process forms in relation to the teeth (Fig. 2-26). When teeth are lost, so also gradually is the alveolar process, creating the characteristic facial profile of the edentulous person whose chin and nose approximate because of a reduction in facial height. Although the histologic structure of the alveolar process is essentially the same as that of the basal bone, practically it is necessary to make a distinction between the two. The position of teeth and supporting tissues, which include the alveolar process, can be modified rather easily by orthodontic therapy. It is much more difficult, however, to modify the position of basal bone; usually this can be achieved only by influencing its growth. The way these bones grow is thus important in determining the position of the jaws and teeth, as will be discussed in detail in Chapter 8.

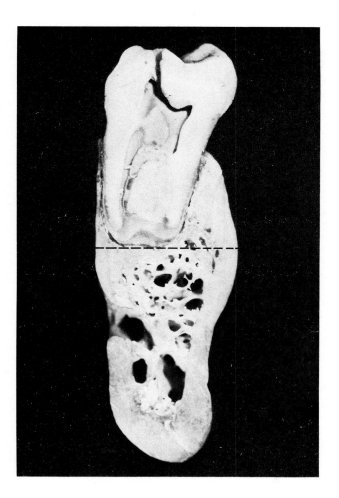

FIG. 3-10 Section through the jaw showing a tooth in situ. The distinction between basal bone and the alveolar process is indicated by the *dotted line*.

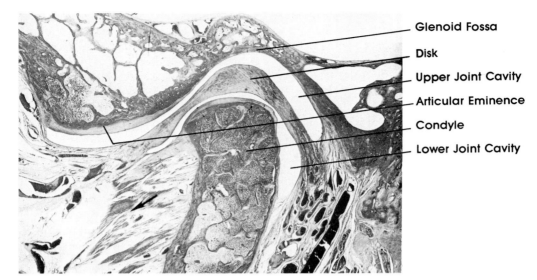

Glenoid Fossa

Disk

Upper Joint Cavity

Articular Eminence

Condyle

Lower Joint Cavity

FIG. 3-11 Sagittal section through the temporomandibular joint. The disk (dividing the joint cavity into upper and lower compartments) is apparent. The muscle attachment to the condyle of the lateral pterygoid muscle and the direction of its pull *(arrow)* to open the jaw and bring the disk and condyle onto the articular eminence (Fig. 9-13) are indicated (From Griffin CJ, et al: *Monogr Oral Sci* 4:1, 1975.)

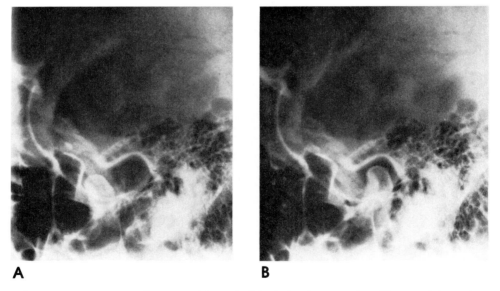

A   B

FIG. 3-12 Movement of the condyle and disk during jaw opening. The condyle and disk are pulled forward onto the articular eminence as the jaw opens. These two radiographs show the translation of the condyle during opening. **A,** With the jaw open the condylar head is close to the articular eminence. **B,** With the jaw closed it is situated in the glenoid fossa. (**A** and **B** courtesy Dr. D.W. Stoneman.)

TEMPOROMANDIBULAR JOINT

The relationship between the bones of the upper and lower jaws is maintained by the articulation of the condylar process of the mandible with the glenoid fossa of the temporal bone. This articulation, the temporomandibular joint (TMJ), is a synovial joint displaying special features that permit the complex movements associated with mastication. Its specialization is reflected in its histology (Fig. 3-11). A typical synovial joint consists of two bones covered by hyaline cartilage and separated by a cavity filled with synovial fluid contained within a capsule lined by a synovial membrane. The joint cavity may or may not be divided by an articular disk. The TMJ is formed by a capsule lined with a synovial membrane and is separated into two compartments by a specialized movable disk. The articular surfaces of the bone are covered not by hyaline cartilage but instead by a fibrous layer that is a continuation of the periosteum covering the individual bones. A simplified way to understand the function of a TMJ is to consider it as a joint with the articular disk, being a movable articular surface (Fig. 3-12).

The histology of the disk is adapted to this unusual function in the following way: The anterior part of the disk consists of collagen fiber bundles and fine elastic fibers intermingling with the tendon of the external or lateral pterygoid muscle. This part of the disk is innervated and vascularized. The central portion of the disk consists of collagen fibers, some fine elastic fibers, and (in older disks) cartilage cells, thus making this part of the disk fibrocartilage. The central portion is not innervated and is avascular. Posteriorly the disk splits into two leaves enclosing a central area of loose neurovascular connective tissue characterized by numerous arteriovenous anastomoses. The upper leaf consists of collagen bundles and thick elastic fibers; the lower leaf consists only of fine elastic fibers intermingled with collagen bundles. This structural arrangement permits a forward movement of the disk, with the elastic fibers being responsible for its recoil.

SUMMARY

This chapter has described the functions of teeth as including (1) mastication, (2) speech, (3) esthetics, and (4) (in animals) attack and defense. The constituent tissues of the tooth—enamel, dentin, and pulp—have been briefly described. The nonvital nature of enamel, making replacement impossible, contrasts with the viability of dentin, making this tissue capable of repair. Dentin and pulp, it is explained, should be considered as a single tissue.

The attachment of the tooth to the jaw (the periodontium) is described as consisting of (1) cementum, (2) the PDL, (3) alveolar bone, and (4) the gingiva. These tissues should be considered together as one functional unit.

The environment of the tooth comprises mainly the oral mucosa, consisting of masticatory, lining, and specialized mucosa. The penetration of oral mucosa by the teeth and the junction between oral mucosa and the tooth are unique anatomic features. This junction represents a weakness in the protective function or oral mucosa and is the site where the periodontal disease most often begins.

The complex nature of saliva and the simple histology of the salivary glands are introduced, along with the substance known as dental plaque. Finally, the anatomy and simple histology of the jawbones and the articulation between them are described.

BIBLIOGRAPHY

Blackwood HJJ: The mandibular joint: development, structure and function. In Cohen B, Kramer IRH (eds): *Scientific foundations of dentistry*, London, 1976, William Heinemann Medical Books.

Carlsson GE, Oberg T: Remodelling of the temporomandibular joints, *Oral Sci Rev* 6:53, 1974.

Collins LMC, Dawes C: The surface area of the adult human mouth and thickness of the salivary film covering the teeth and oral mucosa, *J Dent Res* 66:1300, 1987.

DeBoever JA: Functional disturbances of the temporomandibular joints, *Oral Sci Rev* 2:100, 1973.

Durkin JF, Heeley JD, Irving JT: The cartilage of the mandibular condyle, *Oral Sci Rev* 2:29, 1973.

Griffin CJ, Hawthorn R, Harris R: Anatomy and histology of the human temporomandibular joint, *Monogr Oral Sci* 4:1 1975.

Noble HW: The evolution of the mammalian periodontium. In Melcher AH, Bowen WH (eds): *Biology of the peridontium*, New York, 1969, Academic Press.

Noble HW: Comparative functional anatomy of temporomandibular joint, *Oral Sci Rev* 2:3, 1973.

Poswillo D: Surgery of the temporomandibular joint, *Oral Sci Rev* 6:87, 1974.

Rees LA: The structure and function of the mandibular joint, *Br Dent J* 96:125, 1954.

Worth HM: The role of radiologic interpretation in disease of the temporomandibular joint, *Oral Sci Rev* 6:3, 1974.

CHAPTER 4

Development of the Tooth and Its Supporting Tissues

THE development of the tooth involves many complex biologic processes, including epithelial-mesenchymal interactions, differentiation, morphogenesis, fibrillogenesis, and mineralization (which are discussed in other chapters). This chapter gives a straightfoward account of tooth development, preparatory to the more detailed accounts of dental development that follow.

In Chapter 1 it was explained how the stomatodeum, or primitive oral cavity, is formed. When the stomatodeum is examined under a light microscope, it can be seen to be lined by a primitive two- or three-cell-thick layered epithelium covering an embryonic connective tissue that, because of its origin from neural crest, is termed ectomesenchyme. In hematoxylin and eosin (H&E)–stained sections the epithelial cells appear empty; however, they were once filled with glycogen that was washed out of the cells during tissue preparation. The ectomesenchyme consists of a few spindle-shaped cells separated by a gelatinous ground substance.

PRIMARY EPITHELIAL BAND

In Chapter 2 it was explained how, after 37 days of development, a continuous band of thickened epithelium forms around the mouth in the presumptive upper and lower jaws from the fusion of separate plates of thickened epithelium. These bands are roughly horseshoe shaped and correspond in position to the future dental arches of the upper and lower jaws (Figs. 4-1 and 4-2, A and B). The formation of these thickened epithelial bands is the result not so much of increased proliferative activity within the epithelium as of a change in orientation of the cleavage plane of dividing cells (Fig. 4-2, C). Each band of epithelium, called the primary epithelial band, very quickly gives rise to two subdivisions: the *vestibular lamina* and the *dental lamina*. Indeed, so rapidly does this distinction take place that some authors consider the laminae to originate as separate entities.

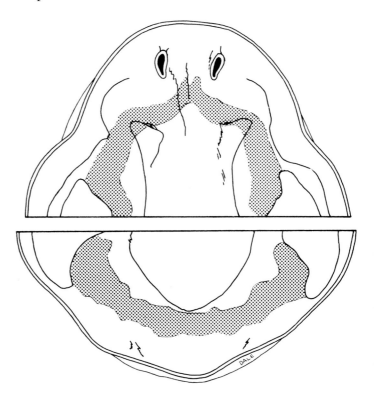

FIG. 4-1 Reconstructed early oral cavity. The position of the primary epithelial band *(shaded areas)* is indicated. (Adapted from Nery EB, et al: *Arch Oral Biol* 15:1315, 1970.)

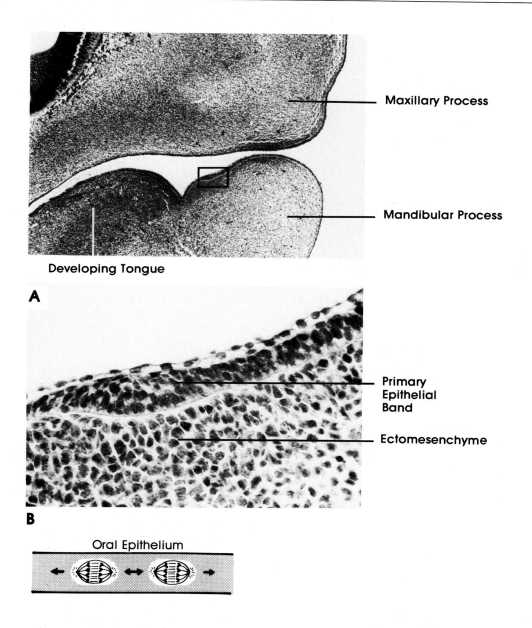

Maxillary Process

Mandibular Process

Developing Tongue

A

Primary Epithelial Band

Ectomesenchyme

B

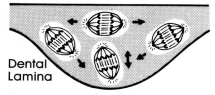

Oral Epithelium

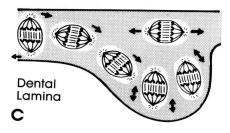

Dental Lamina

Dental Lamina

C

FIG. 4-2   Sagittal section through the head of an embryo. **A** shows the thickened epithelium of the primary epithelial band. **B** is the same structure at higher magnification. **C** shows the change in plane of cleavage. (**A** and **B** from Nery EB, et al: *Arch Oral Biol* 15:1315, 1970; **C** from Ruch JV: In Linde A [ed]: *Dentin and dentinogenesis,* Boca-Raton Fla, 1984, CRC Press, vol 1.)

Vestibular Lamina

If a coronal section through the developing head region of an embryo at 6 weeks of development is examined carefully, no vestibule or sulcus can be seen between the cheek and tooth-bearing areas (Fig. 4-3). The vestibule forms as a result of the proliferation of vestibular lamina into the ectomesenchyme. Its cells rapidly enlarge and then degenerate to form a cleft that becomes the vestibule between the cheek and the tooth-bearing area.

Dental Lamina

Within the dental lamina continued and localized proliferative activity leads to the formation of a series of epithelial ingrowths into the ectomesenchyme at sites corresponding to the positions of the future deciduous teeth. At this time the mitotic index, the labeling index, and the growth of the epithelial cells are significantly lower than corresponding indices in the underlying ectomesenchyme, which suggests that part of the "ingrowth" is achieved by ectomesenchymal upgrowth. From this point tooth development proceeds

in three stages: the bud, cap, and bell. These terms are descriptive of the morphology of the developing tooth germ; they do not properly describe the significant functional changes that occur during development, such as morphogenesis and histodifferentiation. It should also be noted that, because development is a continuous process, clear distinction between the transition stages is not possible. A further problem for the beginning student is that in examining sections of human embryos it is possible to section a tooth germ at a particular stage of development in such a way that it mimics another (Fig. 4-4).

BUD STAGE

The bud stage is represented by the first epithelial incursion into the ectomesenchyme of the jaw (Fig. 4-5). The epithelial cells show little if any change in shape or function. The supporting ectomesenchymal cells are closely packed beneath and around the epithelial bud.

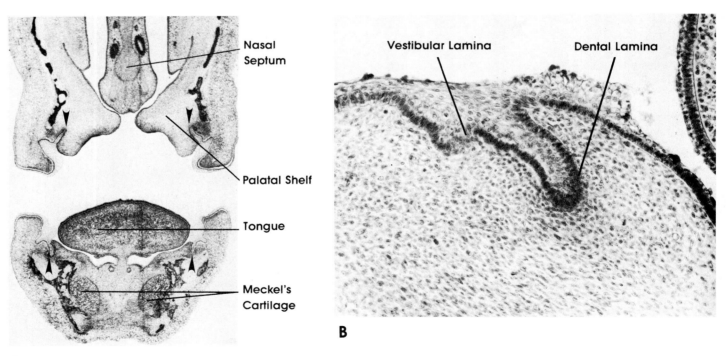

FIG. 4-3   Coronal section through the anterior portion of the developing head. **A,** The positions of the dental and vestibular laminae in the four quadrants are marked with *arrows.* **B,** The two laminae at higher magnification.

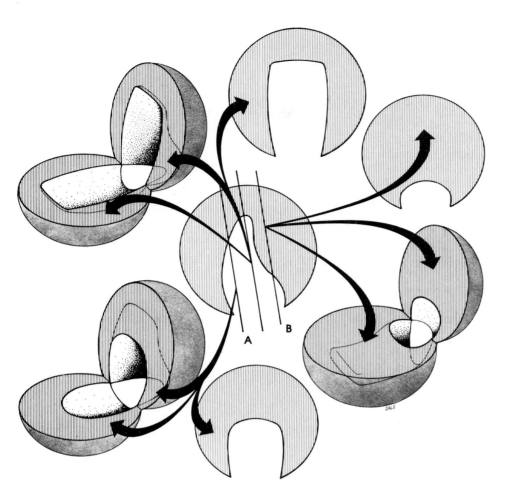

FIG. 4-4 Manner in which different histologic appearances can be created by cutting through a single tooth germ. Off-center sections (*A* and *B*) may mimic other stages of tooth development.

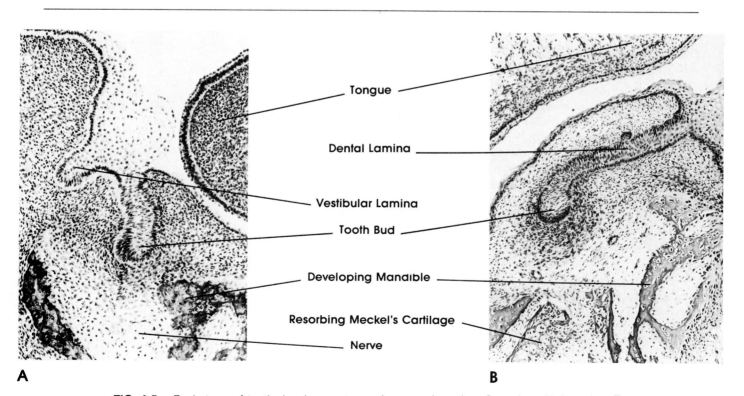

Tongue

Dental Lamina

Vestibular Lamina

Tooth Bud

Developing Mandible

Resorbing Meckel's Cartilage

Nerve

A

B

FIG. 4-5 Bud stage of tooth development seen in coronal section, **A,** and sagittal section, **B.**

CAP STAGE (PROLIFERATION)

As the epithelial bud continues to proliferate into the ectomesenchyme, cellular density increases immediately adjacent to the epithelial ingrowth. This process, classically referred to as a *condensation* of the ectomesenchyme, results from a local grouping of cells that have failed to produce extracellular substance and have thus not separated from each other (Fig. 4-6). At this early stage of tooth development it is already possible to identify the formative elements of the tooth and its supporting tissues. The epithelial ingrowth, which superficially resembles a cap sitting on a ball of condensed ectomesenchyme, is called the *dental organ**; among other functions it eventually forms the enamel of the tooth.

The ball of condensed ectomesenchymal cells, called the *dental papilla*, forms the dentin and pulp. The condensed ectomesenchyme limiting the dental papilla and encapsulating the dental organ—the *dental follicle*—gives rise to the supporting tissues of the tooth. Because the dental organ sits over the dental papilla like a cap, this stage of tooth development is known as the cap stage (Fig. 4-7).

The dental organ, dental papilla, and dental follicle together constitute the tooth germ. It is worth noting that early in the ontogeny (life history) of the tooth those structures giving rise to the dental tissues (enamel, dentin-pulp, and supporting apparatus of the tooth) can be identified as discrete entities.

BELL STAGE (HISTODIFFERENTIATION AND MORPHODIFFERENTIATION)

Continued growth of the tooth germ leads to the next stage of tooth development, the bell stage (Fig. 4-8), so called because the dental organ comes to resemble a bell as the undersurface of the epithelial cap deepens. Important developmental changes begin late in the cap stage and continue during the transition of the tooth germ from cap to bell. Through these changes, termed *histodifferentiation*, a mass of similar epithelial cells transforms itself into morphologically and functionally distinct components. The cells in the center of the dental organ continue to synthesize and secrete glycos-

---

*Enamel organ was first used to describe this structure. Some years ago an attempt was made to change the term to dental organ, to reflect more accurately the wider functions of this structure, which is responsible for determining the shape of the crown, initiating dentin formation, establishing the dentogingival junction, and forming enamel. The components of the organ were, likewise, renamed; internal enamel epithelium, for example, became internal dental epithelium. The author prefers the term dental organ, but it should be understood that this designation is not universally accepted.

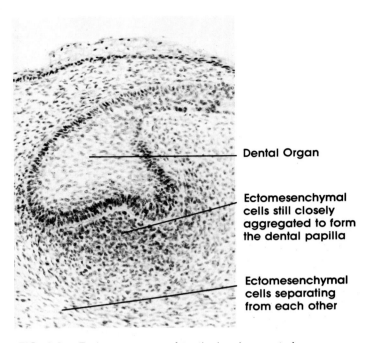

Dental Organ

Ectomesenchymal cells still closely aggregated to form the dental papilla

Ectomesenchymal cells separating from each other

FIG. 4-6 Early cap stage of tooth development. A condensation of the ectomesenchyme associated with the epithelial cap is easily identified (Fig. 4-7).

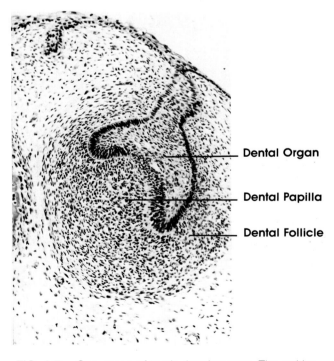

Dental Organ

Dental Papilla

Dental Follicle

FIG. 4-7 Cap stage of tooth development. The epithelial dental organ sits over a ball of ectomesenchymal cells, the dental papilla, that extend around the rim of the dental organ to form the dental follicle.

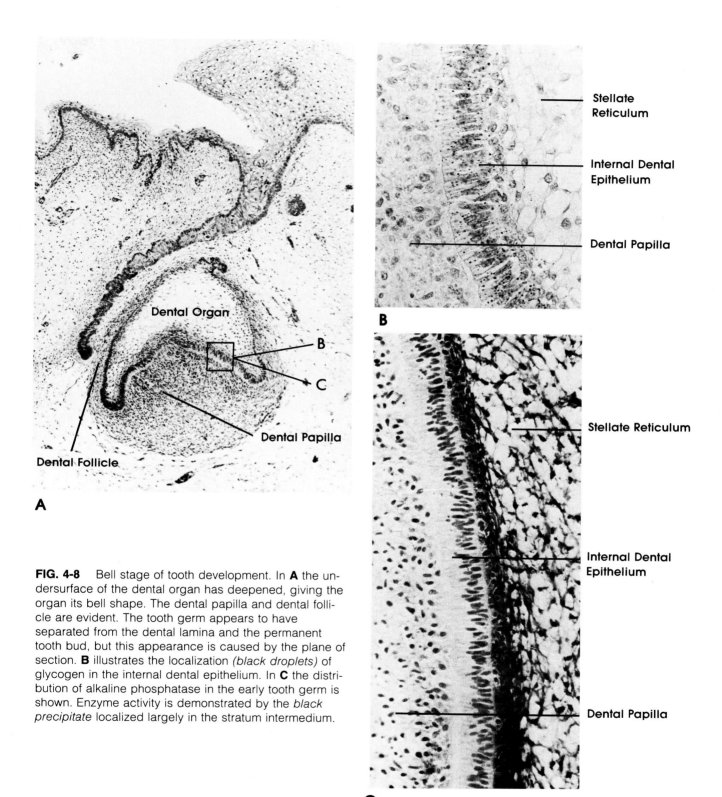

Stellate
Reticulum

Internal Dental
Epithelium

Dental Papilla

B

Dental Organ

B

C

Dental Papilla

Dental Follicle

A

Stellate Reticulum

Internal Dental
Epithelium

Dental Papilla

C

FIG. 4-8 Bell stage of tooth development. In **A** the undersurface of the dental organ has deepened, giving the organ its bell shape. The dental papilla and dental follicle are evident. The tooth germ appears to have separated from the dental lamina and the permanent tooth bud, but this appearance is caused by the plane of section. **B** illustrates the localization *(black droplets)* of glycogen in the internal dental epithelium. In **C** the distribution of alkaline phosphatase in the early tooth germ is shown. Enzyme activity is demonstrated by the *black precipitate* localized largely in the stratum intermedium.

aminoglycans into the extracellular compartment between the epithelial cells. Glycosaminoglycans are hydrophilic and so pull water into the dental organ. The increasing amount of fluid increases the volume of the extracellular compartment of the dental organ, and the cells of the organ are forced apart. Since the cells retain connections with each other through their desmosomal contacts, they become star shaped (Fig. 4-9). The center of the dental organ is thus termed the *stellate reticulum*.

At the periphery of the dental organ the cells assume a cuboidal shape and form the *external*, or *outer*, *dental epithelium*. The cells bordering on the dental papilla differentiate into two histologically distinct components. Those immediately adjacent to the dental papilla assume a short columnar shape and are characterized by high glycogen content (Fig. 4-8, *B*); together they form the *internal (or inner) dental epithelium*. Between the internal dental epithelium and the newly differentiated stellate reticulum some epithelial cells differentiate into a layer called the *stratum intermedium*. The cells of this layer are soon characterized by an exceptionally high activity of the enzyme alkaline phosphatase (Fig. 4-8, *C*). Although the cells of this layer are histologically distinct from the cells of the internal dental epithelium, both layers should be considered as a single functional unit responsible for the formation of enamel. The internal dental epithelium meets the external dental epithelium at the rim of the dental organ; this junctional zone is known as the *cervical loop*.

ENAMEL KNOT, ENAMEL CORD, AND ENAMEL NICHE

During the stages of tooth development described so far, some transient structures occur that are not necessarily present in every tooth germ or present at the same time. The first such structure is the *enamel knot* (Fig. 4-10), a localized thickening in the internal dental epithelium at the center of the tooth germ. The knot is often continuous with the *enamel cord*, or *septum*, which is a strand of cells running from the knot to the external dental epithelium that seems to divide the dental organ in two (Fig. 4-11). The function of these two structures is not known, but evidence is emerging that these structures are involved in determining the initial position of the first cusp of the tooth during crown pattern formation. Finally, the *enamel niche* is an apparent structure in histologic sections, created because the dental lamina is a sheet rather than a single strand and often contains a concavity filled with connective tissue. A section through this arrangement creates the impression that the tooth germ has a double attachment to the oral epithelium by two separate strands (Fig. 4-12).

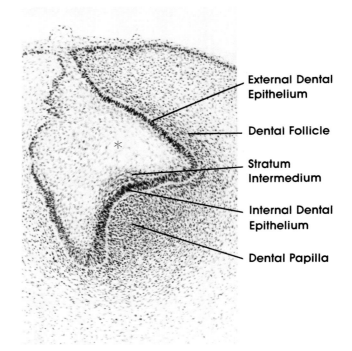

External Dental Epithelium

Dental Follicle

Stratum Intermedium

Internal Dental Epithelium

Dental Papilla

FIG. 4-9 Beginning of histodifferentiation within the dental organ forming the stellate reticulum *(asterisk)*. The peripheral epithelial cells are differentiating into the internal and external dental epithelia.

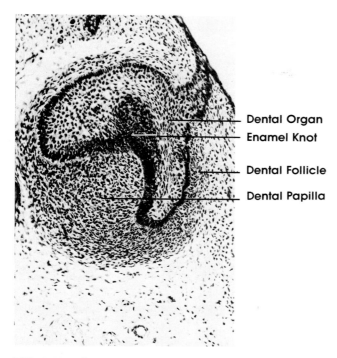

FIG. 4-10 Cap stage tooth germs showing the position of the enamel knot.

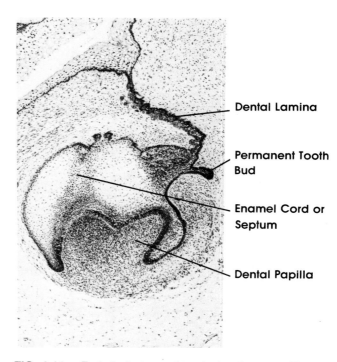

FIG. 4-11 Early bell stage of tooth development. The dental organ seems to be divided by the enamel septum or cord.

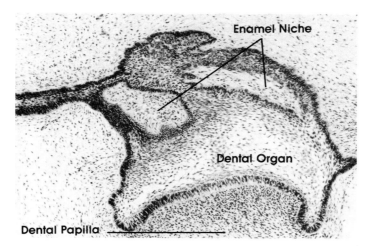

FIG. 4-12 Enamel niche. This structure is created by the plane of section cutting through a curved dental lamina so that mesenchyme appears to be surrounded by dental epithelium.

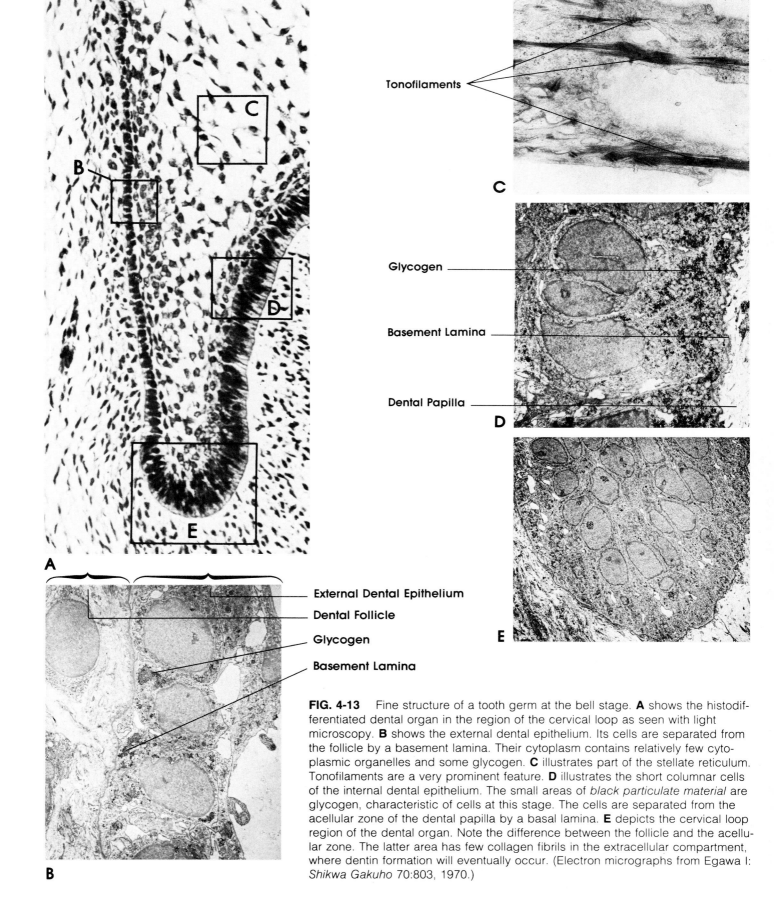

Tonofilaments

C

Glycogen

Basement Lamina

Dental Papilla

D

E

External Dental Epithelium
Dental Follicle
Glycogen
Basement Lamina

A

B

FIG. 4-13 Fine structure of a tooth germ at the bell stage. **A** shows the histodifferentiated dental organ in the region of the cervical loop as seen with light microscopy. **B** shows the external dental epithelium. Its cells are separated from the follicle by a basement lamina. Their cytoplasm contains relatively few cytoplasmic organelles and some glycogen. **C** illustrates part of the stellate reticulum. Tonofilaments are a very prominent feature. **D** illustrates the short columnar cells of the internal dental epithelium. The small areas of *black particulate material* are glycogen, characteristic of cells at this stage. The cells are separated from the acellular zone of the dental papilla by a basal lamina. **E** depicts the cervical loop region of the dental organ. Note the difference between the follicle and the acellular zone. The latter area has few collagen fibrils in the extracellular compartment, where dentin formation will eventually occur. (Electron micrographs from Egawa I: *Shikwa Gakuho* 70:803, 1970.)

Fine Structure of the Tooth Germ

The fine structure of the tooth germ at the bell stage (Fig. 4-13) is relatively uncomplicated but must be understood to appreciate the ultrastructural changes occurring in preparation for the formation of the dental hard tissues, enamel, and dentin. The dental organ is supported by a basal lamina around its periphery. The external dental epithelial cells are cuboidal and have a high nuclear/cytoplasmic ratio (little cytoplasm). Their cytoplasm contains free ribosomes, a few profiles of endoplasmic reticulum, some mitochondria, and a few scattered tonofilaments. Adjacent cells are joined by junctional complexes. The star-shaped cells of the stellate reticulum are connected to each other, to the cells of the external dental epithelium, and to the stratum intermedium by attachment plaques known as desmosomes. (See Chapter 5.) Their cytoplasm contains all the usual cytoplasmic organelles, but these are sparsely distributed. The cells of the stratum intermedium are connected to each other and to the cells of the stellate reticulum and internal dental epithelium by desmosomes. Their cytoplasm also contains the usual complement of organelles and tonofilaments. The cells of the internal dental epithelium have a centrally placed nucleus and a cytoplasm that contains free ribosomes, a few scattered profiles of rough endoplasmic reticulum, mitochondria evenly dispersed, some tonofilaments, a Golgi complex situated toward the stratum intermedium, and a high glycogen content.

Dental Papilla at the Bell Stage

The dental papilla is separated from the dental organ by a basement membrane from which a mass of fine aperiodic fibrils depends into what is usually termed a cell-free zone. This term is confusing, however, since the cell-free zone of Weil also exists below the odontoblasts in the mature dental pulp. To prevent confusion, the cell-free zone in the papilla will be referred to here as the *acellular zone*. The cells of the dental papilla appear as undifferentiated mesenchymal cells having a relatively uncomplicated structure with all the usual organelles. A few fine scattered collagen fibrils occupy the extracellular spaces. The dental follicle is clearly distinguished from the dental papilla, in that many more collagen fibrils occupy the extracellular spaces between the follicular fibroblasts; these are generally oriented in a radial pattern around the dental organ and dental papilla.

Breakup of the Dental Lamina and Crown Pattern Determination

Two other important events take place during the bell stage. First, the dental lamina joining the tooth germ to the oral epithelium breaks up into discrete islands of epithelial cells, thus separating the developing tooth from the oral epithelium. Second, the internal dental epithelium folds, making it now possible to recognize the shape of the future crown pattern of the tooth (Fig. 4-14). Note that the crown pattern of the tooth is determined very early in its development, suggesting that aberrant crown patterns result from factors operating at this time. (For further discussion, see Chapter 6.)

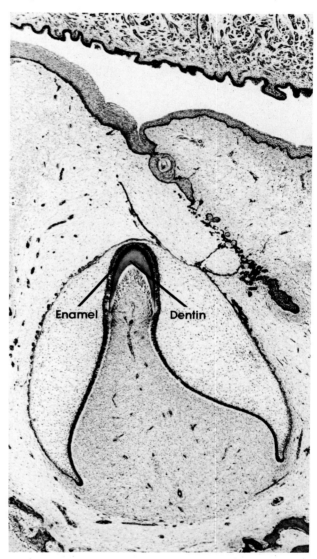

Enamel   Dentin

FIG. 4-14 Late bell stage (early crown stage) of tooth development. The dental lamina is disintegrating, so the tooth now continues its development divorced from the oral epithelium. The crown pattern of the tooth has been established by folding of the internal dental epithelium. Note that this folding has reduced the amount of stellate reticulum over the future cusp tip. Dentin and enamel have begun to form at the crest of the folded internal dental epithelium.

Fragmentation of the dental lamina results in the formation of discrete clusters of epithelial cells that normally degenerate and are resorbed. If any persist, they may form small cysts (eruption cysts) over the developing tooth and delay eruption. An important consequence of the fragmentation of the dental lamina is that the tooth continues its development within the tissues of the jaw divorced from the oral epithelium. This means that before the tooth can function it must reestablish a connection with the oral epithelium, and penetrate it, to reach the occlusal plane. As discussed in Chapter 3, this penetration of the lining epithelium by the tooth is a unique example of a natural break in the epithelium of the body. The etiologic factors responsible for gingivitis, and most likely periodontal disease, pass through this junction between epithelium and tooth.

NERVE AND VASCULAR SUPPLY DURING EARLY DEVELOPMENT

Much attention has been directed to the vascular and nerve supplies to the developing tooth, since it has been suggested that either or both may somehow be involved in the induction of teeth. There is evidence that discrete areas of increased capillary density in the ectomesenchyme are where the tooth buds develop; also nerve terminals seem to determine where other epithelial appendages, such as whiskers and taste buds, develop. The few existing studies on the development of vascular and nerve supplies to teeth in primates tend to agree with similar studies on smaller mammals. Thus the ensuing account is a generalized one.

Vascular Supply

Clusters of blood vessels are found ramifying around the tooth germ in the dental follicle and entering the dental papilla (or pulp) during the cap stage. Their number in the papilla increases during histodifferentiation, reaching a maximum at the onset of the crown stage of tooth development. Interestingly, the vessels entering the papilla are clustered into groups that coincide with the position where the roots will form. With age, the volume of pulpal tissue diminishes and the blood supply becomes progressively reduced, affecting the tissue's viability.

The dental organ, derived solely from epithelium, is avascular, although a heavy concentration of vessels in the follicle exists adjacent to the outer dental epithelium.

Nerve Supply

Pioneer nerve fibers approach the developing tooth during the bud-cap stage of development. Their target clearly is the dental follicle; nerve fibers ramify and form a rich plexus around the tooth germ in that structure. Not until dentinogenesis begins, however, do they penetrate the dental papilla. Although a possible relationship has been assumed between the developing nerve and blood supplies (i.e., that the nerves might supply the vessels), this clearly is not the case: the timing differs in establishment of the papillary vascular and neural supplies. Furthermore, histochemical studies show that autonomic nerve fibers are absent from the makeup of the pioneer nerve fibers approaching the tooth germ. This means that the initial innervation of the developing teeth is concerned with the sensory innervation of the future periodontal ligament and pulp. At no time do nerve fibers enter the dental organ.

FORMATION OF THE PERMANENT DENTITION

So far, only the initial development of the deciduous (or primary) dentition has been described. The permanent (secondary) dentition also arises from the dental lamina. The tooth germs that will give rise to the permanent incisors, canines, and premolars form as a result of further proliferative activity within the dental lamina at a point where it joins the dental organs of the deciduous tooth germs. This increased proliferative activity leads to the formation of another epithelial cap and associated ectomesenchymal response on the lingual aspect of the deciduous tooth germ (Fig. 4-15).

The molars of the permanent dentition have no deciduous predecessors, so their tooth germs do not originate in the same way. Instead, when the jaws have grown long enough, the dental lamina burrows posteriorly beneath the lining epithelium of the oral mucosa into the ectomesenchyme. This backward extension successively gives off epithelial ingrowths that, together with the associated ectomesenchymal response, form the tooth germs of the first, second, and third molars (Fig. 4-16). It is because of this backward extension of the dental lamina into the flattened ramus of the forming mandible that, on occasion, teeth occur in the bony ramus of the adult mandible.

Thus the teeth of the primary and secondary dentitions all form in essentially the same manner, though at different times (Fig. 4-17). The entire primary dentition is initiated between the sixth and eighth weeks of embryonic development, the successional permanent teeth between the twentieth week in utero and the tenth month after birth, and the permanent molars between the twentieth week in utero (first molar) and the fifth year of life (third molar). Aberrations in this pattern of development result in missing teeth or the formation of extra teeth.

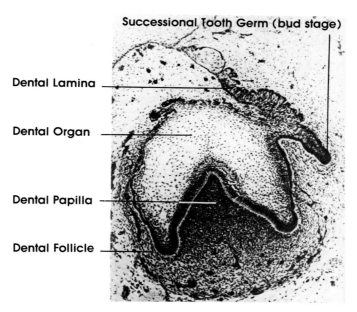

FIG. 4-15 Photomicrograph of the early bell stage of tooth development. Further epithelial proliferation from the dental lamina forms the tooth bud of the successional tooth germ. This situation occurs only in relation to primary or deciduous tooth germs (Courtesy Dr. E.B. Brain. Reprinted from Ten Cate AR: In Melcher AM, Bowen WH [eds]: *Biology of the periodontium,* New York, 1969, Academic Press.)

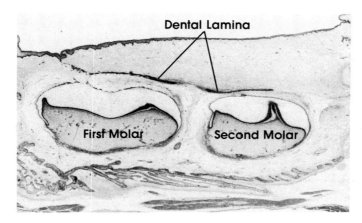

FIG. 4-16 Sagittal section through the distal part of a developing jaw showing the incipient permanent molar tooth germs.

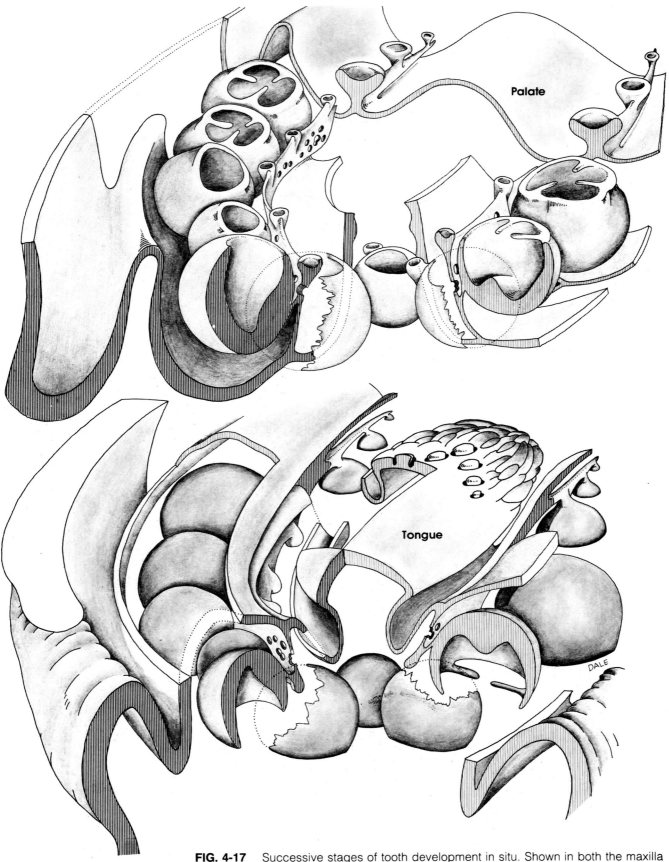

FIG. 4-17 Successive stages of tooth development in situ. Shown in both the maxilla and the mandible are tooth germs of the permanent dentition.

HARD TISSUE FORMATION OR CROWN STAGE

The next step in the development of the tooth, late in the bell stage, is formation of the two principal hard tissues of the tooth: the dentin (that specialized hard connective tissue forming the bulk of the tooth) and the enamel (Fig. 4-18). The formation of dentin, which always precedes enamel formation, marks the onset of the crown stage of tooth development (Fig. 4-19). Until completion of the bell stage, all cells of the internal dental epithelium are continually dividing to permit overall growth of the tooth germ. At the sites of the future cusp tips, where dentin will first be formed, mitotic activity ceases and the small columnar cells of the internal dental epithelium elongate, becoming tall and columnar with their nuclei aligned adjacent to the stratum intermedium and away from the dental papilla.

As these morphologic changes occur in the cells of the internal dental epithelium, changes also occur within the adjacent dental papilla. The undifferentiated ectomesenchymal cells increase rapidly in size and ultimately differentiate into odontoblasts, the dentin-forming cells. This increase in size of the papillary cells eliminates the acellular zone between the dental papilla and the internal dental epithelium. Tissue culture experiments have established that the differentiation of odontoblasts from the undifferentiated ectomesenchyme of the dental papilla is initiated by an organizing influence from the cells of the internal dental epithelium. In the absence of epithelial cells, no dentin will develop.

As development continues, there is a progressive maturation of the cells of the internal dental epithelium down the cusp slopes and a progressive differentiation of odontoblasts in the papilla. The odontoblasts, as they differentiate, begin to elaborate the organic matrix of dentin, collagen, and ground substance, which ultimately mineralizes. As the organic matrix is deposited, the odontoblasts move toward the center of the dental papilla, leaving behind a cytoplasmic extension around which dentin is formed. In this way the tubular character of dentin is established. Chapter 9 gives a full account of dentin formation, or *dentinogenesis*.

After the first dentin has been formed, and only then, the cells of the internal dental epithelium differentiate further, assuming a secretory function and producing an organic matrix against the newly formed dentinal surface. Almost immediately, this organic matrix is partially mineralized and becomes the enamel of the crown. The enamel-forming cells (or ameloblasts) move away from the dentin, leaving behind an ever-increasing thickness of enamel. Chapter 11 deals fully with the process of enamel formation, or *amelogenesis*.

It has been stated that odontoblasts differentiate under an organizing influence stemming from the cells of the internal dental epithelium. Likewise, it has been stressed that enamel formation cannot begin until some dentin has formed—an example of reciprocal induction.

Before forming the first dentin, cells of the dental organ and, in particular, those of the internal dental epithelium receive nourishment from two sources:

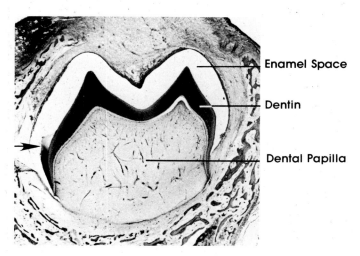

FIG. 4-18 Crown stage of tooth development. The formation of hard tissue is well advanced. Because of demineralization during section preparation, the enamel has been lost from this specimen (except for a small fragment at the cervical margin, *arrow*). The white area shown in section is referred to as the *enamel space*.

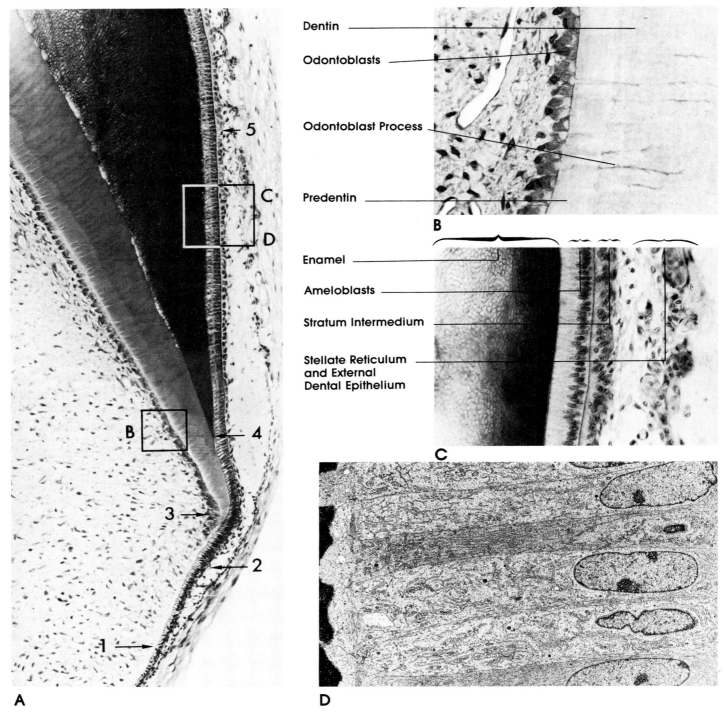

Dentin

Odontoblasts

Odontoblast Process

Predentin

B

Enamel

Ameloblasts

Stratum Intermedium

Stellate Reticulum
and External
Dental Epithelium

C

A

D

FIG. 4-19 Photomicrograph of many key features of tooth development. **A** traces the development of the dental epithelium. At *1* the epithelium is separated from the dental papilla by an acellular zone. At *2* the cells of the dental epithelium have elongated and the acellular zone is eliminated as odontoblasts differentiate from the dental papilla. At *3* the odontoblasts retreat toward the center of the pulp, leaving behind formed dentin, **B**. At *4* the cells of the dental epithelium, now ameloblasts, begin to migrate outward and leave behind formed enamel, **C** and **D**. At *5* the enamel organ has collapsed as the stellate reticulum is lost. **D** is an electron micrograph of functioning human ameloblasts. (**A** to **D** from Matthiessen ME, Romert P: *Scand J Dent Res* 86:67, 1978.)

TABLE 4-1	Time scale of human tooth development

Age	Development characteristics
42 to 48 days	Dental lamina formation
55 to 56 days	Bud stage: deciduous incisors, canines, and molars
14 weeks	Bell stage for deciduous teeth, bud stage for permanent teeth
18 weeks	Dentin and functional ameloblasts in deciduous teeth
32 weeks	Dentin and functional ameloblasts in permanent first molars

blood vessels located in the dental papilla and vessels situated along the periphery of the external dental epithelium. When the dentin is formed, it cuts off the papillary source of nutrients, causing a drastic reduction in the amount of nutrients reaching the dental organ. This reduction occurs at a time when the cells of the internal dental epithelium are about to secrete enamel, and thus there is an increased demand for nutrients. The demand is satisfied by an apparent collapse of the stellate reticulum, through which the ameloblasts are approximated to the blood vessels lying outside the external dental epithelium. Until this point the ameloblasts meet their metabolic requirements by using the glycogen stored in their cytoplasm and probably also by using some of the extracellular components of the stellate reticulum. Figure 4-19 summarizes the formation of hard tissue; and Table 4-1 gives an approximate time scale of tooth development up to the crown stage.

ROOT FORMATION

The root of the tooth consists of dentin. Two aspects of dentinogenesis have been explained: (1) how the differentiation of odontoblasts from cells of the dental papilla is initiated by cells of the internal dental epithelium and (2) how these cells form the dentin of the crown. It follows that epithelial cells are also required to initiate the odontoblasts, which will eventually form the dentin of the root. Odontoblasts are formed as epithelial cells of the external and internal dental epithelium proliferate from the cervical loop of the dental organ to form a double layer of cells known as *Hertwig's epithelial root sheath*. This sheath of epithelial cells grows around the dental papilla between the papilla and the dental follicle until it encloses all but the basal portion of the papilla. The rim of this root sheath, the epithelial diaphragm, encloses the primary apical foramen. As the inner epithelial cells of the root sheath

progressively enclose more and more of the expanding dental papilla, they initiate the differentiation of odontoblasts from cells at the periphery of the dental papilla. These cells eventually form the dentin of the root. In this way a single-rooted tooth is formed (Fig. 4-20).

Multirooted teeth are formed in essentially the same way. To picture multiple root formation, imagine the root sheath as a collar or skirt hanging from the enamel organ. By visualizing two tongues of epithelium growing toward each other from this collar, you may be able to appreciate how a primary apical foramen is converted into two secondary apical foramina, and how, if three tongues are formed, three secondary apical foramina will arise (Fig. 4-21). Aberrations in this splitting of the primary apical foramen can lead to the formation of pulpoperiodontal canals at the sites of fusion of the epithelial tongues.

An intact root sheath extending from the cervical loop to the apical foramen can rarely be demonstrated in histologic sections; and when it can, it is evident only at the initial stages of root formation. Once the root sheath forms, it rapidly initiates root formation and then becomes fragmented. In the case of mandibular teeth the tip of the forming root remains in a basically stationary position relative to the inferior border of the mandible, which means that the free border of the root sheath must be in a stable position. With the onset of root formation the crown of the tooth is growing away from the bony base of the crypt and the root sheath is not actually growing into the jaw. Because of these growth changes, the root sheath is stretched; although cell division occurs within it, eventually it fragments to form a fenestrated network around the tooth. In longitudinal section this fenestrated network is seen as a discrete cluster of epithelial cells known as the *epithelial cell rests of Malassez* (Fig. 4-22). In adults these epithelial cell rests persist next to the root surface within the periodontal ligament. Although functionless, they are the source of the epithelial lining of dental cysts that develop in reaction to inflammation of the periodontal ligament (PDL).

TOOTH ERUPTION

It has been stressed that tooth development occurs within the bone of the developing jaw in bony crypts separate from the oral epithelium. Soon after formation of the root is initiated, the tooth begins to erupt (i.e., move in an axial direction) until it assumes its final position in the mouth with its occlusal surface in the occlusal plane. The possible mechanisms of tooth eruption will be discussed extensively in Chapter 15; for the moment, it is necessary only to recognize that an axial movement of the tooth occurs.

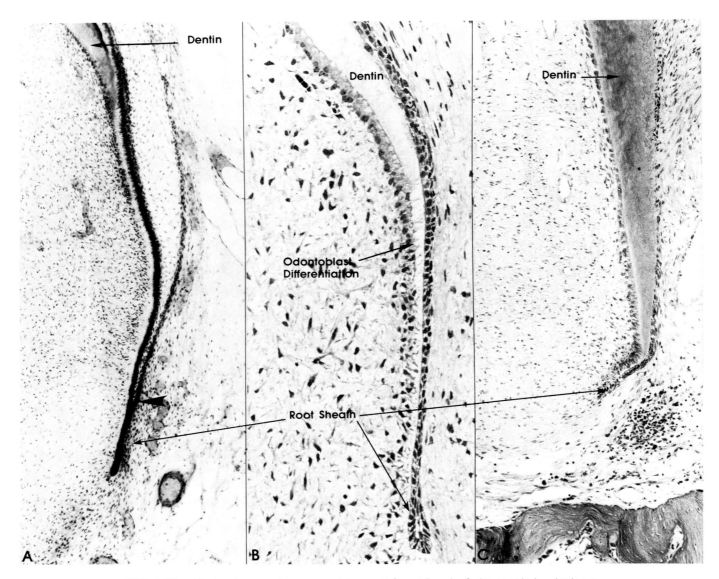

FIG. 4-20 Photomicrographs summarizing root formation. In **A** the root is beginning to form and can be seen as an extension of epithelium (the root sheath) from the cervical loop *(arrow head)*. The epithelium will initiate the differentiation of odontoblasts from the dental papilla. This is shown in **B,** as is the formation of root dentin. In **C** root formation is almost complete. The root sheath is now a small tag of epithelium that is initiating the final differentiation of odontoblasts at the rim of the future apical foramen.

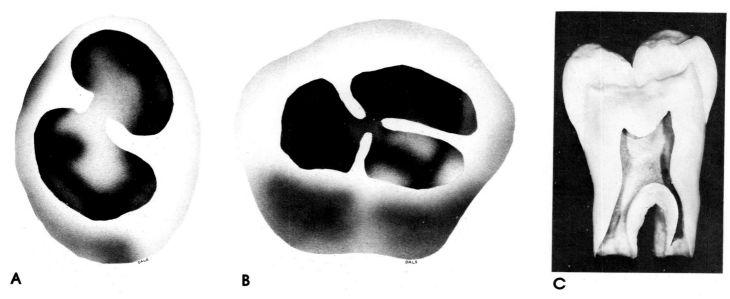

FIG. 4-21 Root formation in the undersurfaces of developing tooth germs. **A,** Two-rooted tooth. **B,** Three-rooted tooth. **C,** Section of a developing tooth. The roots have not finished forming, and the division into two roots is clearly seen. (Redrawn from Oöe T: *Human tooth and dental arch development,* Tokyo, 1981, Ishiyaka.)

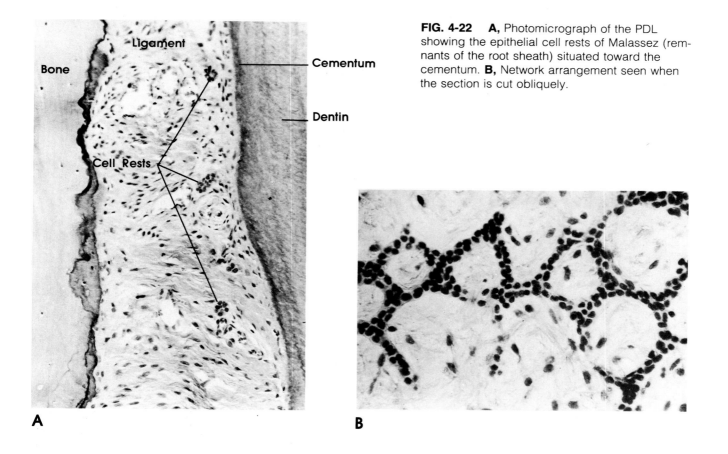

FIG. 4-22 **A,** Photomicrograph of the PDL showing the epithelial cell rests of Malassez (remnants of the root sheath) situated toward the cementum. **B,** Network arrangement seen when the section is cut obliquely.

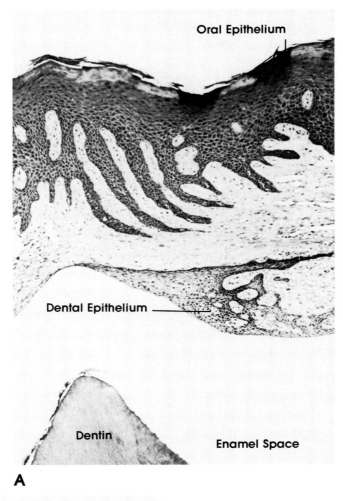

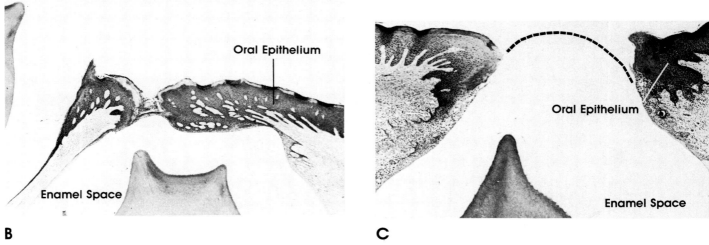

FIG. 4-23 Erupting tooth. **A,** As the tooth approaches the oral epithelium, the dental epithelium and oral epithelium are both supported by the same connective tissue. The connective tissue is lost in **B,** and the two epithelia fuse. The epithelia over the tooth break down to form an epithelium-lined canal through which the tooth erupts, **C.** Epithelial continuity is maintained at all times. The *dotted line* in **C** represents the enamel surface.

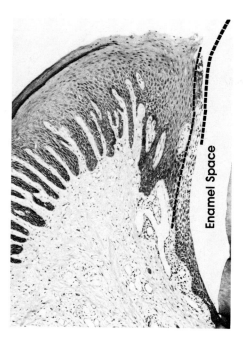

FIG. 4-24 Formation of the dentogingival junction from the oral and dental epithelia. The *thick dotted line* delineates the enamel surface; the *thin dotted line* separates junctional epithelium from oral epithelium.

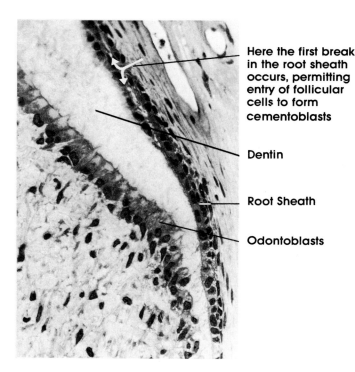

Here the first break in the root sheath occurs, permitting entry of follicular cells to form cementoblasts

Dentin

Root Sheath

Odontoblasts

FIG. 4-25 Fragmentation of the root sheath and the initial formation of cementum. Follicular cells migrate through a break in the epithelium *(arrow)* to lie against the surface of newly formed dentin.

In erupting, the crown of the tooth must escape from its bony crypt and pass through the lining mucosa of the oral cavity. As eruptive movement begins, the enamel of the crown is still covered by a layer of ameloblasts and remnants of the dental organ, which now form several layers of uniform cuboidal cells. Together the ameloblast layer and the adjacent cuboidal cells form the *reduced dental epithelium*. The bone overlying the erupting tooth is soon resorbed and the crown passes through the connective tissue of the mucosa, which is broken down in advance of the erupting tooth. The reduced dental epithelium and the oral epithelium fuse and form a solid knot of epithelial cells over the crown of the tooth. The central cells in this mass of epithelium degenerate, forming an epithelial canal through which the crown of the tooth erupts (Fig. 4-23). In this way tooth eruption is achieved without exposing the surrounding connective tissue and without hemorrhage. During eruption the cells of the reduced dental epithelium lose their nutritive supply and degenerate, thus exposing the enamel and simultaneously transforming it into a nonvital tissue.

As the tooth pierces the oral epithelium, another significant development occurs: the *dentogingival junction* forms from epithelial cells of both the oral epithelium and the reduced dental epithelium (Fig. 4-24). The importance of this junction has already been stressed. (Its histology is discussed in detail in Chapters 13 and 14.)

FORMATION OF SUPPORTING TISSUES

While roots are forming, the tooth's supporting tissues also develop. Recall that at the bell stage the tooth germ consists of the dental organ, dental papilla, and dental follicle, the last component being a fibrocellular layer investing both the dental papilla and the dental organ. From the dental follicle the supporting tissues of the tooth form. As the root sheath fragments, ectomesenchymal cells of the dental follicle penetrate between the epithelial fenestrations and become apposed to the newly formed dentin of the root (Fig. 4-25). In this situation these cells differentiate into cementumforming cells (or cementoblasts). They elaborate an organic matrix consisting of collagen and ground substance that becomes mineralized and in which collagen fiber bundles of the PDL become anchored. The cells of the PDL and the fiber bundles also differentiate from the dental follicle. There is some recent evidence that the bone in which the ligament fiber bundles are embedded is also formed by cells that differentiate from the dental follicle (Fig. 4-26).

In conclusion: This chapter has described the formation of the teeth and their supporting tissues in rel-

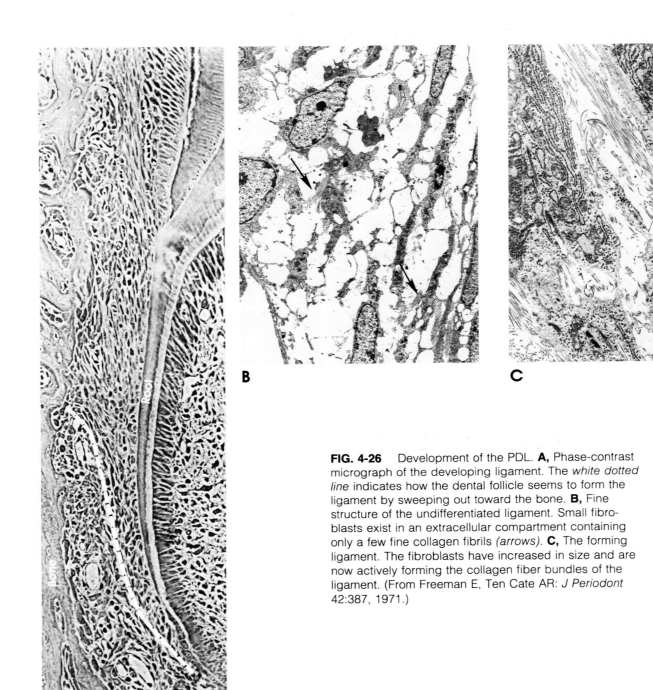

A

B

C

FIG. 4-26 Development of the PDL. **A,** Phase-contrast micrograph of the developing ligament. The *white dotted line* indicates how the dental follicle seems to form the ligament by sweeping out toward the bone. **B,** Fine structure of the undifferentiated ligament. Small fibroblasts exist in an extracellular compartment containing only a few fine collagen fibrils *(arrows)*. **C,** The forming ligament. The fibroblasts have increased in size and are now actively forming the collagen fiber bundles of the ligament. (From Freeman E, Ten Cate AR: *J Periodont* 42:387, 1971.)

atively simple terms. Many of the more important aspects of tooth development will be discussed in other chapters in considerably greater detail. For the time being, an overview of dental development will suffice to relate the information that follows to an overall picture.

BIBLIOGRAPHY

Atkinson ME, Mohamed SS: A histochemical study of the cholinergic and adrenergic innervation of the developing teeth and oral tissues in the mouse, *Arch Oral Biol* 28:353, 1983.

Baume LJ, Becks H: Development of the dentition of *Macaca mulatta, Am J Orthod* 36:723, 1950.

Brady CL, Browne RM, Calverly BC, et al: Symposium on odontogenic epithelium, *Br J Oral Surg* 8:1, 1970.

Carlsen O: Odontogenetic morphology, *Odontol Tidskr* 75:499, 1967.

Coslet JG, Cohen DW: Observations on the development of the vestibular trough in the human fetus. I. The anterior portion of the mouth, *J Periodontol* 40:320, 1969.

Decker JD: A light and electron microscope study of the rat molar enamel organ, *Arch Oral Biol* 8:301, 1963.

Decker JD: The development of a vascular supply to the rat molar enamel organ, *Arch Oral Biol* 12:453, 1967.

Egawa I: Electron microscopy of human enamel organ, *Shikwa Gakuho* 70:803, 1970.

Freeman E, Ten Cate AR: Development of the periodontium: an electron microscopic study, *J Periodontol* 42:387, 1971.

Gaunt WA: The vascular supply to the dental lamina during early development, *Acta Anat* 37:232, 1959.

Gaunt WA: The vascular supply in relation to the formation of roots of the cheek teeth of the mouse, *Acta Anat* 43:116, 1960.

Gaunt WA, Miles AEW: Fundamental aspects of tooth morphogenesis. In Miles AEW (ed): *Structural and chemical organization of teeth*, New York, 1967, Academic Press, vol 1.

Hixon EH: Growth of the dentition and its supporting structure, *J Am Dent Assoc* 82(4):782, 1971.

Kollar EJ, Lumsden AGS: Tooth morphogenesis: the role of the innervation during induction and pattern formation, *J Biol Buccale* 7:49, 1979.

Kraus BS: Calcification of the human deciduous teeth, *J Am Dent Assoc* 59(6):1128, 1959.

Kraus BS, Jordan EE: *The human dentition before birth*, Philadelphia, 1965, Lea & Febiger.

Lumsden AGS: Pattern formation in the molar dentition of the mouse, *J Biol Buccale* 7:77, 1979.

Lunt RC, Law DB: A review of the chronology of eruption of deciduous teeth, *J Am Dent Assoc* 89:872, 1974.

McFall WT Jr, Kraus BS: Notations on surface morphology of prenatal oral mucous membranes, *Periodontics* 3:141, 1965.

Mohamed SS, Atkinson ME: A histological study of the innervation of developing mouse teeth, *J Anat* 136:735, 1983.

Nery EB, Kraus BS, Croup M: Timing and topography of early human tooth development, *Arch Oral Biol* 15:1315, 1970.

Oöe T: On the early development of human dental lamina, *Okajimas Folia Anat Jpn* 30:197, 1957.

Oöe T: On the development of position of the tooth germs in the human deciduous molar teeth, *Okajimas Folia Anat Jpn* 32:97, 1959.

Oöe T: À propos de la formation de la bifurcation ou tripartition des racines dans les molaires humaines, *Acta Anat* 82:512, 1973.

Oöe T: *Human tooth and dental arch development*, Tokyo, 1981, Ishyaku.

Orban E, Mueller E: The development of the bifurcation of multirooted teeth, *J Am Dent Assoc* 16:297, 1929.

Osborn JW: A realistic interpretation of morphogenesis, *J Biol Buccale*, 6:327, 1979.

Pannese E: Observations on the ultrastructure of the enamel organ. I. Stellate reticulum and stratum intermedium, *J Ultrastruct Res* 4:372, 1960.

Pannese E: Observations on the ultrastructure of the enamel organ. II. Involution of the stellate reticulum, *J Ultrastruct Res* 5:328, 1961.

Pannese E: Observations on the ultrastructure of the enamel organ. III. Internal and external enamel epithelia, *J Ultrastruct Res* 6:186, 1962.

Pearson AA: The early innervation of the developing deciduous teeth, *J Anat* 123:563, 1977.

Provenza DV, Sisca RF: Electron microscope studies of human dental primordia, *Arch Oral Biol* 16:121, 1971.

Saunders RLCH, Rockert HOE: Vascular supply of dental tissues, including lymphatics. In Miles AEW (ed): *Structural and chemical organization of teeth*, New York, 1967, Academic Press, vol 1.

Schour I, Massler M: Studies in tooth development: the growth pattern of human teeth, *J Am Dent Assoc* 27:1785, 1918, 1940.

Scott JH: The development and function of the dental follicle, *Br Dent J* 85:193, 1948.

Scott J: The development, structure and function of the alveolar bone, *Dent Pract Dent Rec* 19:19, September 1968.

Silva DG, Kailis DG: Ultrastructural studies on the cervical loop and the development of the amelodentinal junction in the cat, *Arch Oral Biol* 17:279, 1972.

Sisca RF, Provenza DV: Electron microscopic studies of human tooth development: prospective gingival epithelium, *J Periodont Res* 5:293, 1970.

Slavkin HC: *Developmental aspects of oral biology*, New York, 1972, Academic Press.

Slavkin HC: Embryonic tooth formation: a tool for developmental biology, *Oral Sci Rev* 4:7, 1974.

Ten Cate AR, Mills C, Solomon G: The development of the periodontium: a transplantation and autoradiographic study, *Anat Rec* 170:365, 1971.

Thesleff I, Barrach HJ, Foidart JM, et al: Changes in the distribution of type IV collagen, laminin, proteoglycan, and fibronectin during mouse tooth development, *Develop Biol* 81:182, 1981.

Thesleff I, Stenman S, Vaheri A, Timpl R: Changes in the matrix proteins, fibronectin and collagen during differentiation of mouse tooth germs, *Develop Biol* 70:116, 1979.

Thomas MJ: Observations on the development and function of the enamel organ, *J Am Dent Assoc* 12:255, 1925.

Tongue CH: The time-structure relationship of tooth development in human embryogenesis, *J Dent Res* 48:745, 1969.

Van der Linden FPGM, Duterloo HS: *Development of the human dentition,* New York, 1976, Harper & Row.

West CM: The development of the gums and their relationship to the deciduous teeth in the human fetus, *Contrib Embryol* 79:25, 1924.

CHAPTER 5

Fibroblasts and Their Products

S O FAR, the development and structure of teeth and their supporting tissues have been described in a straightforward manner to give the beginning student an understanding and vocabulary that will permit a more detailed study of the dental tissues discussed in subsequent chapters. Before we embark on a consideration of these subjects, however, three additional chapters need to be presented dealing with basic biologic concepts and problems that have a direct bearing on the development, structure, and function of dental tissues. In this chapter we consider the fibroblast and its products, and in Chapters 6 and 7 we will take up the subjects of epithelial mesenchymal relationships and the principles of hard tissue formation and destruction.

THE FIBROBLAST

Fibroblasts are the predominant cell of connective tissue; and, because all tissues of the tooth (except enamel) and its supporting apparatus are connective, fibroblasts play an important role in the development, structure and function of the tooth. As their name suggests, fibroblasts function to form the (extracellular) fibers of connective tissue, that is, *collagen* and *elastin* (together with the latter's variants, *oxytalan* and *eluanin*). Their name is misleading, however, since fibroblasts have many other, equally important, functions. Thus they produce and maintain the ground substance in which they and their fibrous products are enmeshed. They also exhibit contractility and motility, which are utilized in determining the structural organization of connective tissue, especially during embryogenesis. Fibroblasts therefore may be aptly described as the architect, builder, and caretaker of connective tissue.

Structure of the Fibroblast

Fibroblasts are normally recognized under the light microscope by their association with collagen fiber bundles (Fig. 5-1). The resting fibroblast (e.g., in tendons) has a flattened, dark-staining, closed nucleus and little cytoplasm. The active fibroblast (e.g., in the PDL) has a pale staining open-faced nucleus and much more cytoplasm (Fig. 5-2, *A*). Under the electron microscope (Fig. 5-2, *B*), active fibroblasts are seen to have the usual complement of cytoplasmic organelles, but in exaggerated amounts, so that there are a number of Golgi complexes and many profiles of rough endoplasmic reticulum, mitochondria, and secretory vesicles, all indicative of these cells' synthetic and secretory function.

Cytoskeleton

The fibroblast possesses a cytoskeleton, demonstrable with special staining techniques (Fig. 5-3), that consists of microtubules and filaments.

Microtubules are long gently curving cylindrical protein structures with an average diameter of 240 nm (Fig. 5-4). The major protein making up the tubule is called *tubulin* and is very similar to the muscle protein actin. The function of microtubules is associated with maintaining the shape of the cell and the position of its intracellular structures as well as determining secretory pathways.

Filaments are of two types, distinguished on the basis of their diameter—microfilaments (less than 80 nm diameter) and intermediate filaments (80 to 120 nm). *Microfilaments*, composed of the contractile proteins actin and myosin, serve as intracellular "muscles"; they are concerned with the maintenance of cell shape and with cytoplasmic movement and cell motility. They are normally organized in one of two configurations: long

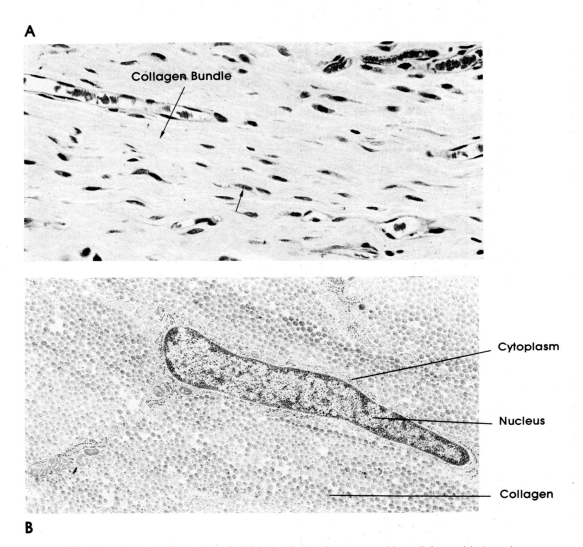

FIG. 5-1 Inactive fibroblast. **A,** With the light microscope this cell *(arrow)* is largely identified by (1) its relationship to the collagen fiber bundles, (2) its dark-staining nucleus, and (3) its sparse cytoplasm. **B,** With the electron microscope the cytoplasm is seen to possess few cytoplasmic organelles.

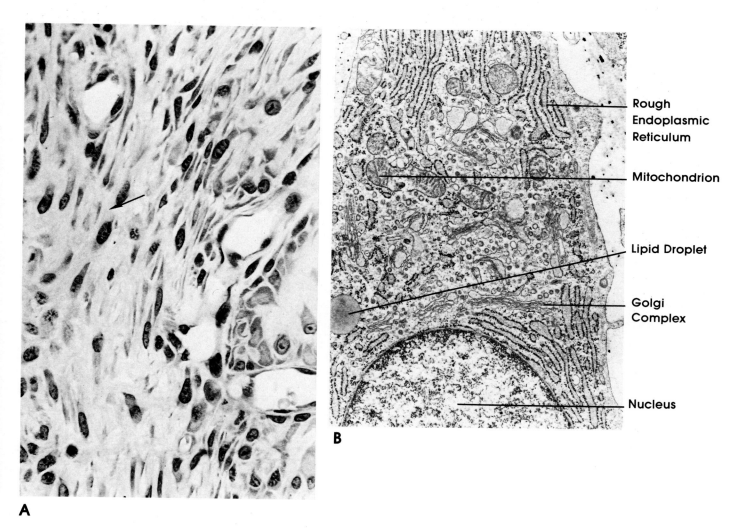

Rough
Endoplasmic
Reticulum

Mitochondrion

Lipid Droplet

Golgi
Complex

Nucleus

B

A

FIG. 5-2 Active fibroblast. **A,** This cell *(arrow)* as seen with the light microscope has an open-faced nucleus and much cytoplasm that, when viewed with the electron microscope, **B,** is seen to be filled with numerous cytoplasmic organelles.

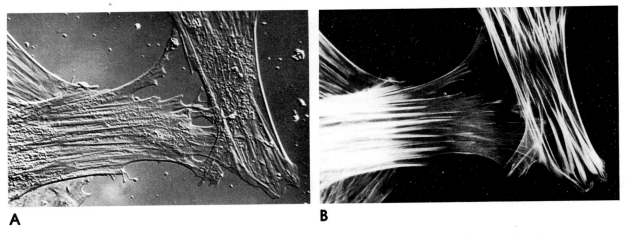

FIG. 5-3   Differing techniques to demonstrate the cytoplasmic skeletal system in pig PDL fibroblasts. **A,** Cell viewed by the Nomarski technique of microscopy. Raised elements are bundles of microfilaments. **B,** Same cells labeled with a highly specific antibody for actin, which is a constituent of microfilaments. (**A** and **B** courtesy Dr. J. Aubin.)

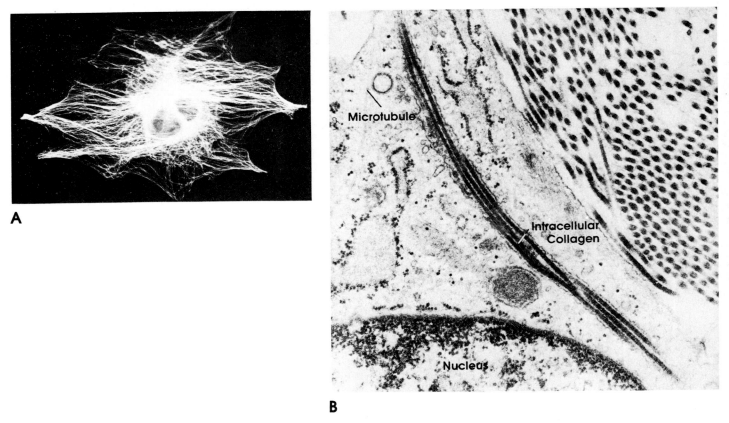

FIG. 5-4   **A,** Pig PDL fibroblast labeled with antibody against tubulin. **B,** Electron microscope appearance of a microtubule. (**A** courtesy Dr. J. Aubin.)

straight bundles of closely apposed microfilaments or individual filaments forming a cross-linked three-dimensional network (Fig. 5-5). *Intermediate filaments*, composed of another protein (vimentin), help form the cytoskeleton and are concerned with maintaining cell shape and the contact between adjacent cells. They often appear as slender gently curving structures (Fig. 5-6) and are not contractile. The ultrastructural appearance of the filamentous system in a fibroblast is depicted in Figure 5-7.

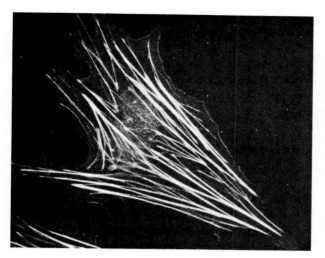

FIG. 5-5 Pig PDL fibroblast labeled with antibody against actin to show microfilaments. (Courtesy Dr. J. Aubin.)

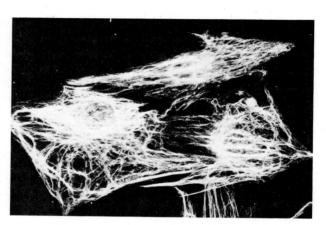

FIG. 5-6 Pig PDL fibroblasts labeled with antibody against vimentin to show intermediate filaments. (Courtesy Dr. J. Aubin.)

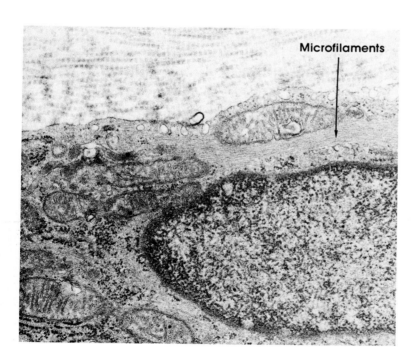

Microfilaments

FIG. 5-7 Electron micrograph of a fibroblast illustrating the ultrastructural appearance of microfilaments.

Contraction and motility

The cytoskeleton of the fibroblast, containing as it does contractile proteins, enables the fibroblast to contract. This ability to contract is expressed in a number of ways, but in particular it manifests itself as an ability of the cell to move. A fibroblast grown in a culture dish "crawls" about by extending a leading edge, attaching that edge to the substratum by means of an attachment plaque, and then contracting and pulling itself forward—as a sailor climbing a rope. The fibroblast can also influence its immediate environment if it remains stationary and utilizes its contractile properties to pull on adjacent structural elements—just as a sailor hauling in a sail. An intermediate situation exists that involves both fibroblast movement and the influence of this movement on the immediate environment. Fibroblasts crawling about on a collagen gel cause the gel to wrinkle. The analogy here is the sailor running on the beach—with each step forward leaving a heap of sand behind the footprint.

Junctions

When fibroblasts come into contact with each other (which is not the normal circumstance but does occur in the PDL), their plasma membranes develop junctional arrangements. Junctional arrangements between cells are usually described in the context of contacts between epithelial cells (where they are most frequent, given the functions of epithelium to protect and seal).

Three types of junctions are described: (1) *tight* or *occluding*, (2) *adhering*, and (3) *gap*. Further descriptive breakdown of junctions is made on the basis of their extent and shape. Thus, if a junction encircles or girdles the cell, it is prefixed by the term *zonula* (e.g., zonula adherens or zonula occludens); and if it is more circumscribed, the prefix *macula* is used (macula occludens).

In tight junctions the fusion of adjacent cell membranes occurs much as the teeth of a zipper intermesh, and generally such junctions prevent any movement of material between cells, but, as we shall see in the discussion of enamel formation, they may alternate between being tight and leaky. Tight junctions encircle the cell and therefore exist as zonulae occludentes.

Junctions of the adherens type may be zonular or macular in form. In the zonula adherens a gap of some 20 nm is maintained between the opposing cell membranes that is filled with filamentous material. Microfilaments anchor themselves to the cytoplasmic face of this junction. In the macula adherens, also commonly known as the *desmosome*, a gap is maintained between the cells of some 30 nm whose center is occupied by a dark line (thought to represent a region where trans-

membrane linkers fuse). The adjacent cell membranes are somewhat thickened and, again, internal filaments anchor themselves to the cytoplasmic portion of the membrane. Another form of the macula adherens is the *hemidesmosome*, which is found on the surface of epithelial cells in contact with noncellular surfaces such as the basal lamina or enamel in the case of the dentogingival junction. Morphologically the hemidesmosome resembles exactly half a desmosome, but differences in protein structure between the desmosome and hemidesmosome have been described.

A gap junction (Fig. 10-33) is spotlike in outline and is a region where the two apposing cell membranes come close together but maintain a gap of about 3 nm. Across this gap run numerous tubular structures with lumina some 2 nm in diameter that directly link the interiors of contiguous cells. Ions and small water-soluble molecules pass unimpeded through these gaps.

Fibroblasts exhibit junctions of both the gap and the adherens type. As well as forming junctions between themselves, fibroblasts have the ability to adhere to their external environment through a series of transmembrane molecules (integrins, syndecan, CD44) that have an intracellular domain binding to cytoskeletal elements, a transmembrane domain, and an extracellular domain that binds to any number of extracellular matrix components. Such transmembrane molecules may also serve as membrane receptors. Morphologically this coupling arrangement has been described as a fibronexus (Figs. 5-8 and 14-11).

It has already been explained why the ability of fibroblasts to form attachments to the external environment is important: Such attachments are required for the cells to move or influence their immediate environment.

Heterogeneity

Although fibroblasts generally look alike under the microscope—distinguishable only as being active or quiescent, on the basis of a diversity of synthetic products, rate of synthesis, response to regulatory molecules, and cellular turnover rates—it is now recognized that heterogeneity exists within fibroblast populations (e.g., as found in the PDL).

Aging

Fibroblasts originate from mesenchymal cells. Once differentiated, fibroblasts can replicate by mitotic cell division (as seen in wound repair and in-vitro cultures of fibroblast populations). When fibroblasts from embryonic tissue are cultured, however, they are able to undergo about 50 divisions before they become senescent and die. This number is reduced to 20 when fi-

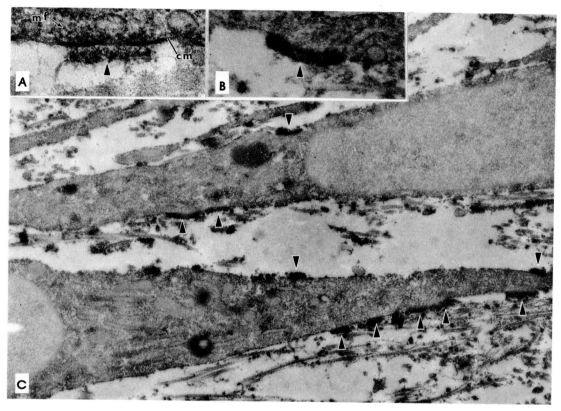

FIG. 5-8 **A,** Electron micrograph demonstrating the ultrastructural components of a fibronexus after fixation with glutaraldehyde containing tannic acid. A fibronexus is composed of intracellular microfilaments (in cross section), a portion of the cell membrane, and an extracellular matrix component *(arrowhead).* **B,** Immunocytochemical demonstration of fibronectin *(arrowhead)* as the major structural component of extracellular matrix. **C,** Distribution of fibronexi on the membrane of the differentiating PDL fibroblasts. (**A** to **C** courtesy Dr. Moon-II Cho.)

broblasts from adult tissue are cultured. Fibroblasts from long-lived species, such as the tortoise, can replicate more often than similar cells from short-lived species such as the mouse. This suggests that there is a correlation between age and life-span of the fibroblast; but there is need for caution in making this interpretation since it is possible that undifferentiated mesenchymal cells situated perivascularly can replicate an infinite number of times, which would give rise to a persistent fibroblast population.

SECRETORY PRODUCTS

Fibroblasts have the ability to synthesize and secrete a wide range of extracellular molecules. Four are of particular interest here: (1) collagens, (2) elastins, (3) proteoglycans, and (4) glycoproteins.

Collagens

At last count, 15 genetically, chemically, and immunologically distinct types of collagen (listed as types 1 to 15) have been identified and described.* All collagens are composed of three polypeptide alpha chains coiled around each other to form the typical triple helix configuration (Fig. 5-9). Common features include an amino acid composition with high proportions of glycine and always containing hydroxyproline and hydroxylysine.

Variations are brought about by (1) differences in the assembly of the basic polypeptide chains, (2) different lengths of the helix, (3) various interruptions in the helix, and (4) differences in the terminations of the helical domains. In spite of these differences, collagens can be grouped into three domains according to their molecular size and whether the molecules are assembled in a fibrous form.

First domain (collagens I, II, III, V, and XI). These collagens have a molecular weight of 95,000 kD (kiloDaltons). They aggregate by the thousands in a regular way in the extracellular compartment to form fibrils with a typical 67 nm banding pattern.

In most connective tissues type I is the major collagen, although some type III and type V collagens are also present.

Second domain (collagens IV, VI, VII and XII). These collagens also consist of chains of molecular weight of 95,000 kD or above, but they do not assemble as fibrils in the extracellular compartment. Of particular interest are type IV and type VII collagens. Type IV collagen contains frequent nonhelical sequences and aggregates in a chicken wire sheetlike configuration; it is an essential component of the basement membrane and is a characteristic gene product of epithelial cells. Type VII collagen has unusually large nonhelical ends comprising two thirds of the molecule's size; it forms the anchoring fibrils dependent from the basement membrane. Although the term *anchoring fibril* is used, remember that this collagen is not assembled in a fibrous form.

---

*It is of interest that when the first edition of this book was produced, in 1980, only five collagens were recognized.

Third domain (collagens VIII, IX, X, and XIII). These collagens consist of chains with a molecular weight less than 95,000 kD. They exhibit several interruptions in the triple helix.

• • •

Figure 5-10 gives a summary of some of the known collagens. Type I and type III are important for understanding the function of dental tissues, and their synthesis and assembly will be described now in some detail.

Collagen synthesis and assembly

Fibrous collagen is synthesized in the following way (Fig. 5-11): Individual polypeptide chains are formed by the assembly of specific amino acids on ribosomes associated with the rough endoplasmic reticulum (RER). These chains are some 50% longer than the chains found in the final molecule, because they possess sequences of amino acids at each end (designated as "N" and "C" terminal peptides) that play an important role in collagen synthesis but are eventually removed. Before helix formation can occur, however, there is a requirement for hydroxylation of some of the proline and lysine residues within the polypeptide chains to form hydroxyproline and hydroxylysine. This step demands activity of the enzymes prolylhydroxylase and lysylhydroxylase, both of which are vitamin C dependent; in other words, without the vitamin, collagen cannot form. This explains why an early symptom of scurvy is a loosening of the teeth: with diminished formation and no diminution in the rate of turnover, the collagen content of the PDL is lessened. As hydroxylation occurs, sugar residues are added to the newly hydroxylated groups and this addition also requires enzymatic assistance (glucosyltransferase and galactolysyltransferase). Once hydroxylated and glycosylated, the three polypeptide chains are assembled into the classic triple helix configuration. For helix formation to occur, it is essential that the chains be properly aligned, and this is achieved by disulfide bonding at the C-terminal extension. Once aligned and assembled into the helix configuration, the molecule is transported to the Golgi apparatus, where further remodeling of the C-terminal end occurs to form the procollagen molecule. Procollagen molecules are aligned in a nonstaggered configuration for further transit to the cell surface. The formation and secretion of the collagen molecule take about 35 to 60 minutes (known as the transit time). Fibroblasts synthesize more polypeptide chains than needed, and excess chains are segregated and destroyed by the cell's lysosomal system.

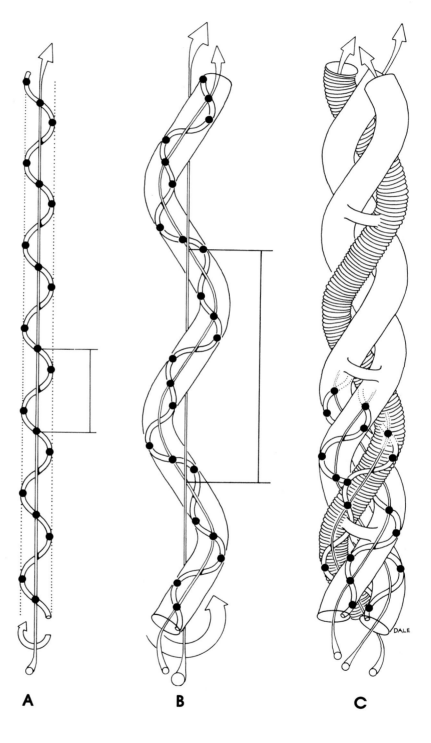

FIG. 5-9 Structural organization of fibrous collagen. **A,** Chain of amino acids assembled with a left-handed helix. **B,** Same chain assuming a secondary spiral in the opposite direction to form a compound helix. **C,** Three such chains combined to give a superhelix arrangement.

A   B   C

TYPE	CHAINS	TRIMETRIC	LENGTH	AGGREGATION	LOCATION
I	α1 (I) α2 (I)	α1 (I)$_2$α2 (I)	300 nm	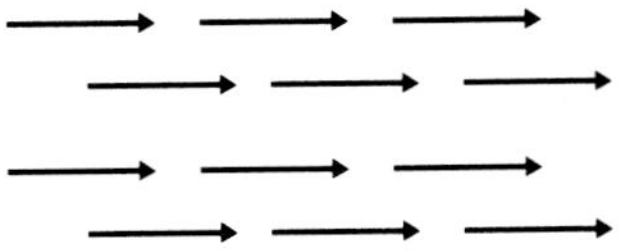 Fibrous	Abundant in skin, bone, gingiva, periodontal ligament, cementum and most other connective tissues
II	α1 (II)	α1 (II)$_3$	300	Fibrous	Cartilage, vitreous humor
III	α1 (III)	α1 (III)$_3$	300	Fibrous	Embryonic connective tissue, pulp, periodontal ligament, skin
IV	α1 (IV) α2 (IV)	α1 (IV)$_2$α(IV)	390	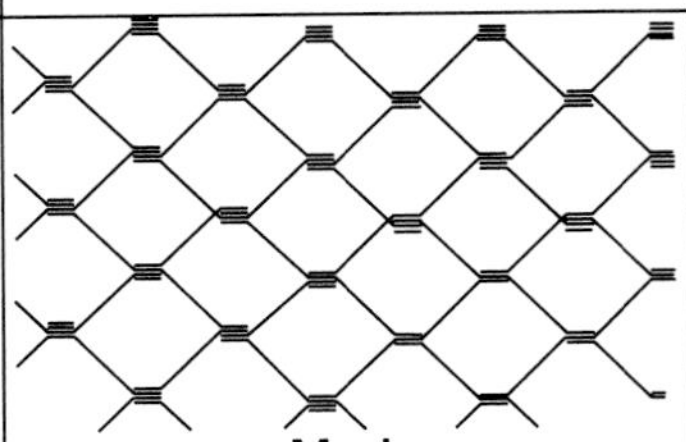 Mesh	Basement membrane
V	α1 (V) α2 (V) α3 (V)	α1 (V)$_2$α2(V) α1 (V)α2(V)α3(V)	300		Widely distributed: basement membranes, blood vessels, ligaments, skin, dentin, gingiva, periodontal ligament
VI	α1 (VI) α2 (VI) α3 (VI)	α1 (VI)α2 (VI)α3 (VI)	105	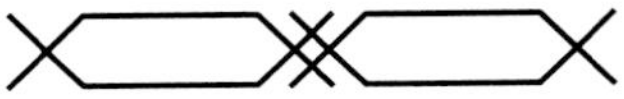 Microfibril	Widely distributed: ligaments, skin, bone cartilage
VII	α1 (VII)	α1 (VII)$_3$	450	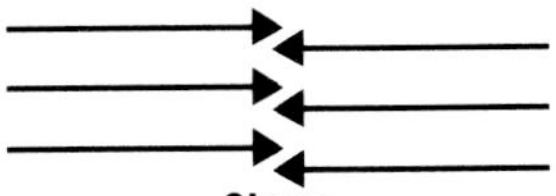 Strap	Anchoring fibrils of basement membrane
VIII	α1 (VIII)	Unknown			Endothelial cells, cartilage, junctional epithelium
IX	α1 (IX) α2 (IX) α3 (IX)	α1 (IX)α2 (IX)α3 (IX)	200		Cartilage
X	α1 (X)	α1 (X)$_3$	150		Cartilage, bone
XI	α1 (XI) α2 (XI) α3 (XI)	α1 (XI)α2 (XI)α3 (XI)			Cartilage, bone
XII	α1 (XIII)	α1 (XIII)$_3$			Calvaria, tendon, periodontal ligament, cartilage
XIII					Epidermis, cartilage

FIG. 5-10 Some of the 13 types of collagen so far described. The *second column* lists the chains found in a given collagen type. The *third column* (trimeric form) details how these chains are assembled. The *fourth column* indicates how trimeric chains aggregate.

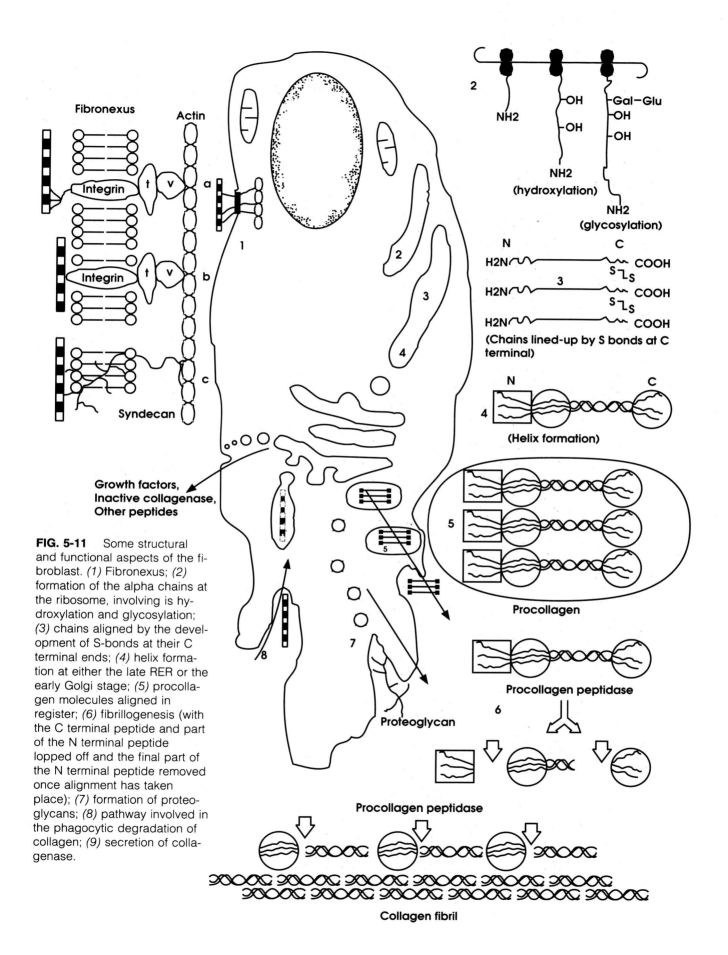

Fibronexus

Actin

Integrin

t v a

Integrin

t v b

c

Syndecan

2

NH2

—OH

—OH

Gal—Glu
—OH
—OH

NH2
(hydroxylation)

NH2
(glycosylation)

N   C
H2N⌇⌇⌇⌇⌇COOH
                  S⌐S
H2N⌇⌇⌇⌇⌇COOH   3
                  S⌐S
H2N⌇⌇⌇⌇⌇COOH
(Chains lined-up by S bonds at C
terminal)

N   C
4
(Helix formation)

5

Procollagen

Procollagen peptidase

6

Procollagen peptidase

Collagen fibril

Growth factors,
Inactive collagenase,
Other peptides

1
2
3
4
5
7
8

Proteoglycan

FIG. 5-11 Some structural and functional aspects of the fibroblast. *(1)* Fibronexus; *(2)* formation of the alpha chains at the ribosome, involving is hydroxylation and glycosylation; *(3)* chains aligned by the development of S-bonds at their C terminal ends; *(4)* helix formation at either the late RER or the early Golgi stage; *(5)* procollagen molecules aligned in register; *(6)* fibrillogenesis (with the C terminal peptide and part of the N terminal peptide lopped off and the final part of the N terminal peptide removed once alignment has taken place); *(7)* formation of proteoglycans; *(8)* pathway involved in the phagocytic degradation of collagen; *(9)* secretion of collagenase.

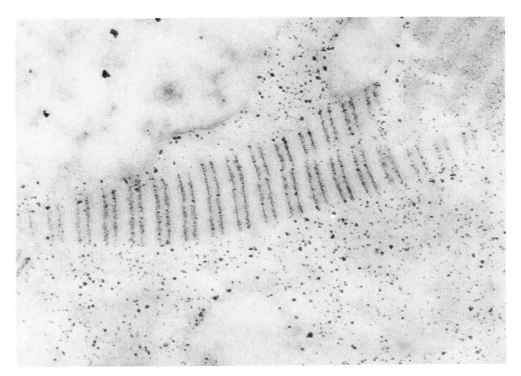

FIG. 5-12 Aggregation of collagen molecules to form a fiber. (From Goose DH, Appleton J: *Human dentofacial growth,* New York, 1982, Pergamon Press, Chap. 2.)

Fibrillogenesis

So far, the synthesis of procollagen molecules has been described. These molecules are now secreted and, when sufficient numbers have been attained, are assembled extracellularly so that they can be observed in the form of the typical banded collagen fibril (Fig. 5-12).

The entire process of assembly is known as fibrillogenesis, but how it occurs is not yet fully understood. It has been suggested that there is selective removal at the cell surface of the entire C-terminal extension and a portion of the N-terminal extension of procollagen molecules as a result of the activity of procollagen peptidase. This permits an initial alignment of five-unit staggered microfibrils. These microfibrils, in turn, become aligned parallel to each other (could this be the function of the remaining portion of the N terminal peptide?) and staggered, giving rise to a regular series of *gaps* within the fibrils. The nature and size of the spaces within the collagen fibril and within the collagen molecule are important, for it is here that much of the mineral of hard connective tissues, bone, dentin, and cementum is located (Fig. 5-13). Once aligned in this way, the microfibrils lose the final remnant of their N-terminal extension through further action of procollagen peptidase.

When polypeptide chains are assembled into the triple helix, intramolecular hydrogen bonds fix their arrangement. At the time of extrusion of the procollagen molecule, an enzyme (lysylhydroxylase) initiates the synthesis of additional cross-links in the collagen molecule. The activity of this enzyme is inhibited by lathyrogens, drugs that have been used experimentally to determine the relationship, if any, between collagen synthesis and tooth eruption. The stability of the collagen fibril arrangement is further solidified with time as covalent bonds form cross-links between the individual collagen macromolecules. Although such cross-links are few, they significantly increase the stability of the collagen fibril so that it becomes chemically more insoluble.

Collagen degradation

The synthesis of collagen types I and III and their assembly into fibrils have been described. It is now recognized that many connective tissues remodel, albeit at differing rates and in different locations, which implies that both collagen and ground substance are being synthesized and degraded continuously, with the rate for each process the same if tissue architecture is to be preserved. Two mechanisms are associated with the degradation of collagen: (1) the selective ingestion

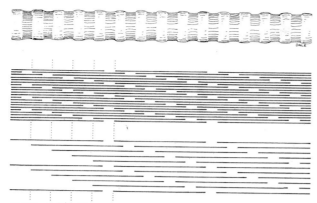

Approx. 1/4 Stagger

|__ 300nm __| Overlap Region — — Lacunae Region

FIG. 5-13 Collagen molecules aggregating to form a banded fibril. The lacunae or "holes" contain more stain and create the banded appearance seen on electron micrographs. These holes are filled with minerals in hard connective tissues.

TABLE 5-1	Matrix metalloendoproteinases (MMPs) involved in the degradation of collagen		
Collagenase	MMP-I	Native collagen	
Gelatinase	MMP-II	Denatured collagen	
Stromelysin	MMP-III	Fibronectin-proteogly-can core	
Telopeptidase	MMP-IV	C-terminal telopeptide	
¾-collagen endopeptidase	MMP-V	Collagen TCA and TCB (gelatin)	

of collagen fibrils by fibroblasts and their degradation *intracellularly* (Fig. 5-14) and (2) the secretion by cells of a number of enzymes that sequentially degrade collagen *extracellularly*.

Intracellular degradation. The steps in this process involve (1) recognition of the collagen fibrils to be degraded, (2) cleavage of the fibrils, (3) phagocytosis of the cleaved fibrils, (4) formation of a phagolysosome, and (5) intracellular digestion of collagen fibers within the phagolysosome by lysosomal enzymes (particularly cathepsin).

Extracellular degradation. *Matrix metalloendoproteinase* (MMP) is the name given a group of enzymes secreted by some cells, including fibroblasts, that can degrade collagen and other matrix macromolecules into small peptides (Table 5-1). Collagenase is the best characterized of these enzymes. It plays a pivotal role in collagen degradation, for it is the only enzyme that at a neutral pH can cleave the triple helix of the collagen molecule. This activity, however, achieves only the initial fragmentation of the fibril; other enzymes are required for continued degradation. Figure 5-15 describes the likely sequence and combination of enzymatic events involved in the extracellular degradation of collagen.

Control mechanisms

With respect to intracellular digestion, it is not too difficult to imagine how a selective and precise degradation of collagen can be achieved by individual fibroblasts. Furthermore, the ability of the fibroblast to synthesize and degrade collagen simultaneously pro-

vides added finesse in the control of connective tissue makeup.

What is not understood is how fibroblasts select a particular collagen fibril, or group of fibrils, for ingestion and how they achieve the initial fragmentation of such fibrils. A suggestion with respect to identification depends on the close association of fibroblasts with collagen fibers through cell surface receptors which may signal to the cell a change in the external environment (e.g., tensile or compressive forces altering fiber structure). With respect to initial fragmentation of the fibril, nothing is known although, again, it has been speculated that extracellular fibril degradation acting locally at the cell surface may be involved; however, there is considerable evidence against such speculation. For example, collagen phagocytosis is not impaired in the presence of a neutralizing antibody to collagenase or in the presence of proteinase inhibitors. Furthermore, in the normal PDL, where there is a very high rate of collagen turnover involving the phagocytic mechanism, the presence of collagenase cannot be detected.

Regulation of extracellular collagen degradation is less precise. Clearly, there must be some form of control; otherwise, the indiscriminate release of MMPs would have serious consequences for the well-being of the organism. Three possible control mechanisms are known to exist: (1) the inhibition of collagenase activity by some of the normal components of serum, especially alpha 2 macroglobulin, (2) the need for proenzyme activators for the MMPs, and (3) the existence of specific tissue inhibitors of metalloendoproteinase activity (TIMPs). The latter two are products of fibroblasts, which suggests the possibility of some local control even if not as precise as that achieved by the phagocytic mechanism. This form of collagen destruction is usually described in association with inflammatory lesions, wherein precision is not a factor, and in relation to the remodeling of bone, wherein precision is introduced by the osteoclast's defining and controlling a limited environment associated with the bone surface. (See Chapter 7.)

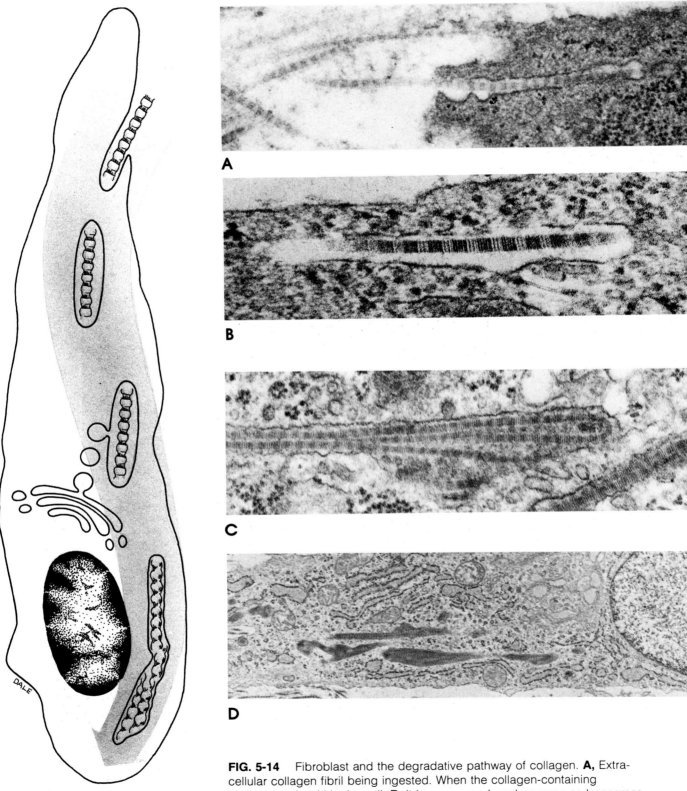

FIG. 5-14   Fibroblast and the degradative pathway of collagen. **A,** Extra-cellular collagen fibril being ingested. When the collagen-containing phagosome is within the cell, **B,** it becomes a phagolysosome as lysosomes fuse with it, **C.** Digestion of the collagen continues in this structure, **D.** (**A, C,** and **D** from Ten Cate AR, et al: *Am J Orthod* 69: 155, 1976.)

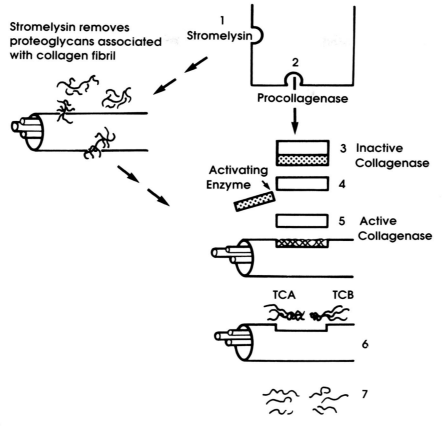

FIG. 5-15   Sequence of events leading to the degradation of collagen fibrils by colla-genase. Numerous factors have been described that stimulate connective cells to synthesize procollagenase, glycosydases, and neutral proteases. *(1)* The proteoglycan-degrading enzymes protoglycanase and stromelysin (MMP III) remove proteoglycans that surround the collagen fibers and expose them to collagenase (MMP I); *(2)* inactive collagenase is secreted; *(3)* the enzyme is usually found in the intracellular space bound to an inhibitor; *(4)* an activating enzyme removes the inhibitor; *(5)* the active col-lagenase binds to fibrillar collagen and splits the molecule into two fragments (TCA and TCB), so that it denatures and begins to unfold at body temperature *(6);* the denatured collagen fragments are finally degraded *(7)* by gelatinase (MMP II) and 3,4-collagen endopeptidase (MMP V). (From Nimni ME: In Nimni ME [ed]: *Collagen.* Vol 1, *Biochem-istry,* Boca Raton Fla, 1988, CRC Press.)

Elastin, Oxytalan, Eluanin, and Reticulin

Elastin and its intermediate forms oxytalan and elu-anin are closely related. All are products of fibroblasts; and their formation involves a synthetic pathway similar to that described for collagen, with the secretion of tropoelastin and its assembly outside the cell. Elastin is a protein with an amorphous structure that, when it occurs alone (as in the walls of blood vessels), is de-posited in sheets or laminae. To form an elastic fiber, a tubular glycoprotein must first be secreted in a mi-crofibrillar form, and these microfibrils then provide a

scaffold for the assembly of elastin in a fibrous form. As elastin is added to this scaffold, the microfibrils are displaced peripherally so that the elastic fiber has a final structure of a central core of elastin containing some embedded microfibrils enveloped by a peripheral sleeve of microfibrils.

Because microfibrils must be formed first, they are most evident in forming elastic tissue; and it is believed that the oxytalan fiber, a normal constituent of the PDL, represents these microfibrils. As elastin is added, how-ever, another intermediate form of elastic fiber is rec-

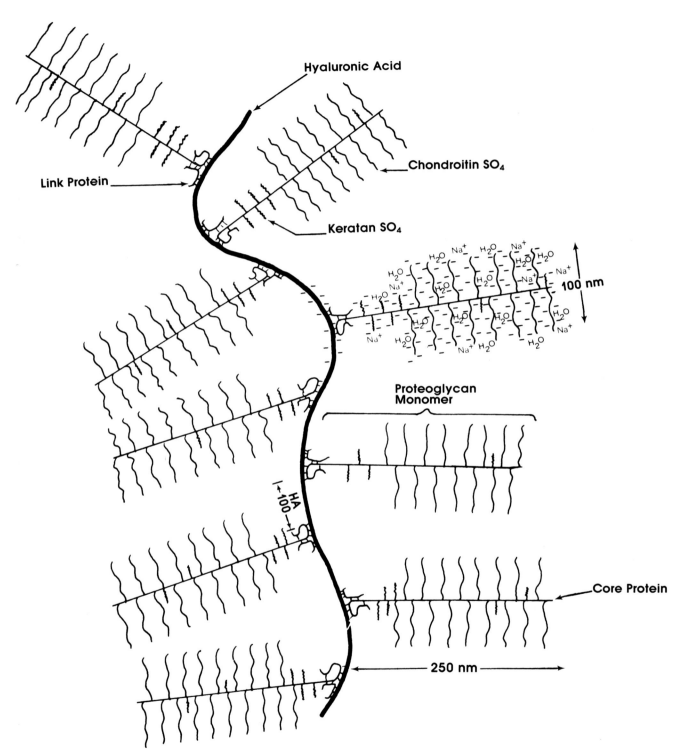

FIG. 5-16 Model of a proteoglycan aggregate. (From Daniel JC: In Meyer J et al [eds]: *The structure and function of oral mucosa,* New York, 1984, Pergamon Press.)

ognized (known as eluanin) whose microfibrils are simply scattered throughout the elastin and not yet formed in a peripheral sleeve. Little if anything is known about the turnover of elastic tissue, although an enzyme (elastase) has been described.

Ground substance

Fibroblasts are also responsible for the formation of the nonfibrous components of the extracellular matrix that surrounds them, usually referred to as ground substance. Ground substance is amorphous when studied with both light and conventional electron microscopy and consists of a biochemically complex, highly hydrated, semisolid gel. The hydrated nature of the ground substance is of some importance, for it provides a mechanism of regulating tissue water. The macromolecules making up the ground substance include proteoglycans and adhesive glycoproteins.

Proteoglycans

Proteoglycans are a large group of extracellular and cell surface–associated macromolecules that consist of a protein core to which are attached glycosaminoglycan chains (Fig. 5-16). Previously proteoglycans were classified into three groups depending on the glycosaminoglycan chains associated with the protein core—dermatan sulfate, heparan sulfate, and chondroitin sulfate—the assumption being that there was no admixture. Now it is recognized that admixture occurs, making classification difficult.

Five proteoglycans are of particular interest. The first is *decorin,* so called because it binds to collagen and is visualized as "decorations" on the collagen fibril. It is of importance because it is thought to play a role in regulating growth of collagen fibrils. The second is *versican,* a large proteoglycan that is thought to assist in bonding cell surface glycoproteins to the extracellular matrix. The third is *perlecan,* a cell surface proteoglycan. The name perlecan arises because the large core protein contains a number of globular domains forming a pearl necklace–like structure. It binds to fibronectin and helps anchor the fibroblast to the extracellular matrix. The fourth is *syndecan,* which is distinguished in that it has an extracellular domain, a membrane-spanning domain, and a cytoplasmic domain and is known to bind to collagen and other extracellular glycoproteins (e.g., fibronectin and tenascin). The fifth proteoglycan, similar to syndescan, is named *CD44.* It also has intracellular, transmembrane, and extracellular domains capable of binding to fibronectin, laminin, and collagen.

Glycoproteins

The final group of extracellular molecules is glycoproteins, two of which have adhesive properties (i.e., fibronectin and tenascin). The primary function of these molecules is to bind cells to extracellular elements.

Fibronectin is composed of S-S linked polypeptide chains that have several structural domains capable of reacting with both cells and extracellular matrix components and, through this linkage, capable of being involved in the attachment, spreading, and migration of cells.

Tenascin is an adhesive glycoprotein synthesized at specific times and locations during embryogenesis. In adults its distribution is specific and restricted. It binds to fibronectin and to proteoglycans; hence its description as an adhesive glycoprotein. In particular, tenascin is known to bind to syndecan, which means that it blocks the binding capacity of this cell surface molecule and thereby enables the cell to move more freely. It is of interest that the migratory pathway for neural crest cells is forecast by the expression of tenascin along that pathway.

Integrins

Some of the more important molecules of the ground substance have now been described. It has been pointed out that two proteoglycans are distinct—syndecan and CD44—in that they cross the cell membrane to connect extracellular matrix molecules to the cell's cytoskeleton and thus ultimately affect the cell's be-

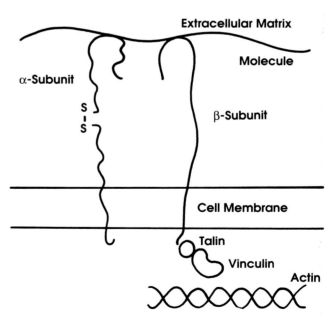

FIG. 5-17 Integrin structure. The β subunit is well conserved among species and is involved primarily in linkage to the cytoskeleton of the cell. The α subunit confers binding specificity. (Redrawn from Milam SB, et al: *Crit Rev Oral Biol Med* 2:451, 1991.)

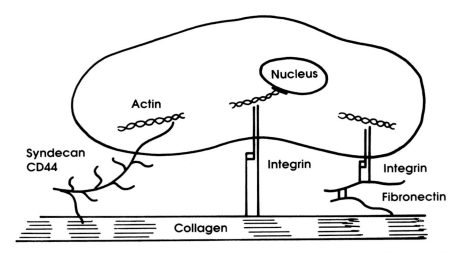

FIG. 5-18   Various forms of cell-matrix interaction. (Redrawn from Uitto VJ, Larjava H: *Crit Rev Oral Biol Med* 2(2):323, 1991.)

havior. There also exists, however, a whole superfamily of glycoproteins that serve as transmembrane receptors and are collectively known as the integrins. Integrins have a large extracellular domain, a small transmembrane domain and an intracellular domain and consist of two polypeptide units (α and β). The alpha unit confers ligand specificity. The beta unit interacts with the cytoskeleton by a sequential series of linked proteins beginning with talin, which is attached to vinculin, which in turn is attached to actin filaments of the cytoskeleton (Fig. 5-17).

The various connections possible between fibroblasts and the extracellular matrix are summarized in Figure 5-18.

Fibroblasts also secrete many other proteins, including growth factors (Chapter 6) and enzymes such as collagenase. This fact, taken alone, indicates that the fibroblast, as well as producing the structural elements of connective tissue, is busily engaged in monitoring and responding to the external environment it has itself created.

SUMMARY

The point has been made that fibroblasts are cells with differing phenotypes and many different functions. They synthesize, secrete, and maintain the fibers and ground substance of connective tissue, including collagen and elastin and its variants. Collagen is the most frequent fiber found in connective tissue, with at least 15 genetically distinct types now identified. By varying the composition, aggregation patterns, and quantity of

collagen, as well as the composition of ground substance, fibroblasts can generate many varied permutations that allow maximum functional flexibility of connective tissues. At the same time fibroblasts possess a series of transmembrane receptors that enable them to monitor and respond to the environment they have created. One response is their ability to remodel that environment by simultaneously synthesizing and degrading their products to bring about turnover without distortion of architecture.

BIBLIOGRAPHY

Aubin JE, Zimmerman AM, Forer A (eds): *Immunofluorescence studies of cytoskeletal proteins during cell division,* New York, 1981, Academic Press.

Aubin J, Opas M: Cell adhesion and motility. In Davidovitch Z, (ed): *The biological mechanisms of tooth eruption and root resorption,* Birmingham, AL, 1988, EBSCO Media, pp 43-51.

Bertold PM: Proteoglycans of the periodontium: structure, role, and function, *J Periodont Res* 22:431, 1987.

Birkedal-Hansen H: From tadpole collagenase to a family of matrix metalloproteinases, *J Oral Pathol* 17:445, 1988.

Gross J, Lapiere CM: Collagenolytic activity in amphibian tissue: a tissue culture assay, *Proc Natl Acad Sci USA* 48:1014, 1962.

Heath J: Finding the missing links, *Nature* 320:484, 1986.

Jones JCR, Yokoo KM, Goldman RD: Is the hemidesmosome a half desmosome? An immunological comparison of mammalian desmosomes and hemidesmosomes, *Cell Motil Cytoskeleton* 6:560, 1986.

Leblond CP: Synthesis and secretion of collagen by cells of connective tissue, bone, and dentin, *Anat Rec* 224:123, 1989.

Lewis J: Morphogenesis by fibroblast traction, *Nature* 307:413, 1984.

Martin GR, Timpl R, Muller PK, Kuhn K: The genetically distinct collagens, *Trends Biochem Sci* 10:285, 1985.

McCulloch CAG, Borden S: Role of fibroblast sub-populations in periodontal physiology and pathology, *J Periodont Res* 26:144, 1991.

Milam SB, Haskin C, Zardeneta JS, et al: Cell adhesion proteins in oral biology, *Crit Rev Oral Biol Med* 2:451, 1991.

Nimni ME,: Collagen. In Nimni ME (ed): *Collagen*. Vol 1, *Biochemistry*, Boca Raton Fla, 1988, CRC Press, pp 1-75.

Rahemutulla F: Proteoglycans of oral tissues, **Crit Rev Oral Biol Med** 3:135, 1992.

Ruoslahati E, Pierschbacher MD: New perspectives in cell adhesion: RGD and Integrins, *Science* 238:491, 1987.

Singer II: The fibronexus: a transmembrane association of fibronectin containing fibres and bundles of 5nm microfilaments in hamster and human fibroblasts, *Cell* 16:675, 1979.

Sodek J: A comparison of the rates of synthesis and turnover of collagen and noncollagen proteins in adult rat periodontal tissues and skin using a microassay, *Arch Oral Biol* 22:655, 1977.

Ten Cate AR: Morphological studies of fibrocytes in connective tissue undergoing rapid remodelling, *J Anat* 112:401, 1972.

Ten Cate AR, Deporter DA: The degradative role of the fibroblast in the remodelling and turnover of the collagen in soft connective tissue, *Anat Rec* 182:1, 1975.

Uitto V-J, Larjava H: Extracellular matrix molecules and their receptors: An overview with special emphasis on periodontal tissues, *Crit Rev Oral Biol Med* 2(2):323, 1991.

Weinstock M, Leblond CP: Synthesis, migration, and release of precursor collagen by odontoblasts as visualized by radioautography after ^{3}H-proline administration, *J Cell Biol* 60:92, 1974.

Weinstock M, Leblond CP: Formation of collagen, *Fed Proc* 33:1205, 1974.

CHAPTER 6

Epithelial-Mesenchymal Relations

I N the developing embryo a functional relationship exists between epithelium and the mesenchyme that supports it, and the proper interplay between these tissues is essential for orderly development. To illustrate this point, consider the following: teeth cannot form until mesenchyme establishes contact with the first branchial arch epithelium; the shape of the tooth is determined by folding of the dental epithelium, and this folding is dictated by the mesenchyme of the dental papilla; odontoblast differentiation requires the presence of epithelium; the anatomy of the dentogingival junction is determined by its supporting connective tissue; and the list goes on. Although the above examples represent developmental situations, the same relationship persists in mature tissue. For example, connective tissue continues to control expression of the oral epithelium (Fig. 6-1).

EXPERIMENTAL STUDIES

Improved techniques in tissue, organ, and cell culture, combined with the ability to separate epithelium from mesenchyme, have permitted detailed study of the relationships between these two tissues. Simply stated, epithelium and mesenchyme can be separated from each other and then recombined in differing combinations and permitted to continue development in a culture dish (or in the anterior chamber of the eye, as a natural culture dish). Another significant advance has been the development of immunocytochemical staining techniques, which permit the precise identification and localization of a whole host of molecules within cells, at cell surfaces, and related to the extracellular compartment (Fig. 5-3, B). Finally, the development of in-situ hybridization has been useful. This technique enables researchers to localize messenger RNA in cells from histologic sections and thus determine which gene product is being synthesized by a particular cell at a given time

How Cells and Tissues Communicate with Each Other

Communication is possible between cells through either (1) direct cell-to-cell contact or (2) the transmission of molecules synthesized and secreted by one cell and then captured by surface receptors of another cell.

Cell-to-cell contact

When cells come into contact with each other, junctional arrangements are established that take several forms (as described in Chapter 5). Most are concerned with adherence; but one form of junction, the gap junction, permits direct communication between cells. Gap junctions occur frequently between embryonic cells of the same population, which suggests that they likely have some role to play in development. No evidence exists, however, for the occurrence of cell-to-cell contact between epithelial and mesenchymal cells during the early stages of tooth development; and, indeed, the presence of a basal lamina between the two tissues precludes direct contact.

Cell surface receptors

Cells can communicate with each other, and can influence their own behavior, by synthesizing and secreting various molecules (cytokines) coincident with the development of cell surface receptors. They then recognize and capture these molecules, which, once captured, go on to influence cell behavior and phenotype. *Endocrine* communication is a well-recognized phenomenon involving the secretion by a group of cells (e.g., the islets of Langerhans) of a cytokine, which exerts its influence in a widespread way. By contrast, a more localized communication system involves au-

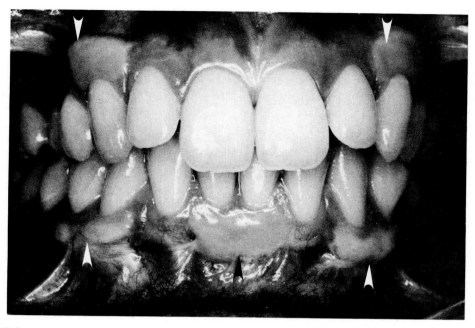

FIG. 6-1 Severe recession of the attached gingiva. Nonkeratinized alveolar mucosa almost approaches the gingival margin. Grafts of keratinized palatal mucosa were placed adjacent to the teeth *(arrows)*. Because the grafts consisted of palatal epithelium and palatal connective tissue, the epithelium retains the characteristics of palatal epithelium.

Growth Factor Families
Transforming growth factor β (TGF β)
TGF β1 to β5
Activins and inhibins
BMP (bone morphogenic protein) 2 to 7
Fibroblast growth factor (FGF)
Epidermal growth factor (EGF)
Nerve growth factor (NGF)
Platelet-derived growth factor (PDGF)
Insulinlike growth factor (IGF)

tocrine and paracrine regulation. *Autocrine* regulation involves the cell's expressing a cytokine, which is then captured by the surface receptors of that same cell. If the cytokine is captured by the receptors of an adjacent cell, however, this is described as *paracrine* regulation (Fig. 6-2). Increasing numbers of cytokines are being identified, and one important family is growth factors (box). Growth factors, once captured, can selectively stimulate the production and secretion of extracellular matrix molecules (e.g., fibronectin and tenascin). Such

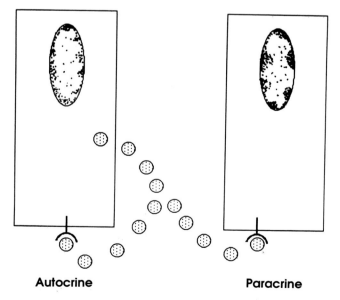

Autocrine   **Paracrine**

FIG. 6-2 Autocrine and paracrine regulation.

induced changes affect the composition and three-dimensional structure of the extracellular matrix, which, in turn, influences the proliferative and migratory capacity of the cells. If, for example, a cell is stimulated following the capture of growth factor to produce tenascin, this glycoprotein can then bind with syndecan and block the cell's ability to bind to fibronectin which in turn facilitates its migration.

Basal Lamina

A structure known as the basal lamina supports epithelium and separates it from mesenchyme (Figs. 6-3 and 18-22). It is essentially an epithelial product consisting of two layers, a lamina lucida and a lamina densa. Its main constituents are type IV collagen, the adhesive glycoproteins laminin and fibronectin, and the proteoglycan heparan sulfate. Type IV collagen forms a flexible sheet with a chicken-wire configuration in the lamina densa and has specific binding sites for laminin, fibronectin, and heparan sulfate. Laminin in the lamina lucida binds with the same molecules, but it also binds with epithelial cells, thereby fixing these cells to the sheet of type IV collagen.

What is important in the present context is that the basal lamina, in addition to providing for attachment, contributes to epithelial-mesenchymal communication. It does this in two ways: first, it is a dynamic sieve that can control the passage of molecules between the two tissues and, second, it provides a spatial configuration to which mesenchymal cells can react. This dynamism

is exemplified as follows: Heparin sulfate is lost temporarily from the basal lamina supporting the internal dental epithelium as this epithelium folds during crown pattern formation, and it reappears once the shape of the crown has been determined. Isolated basal lamina, produced by the internal dental epithelium, when combined with dental papillary cells causes differentiation of odontoblasts. Apparently what is happening here is that preodontoblasts develop receptors to fibronectin, bind to the basal lamina, and achieve the spatial orientation necessary for further differentiation.

It can therefore be argued that, because the basal lamina is largely a product of epithelial cells, this inductive relationship represents direct contact between epithelium and mesenchyme.

Migration and Determination of Neural Crest Cells

The above principles recognized, we can now consider specific situations. Recall (from Chapter 1) that neural crest cells separate from neurectoderm, migrate extensively, and differentiate into a number of specific tissues. Two questions arising then are (1) How is the migratory pathway determined? and (2) When do these cells acquire specificity?

The pattern of migration is determined largely by factors resident in the tissues through which the cells will migrate. In this regard the glycoprotein tenascin plays a significant role because the spatial and temporal patterns of its expression in the embryo correlate with the pathways of neural crest migration. Tenascin is believed to exert its influence in two ways. It binds with the adhesive glycoprotein fibronectin to lessen the latter's "sticky" effect, and it unites with syndecan to block that molecule's ability to bind with fibronectin. Both reactions enhance the mobility of migrating cells.

There is considerable evidence that migratory neural crest cells are uncommitted until they reach their final site of residence and influence. For instance, when mammalian neural crest tissue from the head region is combined with various epithelia and development is permitted to continue in the anterior chamber of the eye, teeth and their supporting tissues form only if first-arch epithelium is available (Table 6-1). Furthermore, it does not matter whether head or trunk neural crest tissue is used (Fig. 6-4). This evidence reinforces the conclusion that local epithelial influences activate the potential for tooth development from ectomesenchyme. When this initiative step has been achieved, however, it is clear that ectomesenchyme then assumes a dominant role in the ensuing epithelial-mesenchymal reactions associated with dental development. For example, when ectomesenchyme of the early dental papilla is combined with presumptive skin epithelium,

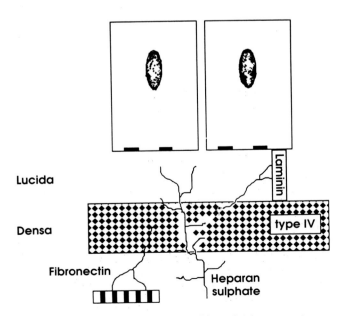

FIG. 6-3 Structure and composition of a basement membrane.

the skin epithelium changes its developmental direction and assumes the characteristics of a dental organ (Fig. 6-5). Conversely, if a dental organ is recombined with skin mesenchyme, it loses its dental characteristics and assumes those of epidermis. These results indicate that the determinants (inducers) of tooth development reside in ectomesenchyme rather than within epithelium.

TABLE 6-1 Outcome of various recombinations of epithelium and neural crest

	Teeth	Bone	Cartilage	Neural
Neural crest and mandibular epithelium	+	+	+	+
Neural crest and limb epithelium	−	+	+	+
Neural crest alone	−	−	+	+
Mandibular epithelium alone	−	−	−	−

From Lumsden AGS. In Mederson PFA (ed): *Development and evolutionary biology of the neural crest,* New York, 1987, John Wiley & Sons.

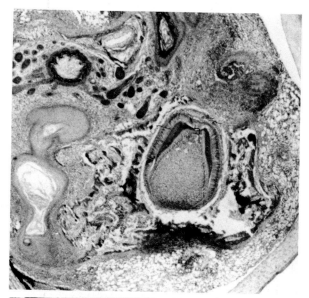

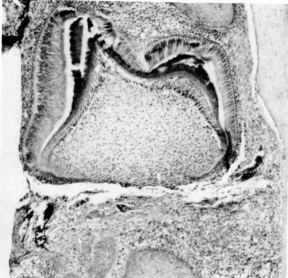

FIG. 6-4 Intraocular recombination of neural crest and dental epithelium. **A,** Tooth formed from the combination of cranial neural crest and mandibular epithelium. **B,** Tooth formed from the combination of trunk neural crest and mandibular epithelium. (Courtesy Dr. A.G.S. Lumsden.)

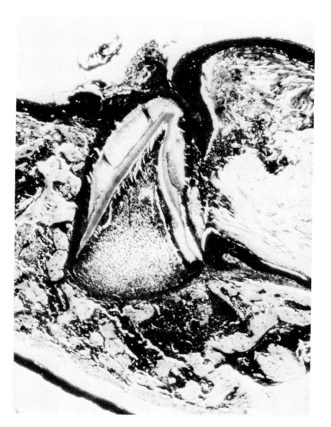

FIG. 6-5 Tooth that has developed from skin epithelium. Molar ectomesenchyme combined with plantar epithelium to produce this anomaly. (From Kollar EJ, Baird GR: *J Embryol Exp Morphol* 24:173, 1970.)

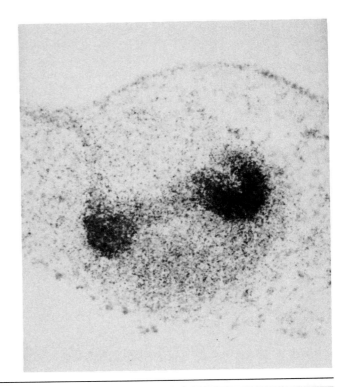

FIG. 6-6 In situ hybridization revealing the intense expression of transforming growth factor β1 in the cervical loop region during the cap stage of tooth development. (From Thesleff I, Vaahtokari A: *Proc Finn Dent Soc* 88:357, 1992.)

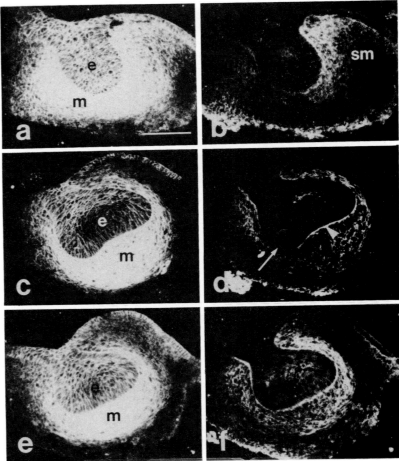

FIG. 6-7 Immunohistochemical localization of syndecan (*a*, *c*, and *e*) with tenascin (*b*, *d*, and *f*) in different regions of the same tooth germ during transition from the bud to the cap stage showing the shifts in distribution. *e*, Epithelium; *m*, mesenchyme; *sm*, mesenchymal cells surrounding the tooth germ. (Bar = 100μm.) (From Vainio S, Thesleff I: *Differentiation* 50:97, 1990.)

Role of Extracellular Matrix, Growth Factors, and Cell Surface Receptors in Tooth Morphogenesis

It is clear that (1) epithelial-mesenchymal interactions represent a local control mechanism that initiates and regulates the development of the tooth and (2) this influence resides in the sequential expression of cytokines and associated transmembrane receptors that can capture and transduce the cytokine as an intracellular second messenger, resulting in a change of phenotype. The mapping alone, however, of such molecules as tenascin, syndecan, epidermal growth factor, transforming growth factor, and fibronectin during tooth development (Figs. 6-6 and 6-7), other than indicating a spatial and temporal relationship, has not yet revealed the precise functions of these molecules in dental development. Nevertheless, their recognition has greatly improved our understanding of the cascade of events taking place during tooth development.

Long-term Potential for Tooth Development

Once the ability to initiate tooth development has been acquired by ectomesenchyme, it is maintained by dental papillary cells. Thus, if early tooth germs are cultured for an extended period, the cells dedifferentiate and the morphology of the germs is completely lost; yet, if these dedifferentiated epithelial and ectomesenchymal cells are harvested and recombined in vivo, they form a tooth (the program for tooth formation is not lost). Of particular interest in this regard is the finding that, if mouse tooth ectomesenchyme is combined with chick epithelium, teeth develop. Avian oral epithelium has maintained the competence to form a dental organ, a competence last expressed some 100,000 years ago!

TEETH

As already stated, the evidence is firm that first arch epithelium is obligated to induce the dental potential of neural crest–derived ectomesenchyme. Although in many animals teeth are all the same shape (homodont), in most mammals they are different (heterodont), falling into three families—incisoriform, caniniform, and molariform. Thus the mechanism or mechanisms that initiate tooth development must also accommodate the development of different-shaped teeth.

Using the experimental systems already described, researchers have been able to switch dental papillae with dental organs from different tooth families and vice versa. When the dental papilla of an incisor tooth germ is recombined with the dental organ of a molar tooth germ, the dental organ assumes the shape of the incisor. Likewise, a molar dental papilla can cause an incisor dental organ to become molariform (Fig. 6-8). These experiments, together with experiments that induce

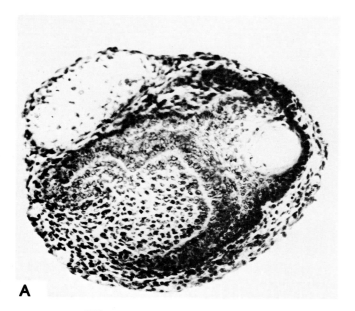

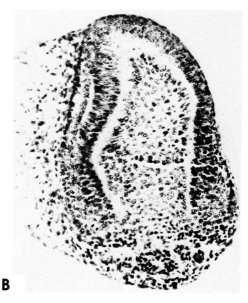

FIG. 6-8 Recombination of dental epithelium and ectomesenchyme. **A,** Incisor epithelium combined with molar papilla results in a molariform tooth. **B,** Molar epithelium combined with incisor papilla results in an incisiform tooth. (From Kollar EJ, Baird GR: *J Embryol Exp Morphol* 21:131, 1969.)

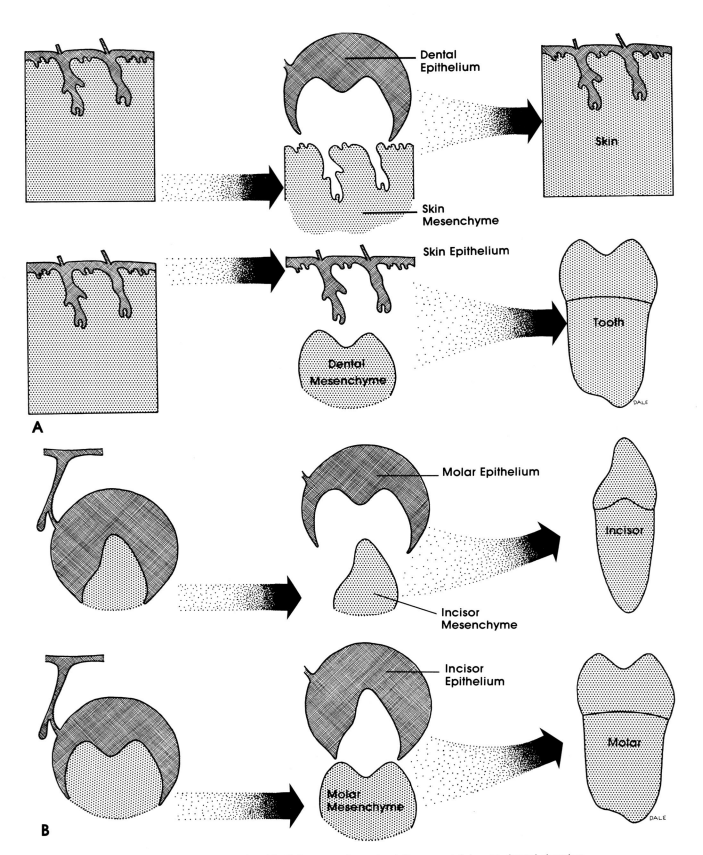

FIG. 6-9 Summary of epithelial-mesenchymal relations pertaining to dental development. Dental ectomesenchyme determines not only that the epithelium becomes "dental" but also that it is responsible for the shape of the tooth crown. **A,** Skin mesenchyme combined with dental organ results in skin; dental ectomesenchyme combined with skin epithelium results in a tooth. **B,** Incisor ectomesenchyme converts a molar enamel organ to an incisor, and vice versa.

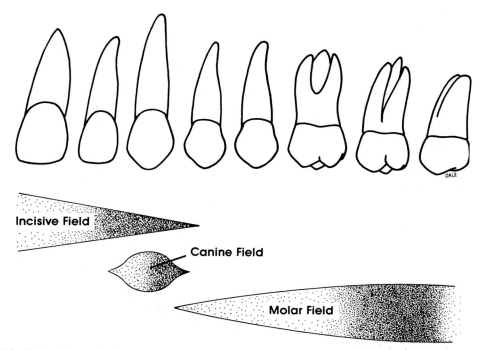

FIG. 6-10 Hypothetical differentiation of the mammalian dentition. Morphogenetic fields are thought to influence tooth germs to differentiate into incisors, canines, and molars. (Modified from Osborn JW, Ten Cate AR: *Advanced dental histology*, ed 3, Bristol UK, 1983, John Wright & Sons.)

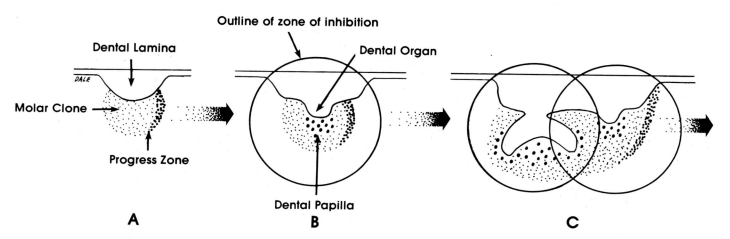

FIG. 6-11 Clone theory. The molar clone, **A,** has induced the dental lamina to begin tooth development. At its posterior border the clone and dental lamina grow posteriorly by means of the progress zone. When a clone reaches the critical size, a tooth bud is initiated at its center, **B.** A zone of inhibition surrounds the tooth bud and the next tooth bud, **C,** is not initiated until the progress zone of the clone has escaped its influence. (From Osborn JW, Ten Cate AR: *Advanced dental histology,* ed 3, Bristol UK, 1983, John Wright & Sons.)

the dental organ to form from skin, indicate that ectomesenchyme, once determined, not only can induce the development of a tooth but also determines its shape (Fig. 6-9).

The question now becomes (1) are neural crest cells, as they migrate and form ectomesenchyme, programmed to form teeth all of one family that subsequently become modified in shape by local external factors (field theory)? or (2) is the tooth-forming ectomesenchyme differentiated to form teeth of different families (clade theory)?

The field theory proposes three graded fields in the jaw for the three families of teeth (Fig. 6-10); thus a tooth bud forming at a given location develops according to its position within the field. The clade theory states that the ectomesenchyme, as it migrates into the jaws, becomes segregated into three clades, incisor, canine, and molar. Taking the molar clade as an example, we can suppose that this group of cells (Fig. 6-11) initiates the development of a deciduous first molar, at the same time creating a zone of inhibition around itself that prevents further dental development; only when posterior growth of the ectomesenchyme escapes the zone of inhibition does the next tooth germ differentiate.

There is some experimental evidence to support both claims. The experiment already referred to in which neural crest tissue is recombined with oral epithelium suggests that these cells are not determined until they reach the first arch. When the tooth bud of the first molar, however, is dissected out and permitted to continue development in the anterior chamber of the eye, first, second, and third molars develop. (This result also indicates that neural and vascular elements are not determinants of tooth development.) It is likely, therefore, that a field initiates a clone.

Determination of Tooth Shape

Recall that the crown pattern of a tooth is determined during the bell stage of tooth development (Fig. 4-12). At this stage the tooth germ can be likened to a fluid drop with a partition (the internal dental epithelium) across its middle. The stellate reticulum cells are separated from each other by ground substance (consisting largely of glycosaminoglycans, which attract water) so that the dental organ is turgid and exerts pressure on both the internal and the external dental epithelia. The growing dental papilla also exerts pressure on the internal dental epithelium, because it is contained within the dental follicle. Thus the internal dental epithelium lies between two opposing pressures, which cancel each other, and is therefore in a state of equilibrium; the folding that occurs as the crown develops results not from growth pressures within the dental papilla but from intrinsic growth caused by differential rates of mitotic division within the internal dental epithelium.

Actually, it is the cessation of mitotic division within cells of the internal dental epithelium that determines the shape of a tooth. When the tooth germ is growing rapidly during the early bell stage, cell division occurs throughout the internal dental epithelium. As development continues, cell division ceases at a particular point because the cells are beginning to differentiate and assume their eventual function of producing enamel. The point at which internal dental epithelial cell maturation first occurs represents the site of future cusp development, or the growth center. Because the internal dental epithelium is constrained at the cervical loop and because there is continued proliferation of cells on each side of the zone of maturation, the epithelium buckles and forms a cuspal outline (Fig. 6-12). Thus the future cusp is pushed up toward the external dental epithelium. This account contrasts sharply with accounts in older texts, which referred to collapse of the stellate reticulum as a way of explaining the approximation of internal dental and external dental epithelia.

Eventually the zone of maturation sweeps down the cusp slopes and is followed by the deposition of dentin and enamel, which fixes as the outline of the amelodentinal junction. A zone of maturation always precedes the zone of maturation on the flanks of the cusp, however, resulting in an emphasis of cusp outline (Fig. 6-13). The occurrence of a second zone of maturation within the internal dental epithelium leads to the formation of a second cusp, a third zone leads to a third cusp, and so on until the final cuspal pattern of the tooth is determined.

It would seem therefore that the crown pattern of the tooth is determined by differential cell division within the internal dental epithelium, contradicting the results of earlier recombination experiments. These experiments indicated, however, that the factors causing maturation and the cessation of cell division in the internal dental epithelium reside in the ectomesenchyme of the dental papilla. Thus it is clear that (1) the shape of the crown results from the interaction between dental papillary ectomesenchyme and the internal dental epithelium of the dental organ and (2) this interaction influences the growth pattern of the epithelium so that it folds to produce the outline of the crown pattern.

You can easily appreciate that the shape of teeth is remarkably consistent. Where aberrations occur (most commonly in the third molar and the maxillary lateral incisor), it is as a result of some effect exerted early in the developmental history of the tooth.

By way of summarizing what is known about the contribution of neural crest and first arch epithelium

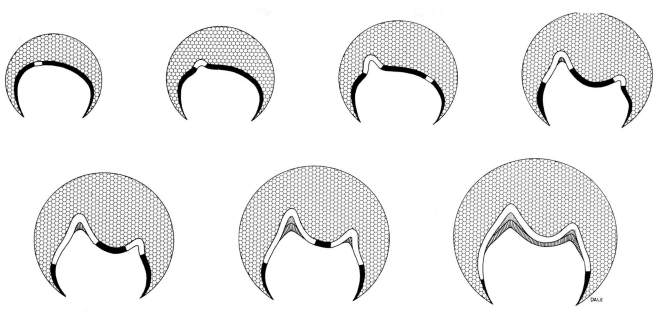

FIG. 6-12 Summary of crown pattern formation in the internal dental epithelium. The zone of cell division is indicated by the *darkened area* in the internal dental epithelium, and the zone of maturation by the *white area*.

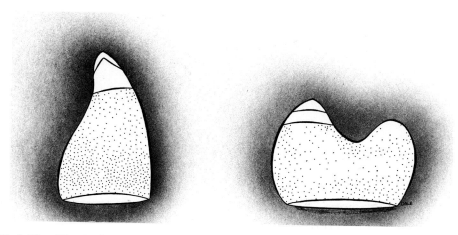

FIG. 6-13 Distribution of dividing cells in the internal dental epithelium in a single-cusped and a bicusped tooth. In a single-cusped tooth cell division is concentrated in the rim of the tooth as the epithelium thrusts upward. In the bicusped tooth there is an additional concentration of dividing cells between the cusps. (Modified from Osborn JE, Ten Cate AR: *Advanced dental histology*, ed 3, Bristol UK, 1983, John Wright & Sons.)

to the initiation and development of teeth, the following should be helpful:

1. It is known that neural crest cells migrate into the first arch and there form a band of ectomesenchyme beneath the epithelium of the stomatodeum.
2. It is known that these cells need to come into approximation with oral epithelium of the first arch before they can express their dental potential.
3. It is known that after this epithelial influence is exerted the ectomesenchyme of the dental papilla assumes a dominant role in further tooth development. Thus it is now able to (a) induce other nondental epithelium to form dental tissue and (b) determine the crown pattern of the tooth. We do not know how it does this.
4. It is known that the basal lamina plays a role in communication between epithelium and mesenchyme.
5. It is known that extracellular matrix molecules play a significant role.
6. It is known that the expression of various cytokines and associated cell surface receptors is critical.

BIBLIOGRAPHY

Billingham RE, Silvers WK: The origin and conservation of epidermal specificities, *N Engl J Med* 288:537, 1963.

Butler PM: The ontogeny of molar pattern, *Biol Rev Camb Philos Soc* 31:30, 1956.

D'Souza RN, Happonen RP, Flanders KC, Butler WT: Histochemical localization of transforming growth factor b1 in developing rat molars using antibodies to different epitopes, *J Biol Buccale* 18:299, 1990.

D'Souza RN, Happonen RP, Ritter NM, Butler WT: Temporal and spatial patterns of transforming growth factor b1 expression in developing rat molars, *Arch Oral Biol* 35:957, 1990.

Fleischmajer R, Billingham RE: *Epithelial-mesenchymal interactions,* Baltimore, 1968, Williams & Wilkins.

Grobstein C: Epithelio-mesenchymal specificity in the morphogenesis of mouse submandibular rudiments in vitro, *J Exp Zool* 124:383, 1953.

Grobstein C, Cohen J: Collagenase effect on the morphogenesis of embryonic salivary epithelium in vitro, *Science* 150:626, 1965.

Koch WE: Tissue interaction during in vitro odontogenesis. In Slavkin HS, Bavetta LA (eds): *Developmental aspects of oral biology,* New York, 1972, Academic Press.

Kogaya Y, Kim S, Akisaka T: Changes in the ultrastructural distribution of dental basement heparan sulfate during early mouse tooth development, *J Biol Buccale* 18:109, 1990.

Kollar EJ: Histogenetics of dermal-epidermal interactions. In Slavkin HS, Bavetta LA (eds): *Developmental aspects of oral biology,* New York, 1972, Academic Press.

Kollar EJP: Epithelial-mesenchymal interactions in the mammalian integument: tooth development as a model for instructive interaction. In Sawyer RH, Fallon JF (eds): *Epithelial mesenchymal interactions in development,* New York, 1983, Praeger.

Kollar EJ, Baird GR: The influence of the dental papilla on the development of tooth shape in embryonic mouse tooth germs, *J Embryol Exp Morphol* 21:131, 1969.

Kollar EJ, Baird GR: Tissue interactions in embryonic mouse tooth germs. I. Reorganization of the dental epithelium during tooth-germ reconstruction, *J Embryol Exp Morphol* 24:159, 1970.

Kollar EJ, Baird GR: Tissue interactions in embryonic mouse tooth germs. II. The inductive role of the dental papilla, *J Embryol Exp Morphol* 24:173, 1970.

Kollar EJ, Fischer C: Tooth induction in chick epithelium: expression of quiescent genes for enamel synthesis, 207:993, 1980.

Lumsden AGS: The neural crest contributions to tooth development. In Mederson PFA (ed): *Development and evolutionary biology of the neural crest,* New York, 1987, John Wiley & Sons.

Main JHP: Retention of potential to differentiate in long-term culture of tooth germs, *Science* 152:778, 1966.

Mina M, Kollar EJ: The induction of odontogenesis in nondental mesenchyme combined with early murine mandibular arch epithelium, *Arch Oral Biol* 32:123, 1987.

Mina M, Kollar EJ, Bishop JA, Rohrbach DH: Interaction between the neural crest and extracellular matrix proteins in craniofacial skeletogenesis, *Crit Rev Oral Biol Med* 1:79, 1990.

Osborn JW: Morphogenetic gradients: fields versus clones. In Butler PM, Joysey KA (eds): *Development, function, and evolution of teeth,* New York, 1978, Academic Press.

Rahemtulla F: Proteoglycans of oral tissues, *Crit Rev Oral Biol Med* 3:135, 1992.

Ruch JV: Determinisms of odontogenesis, *Cell Biol Rev* 14:1, 1987.

Singer SJ: Intercellular communications and cell-cell adhesion, *Science* 255:1671, 1991.

Slavkin HCP: Embryonic tooth formation: a tool for developmental biology, *Oral Sci Rev* 4:1, 1974.

Slavkin HC: Molecular determinants of tooth development: a review, *Crit Rev Oral Biol Med* 1:2, 1990.

Thesleff I, Harmerinta K: Tissue interactions in tooth development, *Differentiation* 18:75, 1981.

Thesleff I, Partanen AM, Vaniso S: Epithelial-mesenchymal interactions in tooth morphogenesis: the roles of extracellular matrix, growth factors, and cell surface receptors, *J Craniofac Genet Dev Biol* 11:229, 1991.

Vaahtokari A, Vainio S, Thesleff I: Associations between transforming growth factor B1 RNA expression and epithelial-mesenchymal interactions during tooth morphogenesis, *Development* 113:985, 1991.

Van Scott EJ, Reinertson RP: The modulating environment on epithelial cells studied in human autotransplants, *J Invest Dermatol* 36:109, 1961.

CHAPTER 7

Hard Tissue Formation and Destruction

THE hard tissues of the body—bone, cementum, dentin, and enamel—are all associated with the functioning tooth. Since the practice of dentistry involves manipulation of these tissues, a detailed knowledge of them is obligatory (and each is discussed separately in later chapters). The purpose of this chapter is (1) to explain that there are a number of common features associated with hard tissue formation, even though the final products are structurally distinct, (2) to indicate that the functional role of a number of these features is not understood, and (3) to describe the common mechanism of hard tissue breakdown.

HARD TISSUE FORMATION

It is easy to comprehend why three of the four hard tissues in the body (i.e., bone, cementum, and dentin) have many similarities in their formation. They are all specialized connective tissues, and collagen (principally type I) plays a large role in determining their structure. Although enamel is not a connective tissue and has no collagen involved in its makeup, its formation still follows many of the principles involved in the formation of hard connective tissue.

Hard tissue formation may be summarized as the production by cells of an organic matrix capable of accepting mineral, with the activity of the enzyme *alkaline phosphatase* and a good blood supply prerequisites. This rather simple concept, however, embraces a number of complex events, many of which are not properly understood. For example: What is the role of alkaline phosphatase? How is mineralization initiated in the organic matrix? Or, for that matter, how is mineral brought to the mineralization site? Each of these events will be discussed in turn.

Cells

Cells produce the organic matrices of hard tissues. Since hard tissue–forming cells must be synthetic, they all possess the armamentarium for synthesis and secretion: abundant mitochondria, much rough endoplasmic reticulum, and Golgi profiles. The assembly line and secretory pathway for the constituents of the organic matrix are well established and involve (successively) rough endoplasmic reticulum, transport vesicles, Golgi apparatus, and secretory vesicles.

Organic Matrix

In the case of hard connective tissues the organic matrix always consists of a fibrous protein (type I collagen) associated with varying amounts and types of other macromolecules (proteoglycans, phosphoproteins, phospholipids). The organic component of enamel consists of a distinctive family of enamel proteins. Nevertheless, all hard tissue matrices, regardless of their composition, are capable of accepting mineral in the form of hydroxyapatite crystals.

Mineral

The inorganic component of mineralized tissue consists of biologic apatite, which is essentially a calcium phosphate salt approximating in composition calcium hydroxyapatite which is represented $Ca_{10}(PO_4)_6(OH)_2$. It is important to grasp that this formula indicates only the atomic content of a conceptual entity known as the unit cell, which is the least number of calcium, phosphate, and hydroxyl ions able to establish ionic relationships. The unit cell of biologic apatite has the shape of a stubby rhombic prism; when stacked together, these prisms form the lattice of a crystal. The number

A

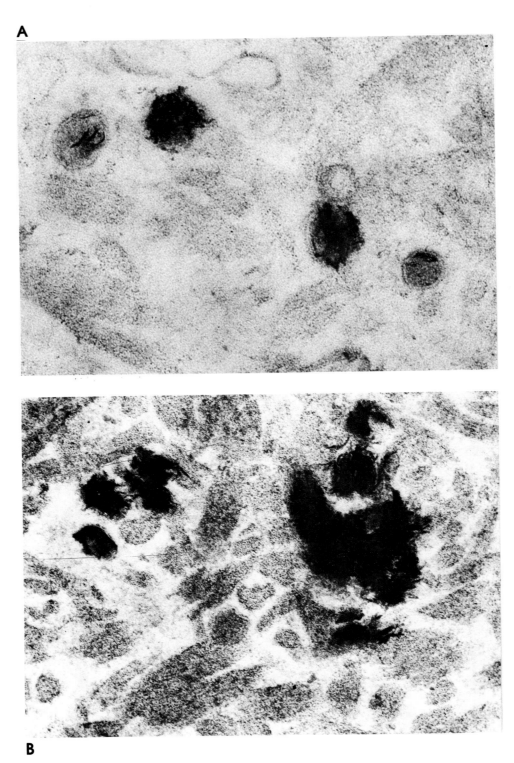

B

FIG. 7-1 Matrix vesicles. **A,** Four vesicles containing rudimentary apatite crystals. **B,** These crystals have ruptured from the vesicles and are joining with others to form mineralized masses. (From Eisenmann DR, Glick PL: *J Ultrastruct Res* 41:18, 1972.)

of repetitions of this arrangement produces crystallites of various sizes. Thus the hydroxyapatite found in mesenchymal hard tissues occurs as crystallites of approximately 100 × 200 × 50 × 50 Å dimensions whereas the hydroxyapatite of enamel forms a considerably larger crystal some 1400 Å long and 800 Å wide.

A layer of water, called the *hydration shell*, exists around each crystallite, which means that there are three surfaces to an apatite crystallite: the crystal interior, the crystal surface, and the hydration shell, all of which are available for the exchange of ions. Thus magnesium and sodium can substitute in the calcium position and fluoride and chloride in the hydroxyl position. Furthermore, ions may be adsorbed to the crystal surface by electrostatic attraction or bound in the hydration layer. The apatite crystallite is able to retain its structural configuration while accommodating these substitutions.

Direct visualization of the detailed structure of the apatite crystallite with the electron microscope is not easy, and there are difficulties in interpretation, but generally the crystals are described as needlelike or platelike.

In summary: Biologic apatite is built on a definite ionic lattice pattern that permits considerable variation in its composition through substitution, exchange, and adsorption of ions. This pattern of ionic variability reflects the immediate environment of the crystal and is used clinically to modify the structure of crystals by exposing them to a fluoride-rich environment.

MINERALIZATION

Tissue fluid is supersaturated with respect to calcium and phosphate ions, and it may be wondered why spontaneous precipitation of a calcium phosphate product does not occur in this circumstance. There are a number of reasons: first, tissue fluid contains other macromolecules, which inhibit crystal formation; and, second, the initial cluster of ions needed to form a lattice structure is unstable and, although a few may form, not enough clusters remain for the critical number of crystals to develop. Furthermore, the formation of a cluster of ions requires the expenditure of energy and an energy barrier must be overcome for crystallization to occur. Inhibitors of mineralization increase the amount of energy required.

Thus a number of conditions must be met, either singly or in combination, for mineralization to occur. Any local increase in the concentration of inorganic ions will permit a sufficient number of ionic clusters and crystallites to form. This is called *homogeneous nucleation*. The presence of a nucleating substance (which has the effect of lowering the energy barrier) also will allow

crystal formation to occur, in the absence of a locally increased ionic concentration. This is called *heterogeneous mineralization*. Finally, mechanisms exist to remove, inactivate, or exclude inhibitors of mineralization. Once the first crystallite has formed, however, a supersaturated solution can readily sustain crystal growth.

Two mechanisms exist to achieve the mineralization of hard connective tissue: the first involves a structure called the *matrix vesicle* (Fig. 7-1) and the second by heterogeneous nucleation (Fig. 7-2).

In the first mechanism the vesicle exists only in relation to initial mineralization. The vesicle is a small membrane-bound structure that buds off from the cell to form an independent unit within the first-formed organic matrix of hard tissue. Within this vesicle the first morphologic evidence of a crystallite is seen, and it is assumed that the vesicle provides within itself a microenvironment that permits the initial formation of a crystal of apatite. The matrix vesicle is characterized by its content of anionic phospholipids able to bind to calcium, a capacity enhanced by the presence of inor-

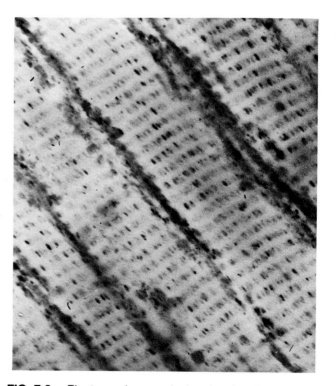

FIG. 7-2 Electron micrograph showing the disposition of crystals in collagen fiber bundles. The gaps in the collagen fibrils are where mineral has been deposited. (From Nylen MV, et al: *Calcification in biological systems,* American Association of Science Publication no. 64, 1960.)

ganic phosphate, thereby forming calcium–inorganic phosphate (CaP$_i$) phospholipid complexes, which so far have been found only in mineralizing situations. Also there is the possibility that membrane lipids (proteolipids) are involved, in that alkaline phosphatase and ATPase seem to be associated with membrane transport and are believed to be linked to the import of calcium and phosphate into the matrix vesicle. Thus, within this microenvironment, all the proposed mechanisms for initial mineralization exist. Although membrane control might selectively increase the local concentrations of inorganic ions to permit homogeneous nucleation, calcium binding lipids certainly seem to function as nucleators (causing the nucleation of hydroxyapatite from metastable solutions of calcium phosphate and, conversely, when selectively removed from matrix vesi-

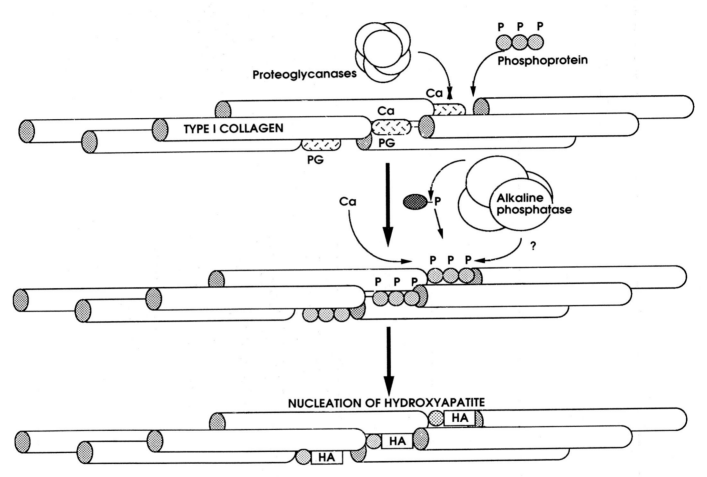

FIG. 7-3 Collagen mineralization. The fibers of collagen are formed along with secreted noncollagenous proteins such as proteoglycans (PGs), some of which occupy the gap zone between the collagen molecules. PGs can also bind to calcium ions and keep them in the gap zones. Enzymes such as proteoglycanases degrade the proteoglycans and allow phosphoproteins to bind to collagen in the gap zones. Phosphoproteins immobilize phosphates in an organized fashion in the gap zones and initiate the first mineral deposits. The enzyme complex alkaline phosphatase also plays a role, primarily by dephosphorylating other organic molecules but also, perhaps, by dephosphorylating some of the phosphoproteins in the gap zones. Localized increases in phosphate ions encourage the precipitation of additional calcium-phosphate complexes in the gap zones. These precipitates rapidly convert to the first hydroxyapatite (HA) crystals. Eventually HA crystals spread between collagen fibrils to fully mineralize the tissue. *Ca*, Calcium; *P*, phosphate. (From Limeback H: *Curr Opin Dent* 1:826, 1991.)

cles, losing their ability to initiate calcification). Enzyme activity associated with the matrix vesicle might also be involved in the selective removal of inhibitors.

In the second mechanism, which is more ordered, the heterogeneous nucleators exhibit a close relationship to collagen.

A number of noncollagenous molecules (phosphoproteins, proteoglycans, phospholipids) have been implicated, but their role in mineralization is complex and not fully understood. Some may act as nucleators, and others to control crystal growth. What follows is a simplified account of how these noncollagenous proteins may be involved in mineralization.

It is in the gap zones at the ends of collagen molecules that the mineral first appears. Initially these gaps are filled with proteoglycans, which bind to calcium. The proteoglycans are removed enzymatically, leaving behind the calcium; and as they are removed phosphoproteins bind to the collagen. Dephosphorylation of the phosphoprotein (as a result of alkaline phosphate activity) provides the additional phosphate ions for nucleation and crystal growth (Fig. 7-3).

Lipids are also involved somehow in the initial mineralization. Anionic phospholipids bind to calcium, and this binding capacity is enhanced by the presence of inorganic phosphate, producing CaP_i-phospholipid complexes. Such complexes have been found only in calcified tissue, at mineralizing fronts, and in matrix vesicles.

The initial mineralization of enamel is thought to be achieved by crystal growth from dentin apatite crystals, with the subsequent shape and size of the enamel crystals being determined by the enamel matrix (Fig. 11-4).

Crystal Growth

Once an apatite crystallite has been initiated, its initial growth is rapid, occurring in minutes or less; and later, slower growth results in crystals that exceed their initial size by 10 to 20 times. Such growth plays an important part in mineralization and is especially important in enamel formation.

A number of factors influence crystal growth and composition, but especially important is the immediate environment of the growing crystal. For example, noncollagenous proteins are able to bind selectively to different surfaces of the crystal, preventing further growth and thereby determining the shape of the crystal. Pyrophosphate accumulation on the crystal surface also blocks further growth.

Secondary Nucleation

Additional crystallites may form by secondary nucleation from mineral-phase particles arising from the collision and fracture of crystals previously formed by heterogenous nucleation.

ALKALINE PHOSPHATASE

The enzyme alkaline phosphatase is always associated with the production of any mineralized tissue. In all cases it exhibits a similar pattern of distribution, being involved with the blood vessels and cell membranes of hard tissue–forming cells. In hard connective tissues it is also found in the organic matrix, associated with matrix vesicles (when present) as well as occurring free within the matrix.

Although alkaline phosphatase has a clearcut function—hydrolyzing phosphate ions from organic radicals at an alkaline pH—its role in mineralization has not been established. A precise description of this role is complicated by at least two factors. First, the term alkaline phosphatase is nonspecific, describing a group of enzymes that all have the capacity to cleave phosphate ions from organic substrates at an alkaline pH. Second, the enzyme may have more than one distinct function in mineralization.

When associated with cell membranes, alkaline phosphatase is thought to play some role in ion transport; for many years its activity was associated with calcium transport. It has now been shown, however, that inhibitors of alkaline phosphatase activity do not interfere with calcium transport, and therefore attention has again shifted to the possibility that the enzyme is associated with providing phosphate ions at mineralization sites—the original role proposed for it some 60 years ago.

The extracellular activity of alkaline phosphatase at mineralization sites occurs where continuing crystal growth is taking place. Here it is thought that the enzyme has the function of cleaving pyrophosphate. Hydroxyapatite crystals in contact with serum or tissue fluids are prevented from growing larger because pyrophosphate ions are deposited on their surfaces, inhibiting further growth. Alkaline phosphatase activity breaks down pyrophosphate, thereby permitting crystal growth to proceed.

HOW MINERAL REACHES THE MINERALIZATION SITE

Even though the subject has been studied extensively, the mechanism(s) whereby large amounts of phosphate and calcium are delivered to calcification sites is still not understood.

There are two ways for mineral to reach a mineralization front: either through or between cells. Tissue fluid is supersaturated, at least with respect to octacalcium phosphate, and it could therefore be supposed that fluid simply needs to percolate between cells to reach the organic matrix, where local factors would then permit mineralization. A number of facts, however, deny such a simple explanation—for example, hormones influence the movement of calcium in and out of bone, and tight junctions exist between the cells that prevent the passage of calcium intercellullarly during enamel formation.

The possibility of transcellular transport is dictated by a particular circumstance: the cytosolic free calcium ion concentration cannot exceed 10^{-6} M since a greater concentration would cause calcium to inhibit critical cellular functions, leading to cell death. Three mechanisms have been proposed that permit transcellular transport of calcium without exceeding this critical threshold concentration. The first suggests that as cal-

cium enters the cell it is sequestered by a calcium-binding protein that, in turn, is transported through the cell to the site of release. The second suggests that a continuous and constant flow of calcium ions occurs across the cell without the concentration of free calcium ions ever exceeding 10^{-6} M (water in a hose pipe is a good analogy here; no matter the rate of flow, the amount of water in the pipe is always constant). The third suggests is that calcium is moved along the surface of the acidic phospholipids making up the cell membrane so that in effect it never properly enters the cell. Finally, a note needs to be added concerning the role of intracellullar compartments (e.g., the endoplasmic reticulum and mitochondria) in mineralization. Although it is generally thought that mitochondrial calcium transport systems are present to regulate internal

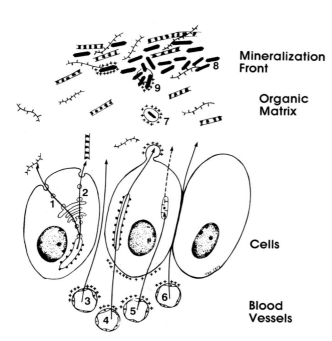

FIG. 7-4 Possible mechanisms associated with the production of a mineralized tissue. *1,* Synthetic pathway for the ground substance (proteoglycans); *2,* synthetic pathway for collagen; *3,* a pathway for inorganic ions between cells; *4,* a pathway for inorganic ions through the cell, presumably bound to macromolecules; *5,* mitochondrial involvement; *6,* a possible route for calcium within the cell membrane; *7,* nitial appearance of an apatite crystal in a matrix vesicle (Fig. 7-1); *8,* first appearance of an apatite crystal, possibly associated with sulfur in the proteoglycan; *9,* crystal growth. The more detailed relation of apatite crystallites to collagen is depicted in Figure 7-2. The sites of alkaline phosphatase activity are indicated by the small plus symbols.

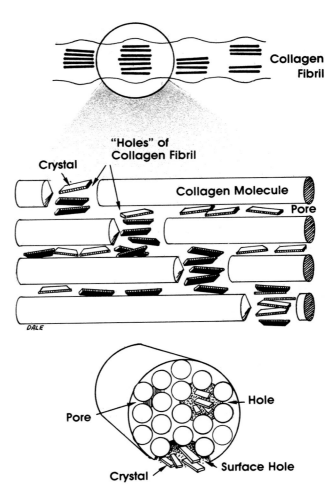

FIG. 7-5 Localization of mineral within the collagen fibril. (Redrawn from Glimcher ML: In Veis A [ed]: *The chemistry and biology of mineralized connective tissues,* New York, 1981, Elsevier–North Holland.)

concentrations of calcium within the mitochondrion, it has been demonstrated that under certain conditions large amounts of calcium can accumulate in the mitochondrion. This has been interpreted as a safety device protecting the calcium concentration of the cytosol; but in reality many studies of hard tissue–forming cells indicate that such cells do not have calcium-transporting systems associated with their mitochondria that are different from those in other cells. Figure 7-4 summarizes what is known and supposed concerning mineralization.

Location of Mineral

Mineral is not simply packed in the ground substance between the collagen fibrils; it is incorporated within the collagen fibril (Fig. 7-5). Indeed in bone 70% to 80% of mineral is located within the collagen fibril. From a number of morphologic studies it is evident that the location of such mineral is the result of heterogeneous nucleation, followed by secondary nucleation, within the gaps of the collagen fibril.

INCREMENTAL LINES IN HARD TISSUES

The production and mineralization of the organic matrix of any hard tissue are phasic—that is, they stop and start. During these alternating periods of activity and quiescence the character of the organic matrix varies slightly, which leads to variations in the degree of mineralization at the boundaries between periods of activity and rest. The phasic formation of hard tissue is thus reflected in its structure; it can be identified as incremental lines both in ground sections (because of variations in mineralization) and in demineralized sections (because of variations in matrix composition). These lines are given various names. For example, they are known as *resting lines* in bone, where they appear as more deeply staining hematoxiphilic lines marking the successive deposition of bone increments, or lamellae. Such lines in bone have been shown to contain less calcium and phosphorus than the rest of bone but significantly more sulfur. Also, the calcium/phosphate ratio in the cement line is significantly greater, suggesting that the mineral here may not be in the form of hydroxyapaptite.

Resting lines are also clearly seen in cementum. Another form of incremental line is the *reversal line*, which is similar to the resting line in composition but is much more wavy. Reversal lines mark the change from bone resorption to bone deposition.

Dentin and enamel also exhibit various incremental lines, indicating phasic deposition. The important point about these two hard tissues is that they do not remodel; thus their incremental line patterns are fixed, providing a permanent record of an individual's metabolic history. For example, in both the enamel and the dentin of teeth that are forming at birth, an accentuated incremental line (the *neonatal line*) records the physiologic changes then occurring. Febrile diseases of childhood and any other minor physiologic disturbances are also recorded permanently in dentin and enamel as accentuated incremental lines. Figure 7-6 shows the consistent pattern of incremental lines in the enamel of two teeth from the same individual. The various patterns will be referred to again as each hard tissue is discussed.

DEGRADATION OF HARD TISSUE

Bone is constantly remodeling and this is achieved by an orchestrated interplay between the removal of old bone and its replacement by new bone. The remaining hard tissues (cementum, dentin, enamel) do not remodel but are degraded and removed during the normal physiologic processes involved in the shedding of deciduous teeth.

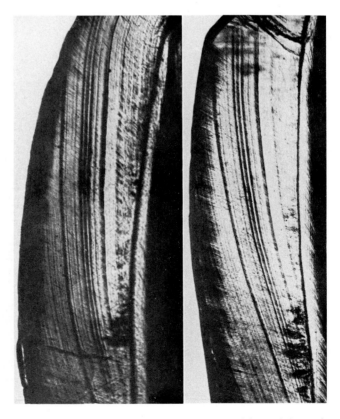

FIG. 7-6　Incremental lines in the enamel from right and left canines of the same person. The similar pattern indicates that a systemic influence has generated these lines. (From Osborn JW: *Oral Sci Rev* 3:3, 1973.)

The degradation and removal of hard tissue are a cellular event brought about by giant multinucleated cells formed through asynchronous fusion of mononuclear cells belonging to the macrophage lineage and originating from the hematopoietic system. They are called *osteoclasts* and are easy to identify under the light microscope because of their size (50 to 100 μm), their multinucleation (2 to 10 nuclei per cell), and their association with the surface of bone (occupying shallow depressions known as *Howship's lacunae* (Fig. 8-21). Under the electron microscope multinucleated osteoclasts exhibit a unique set of morphologic characteristics (Fig. 8-8). Adjacent to the bone surface their cell membrane is thrown into a myriad of deep folds that form a brush border sometimes visible by light microscopy in good preparations. At the periphery of the brush border the plasma membrane is closely apposed to the bone surface (within 0.2 to 0.5 nm), and the adjacent cytoplasm, devoid of cell organelles, is filled with fibrillar contractile proteins. This clear or "sealing" zone not only attaches the cells to the mineralized surface but also (by sealing the periphery of the brush border) isolates a microenvironment between them and the bone surface. The cell organelles consist of many nuclei, each surrounded by multiple Golgi complexes, an array of mitochondria and free polysomes, a rough endoplasmic reticulum, many coated transport vesicles, and numerous vacuolar structures. It has been known for years that osteoclasts are rich in acid phosphatase as well as other lysosomal enzymes. This concentration of enzymes, however, is not associated with lysosomal structures as in most other cells. Instead, it is known that the enzymes are synthesized in the rough endoplasmic reticulum, transported to the Golgi complexes, and from there, in coated transport vesicles, moved to the brush border (where, by a process of exocytosis, their release occurs into the sealed compartment adjacent to the bone surface). Another recently recognized feature of osteoclasts is the presence of a proton pump associated with the ruffled border, pumping hydrogen ions into the sealed compartment. Thus the sequence of resorptive events is considered to be (1)

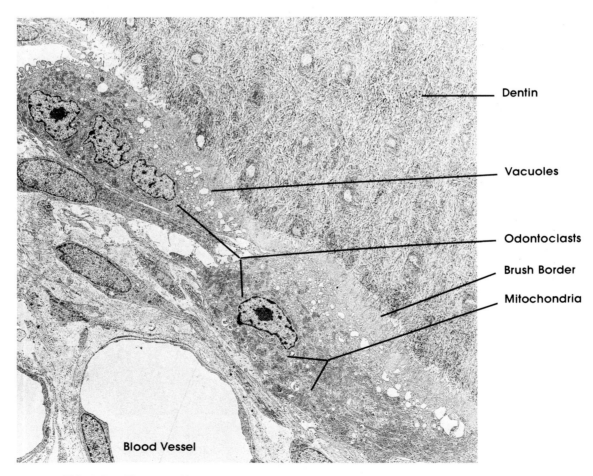

Dentin

Vacuoles

Odontoclasts

Brush Border

Mitochondria

Blood Vessel

FIG. 7-7   Electron micrograph showing odontoclasts eroding dentin. The brush border, many vacuoles, and mitochondria are easily recognizable.

attachment of osteoclasts to the mineralized surface of bone, (2) creation of a sealed acidic environment through action of the proton pump, which demineralizes bone and exposes the organic matrix, (3) degradation of this exposed organic matrix to its constituent amino acids by the action of released enzymes such as acid phosphatase and cathepsin B, and (4) uptake of mineral ions and amino acids by the cell.

The resorptive cells of dental hard tissues are called *odontoclasts* (Fig. 7-7) and are similar in most respects to osteoclasts although maybe somewhat smaller. Odontoclasts possess endocytotic vesicles containing liberated apatite crystals, which suggests that demineralization in the resorptive environment is not as complete as occurs in relation to osteoclasts.

In summary: Hard tissue formation involves cells situated close to a good blood supply, producing an organic matrix capable of accepting mineral (hydroxyapatite). These cells thus have the cytologic features of cells that both synthesize and secrete protein. For all the hard tissues except enamel, this matrix consists of collagen and ground substance and the mineral is located around and within the collagen fibril. In enamel most of the organic matrix is lost once mineralization has been initiated, to accommodate more mineral.

Mineralization in the connective hard tissues entails an initial nucleation mechanism involving a cell-derived matrix vesicle. After initial nucleation, further mineralization is achieved by nucleation related to the collagen fiber. In enamel the mechanism of initial mineralization is thought to be an extension from the apatite crystals of dentin, with further crystal growth dictated by the enamel matrix. Alkaline phosphatase is associated with mineralization, but its role is not understood. How it reaches the mineralization site is also debatable. Mineralization is phasic, which is reflected morphologically by distinguishable incremental lines. The breakdown of hard tissue involves the body's macrophage system, which produces a characteristic multinucleated giant cell, the osteoclast. To break down hard tissue, this cell attaches to mineralized tissue and create a sealed environment that is first acidified to demineralize the hard tissue. Following exposure to the acidic environment, the organic matrix is broken down by the secretion of proteolytic enzymes.

BIBLIOGRAPHY

Ali SY: Analysis of matrix vesicles and their role in the calcification of epiphyseal cartilage, *Fed Proc* 34:135, 1976.

Anderson HC: Vesicles associated with calcification in the matrix of epiphyseal cartilage, *J Cell Biol* 41:59, 1969.

Anderson HC: Matrix vesicle calcification, *Fed Proc* 35:105, 1976.

Anderson HC: Mechanisms of mineral formation in bone, *Lab Invest* 60:329, 1989.

Arsenault AL, Ottensmeyer FP: Quantitative spatial distributions of calcium, phosphorus, and sulfur in calcifying epiphysis by high resolution electronspectroscopic imaging, *Proc Natl Acad Sci USA* 80:1322, 1983.

Arsenault AL, Robinson BW: The dento-enamel junction: a structural and microanalytical study of early mineralization, *Calcif Tissue Int* 45:111, 1989.

Bachra BH: Calcification of connective tissue, *Int Rev Connect Tissue Res* 5:165, 1970.

Bawden JW: Calcium transport during mineralization, *Anat Rec* 224:226, 1989

Becker GL: Calcification mechanisms: roles for cells and mineral, *J Oral Pathol* 6:307, 1977.

Bernard GW: Ultrastructural observations of initial calcification in dentine and enamel, *J Ultrastruct Res* 41:1, 1972.

Bernard GW, Pease DC: An electron microscopic study of initial intramembranous osteogenesis, *Am J Anat* 125:271, 1969.

Boskey AL: The role of extracellular matrix components in dentin mineralization, *Crit Rev Oral Biol Med* 2:369, 1991.

Boyan BD, Schwartz Z, Swain LD, Khare A: Role of lipids in calcification of cartilage, *Anat Rec* 224:211, 1989.

Brighton CT, Hunt RM: Mitochondrial calcium and its role in calcification, *Clin Orthop Rel Res* 100:406, 1974.

Christoffersen J, Landis WJ: A contribution with review to the description of mineralization of bone and other calcified tissues in-vivo, *Anat Rec* 230:435, 1991.

Felix R, Fleisch H: The role of matrix vesicles in nucleation, *Fed Proc* 35:169, 1976.

Fleisch H, Bisaz S: Mechanism of calcification: inhibitory role of pyrophosphatase, *Nature* 195:911, 1962.

Glimcher MJ: Mechanism of calcification: role of collagen fibrils and collagen-phosphoprotein complexes in vitro and in vivo, *Anat Rec* 224:139, 1989.

Katchburian E: Membrane-bound bodies as initiators of mineralization in dentine, *J Anat* 116:285, 1973.

Lehninger AL: Mitochondria and calcium transport, *Biochem J* 119:129, 1970.

Limeback H: Molecular mechanisms in dental hard tissue mineralization, *Curr Opin Dent* 1:826, 1991.

Nylen MU, Scott DB, Mosley VM: Mineralization of turkey leg tendon. II. Collagen-mineral relations revealed by electron and x-ray microscopy. In Sognnaes RF (ed): *Calcification in biological systems*. Washington DC, 1991, American Association for the Advancement of Science, pp 129-142.

Reith EJ: A model for transcellular transport of calcium based on membrane fluidity and movement of calcium carriers within the more fluid microdomains of the plasma membrane, *Calcif Tissue Int* 35:129, 1983.

Salomen CD: Fine structural study on the extracellular activity of alkaline phosphatase and its role in calcification, *Calcif Tissue Res* 15:201, 1974.

Shapiro IM, Greenspan JS: Are mitochondria involved in biological mineralization? *Calcif Tissue Res* 3:100, 1969.

Shapiro IM, Lee NH: Calcium accumulation by chondrocyte mitochondria, *Clin Orthop Rel Res* 106:323, 1975.

Veiss A: *Development and biochemistry.* Vol 22, *The chemistry and biology of mineralized tissues*, New York, 1982, Elsevier–North Holland.

CHAPTER 8

Bone

BONE is a specialized mineralized connective tissue consisting of 33% organic matrix, 28% type I collagen, and 5% noncollagenous protein, including osteonectin, osteocalcin, bone morphogenetic protein, bone proteoglycan, and bone sialoprotein. This organic matrix is permeated by a poorly crystallized calcium-deficient hydroxyapatite $(Ca_{10}(PO_4)_6(OH)_2)$, which makes up the remaining 67% of bone (Fig. 8-1).

In addition to its obvious skeletal functions of support, protection, and locomotion, bone constitutes an important reservoir of minerals. Systemically it is finally controlled by hormonal factors; locally it is controlled by mechanical forces (including tooth movement), growth factors, cytokines, and piezoelectric conditions. Although the figures given above for bone composition are approximate, the ratio between hard and soft components is sufficient to ensure a degree of elasticity. Bone resists compressive forces best and tensile forces least. It also resists forces applied along the axis of its fibrous component; fractures of bone thus occur most readily in response to tensile and slicing stresses.

GROSS BONE HISTOLOGY

Bones have been classified as long or flat on the basis of their gross appearance. Long bones include the bones of the axial skeleton (e.g., tibia, femur, radius, ulna, and humerus). Flat bones include all the skull bones plus the sternum, scapula, and pelvis. Gross inspection of longitudinal or cross sections through long and flat bones shows that, irrespective of different outward appearances, bones have a common inner structure.

Characteristic of all bones are a dense outer sheet of *compact* bone and a central medullary cavity. In living bone the cavity is filled with either red or yellow bone marrow. The marrow cavity is interrupted throughout its length, particularly at the ends of long bones, by a reticular network of *trabecular (alternatively, cancellous or spongy)* bone. These internal trabeculae act as well-banded reinforcement rods to support the outer (thicker) cortical crust of compact bone (Fig. 8-2).

Mature or adult bones, whether compact or trabecular, are histologically identical in that they consist of

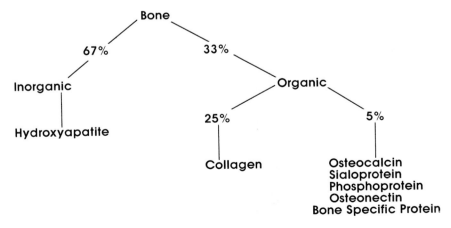

FIG. 8-1 Composition of bone.

microscopic layers or lamellae (that in compact bone are closely packed). Three distinct types of layering are recognized: (1) circumferential, (2) concentric, and (3) interstitial. *Circumferential* lamellae enclose the entire adult bone, forming its outer perimeter. *Concentric* lamellae make up the bulk of compact bone and form the basic metabolic unit of bone, the *osteon*. The osteon is a cylinder of bone, generally oriented in the long axis of the bone. In the center of each osteon the Haversian canal is lined by a single layer of bone cells that cover the bone surface; each canal houses a capillary. Adjacent Haversian canals are interconnected by Volkmann canals, channels that, like Haversian canals, contain blood vessels, thus creating a rich vascular network throughout compact bone. *Interstitial* lamellae are interspersed between adjacent concentric lamellae and fill the spaces between them. They are actually fragments of preexisting concentric lamellae and can take a multitude of shapes (Figs. 8-3 and 8-4).

Surrounding every compact bone is an osteogenic (bone cell–forming) connective tissue membrane, the *periosteum*, that consists of two layers. The inner layer, next to the bone surface, consists of bone cells, their precursors, and a rich microvascular supply. The outer layer, which is more fibrous, gives rise to the Sharpey fibers. These penetrate the cellular layer of the periosteum and extend into the circumferential lamellae. Both the internal surface of compact bone and the entire surface of cancellous bone are covered by a single layer of bone cells, the *endosteum*, which physically separates the bone surface from the bone marrow within (Fig. 8-3).

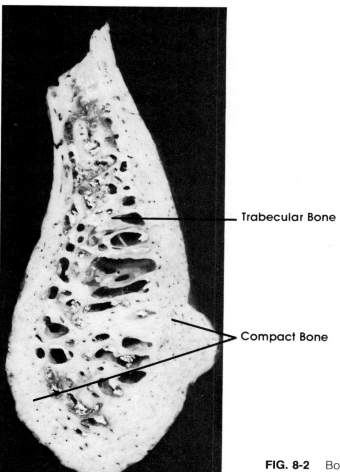

Trabecular Bone

Compact Bone

FIG. 8-2 Body of the mandible. The outer layer of compact bone and an inner supporting network of trabecular bone can be clearly distinguished.

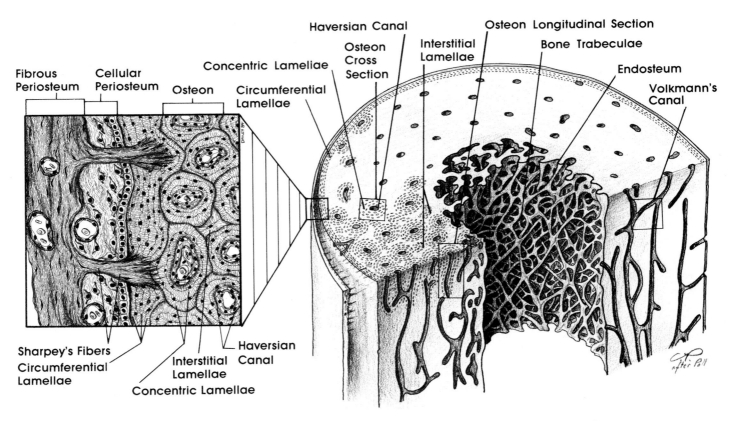

FIG. 8-3 Components of bone. (*Inset:* Compact and trabecular bone within the periosteal surface.)

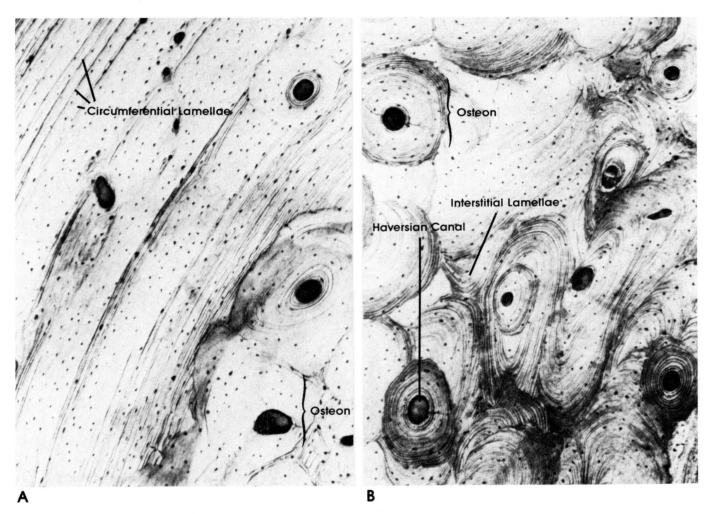

FIG. 8-4 Ground sections of dried bone. **A,** Outer compact bone; **B,** inner compact bone.

EVOLUTION OF BONE TERMINOLOGY

Over the years a number of ways to describe bone have been developed, but the tendency to interchange descriptions has sometimes led to confusion. A simple way to remember each classification is by the order of magnification used: with the naked eye two types of bones can be recognized, compact and spongy or trabecular; with the medium-powered lens more detail can be discerned (Haversian canals, interstitial matrix, circumferential lamellae); finally, with the high-powered lens collagenous matrix can be seen (allowing distinction between the *coarse-fibered woven bone* and the *fine-fibered lamellar bone*). Thus compact bone is seen to contain Haversian systems consisting of fine-fibered lamellar bone.

BONE CELLS

In bone, separate cells are primarily responsible for the formation, resorption, and maintenance of osteoarchitecture. Classically, three types of bone cells are described, each with specific functions: (1) the *osteoblasts*, which forms bone, (2) the *osteocyte*, which (together with inactive osteoblasts [lining cells]) maintains bone, and (3) the osteoclast, which resorbs bone. The

osteoclast is likely aided in the resorption process by wandering macrophages and cytokines emitted by neighboring osteoblasts. Because the osteocyte is derived from the osteoblast, it is more correct to consider bone cells as coming from two lineages only, the first concerned with formation and maintenance and the second with removal. This is an important distinction because large numbers of cells from both sources need to be recruited continuously throughout life to maintain the functional integrity of bone.

Osteoblast

Osteoblasts are uninucleated cells that synthesize both collagenous and noncollagenous bone proteins (the organic matrix, *osteoid*). They are responsible for mineralization and are thought to derive from a multipotent mesenchymal cell or, alternatively, from a perivascular cell. The osteoblast is generally considered to differentiate through a precursor cell, the preosteoblast. Osteoblasts have all the characteristics of hard tissue—forming cells described in Chapter 7 (Fig. 8-5). They constitute a cellular layer over the forming bone surface and have been postulated to form a bone membrane that controls ion flux into and out of the bone. Some support for the idea of a membrane comes from the fact

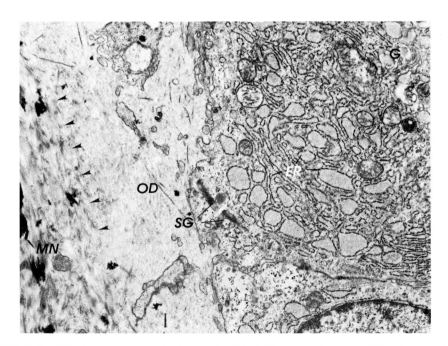

FIG. 8-5 Electron micrograph of an osteoblast. The cytoplasm exhibits abundant rough endoplasmic reticulum *(ER)*. A Golgi complex *(G)* and secretory granules *(SG)* are visible. Newly secreted osteoid *(OD)* is beginning to mineralize *(MN)*. Changes in direction of the collagen fibrils of the osteoid *(arrows)* indicate the end of one lamella and the start of another.

that a filamentous network can be seen within the osteoblast near a cell membrane site adjacent to the bone surface. This network terminates at the lateral cell membrane, where the membrane exhibits an increased electron density coinciding with a parallel density in the membrane of the adjacent cell. Although no junctional complex forms, this arrangement suggests some sort of adherence between adjacent osteoblasts. Gap junctions do form and functionally couple adjacent periosteal cells—preosteoblasts to osteoblasts, osteoblasts to osteoblasts, osteoblasts to osteocytes, and osteocytes to osteocytes. When bone is no longer forming, the surface osteoblasts become inactive and are termed *lining cells*. Such cells have thin flat nuclear profiles with cytoplasm extending along the bone surface, often attenuated to a thickness of less than 0.1 μm. Cytoplasmic organelles are few and include mitochondria, free ribosomes, and isolated profiles of rough endoplasmic reticulum. It has been postulated that these lining cells retain their gap junctions with osteocytes, creating a syncytium that functions to control mineral homeostasis and ensure bone vitality.

Preosteoblasts and, to a lesser extent, osteoblasts (Fig. 8-6) exhibit high levels of alkaline phosphatase on the outer surface of their plasma membranes. This enzyme, which is used experimentally as a cytochemical marker, distinguishes the osteoblast from the fibroblast. Functionally it is believed to cleave organically bound phosphate. The liberated phosphate either (1) contributes to the initiation and progressive growth of bone mineral crystals in hydroxyapatite or (2) stimulates the production or maturation of bone matrix itself. A third possible function, entering the cell and providing maximal phosphorylation of the several phosphoproteins of bone, remains largely untested.

Osteoblasts secrete, in addition to type I and type V collagen and small amounts of several noncollagenous proteins (some of which [the phosphoproteins] are critical to bone mineralization [Chapter 7]), a variety of cytokines. These autocrine or paracrine factors, which include growth factors, help regulate cell metabolism. The kinds and quantities of cytokines vary with the physiologic state of the osteoblast or its osteogenic precursors.

A key factor in the rate of bone cell development is the elaboration by osteoblasts and/or their precursors of a number of growth factors. Osteoblasts secrete several members of the bone morphogenetic protein (BMP) superfamily, including BMP 2, BMP 7, and transforming growth factor beta (TGF-β), in addition

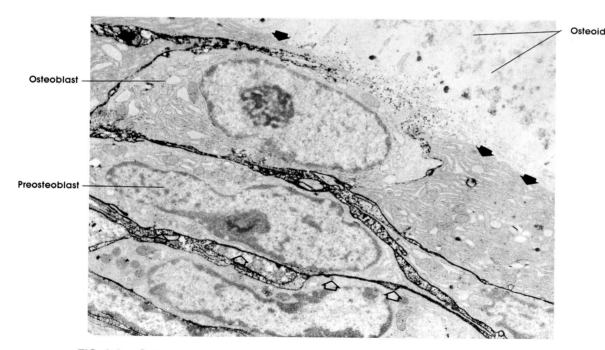

Osteoid

Osteoblast

Preosteoblast

FIG. 8-6 Calvarial preosteoblasts and osteoblasts demonstrating histochemical localization of alkaline phosphatase *(open arrows)* along the plasma membrane. Note that the amount of enzyme on the secretory surface of the osteoblasts *(solid arrows)* is significantly less than that on preosteoblasts, or absent. (Micrograph courtesy Dr. Lorrita Watson.)

to the insulin-like growth factors (IGF-I and IGF-II), platelet-derived growth factor (PDGF-AA), and fibroblastic growth factor beta (FGF-β).

Although the timing of secretion and the complex interactions of these growth factors are unclear, the combinations IGF-I and TGF-β and another platelet-derived growth factor (PDGF-BB) remarkably increase the rapidity of bone formation and bone repair and will likely be very important in future dental therapy. For instance, these combinations may be used to speed healing and bone growth following periodontal surgery or to prevent periodontal disease by the early treatment of periodontal pockets. Likewise, they may be used to enhance osseous integration following the placement of dental implants.

Under physiologic conditions that support resorption rather than formation, osteoblasts can be stimulated by lymphokines (e.g., interleukin 1, tumor necrosis factor alpha) and by prostaglandins (E2) to produce interleukin 6, a factor that clearly increases the resorbing activity of the osteoclast.

The hormones most important in bone metabolism are parathyroid hormone, 1,25-dihydroxyvitamin D, calcitonin, estrogen, and the glucocorticoids. Parathyroid hormone and vitamin D are biphasic in their actions, enhancing bone resorption at high (pharmacologic) concentrations but supporting bone formation at lower (physiologic) concentrations. Calcitonin and estrogen inhibit resorption whereas the glucocorticoids inhibit both resorption and formation (but primarily formation). It is most likely that the hormones affecting bone work primarily through altering the secretion of the abovementioned cytokines.

Osteocyte

As osteoblasts secrete bone matrix, some of them become entrapped in lacunae and are then called osteocytes. The number of osteoblasts that become osteocytes varies depending on the rapidity of bone formation: the more rapid the formation, the more osteocytes are present per unit volume. As a general rule embryonic (woven) bone and repair bone have more osteocytes than does lamellar bone (Fig. 8-17).

After their formation, osteocytes gradually lose most of their matrix-synthesizing machinery and become reduced in size. During their lifespan osteocytes may slowly resorb the immediate surrounding matrix, creating around the osteocytic cell body a space called the *osteocytic lacuna.* Narrow extensions of these lacunae form enclosed channels, or canaliculi, that house radiating osteocytic processes (Fig. 8-7). Thus osteocytes maintain contact with adjacent osteocytes and with the osteoblasts or lining cells on the bone surfaces—the

endosteum, periosteum, and Haversian canals. As previously discussed, processes from adjacent osteocytes and lining cells are joined together by gap junctions, forming the osteoblast-osteocyte complex necessary to bone matrix maintenance and vitality.

Perhaps the most important function of the osteoblast-osteocyte complex is to prevent hypermineralization of bone by continually pumping calcium back into the bloodstream. Hormonal control of this calcium-pumping syncytium is believed to aid in the fine control of serum calcium. Failure of any part of the syncytium results in hypermineralization (sclerosis) and death of the bone maintained by that segment of the syncytium. This nonvital bone is resorbed and replaced during the process of bone turnover.

Osteoclast

Compared to all other bone cells and their precursors, the multinucleated osteoclast is a much larger cell. How many nuclei an osteoclast contains and how large it becomes are roughly related to how well the bone matrix being resorbed has been mineralized. Thus, in the resorption of mature lamellar bone, osteoclasts become much larger than in immature woven bone.

Because of their size, osteoclasts can easily be identified under the light microscope; they are generally seen in a cluster rather than singly (Figs. 8-17, 8-20, and 8-21). The osteoclast is characterized cytochemically by possessing tartrate-resistant acid phosphatase within its cytoplasmic vesicles and vacuoles, which distinguishes it from other giant cells and macrophages.

Typically osteoclasts are found against the bone surface, occupying shallow hollowed-out depressions, called Howship lacunae, that they themselves have created. Scanning electron microscopy of bone-resorbing surfaces shows that Howship lacunae are not merely small focal divots but rather long shallow troughs. This observation attests to both the activity and the mobility of osteoclasts during active resorption.

The ultrastructural features of the osteoclast and its functional activity have already been described (Chapter 7).

Origin of Bone Cells

To maintain the structural integrity of bone, large numbers of cells must be continuously recruited. Interference with recruitment mechanisms can be responsible for various pathologic conditions in bone; therefore the origin of bone cells is a subject of some importance.

Generally it can be stated that the origin of bone-forming cells is mesenchymal, whereas the origin of osteoclasts is hematopoietic both demand the existence of a pleuripotent stem cell.

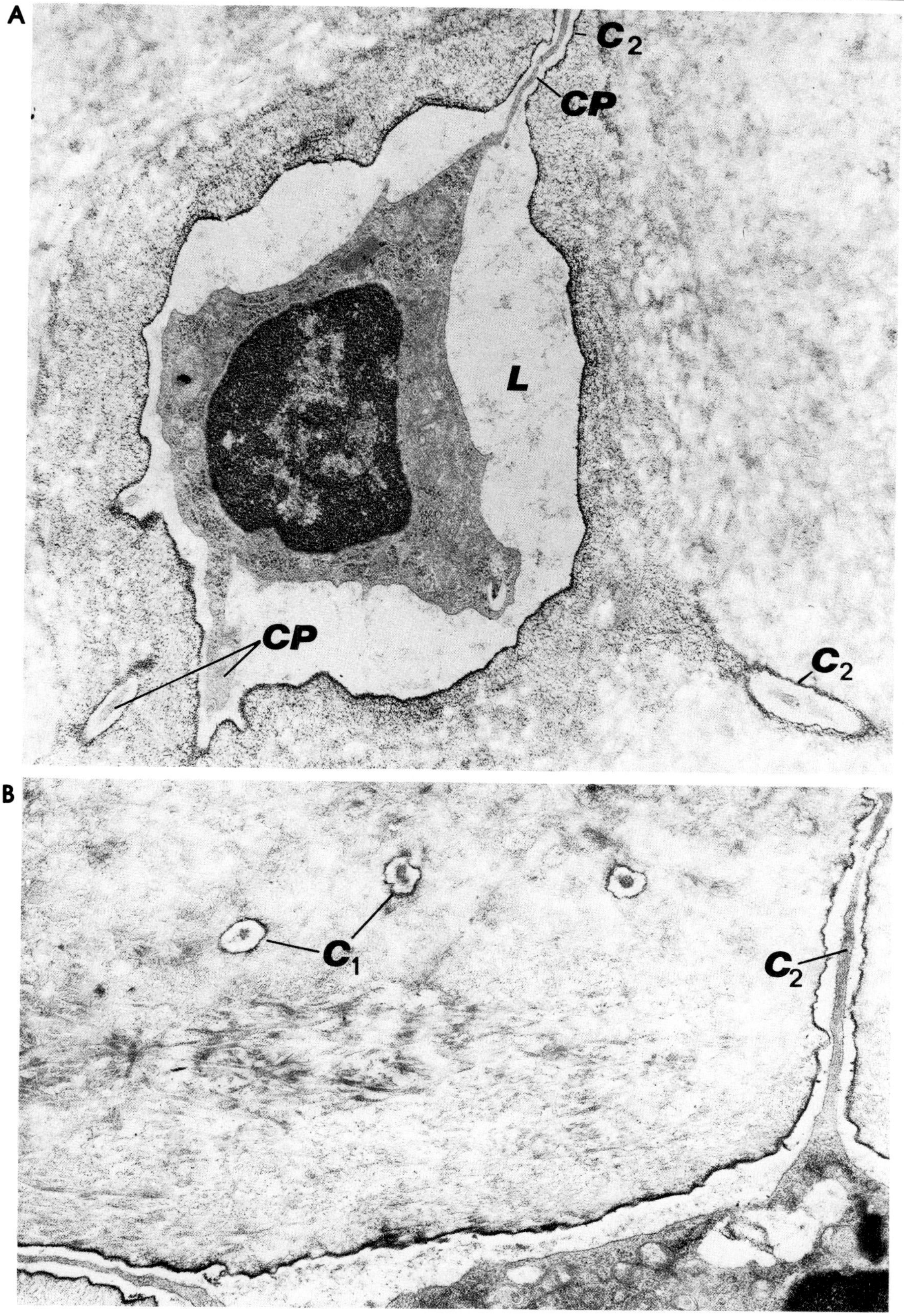

FIG. 8-7 **A,** Electron micrograph of an osteocyte. The cell, housed in its lacuna *(L)*, emits a cytoplasmic process *(CP)*, which exits the lacuna through a canaliculus *(C₂)*. **B,** Cell processes of osteocytes in canaliculi (electron micrograph). Cut in both cross section *(C₁)* and longitudinal section *(C₂)*.

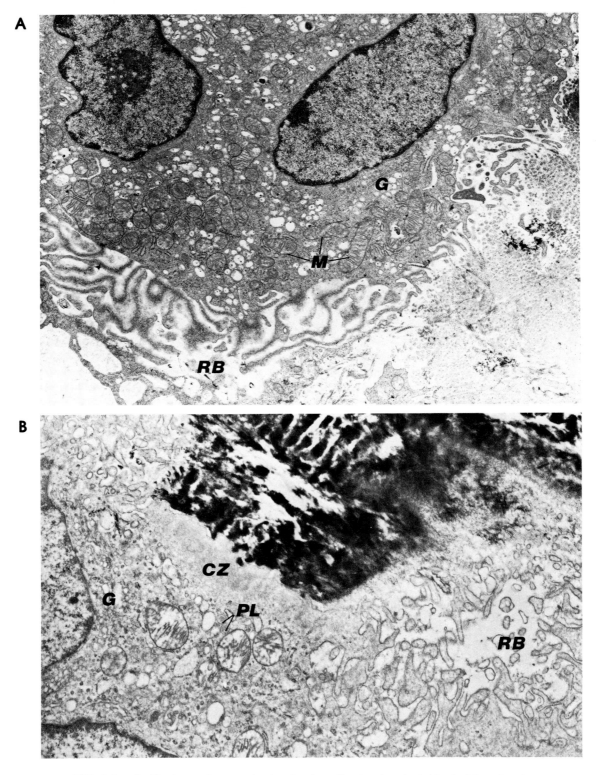

FIG. 8-8   A, Electron micrograph of a demineralized osteoclast. Most of the classic features are evident ruffled border *(RB),* numerous mitochondria *(M),* multinucleation, and tightly arranged Golgi saccules *(G).* **B,** Electron micrograph of an undemineralized osteoclast. The ruffled border *(RB)* is in contact with the mineralized matrix *(black).* A portion of the clear zone *(CZ)* attaches the osteoclast to the mineralized surface; Golgi saccules *(G)* and primary lysosomes *(PL)* are found in the cytoplasm.

It is worth reviewing briefly two classic experiments that have provided the evidence to support these statements:

Fibroblastlike cells from spleen, thymus, and bone marrow stroma have been cloned. When the clones were transplanted under the capsule of a kidney, each formed collagen; but only the clone derived from bone marrow formed bone. Furthermore, this clone was capable of initiating adipose and reticular cell lines. These findings indicate that not only is the bone-forming cell derived from a special source, this source is also pleuripotential.

When cloned endosteal cells were taken from an animal of one sex and implanted under the kidney capsule of an animal of the opposite sex, all the osteoblasts that form have the sex of the second animal, whereas osteoclasts exhibit the sex of the host. This experiment reinforces the specific stromal origin theory for bone-forming cells and indicates a different source for osteoclasts.

Figure 8-8 illustrates the second experiment, which establishes the hematopoietic origin of osteoclasts. Two parabiotic animals with shared circulations were established. One was shielded and the other irradiated to destroy its hematopoietic stem cells. The cross circulation was then temporarily arrested and tritiated thymidine was given to the shielded animal, thereby marking all proliferating cells. Cross circulation was reestablished and fracture repair studied in both animals. In the shielded animal, in which all dividing cells had been labeled, all cells at the fracture repair site (monocytes, macrophages, fibroblasts, chondroblasts, osteoblasts, osteoclasts) were labeled. In the other animal, which had labeled cells only in its hematogenic system, only monocytes, macrophages, and osteoclasts were labeled at the site of fracture repair.

Figures 8-9 and 8-10 summarize current opinion concerning the origin of bone cells.

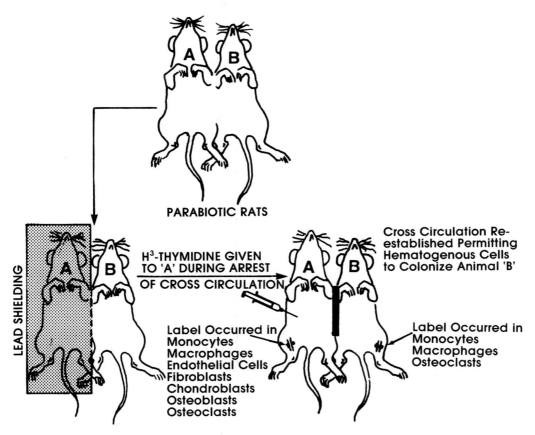

FIG. 8-9 Summary of an experiment indicating the hematopoietic origin of osteoclasts. Parabiotic rats (sharing the same circulation) were used. Rat *A* was shielded from irradiation, which destroyed the hematopoietic tissue in rat *B*. In both rats the femurs were fractured and cross circulation was temporarily arrested. Tritiated thymidine was introduced into rat *A*. When cross circulation was reestablished, only rat *B* had labeled cells in its hematogenous system. Osteoclasts at the fracture site were labeled. (Redrawn from Gothlin G, Ericsson JLE: *Clin Orthop* 120:211, 1976.)

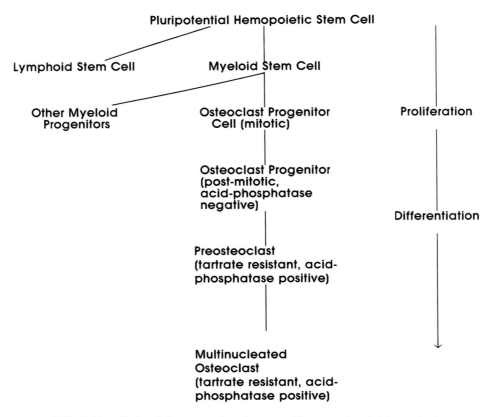

FIG. 8-10   Cells of the osteoclast lineage. (Courtesy Dr. J. Heersche.)

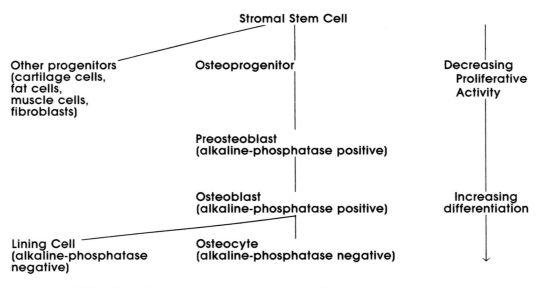

FIG. 8-11   Cells of the osteogenic lineage. (Courtesy Dr. J. Heersche.)

BONE DEVELOPMENT

Although histologically one bone is no different from another, bone formation occurs by three methods: (1) endochondral, (2) intramembranous, and (3) sutural. Endochondral bone formation takes place on a cartilage matrix model, the cartilage immediately preceding bone in development. Intramembranous bone formation occurs directly within a connective tissue membrane. Sutural bone formation is a special case, the bone forming along sutural margins.

Endochondral Bone Formation

Endochondral bone formation occurs at the ends of all long bones, vertebrae, and ribs and at the head of the mandible and base of the skull. Early in embryonic development there is a condensation of mesenchymal cells that takes the general shape of the bone to be formed. Cartilage cells differentiate from these mesenchymal cells, beginning in the diaphysis, and a perichondrium forms around the periphery. Rapid growth of the cartilage anlage ensues—by interstitial growth within the core of the anlage (as more and more cartilage matrix is secreted by each chondroblast) and by appositional growth through cell proliferation and matrix secretion within the expanding perichondrium. This ongoing growth of cartilage is the primary source of growth in these bones (Fig. 8-11).

As differentiation of cartilage cells proceeds toward the metaphysis, the cells organize themselves roughly into longitudinal columns. The longitudinal columns of cells can be subdivided into three functionally different zones: the zone of proliferation, the zone of hypertrophy and maturation, and the zone of provisional mineralization (Figs. 8-12 and 8-13). In the zone of proliferation the cells (which are small and somewhat flattened) primarily constitute a source of new cells.

The zone of hypertrophy and maturation is the broadest zone. As the chondroblasts hypertrophy, the secretory machinery of the chondroblasts increases. In the early stages of hypertrophy the chondroblasts secrete mainly type II collagen, which forms the primary structural component of the longitudinal matrix septa (Figs. 8-12 and 8-13). As hypertrophy proceeds, mostly proteoglycans are secreted. The combination of increased cell size and increased cell secretion leads to an increase in the size of the cartilaginous end of the bone. As the chondroblast reaches maximum size, it secretes type X collagen and chondrocalcin, which, together with partial proteoglycan breakdown, create a matrix environment with the potential to mineralize. Matrix mineralization begins in the zone of mineralization by elaboration of matrix vesicles. (See Chapter 7.) When the fully hypertrophied chondroblasts become sufficiently encased in mineral, they die.

Within the perichondrium in the diaphysis there is increased vascularization. As a result, the perichondrium converts to a periosteum and intramembranous bone begins to form. Concurrently vascularization of the middle of the cartilage occurs, and multinucleated cells called *chondroclasts* (identical to osteoclasts) resorb most of the mineralized cartilage matrix, making room for further vascular ingrowth (Figs. 8-12 and 8-13). The successive steps of cartilage cell proliferation—cartilage matrix production, chondroblast hypertrophy and maturation, cartilage matrix mineralization and chondrocyte death, vascular invasion, and partial cartilage removal—proceed from the diaphysis toward each end of a long bone until bone growth ceases.

Mesenchymal (perivascular) cells accompany the invading blood vessels, proliferating and migrating onto the remains of the mineralized cartilage matrix. This mineralized cartilage is generally all that is left of the longitudinal septa, the horizontal septa having been completely resorbed (Figs. 8-12 to 8-14). The mesenchymal cells differentiate into osteoblasts and begin to deposit osteoid on the mineralized cartilage columns and then to mineralize it. As the bone matrix is produced, the mineralized cartilage matrix becomes an irregularly shaped central zone core or column for a circular rim of new bone matrix (Figs. 8-12 and 8-14). Some of the osteoblasts are surrounded by bone matrix and become osteocytes. This mineralized cartilage core–bone matrix is collectively termed the *primary spongiosa*. With time the space created by the invading vascular system develops into red bone marrow. As the bone continues to grow in length, the marrow continues to expand, at the expense of the mineralized cartilage and bone. Osteoclasts progressively remove both the core of mineralized cartilage and the surrounding bone. This process occurs at approximately the same rate as cartilage formation, so that the volume of the primary spongiosa remains relatively constant during growth (Fig. 8-13).

In some bones (e.g., the tibia, but not the mandible) a secondary invasion of blood vessels into the head (end) of the bone creates a secondary ossification center. This secondary bone growth proceeds in a fashion identical to that occurring in primary bone growth and creates a plate of growing cartilage between the diaphysis and the end (epiphysis) of the bone. This plate is termed the *epiphyseal growth plate* (Fig. 8-11), acknowledging its important contribution to longitudinal bone growth. As bone growth ceases, the cartilage cells fail to proliferate and they then hypertrophy and die; the growth plate disappears, being totally replaced by bone. In addition, as longitudinal bone growth slows and ceases, so does the expansion of the marrow cavity. The bone-

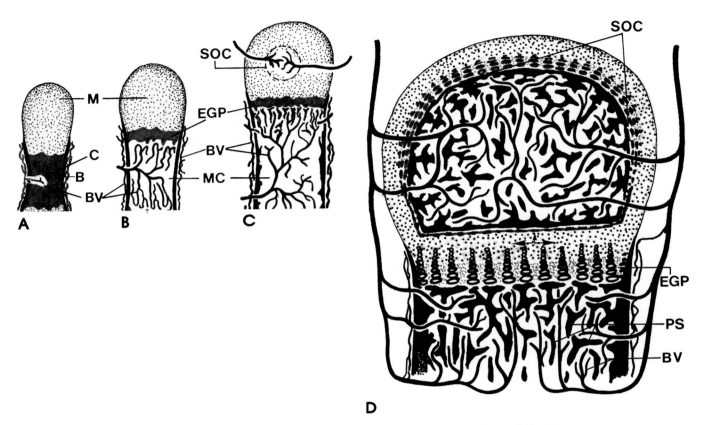

FIG. 8-12 Endochondral bone formation. **A,** Some of the mesenchyme *(M)* of the bone anlage is differentiating into cartilage cells *(C),* which mineralize as the blood vessels *(BV)* grow into the bone center. Blood vessels in the periosteum have begun to induce the formation of intramembranous bone as a bony collar *(B).* **B,** Blood vessels expand and migrate toward the ends of the bone to form a marrow cavity *(MC)* and an epiphyseal growth plate of cartilage cells *(EGP).* **C,** Secondary ingrowth of blood vessels in the head of the bone creates a secondary ossification center *(SOC).*
D, Longitudinal bone growth results as columns of cartilage cells in the epiphyseal growth plate *(EGP)* continue to proliferate, hypertrophy, and secrete matrix (interstitial growth, *arrows*). The chondrocytes mineralize the matrix, which is partially resorbed by chondroclasts. The bone cells that accompany the blood vessels *(BV)* produce bone around the remaining mineralized cartilage matrix, forming the primary spongiosa *(PS)* (Modified from Bloom W, Fawcett DW: *A textbook of histology,* Philadelphia, 1975, WB Saunders.)

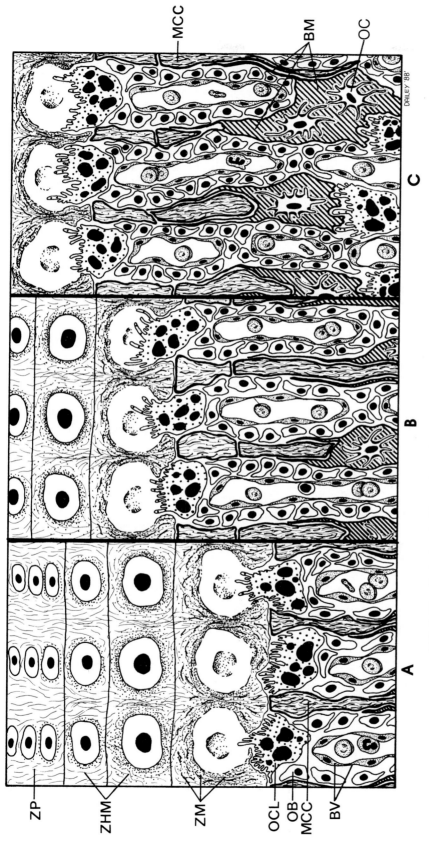

FIG. 8-13　Endochondral bone formation. **A,** Progressive mitosis of cartilage cells in the zone of proliferation (*ZP*), growth and matrix synthesis in the zone of hypertrophy and maturation (*ZHM*), and calcification of longitudinal septa in the zone of provisional mineralization (*ZM*) all lead to increased bone length, in **B.** Death of chondrocytes in the mineralization zone (*ZM*) is followed by chondroclast (*CCL*) invasion and partial cartilage matrix removal. Vascular invasion (*BV*) is accomplished by osteoblasts (*OB*), which secrete bone matrix (*BM*) on the mineralized cartilage core model (*MCC*). **C,** Osteoblasts (*OB*) continue to secrete bone matrix (*BM*) on the mineralized cartilage (*MCC*), and some become osteocytes (*OC*). The result is a primary spongiosa (young trabecular bone). Expansion of the marrow cavity causes resorption of the bone and cartilage matrix by osteoclasts (*OCL*).

covered cartilage remaining in the primary spongiosa and in the secondary ossification centers is replaced by lamellar bone, thus creating the secondary spongiosa found throughout adult bone.

Intramembranous Bone Formation

Intramembranous bone formation was first recognized when early anatomists observed that the fontanelles of fetal and newborn skulls were filled with a connective tissue membrane that was gradually replaced by bone during development and growth of the skull. In intramembranous bone formation, bone develops directly with a soft connective tissue membrane rather than on a cartilaginous model. Embryonically,

at multiple sites within each bone of the cranial vault, maxilla, body of the mandible, and midshaft of long bones, mesenchymal cells proliferate and condense. As vascularity increases at these sites of condensed mesenchyme, osteoblasts differentiate and begin to produce bone matrix de novo.

Once begun, intramembranous bone formation proceeds at an extremely rapid rate. Consequently some of the resident soft connective tissue is not resorbed but intermingles with the newly formed osteoid, creating a highly disoriented and crosshatched bone matrix. This ill-organized matrix mineralizes poorly; because of the rapidity of formation, many osteoblasts are surrounded by bone matrix and become osteocytes,

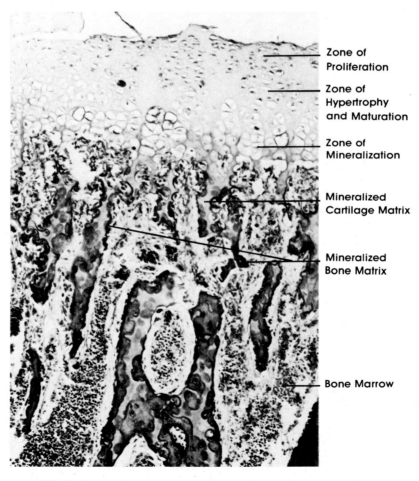

Zone of Proliferation

Zone of Hypertrophy and Maturation

Zone of Mineralization

Mineralized Cartilage Matrix

Mineralized Bone Matrix

Bone Marrow

FIG. 8-14　Light micrograph of endochondral bone formation.

resulting in a very cellular bone. This first embryonic bone is termed coarse-fibered woven bone (Figs. 8-15 and 8-16). At first the woven bone takes the form of radiating spicules, but progressively the spicules fuse into thin bony plates. In the cranium more than one of these plates may fuse to form a single bone. Early plates of intramembranous bone are structurally unsound, not only because of poor fiber orientation and mineralization but also because many islands of soft connective tissue remain within the plates, never being converted to woven bone.

For two important reasons the coarse-fibered woven bone of the early embryo and fetus turns over very rapidly: First, the developing bone marrow expands, inducing endosteal osteoclastic bone resorption around the ever-expanding medullary cavity. Second, rapidly growing soft tissues (including muscle, brain, and tongue) and the developing teeth induce bone resorption or different rates of bone formation on the immediately adjacent periosteal surfaces. As fetal bones begin to assume their adult shape, continued proliferation of soft connective tissue between adjoining bones brings about the formation of sutures and fontanelles. (A more complete discussion of the specific growth patterns in the development of bones of the head can be found in Chapter 21.)

From early fetal development to full expression of the adult skeleton, there is a continual slow transition

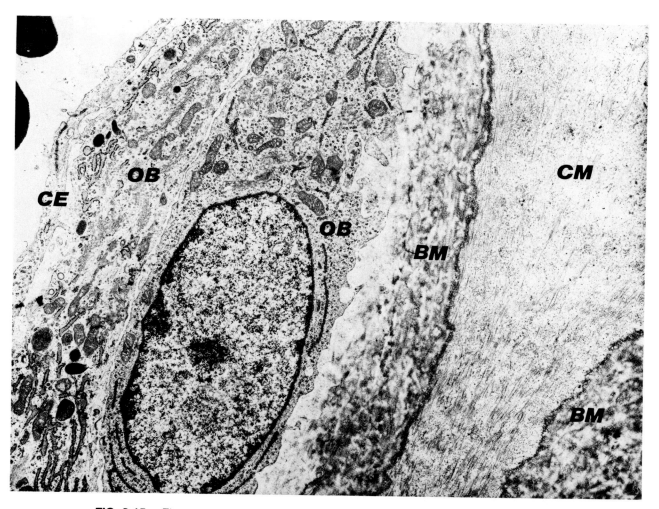

FIG. 8-15 Electron micrograph of endochondral bone formation (demineralized). The cartilage matrix *(CM)* is surrounded by bone matrix *(BM)*. Osteoblasts *(OB)* are sandwiched between the bone matrix and the capillary endothelium *(CE)*.

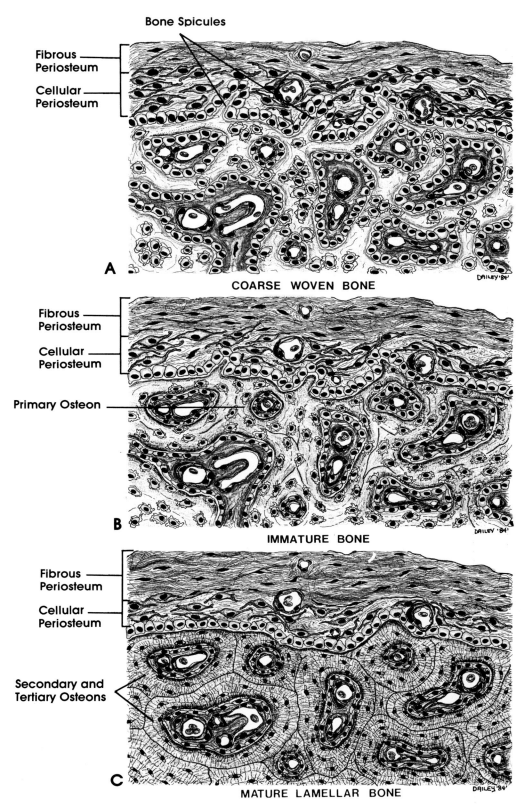

Bone Spicules

Fibrous Periosteum

Cellular Periosteum

A

COARSE WOVEN BONE

DAILEY '84

Fibrous Periosteum

Cellular Periosteum

Primary Osteon

B

IMMATURE BONE

DAILEY '84

Fibrous Periosteum

Cellular Periosteum

Secondary and Tertiary Osteons

C

MATURE LAMELLAR BONE

DAILEY '84

FIG. 8-16 Intramembranous bone formation. **A,** Coarse woven bone. The periosteal surface is very undulating, the bone very cellular and disorganized. **B,** Immature bone. The periosteal surface is less undulating, the bone somewhat less cellular and slightly more organized; some primary osteons are forming. **C,** Mature bone. The surface is less undulating; tightly packed osteons create an organized bone matrix. There are fewer cells and little loose connective tissue.

from woven bone to lamellar bone. This transition is relatively rapid during late fetal development and the first years of life. Bone formed during the transition is called immature bone (Figs. 8-15 and 8-16).

The single most important factor in this conversion is time. The collagen fibrils of lamellar bone are highly organized. In fact, as one lamella succeeds another, the collagen fibrils are laid down at an approximately 90-degree angle to those of the previous lamella. Time is required for this orientation to take place; therefore, the rate of bone formation is necessarily slower with increasing maturation. Histologically, this can be noted in several ways: (1) the periosteal surface, which is extremely irregular and undulating during early bone development, becomes less so, thus bringing about tissue order, including vascular order; (2) the bone is much less cellular because fewer osteoblasts are converted into osteocytes, giving the osteoblasts time to retreat; (3) the collagen fibrils of the soft tissue undergo resorption before osteoid synthesis; and (4) the soft tissue islands encountered in woven bone become much less extensive, eventually disappearing altogether, except for that soft tissue present in the Haversian and Volkmann canals.

The first phase of this transition is the formation of primary osteons. Blood vessels orient themselves along the bone. Because of the slower rate of bone growth, the periosteal surface takes the form of a growing sheet of bone rather than bone spicules. As the sheet approaches blood vessels and the soft tissue of the periosteum, it overgrows and buries these elements. The osteoblasts progressively secrete osteoid at the periphery and migrate toward the central capillary, the soft tissue being removed as the space is filled. The primary osteon tends to be relatively small, with lamellae that are neither numerous nor well delineated. The collagen fibers are slightly better organized; soft tissue–derived fibrils are absent; and the degree of mineralization is greater. As more osteons are formed at the periosteal surface, they become more tightly packed so that eventually a higher percentage of compact bone takes the form of an osteon.

Sutural Bone Growth

Sutures play an important role in the growing face and skull. Found exclusively in the skull, they are the fibrous joints between bones; however, they allow only limited movement. Their function is to permit the skull and face to accommodate growing organs such as the eyes and brain.

To understand the structure of a suture, recall that the periosteum of a bone consists of two layers, an outer fibrous layer and an inner cellular or osteogenic layer. At the suture the outer layer splits, the outermost leaf

running across the gap of the suture to form a uniting layer with the outermost leaf from the other side. The innermost leaf, together with the osteogenic layer of the periosteum, runs down through the suture along with the corresponding layer from the other bone involved in the joint. The osteogenic layer of the suture is called the *cambium*, and the inner leaf the *capsule*. Between these two layers is a loose cellular and vascular tissue (Fig. 8-17).

Sutures are best regarded as having the same osteogenic potential as periosteum. When two bones are separated—for example, the skull bones forced apart by the growing brain—bone forms at the sutural margins, with successive waves of new bone cells differentiating from the cambium. Thus the histologic structure of the suture permits a strong tie between bones while providing a site for new bone formation. The two cambial layers are separated by a relatively inert middle layer, so that growth can occur independently at each bony margin (Fig. 8-17).

BONE TURNOVER

During both embryonic bone development and the entire preadult period of human growth, bone is being formed very rapidly, primarily (but not exclusively) on the periosteal surface. Simultaneously bone is being destroyed along the endosteal surface, at focal points along the periosteal surface (bone modeling), and within the osteons of compact bone. Since bones increase greatly in length and thickness during bone growth, bone formation is occurring at a much greater rate than bone resorption; and despite the fact that all bone surfaces have the potential for resorption, the major activity over the growth period of a bone is formation. This replacement of old bone by new is called *bone turnover*. Bone turnover rates of 30% to 100% per year are common in rapidly growing children: most of the bone present today in a child will not be present a year from now.

Bone turnover does not stop when adulthood is reached, however, although its rate slows. The rate of cortical bone turnover is approximately 5% per year whereas turnover rates of trabecular bone and the endosteal surface of cortical bone can approach 15% per year. In general, when bone turnover occurs beyond 25 years of age, the amount of bone resorbed slightly exceeds the amount formed, particularly trabecular bone and the endosteal surface of the cortex. Slowly, over time, the marrow cavity expands at the expense of both trabecular and cortical bone. The adjacent endosteum undulates, making deep excursions into the cortex. The result is a thinning of the cortex and a net loss of bone.

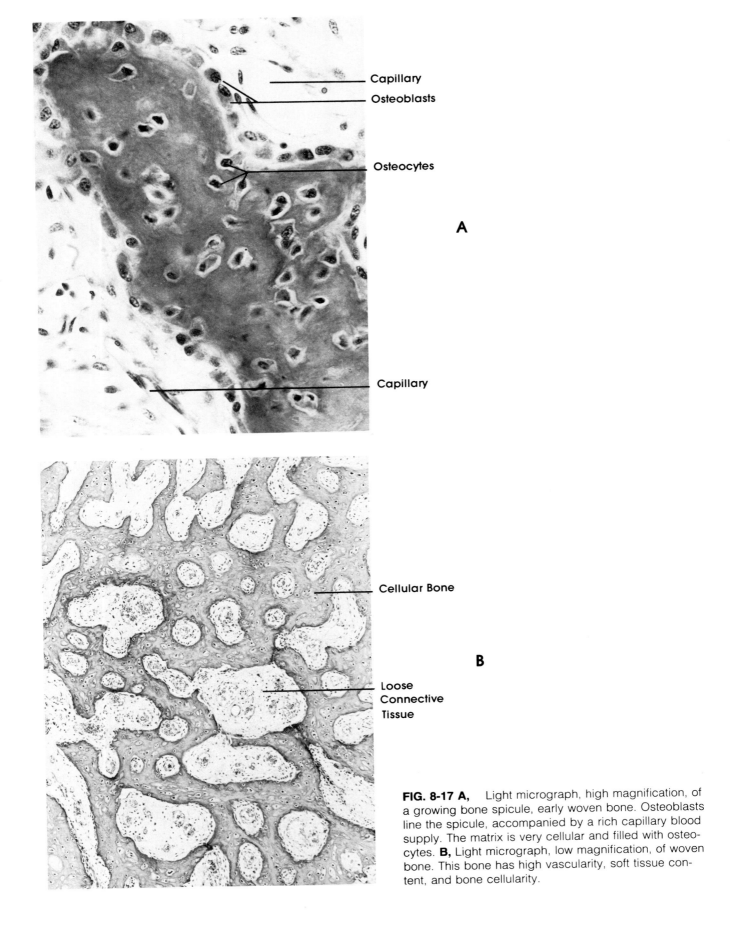

Capillary

Osteoblasts

Osteocytes

A

Capillary

Cellular Bone

B

Loose
Connective
Tissue

FIG. 8-17 A, Light micrograph, high magnification, of a growing bone spicule, early woven bone. Osteoblasts line the spicule, accompanied by a rich capillary blood supply. The matrix is very cellular and filled with osteocytes. **B,** Light micrograph, low magnification, of woven bone. This bone has high vascularity, soft tissue content, and bone cellularity.

A lifelong exercise program and proper nutrition can minimize bone loss in the skeleton. Good oral hygiene also contributes to the health and retention of alveolar bone within the mandible and maxilla.

Primary osteons of fetal bone either are eventually resorbed by osteoclasts to make room for the expanding marrow cavity or undergo turnover—that is, a primary osteon is replaced by succeeding generations of osteons (secondary and tertiary osteons). Each succeeding generation is slightly larger and functionally more mature, and therefore more lamellar (Fig. 8-18).

Exactly what induces turnover in the osteon is poorly understood. As previously stated, the osteocytes and osteoblasts within osteons probably die, bringing about both an influx of blood-borne cells and a proliferation of perivascular cells as the activation step of bone turnover. Next, osteoclasts formed from the fusion of uninucleated cells ream out most of the old osteon and some of the surrounding bone matrix. As the osteoclasts move through bone, the leading edge of resorption is termed the *cutting cone;* it is characterized in cross section by a scalloped array of Howship's lacunae, each housing an osteoclast. The more mature and mineralized the bone, the larger will be the osteoclasts (Figs. 8-19 to 8-21).

During resorption there is a tendency for the cutting cone to drift toward the endosteal surface. This means that secondary and tertiary osteons tend to be nearer

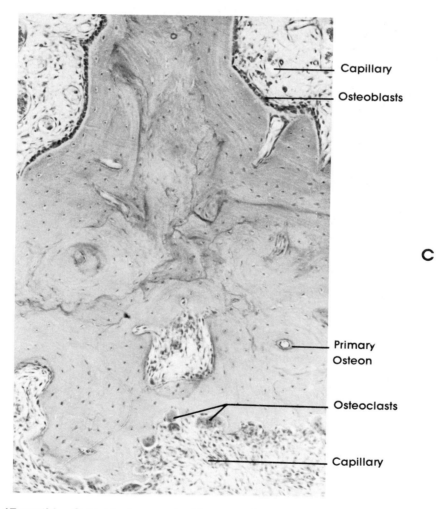

C

Capillary

Osteoblasts

Primary Osteon

Osteoclasts

Capillary

FIG. 8-17 cont'd   C, Light micrograph of immature bone. This section of growing alveolar bone exhibits primary osteons, less bone cellularity and loose connective tissue, a forming surface covered by osteoblasts, and a resorbing surface covered by osteoclasts. (Compare **B** and **C** with mature bone in Figure 8-21, *C.*)

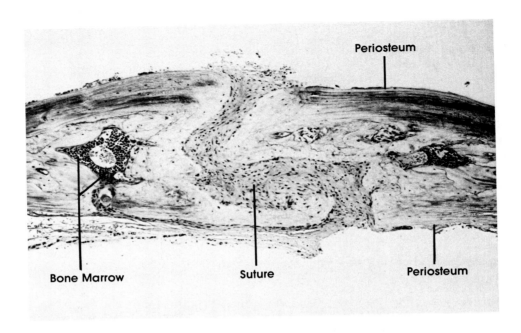

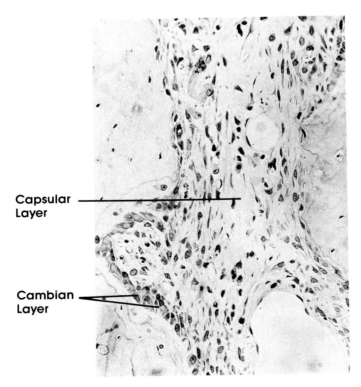

FIG. 8-18 Sutural growth. **A,** A low-magnification light micrograph shows that the suture connects two periosteal surfaces. The central marrow cavity is ill-defined. **B,** A higher magnification shows the developing inner osteogenic or cambian layer and the central capsular layer.

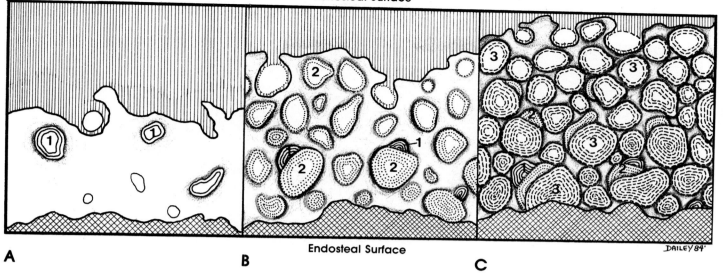

Periosteal Surface

Endosteal Surface

A B C

DAILEY 84'

FIG. 8-19 Progressive bone growth and turnover. **A,** Young immature bone is relatively thin, with few primary osteons *(1)*. Its periosteal surface is very undulating and forms bone rapidly. Its endosteal surface is primarily for resorption. **B,** The immature bone grows (thickens). Its periosteal surface is not as undulating and produces large numbers of secondary osteons *(2)*. The primary osteons are resorbed, and the fragments buried by new bone on the periosteal surface. **C,** The bone becomes nearly mature. It is thicker still, its periosteal surface less undulating, and tertiary osteons *(3)* replace the secondary osteons. Fragments of both primary and secondary osteons form interstitial lamellae. Eventually circumferential lamellae will smooth out the periosteal surface (Fig. 8-2).

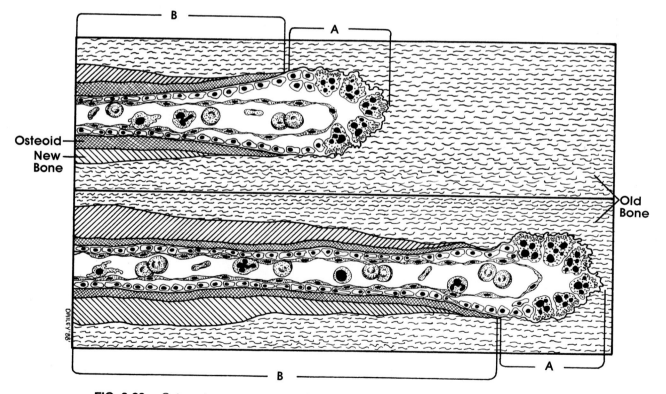

Osteoid
New
Bone

Old
Bone

DAILEY 88'

B

A

B

A

FIG. 8-20 Osteon turnover, compact bone. **A** *(top),* Old bone is being removed in segment *A* by osteoclasts, forming the cutting cone. In segment *B* the osteoblasts begin to synthesize osteoid (filling cone). The osteoid mineralizes, becoming new bone. Turnover of old bone progresses *(bottom),* from left to right as osteoclasts continue to resorb and osteoblasts continue to synthesize and mineralize new osteoid.

Continued.

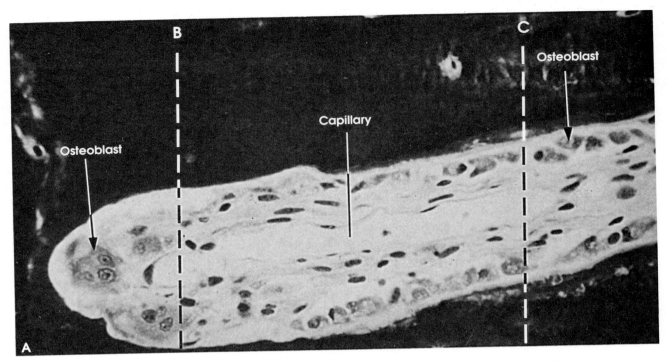

FIG. 8-20, cont'd   B, is a light micrograph showing osteoclasts, osteoblasts, and a central capillary in the same positions as in **A.**

FIG. 8-20, cont'd   C, Demonstration of the constituents of an osteon, cut longitudinally *(top)* and in cross sections *(bottom).* Blood-borne cells *(BBC)* migrate through the endothelial cells and fuse to form osteoclasts *(OCL),* which ream out the old bone, forming both a frontal and a circular array of Howship's lacunae *(HL).* Collectively they make up what is called the cutting cone. Behind the osteoclasts uninucleated cells (preosteoblasts, *POB*) migrate onto the bone surface and differentiate into osteoblasts *(OB).* The osteoblasts are responsible for synthesizing the cement line *(CL)* and the osteoid *(OD)* and for osteoid mineralization. Collectively they form the filling cone, and as they do this they change the orientation of succeeding lamellae *(BL₁, BL₂)* and form osteocytes *(OC). EC* is an ectomesenchymal cell.

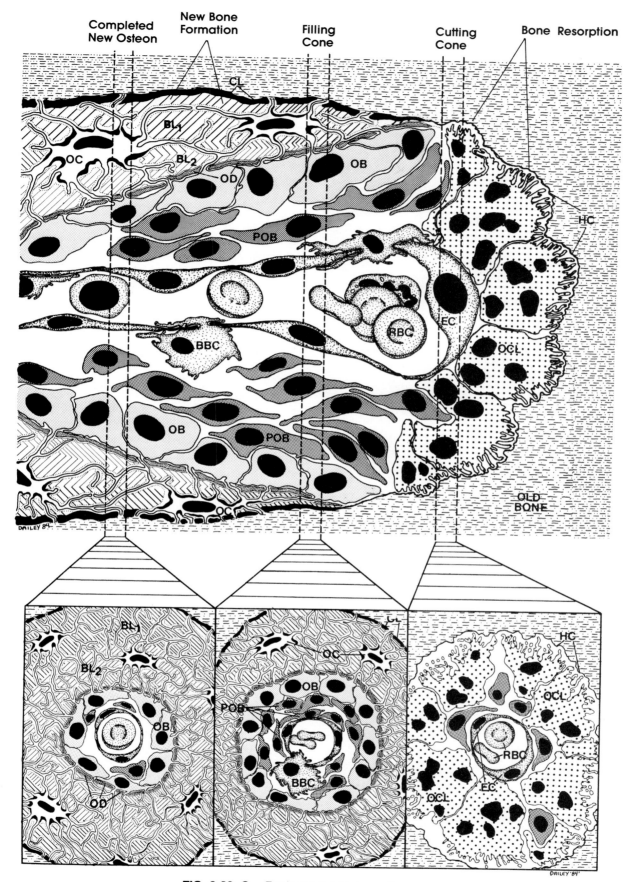

FIG. 8-20, C For legend, see opposite page.

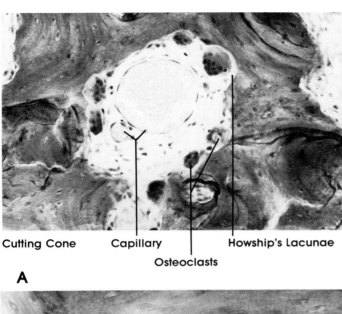

Cutting Cone   **Capillary**   **Howship's Lacunae**

Osteoclasts

A

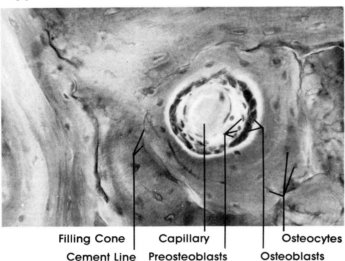

Filling Cone   **Capillary**   **Osteocytes**

Cement Line   **Preosteoblasts**   **Osteoblasts**

B

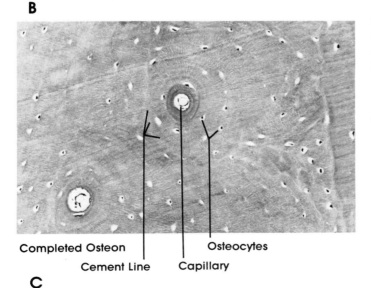

Completed Osteon   **Osteocytes**

Cement Line   **Capillary**

C

the endosteal surface than their predecessors. In addition, a portion of the earlier osteon is left unresorbed and becomes an interstitial lamella (Fig. 8-18).

Behind the cutting cone there is a migration of uninucleated cells onto the roughened cylinder. As these cells differentiate into osteoblasts, they produce a coating termed the *cement* or *reversal line*. On top of the cement line they begin to lay down new bone matrix, mineralizing it from the outside in. The entire area of the osteon where active formation occurs is termed the *filling cone*. As formation proceeds, some osteoblasts become osteocytes. Once formation is complete, the Haversian canal contains a central blood vessel and a layer of inactive osteoblasts, the lining cells, that communicate by means of cell processes with the embedded osteocytes (Figs. 8-19 and 8-20).

Lamellar cancellous or spongy bone (secondary spongiosa) also turns over. A half-moon resorption cavity is created by osteoclasts and then filled in with bone matrix by osteoblasts (Fig. 8-22).

From the above account it is evident, therefore, that a considerable amount of internal remodeling by means of resorption and deposition occurs within bone. How such remodeling is controlled can be an intriguing problem. A key question is How do the osteoclasts become targeted to reach specific sites? As previously stated, osteoblasts, appropriately stimulated by hormones (or perhaps by local environmental changes that occur in situations such as tooth movement), may provide the controlling mechanism for bone resorption. Elevated secretion rates of osteotropic hormones (e.g., parathyroid hormone and 1,25–vitamin D_3) stimulate collagenolysis by the osteoblasts. As a result the nonmineralized osteoid that lines bone surfaces is degraded, exposing the surfaces as osteoblasts are rounded up.

It is then supposed that breakdown products of matrix proteins provide a chemoattractant that directs osteoclasts to the exposed bone surface, to which they attach. In this regard the removal of osteoid is critical because osteoclasts can attach only to a mineralized

FIG. 8-21   Light micrograph of bone turnover. **A,** Cutting cone in cross section. Large multinucleated osteoclasts resorb an old osteon. **B,** Filling cone in cross section. Uninucleated osteoblasts ring the partially formed osteon. The dark cement line, concentric lamellae, and osteocytes *(OC)* can be found at the periphery of the osteon. **C,** End of formation. The small Haversian canal is filled with a single capillary and a layer of squamous lining cells. Concentric lamellae and osteocytes can be seen peripherally.

surface (the same holds true for the resorption of dentin, which does not occur when predentin is present). Once the osteoclasts attach to an exposed mineralized bone surface, osteoclasis occurs (as described in Chapter 7). What needs to be determined is the controlling mechanisms that arrest bone resorption. Such a signal may be hormonal; it is known that calcitonin and leupeptin inhibit both calcium release and collagenolytic activity, presumably by targeting the osteoclasts. Alternatively, the process of resorption may be self-limiting, because mineral dissolution precedes the degradation of organic matrix in the closed environment established by osteoclasts (Fig. 10-3). This means that a porous matrix fringe will develop peripherally and break the marginal seal, resulting in detachment of the osteoclasts.

This ready ability of bone to remodel explains its remarkable plasticity. The repeated deposition and removal of bone tissue accommodate the growth of a bone without changing its shape, function, or relationship to neighboring structures. Thus, for example, a significant increase in size of the mandible is achieved from birth to maturity largely by bone remodeling without any loss in function or change in its position relative to the maxilla. It is most unlikely that any of the bone present in a 1-year-old mandible is present in the same bone 30 years later.

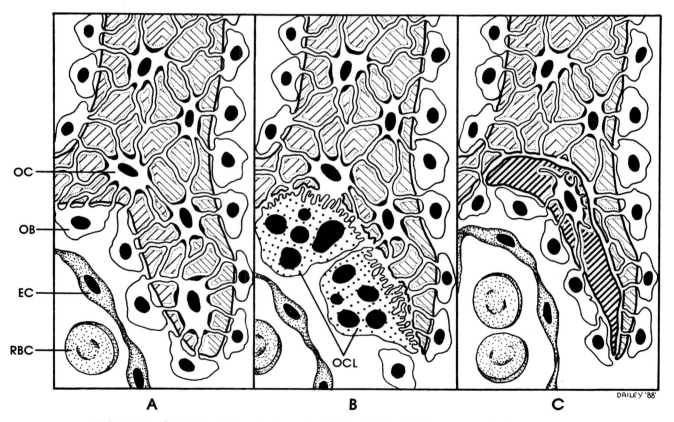

FIG. 8-22   Cancellous bone turnover. In **B** osteoclasts *(OCL)* remove a half-moon segment of trabecula. In **C** osteoblasts *(OB)* displace the osteoclasts and reform the bone. *OC* is an osteocyte, *EC,* an ectomesenchymal cell, and *RBC* an erythrocyte.

BIBLIOGRAPHY

Ash P, Loutit JF, Townsend KMS: Osteoclasts derived from haematogenous stem cells, *Nature* 283:669, 1980.

Atkinson PJ, Wit S: Characteristics of bone. In Smith DC, Williams DP (eds): *Biocompatibility of dental materials,* Boca Raton Fla, 1982, CRC Press, vol 1.

Boyde A: Scanning electron microscope studies of bone. In Bourne GH (ed): *The biochemistry and physiology of bone,* ed 5, New York, 1972, Academic Press, vol 1.

Cameron DA: The ultrastructure of bone. In Bourne GH (ed): *The biochemistry and physiology of bone,* ed 2, New York, 1972, Academic Press, vol 1.

Hancox NS: *Biology of bone,* New York, 1972, Cambridge University Press.

Marks SC Jr, Popoff SN: Bone cell biology: the regulation of development, structure, and function in the skeleton, *Am J Anat* 183:1, 1988.

Owen M: Bone cells: a review, *Radiat Environ Biophys* 17:372, 1980.

Persson M: Structure and growth of facial sutures, *Odontol Rev* 24(suppl 26):1, 1973.

Pritchard JJ, Scott JH, Girgis FG: The structure and development of cranial and facial sutures, *J Anat* 90:73, 1956.

Robinson RA: Bone tissue: composition and function, *Johns Hopkins Med J* 145:10, 1979.

Storey E: Growth and remodeling of bone and bones, *Am J Orthod* 62:142, 1972.

Vaughan JM: *The physiology of bone,* ed 3, Oxford UK, 1981, Clarendon Press.

Walker DG: Bone resorption restored in osteopetrotic mice by transplants of normal bone marrow and spleen cells, *Science* 190:784, 1975.

CHAPTER 9

Dentinogenesis

DENTIN is formed by cells, the odontoblasts, that differentiate from ectomesenchymal cells of the dental papilla following an organizing influence that emanates from cells of the internal dental epithelium. The odontoblasts produce an organic matrix that becomes mineralized to form dentin. Thus the dental papilla is the formative organ of dentin. The dental papilla eventually becomes the pulp of the tooth, but the timing of this activity depends very much on the criteria used to define dental pulp. If pulp tissue is considered to be responsible for dentin formation, the dental papilla becomes the dental pulp at the moment dentin formation begins. If, however, dental pulp is defined as that tissue occupying the pulp chamber of the tooth, the transition of papilla to pulp occurs only after enough dentin has been laid down to enclose a pulp chamber.

PATTERN OF DENTIN FORMATION

Regardless of when the dental papilla becomes the dental pulp, dentin formation begins at the late bell stage of development in the papillary tissue adjacent to the tip of the folded internal dental epithelium (Fig. 9-1). This site, although not actually where the future cusp tip will reside, is where cuspal development begins. From here dentin formation spreads down the cusp slope (i.e., the folded internal dental epithelium) as far as the cervical loop of the dental organ, and the dentin thickens until all the coronal dentin is formed. In multicusped teeth, dentin formation begins independently at the sites of each future cusp tip and again spreads down the flanks of the cusp slopes until fusion with adjacent formative centers occurs. Dentin thus formed constitutes the dentin of the crown of the tooth, or coronal dentin.

Root dentin forms at a slightly later stage of development and requires the proliferation of epithelial cells (Hertwig epithelial root sheath) from the cervical loop of the dental organ around the growing dental papilla to initiate the differentiation of root odontoblasts. The onset of root formation precedes the onset of tooth eruption, and, by the time the tooth reaches its functional position, about two thirds of the root dentin has formed. Completion of root dentin formation does not occur in the deciduous tooth until about 18 months after it has erupted, and in the permanent tooth some 2 to 3 years after it erupts. During this period the tooth is said to have an open apex.

The rate of root coronal dentin deposition is approximately 4 μm per day, with a somewhat slower rate for root dentin deposition. Rates of dentin deposition vary not only within a single tooth but also among different teeth.

Dentin formation continues until the external form of the tooth is completed. Dentin formed to this point is known as primary physiologic dentin. Dentin formation continues once the normal anatomy of the tooth has been established but at a much slower rate. This later-formed dentin is known as secondary physiologic dentin, and its formation results in a gradual but progressive reduction in the size of the pulp cavity.

ODONTOBLAST DIFFERENTIATION

A detailed understanding of how odontoblasts differentiate from undifferentiated ectomesenchymal cells is necessary, not only to understand normal development but also to explain, and perhaps influence, their recruitment when required to initiate repair of dentin.

The differentiation of odontoblasts from the dental papilla in normal development requires the presence of epithelial cells or their products. This inductive role of epithelium in dentinogenesis has been recognized for many years and, as a result, histologic descriptions of dentinogenesis usually begin with the description of morphologic changes occurring in cells of the internal dental epithelium (Fig. 9-2). It should be clearly understood, however, that, apart from this inductive influence, dentin formation is entirely a connective tissue event.

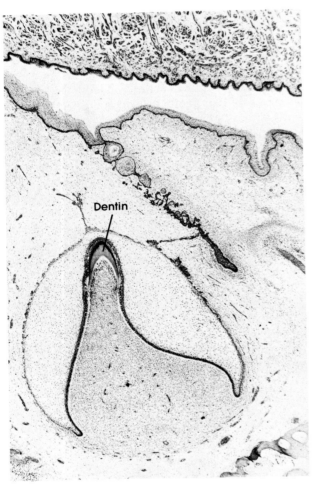

FIG. 9-1 Early dentin formation during the late bell stage of tooth development. From the apex of a dental epithelial fold, dentin formation spreads down the slopes of the cusp.

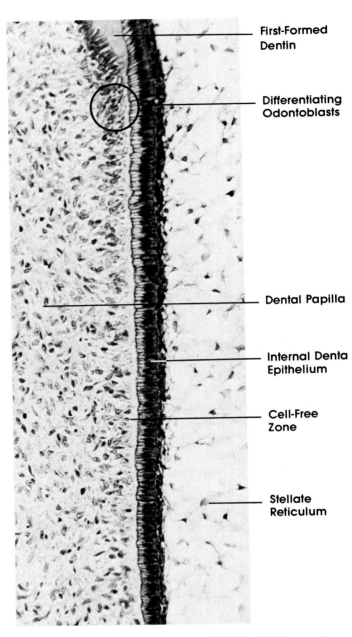

First-Formed Dentin

Differentiating Odontoblasts

Dental Papilla

Internal Denta Epithelium

Cell-Free Zone

Stellate Reticulum

FIG. 9-2 Changes in the internal dental epithelium and dental papilla associated with the formation of dentin. At *bottom*, the internal dental epithelium consists of short columnar cells, many of which are dividing as the tooth germ grows, and is separated from the undifferentiated cells of the dental papilla by an acellular zone. *Higher up*, the cells become tall and columnar and their nuclei migrate to the pole of the cell adjacent to the stratum intermedium. The fine structure of the *circled area* is shown in Figure 9-3.

Before dentinogenesis begins, the cells of the internal dental epithelium are short and columnar, rapidly dividing to accommodate growth of the tooth germ, and supported by a basement membrane that separates the epithelium from the dental papilla. The dental papillary cells at this time are separated from the internal dental epithelium by an acellular zone and are small undifferentiated ectomesenchymal cells with a central nucleus and sparse cytoplasm containing few cytoplasmic organelles dispersed in a relatively structureless ground substance that contains only a small number of fine collagen fibrils. Cell division ceases in the cells of the internal dental epithelium: their shape changes from short cuboidal to tall columnar, and their cell nuclei migrate toward the pole of the cell away from the dental papilla. This change in the position of the nucleus reverses the polarity of the cell. Almost immediately after these changes take place within the internal dental epithelium, changes also occur in the adjacent dental papilla. The ectomesenchymal cells adjoining the acellular zone rapidly enlarge to become, first, preodontoblasts and, then, odontoblasts as their cytoplasm increases in volume to contain increasing amounts of rough endoplasmic reticulum and Golgi complexes (Fig. 9-3). These newly differentiated cells are associated with a good vascular supply. They are further characterized by being highly polarized, with their nuclei positioned away from the internal dental epithelium. The acellular zone between the dental papilla and the internal dental epithelium is gradually eliminated as the odontoblasts differentiate and increase in size and occupy this zone. All these dimensional changes are readily seen in standard hematoxylin and eosin (H&E)–stained sections.

It is only because of the coincidence of these marked histologic changes (seen within both the internal dental epithelium and the dental papilla) and the known requirement for epithelium to initiate differentiation of odontoblasts that the morphologic changes occurring in the dental epithelium have been associated with the differentiation of odontoblasts from the dental papilla. The reality, however, is that these changes do not reflect this function, since similar morphologic changes do not occur within epithelial cells of the Hertwig root sheath, cells that also initiate the differentiation of odontoblasts. The changes occurring within the internal dental epithelium are, in fact, preparatory to and indicative of its cells' assuming an enamel-forming function. In summary, although epithelial cells are required to initiate the differentiation of odontoblasts the morphologic changes exhibited by them as odontoblasts differentiate do not reflect this function.

How then do the epithelial cells initiate odontoblast differentiation? In Chapter 6 reference was made to a whole cascade of determinants to which neural crest cells must be exposed before they assume the characteristics of dental papillary cells; and in any discussion concerning the origin of odontoblasts, it must be assumed that exposure to this cascade is a prerequisite. Here we are concerned only with the final determinants. There is evidence from studies of odontoblast differentiation in the mouse that ectomesenchymal cells of the dental papilla need to undergo a number of cell divisions (cycles) before they attain the capacity to respond to an epithelial influence and differentiate into odontoblasts. During the final division of ectomesenchymal cells adjacent to the dental epithelium, their mitotic spindles are perpendicular to the basement membrane supporting the internal dental epithelium; therefore the resulting daughter cells are superimposed, and it is only those cells next to the basement membrane that differentiate into odontoblasts. As a result, two populations of cells can be distinguished: odontoblasts and a subodontoblastic layer of cells that, because they are removed from the sphere of influence of the internal dental epithelium during the last cell division, represent ectomesenchymal cells exposed to the entire cascade of developmental controls for odontoblast differentiation except the last. In Chapter 6 the role of the basal lamina in epithelial mesenchymal relations was presented, along with the strong evidence that it is the final determinant in odontoblast differentiation. In tissue culture experiments papillary mesenchymal cells have been exposed to the basal lamina alone and induced the differentiation of odontoblasts. Other experimental evidence indicates that what the basal lamina provides is a surface containing fibronectin that permits the preodontoblasts (which have developed receptors for fibronectin) to align themselves along the membrane, assume polarity, and become odontoblasts. It will be explained later (Chapter 20) that reparative odontoblasts are somehow able to differentiate from dental pulp cells in the absence of any epithelial influence. It is thought that such cells derive from cells that have been exposed to all determinants except the final one and that the formation of some type of surface is the key factor in reparative odontoblast differentiation. Figure 9-4 summarizes the determinants for odontoblast differentiation.

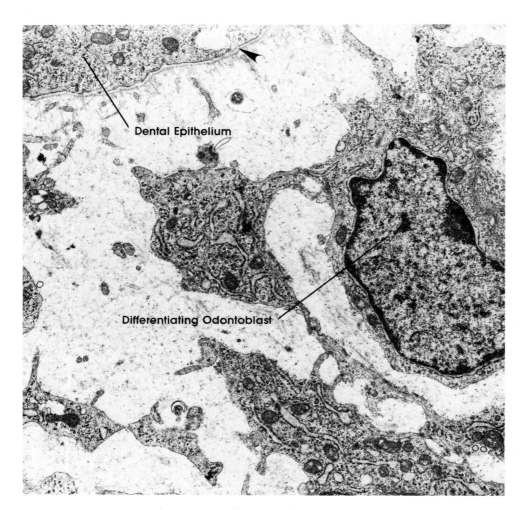

FIG. 9-3 Electron micrograph of differentiating odontoblasts. At *top,* the basal lamina *(arrow)* supporting the internal enamel epithelium can be identified. From this lamina fine aperiodic fibrils extend into the fiber-free extracellular compartment of the dental papilla. The undifferentiated mesenchymal cells have enlarged as their cytoplasm accumulates the necessary organelles for dental synthesis. (From Ten Cate AR, et al: *Anat Rec* 168:491, 1970.)

Dental Epithelium

Differentiating Odontoblast

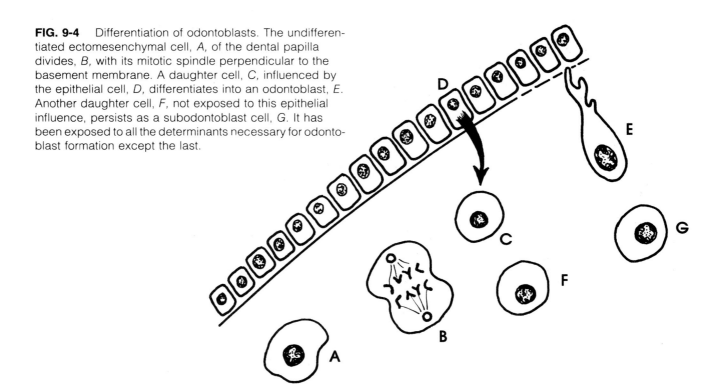

FIG. 9-4 Differentiation of odontoblasts. The undifferentiated ectomesenchymal cell, *A,* of the dental papilla divides, *B,* with its mitotic spindle perpendicular to the basement membrane. A daughter cell, *C,* influenced by the epithelial cell, *D,* differentiates into an odontoblast, *E.* Another daughter cell, *F,* not exposed to this epithelial influence, persists as a subodontoblast cell, *G.* It has been exposed to all the determinants necessary for odontoblast formation except the last.

HISTOLOGY OF THE ODONTOBLAST

Once odontoblasts differentiate, they enter a life cycle related to the formation, maintenance, and repair of dentin and their histology reflects these activities (Fig. 9-5). Under the light microscope two functional states of the odontoblast can be readily recognized: secretory and resting. Under the electron microscope a transitional stage between these two is also visible.

Secretory Odontoblast

By light microscopy the secretory odontoblast is seen to be a large plump cell with an open-faced nucleus situated basally and a basophilic cytoplasm containing a negative Golgi image (Fig. 9-6). By electron microscopy the apical basophilic cytoplasm is found to contain a full complement of organelles required for the synthesis and secretion of extracellular material (Fig. 9-7). Large cisternae of rough endoplasmic reticulum are aligned with the long axis of the cell (Fig. 9-8), and the Golgi apparatus comprises several stacks of saccules; secretory granules are common. Extensive junctional complexes and gap junctions develop between secretory odontoblasts as these cells form a row about 50 μm tall. Although junctional complexes are readily described, their functional status has not yet been properly determined in every instance. At their distal extremity, for example, a junctional complex consists of three types of junctions: a desmosomelike junction, a zonula adherens, and a tight junction. In association with this complex a terminal web of cytoskeletal elements radiates around the peripheral part of the cell, creating a diaphragm configuration with a central open-

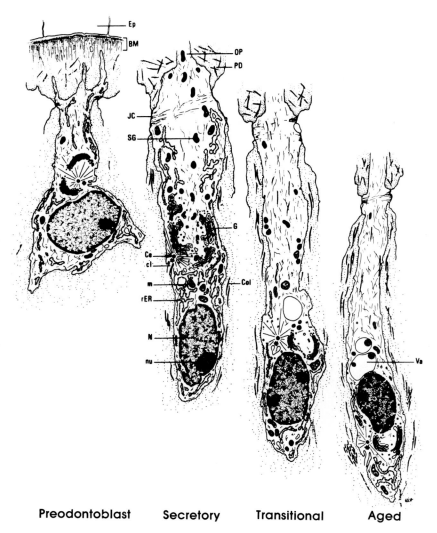

Preodontoblast   Secretory   Transitional   Aged

FIG. 9-5 Various functional stages of the odontoblast. (From Couve E: *Arch Oral Biol* 31:643, 1986.)

ing. Because this structure is part of the cell's cytoskeleton, it is suggested that its relation to the junctional complex may be functional—fastening adjacent odontoblasts together. Another suggested function for the complex is to control the passage of extracellular material (in particular, ionic calcium and phosphorus). Whether this junctional complex is tight or leaky is controversial, since there is evidence arguing for both situations. Finally, numerous gap junctions (maculae communicantes) exist between adjacent odontoblasts and the cells of the subodontoblast layer, but the functional significance of this syncytial relationship is not known. Secretory odontoblasts also exhibit alkaline phosphatase activity along their plasma membranes, probably associated with the transport of inorganic ions and other materials into the cell.

Transitional Odontoblast

The transitional odontoblast stage can be recognized only under the electron microscope. It becomes narrower, and its nucleus is displaced from the basal extremity and exhibits chromatin condensation. The amount of endoplasmic reticulum is reduced and confined to the area around the nucleus; autophagic vacuoles are present and associated with reorganization of the cytoplasm.

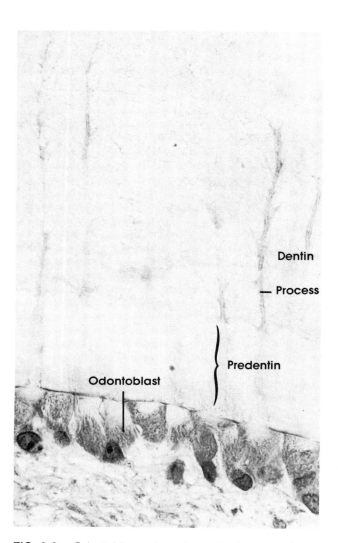

FIG. 9-6 Odontoblasts along the pulp-dentin border. The extracellular compartment between these cells has been eliminated. Note the prominent negative Golgi complex in the odontoblasts, indicating their active status.

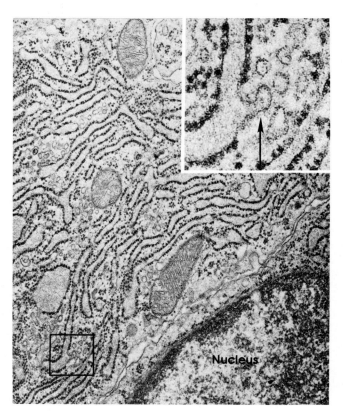

FIG. 9-7 Electron micrograph showing part of the cytoplasm of an active odontoblast. (*Inset*: Higher magnification of the area indicated showing the generation of a transport vesicle from rough endoplasmic reticulum).

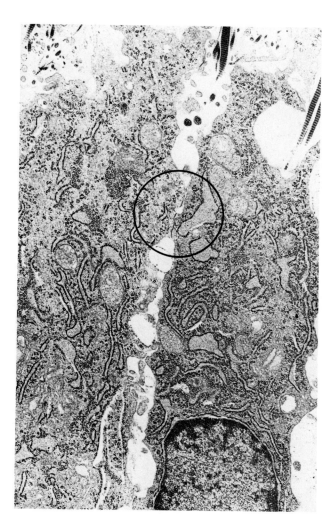

FIG. 9-8 Electron micrograph of newly differentiated and fully functional odontoblasts. A junctional complex *(circle)* has developed between two adjacent cells. (From Ten Cate AR: *J Anat* 125:183, 1978.)

Resting Odontoblast

By light microscopy the resting odontoblast is seen as a small flattened cell (Fig. 10-24) with a closed nucleus, less cytoplasm, and no Golgi image. By electron microscopy the nucleus is found to be situated sufficiently apically to create a prominent infranuclear region where a reduced amount of cytoplasmic organelles are clustered. The supranuclear region is devoid of organelles, except for large lipid-filled vacuoles in a cytoplasm containing tubular and filamentous structures. Secretory granules are absent. It is thought that resting odontoblasts are capable of resuming an active secretory role if appropriately stimulated.

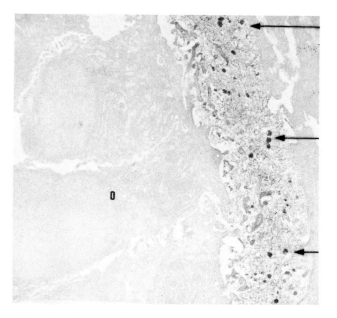

FIG. 9-9 Early dentin formation. This electron micrograph has been specially stained to demonstrate type I collagen, which is seen as fine granular deposits in the dentin matrix completely separated from the odontoblasts *(O)*. Larger deposits *(arrows)* are matrix vesicles. (Courtesy Dr. M.B. Andujar.)

FORMATION OF MANTLE DENTIN

After the differentiation of odontoblasts from undifferentiated ectomesenchymal cells of the papilla, the next step in the production of dentin is formation of its organic matrix, consisting of type I collagen (Figs. 9-9 and 9-11) and associated ground substance. It needs to be appreciated that odontoblasts differentiate in the preexisting ground substance of the dental papilla and that into this ground substance the first dentin collagen synthesized by the odontoblast is deposited. The pathway for collagen synthesis within the odontoblast is identical to that described in the fibroblast (Chapter 6), involving the rough endoplasmic reticulum, Golgi complex, secretory vesicles, and extracellular assembly (Fig. 9-10). The first collagen of dentin appears extracellularly as very distinct large-diameter fibrils (0.1 to 0.2 μm in diameter) that aggregate in the structureless ground substance immediately below the basal lamina supporting the internal dental epithelium. The fibrils are aligned at right angles to the basal lamina and intermingle with the aperiodic fibrils (type VII collagen) dangling from it (Fig. 9-11). These large collagen fibrils, together with the ground substance in which they aggregate, constitute the organic matrix of the first-formed or mantle dentin.

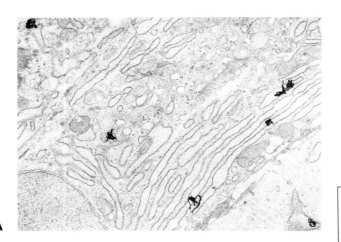

A

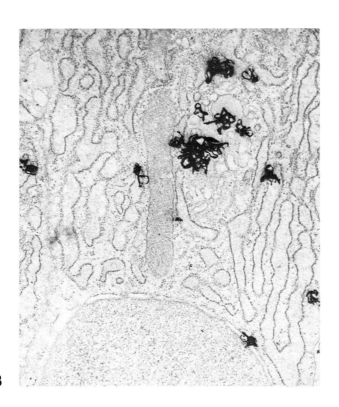

B

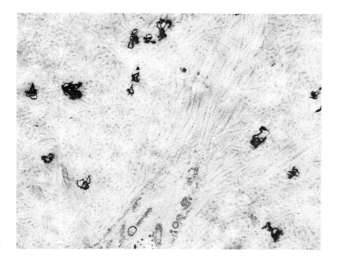

C

FIG. 9-10 Collagen formation in odontoblasts. Tritiated proline (an amino acid incorporated into collagen) can be used to follow the synthesis of collagen in odontoblasts. **A,** The proline is seen as black silver deposits over the cisternae of rough endoplasmic reticulum 5 minutes after being exposed to the cell. After 20 minutes, **B,** it is localized over the Golgi complex; and 4 hours after injection, **C,** it is within collagen of the predentin. (From Weinstock M, LeBlond CP: *Fed Proc* 33:1205, 1974.)

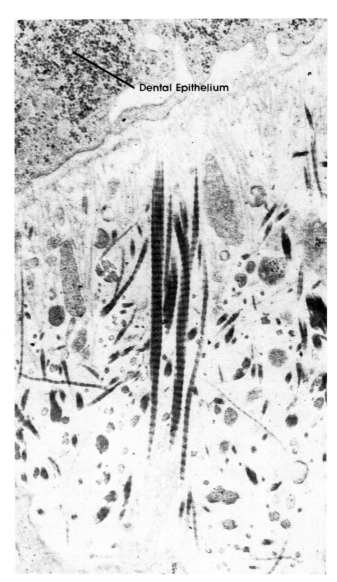

Dental Epithelium

FIG. 9-11 Electron micrograph showing the characteristic deposition of first collagen fibers in the coronal dentin matrix. At *top,* some of the cytoplasm of internal dental epithelium cells is supported by a basal lamina (the black particulate material is glycogen). Large-diameter collagen fibers are aligned at right angles to the lamina, intermingling with aperiodic fibrils. Small scattered vesicles appear throughout this milieu. (From Ten Cate AR: *J Anat* 125:183, 1978.)

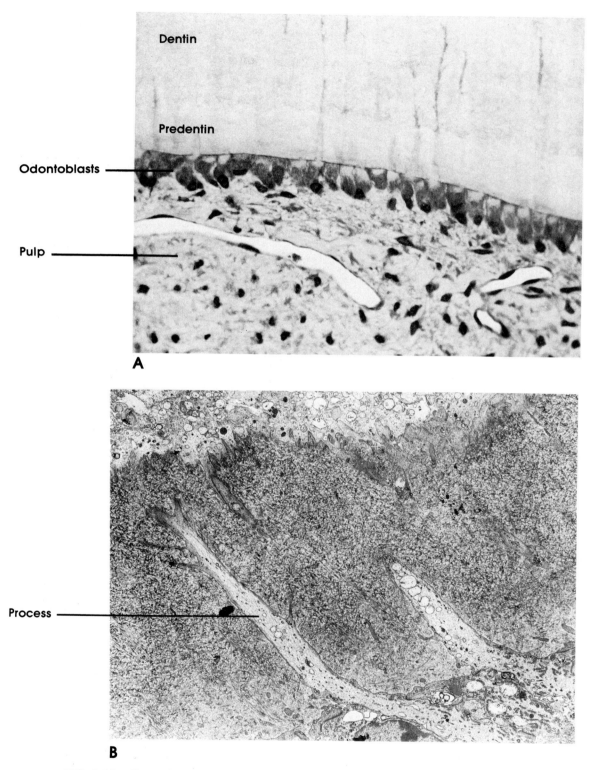

FIG. 9-12 Formation of the odontoblast process. **A,** Photomicrograph showing odontoblasts as they migrate centrally in early dentinogenesis. Note the branching of their processes. **B,** Electron micrograph. At *top left,* the future dentinoenamel junction is seen. Note that the odontoblast process is relatively structureless and fills the tubule. (From Sisca RF, Provenza DV: *Calcif Tissue Res* 9:1, 1972.)

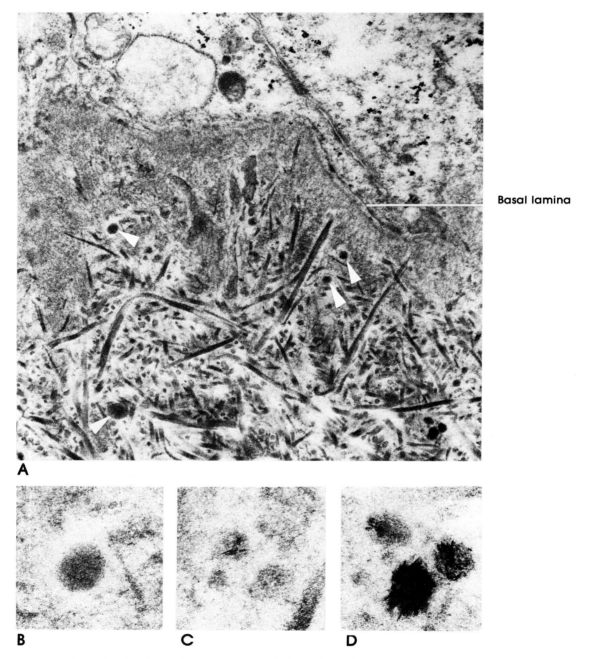

Basal lamina

FIG. 9-13   Electron micrograph of initial dentin formation in a tooth germ at the late bell stage. **A,** Collagen fibrils of the first-formed dentin matrix can be seen, along with the basal lamina supporting ameloblasts. Intermingled between the collagen fibrils are a number of dense bodies *(arrowheads)* in which initial mineralization of the dentin matrix occurs. **B** to **D** show the occurrence and growth of apatite crystals in these vesicles . (From Sisca RF, Provenza DV: *Calcif Tissue Res* 9:1, 1972.)

As the odontoblasts secrete these large-diameter collagen fibers, they continue to increase in size until the extracellular compartment between them is obliterated.

Coincident with this deposition of collagen the plasma membranes of the odontoblasts adjacent to the internal dental epithelium push out short stubby processes. On occasion one of these processes may penetrate the basal lamina and interpose itself between the cells of the internal dental epithelium to form what will later become an enamel spindle. (See Chapter 12.) As the odontoblast forms these processes, it also buds off a number of small membrane-bound vesicles known as matrix vesicles, which come to lie between the large-diameter collagen fibrils.

The odontoblast then begins to move toward the center of the pulp; and as it does, one of its short stubby processes becomes accentuated and is left behind to form the principal extension of the cell, the odontoblast process (Fig. 9-12). Into this milieu the apatite crystallites are introduced. Hydroxyapatite first appears within matrix vesicles as single crystals. These crystals grow rapidly and rupture from the confines of the vesicle to spread as a cluster of crystallites that fuse with adjacent clusters to form the fully mineralized matrix (Fig. 9-13). As the hydroxyapatite crystals are deposited, they obscure the collagen fibrils of the matrix. The deposition of mineral lags behind the formation of the organic matrix so that there is always a layer of organic matrix, called predentin, found between the odontoblasts and the mineralization front. In this way coronal mantle dentin is formed in a layer approximately 150 μm thick.

FORMATION OF PRIMARY PHYSIOLOGIC DENTIN

Once the layer of mantle dentin has formed, dentinogenesis continues in a slightly different manner. First, because of the increase in size of odontoblasts and the fact that the extracellular compartment between them is eliminated, all the organic matrix of dentin is now formed exclusively by the odontoblasts. Second, the collagen component of this matrix now aggregates as much smaller fibrils, which are more closely packed and interwoven with each other and generally aligned at right angles to the tubules. Third, matrix vesicles are no longer generated by the odontoblast, and mineralization involves heterogeneous nucleation (Figs. 9-14 and 9-18). Finally, the odontoblast adds further components to the organic matrix (e.g., lipids, phosphoproteins, phospholipids, and γ-carboxyglutamate proteins) at the mineralization front. One phosphoprotein, phosphophoryn, is of particular interest. It is a highly phosphorylated protein unique to circumpulpal dentin, being absent from predentin and mantle dentin and associated with mineralization. Lesser amounts of it are found in root dentin, which has been linked to the lesser degree of mineralization occurring there. The uniqueness of this protein makes it a phenotypic marker for mature odontoblasts. There is also strong evidence that phospholipid is somehow involved with mineralization, and it can be speculated that the demonstrated absence of both phospholipid and phosphoryn from mantle dentin demands the presence of matrix vesicles at the latter site. The changes in composition of the organic matrix of predentin at the mineralization front are not simply the result of extra material added to the matrix. The occurrence of endocytotic and exocytotic vesicles associated with the odontoblast process as it traverses the predentin indicates that some form of exchange is taking place. The demonstration of proteolytic activity within predentin, coupled with the fact that (1) predentin contains significantly higher amounts of proteoglycans than found in dentin matrix and (2) there is preferential removal of proteoglycans (chondroitin 4 and chondroitin 6 proteoglycans being found in predentin, with only chondroitin 6 occurring in mature dentin), suggests that the breakdown products of proteoglycans are selectively removed and further degraded intracellularly. Such a function for odontoblasts during circumpulpal dentinogenesis also explains in part the need for the lysosomal system in odontoblasts. Another function for this system is the degradation of excess polypeptide chains produced by exuberant collagen synthesis.

PATTERN OF MINERALIZATION

The mineralization of dentin follows a different pattern, which seems to depend on the rate of dentin formation. Basically, mineralization occurs by globular (or calcospheric) calcification, which involves the deposition of crystals in several discrete areas of matrix by heterogeneous capture in collagen at any one time. With continued crystal growth globular masses are formed, that continue to enlarge and eventually fuse to form a single calcified mass. This pattern of mineralization is best seen in the circumpulpal dentin formed just below mantle dentin, where a few large globular masses arise and coalesce. On occasion these large globular masses fail to fuse fully, leaving small areas of uncalcified matrix known as *interglobular dentin*. In the rest of the circumpulpal dentin the size of the globules progressively decreases until the mineralization front appears almost linear. The size of the globules seems to depend on the rate of dentin deposition, with the largest globules occurring where dentin deposition is fastest (Fig. 9-15).

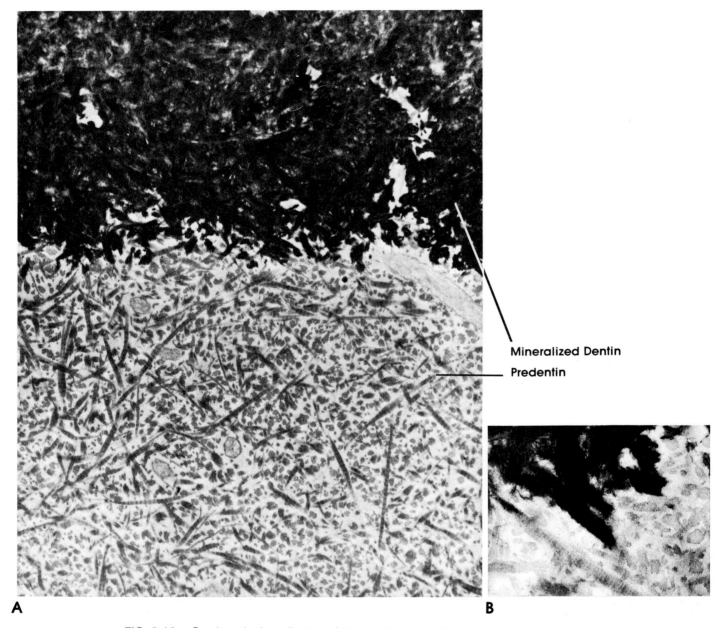

Mineralized Dentin

Predentin

A   B

FIG. 9-14 Continued mineralization of the dentin matrix. **A,** At *bottom,* predentin contains electron-dense crystals of the mineralization front showing a definite relationship to the long dark collagen fibers. **B** presents an example of linear mineralization. (From Eisenmann DR, Glick PL: *J Ultrastruct Res* 41:18, 1972.)

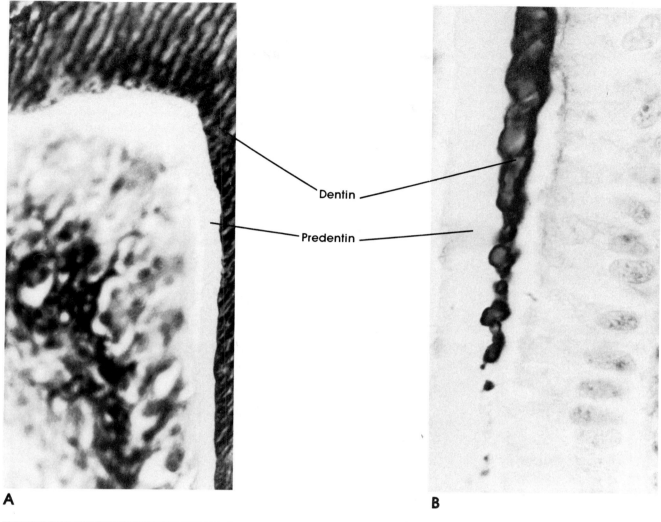

Dentin

Predentin

A

B

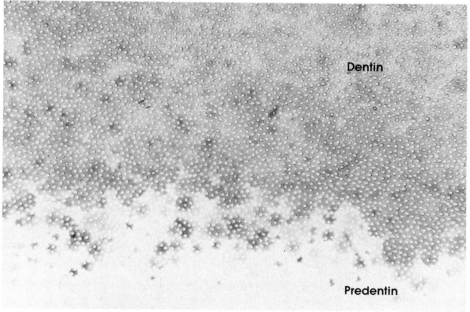

Dentin

Predentin

C

FIG. 9-15 Junction between predentin and dentin. **A** illustrates linear mineralization, and **B** and **C** globular mineralization. **A** and **B** are sections of nondemineralized tooth germs; the black stain is indicative of calcium salts. **C** shows globular mineralization in a decalcified section. Matrix that has mineralized stains more deeply with hematoxylin, and therefore the calcospherites can be seen even though the section has been demineralized.

INCREMENTAL NATURE OF DENTIN FORMATION

The organic matrix of dentin is deposited incrementally at a daily rate of approximately 4 μm; at the boundary between each daily increment, minute changes in collagen fiber orientation can be demonstrated by means of special staining techniques. Superimposed on this daily increment is a further 5-day cycle in which the collagen fiber orientation changes are more exaggerated. This means that the 5-day increment can be readily seen in conventional sections as the *incremental lines of von Ebner* (situated about 20 μm apart). Close examination of globular mineralization shows that the rate in organic matrix is approximately 2 μm every 12 hours (Fig. 9-16). Thus the organic matrix of dentin is deposited rhythmically at a daily rate of 4 μm a day and mineralized in a 12-hour cycle. Deficiencies and irregularities in dentinogenesis are often found and appear as accentuated incremental lines or areas of interglobular dentin.

Dentinogenesis therefore results in the production of an organic matrix, calcified with apatite crystallites, through which run cytoplasmic extensions of the odontoblasts occupying dentinal tubules. Coronal dentin deposition occurs at a rate of about 4 μm per day in a phasic, or incremental, manner.

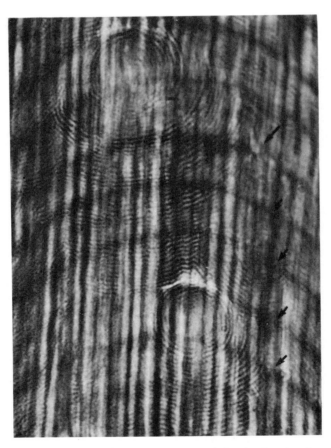

FIG. 9-16   Silver-impregnated section of demineralized dentin showing the striae of von Ebner *(arrows)*. Two globules (concentric rings) can also be seen and represent the incremental mineralization of dentin; 10 to 12 rings occur between each stria of von Ebner. (Courtesy Dr. K. Kawasaki.)

FORMATION OF INTRATUBULAR DENTIN

As new dentin is formed, further changes occur within some of the tubules of previously formed dentin. The odontoblast process shrinks by about a third of its length into the dentin, and a collar of more highly mineralized (40%) dentin is deposited in the space so created. This dentin, called *peritubular dentin* (Fig. 9-17), more properly should be called *intratubular dentin*. (See Chapter 10.) How intratubular dentin forms is not understood. Whereas it has been generally assumed to be the product of odontoblastic activity, there is no evidence for this other than the fact that the odontoblast process contains structural elements needed to permit secretion (e.g., microtubules and vesicular elements); but these could be related to other functions of the process. An alternative and equally valid suggestion is that intratubular dentin forms as a purely physicochemical response involving redistribution of dentin mineral. In support of this contention is the fact that it has been shown that intratubular dentin can form in dentinal tubules present in a slab of dentin mounted on a denture and exposed to the oral environment. It is possible to explain the various forms of intratubular dentin on the basis of this physicochemical response, involving the deposition of mineral around tubule contents. (See Chapter 10.) The differing features of dentin formation are summarized in Figures 9-18 and 9-19.

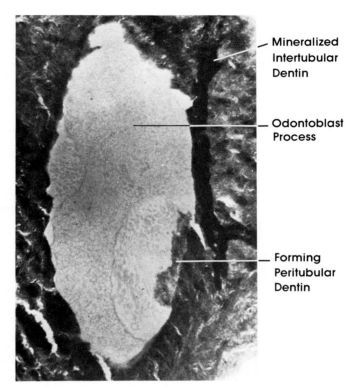

Mineralized Intertubular Dentin

Odontoblast Process

Forming Peritubular Dentin

FIG. 9-17   Electron micrograph showing the formation of intratubular dentin. (Courtesy Dr. H.F. Thomas.)

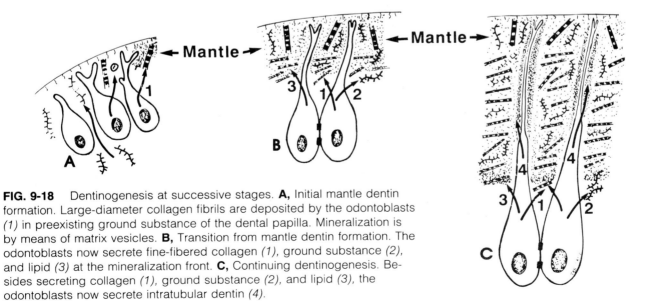

FIG. 9-18   Dentinogenesis at successive stages. **A,** Initial mantle dentin formation. Large-diameter collagen fibrils are deposited by the odontoblasts *(1)* in preexisting ground substance of the dental papilla. Mineralization is by means of matrix vesicles. **B,** Transition from mantle dentin formation. The odontoblasts now secrete fine-fibered collagen *(1)*, ground substance *(2)*, and lipid *(3)* at the mineralization front. **C,** Continuing dentinogenesis. Besides secreting collagen *(1)*, ground substance *(2)*, and lipid *(3)*, the odontoblasts now secrete intratubular dentin *(4)*.

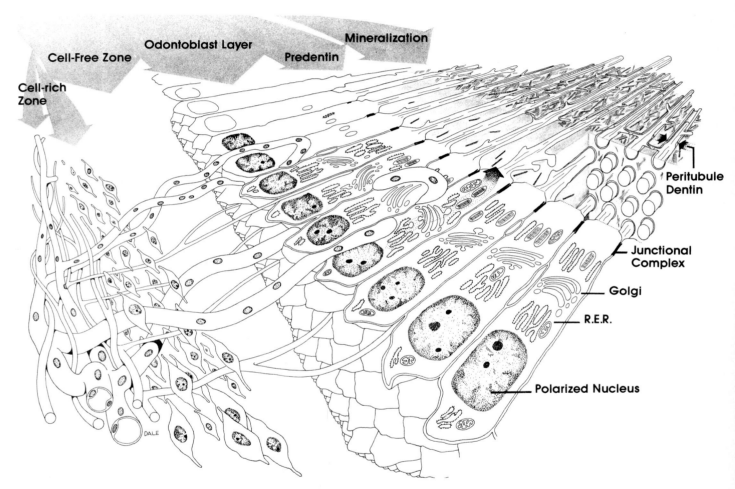

FIG. 9-19 Key features of dentinogenesis.

FORMATION OF ROOT DENTIN

The differentiation of odontoblasts that form root dentin is initiated by epithelial cells of Hertwig's root sheath (Fig. 9-20). It is increasingly being recognized that the product of these root odontoblasts is structurally and compositionally different from coronal dentin. There is the different orientation of collagen fibers in mantle dentin (Fig. 9-21) Also the phosphoryn content of root dentin is less (by almost half in bovine teeth) than that of coronal dentin, and its degree of miner-alization is slightly less. The rate of deposition of root dentin is slower, and in rat molars it has been shown that large interodontoblastic collagen bundles arising from the papillae contribute to the organic matrix of root dentin.

ODONTOBLASTIC MOVEMENT

The odontoblast moves centripetally, leaving behind the formed dentin. How such movement takes place

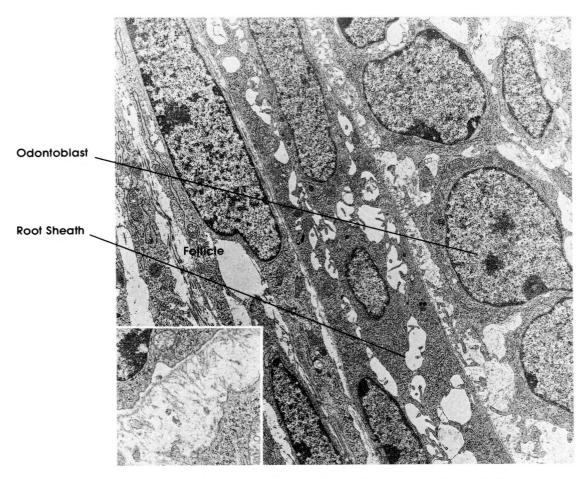

FIG. 9-20 Initial root dentin formation. Epithelial cells of the root sheath have initiated differentiation of odontoblasts that are about to begin the formation of root dentin. (*Inset:* Higher magnification of the milieu in which root dentin matrix will first form. Note the continuity of the basal lamina separating the root sheath from the dental papilla. (From Ten Cate AR: *J Anat* 125:183, 1978.)

Root Sheath

Odontoblast

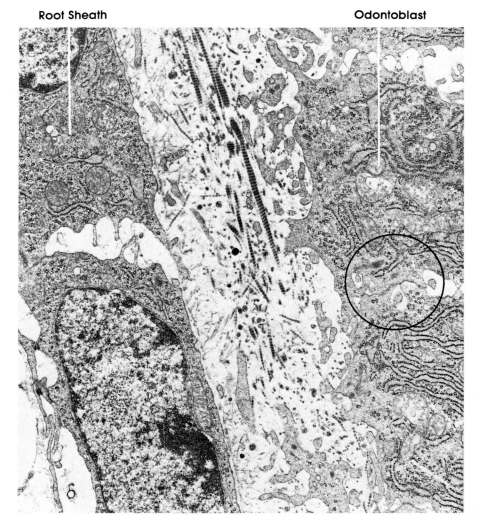

FIG. 9-21   Electron micrograph illustrating initial root dentinogenesis. The epithelial cells of the root sheath are to the left, the odontoblasts to the right. The first collagen fibers of the matrix are aligned parallel to the basement membrane supporting the root sheath cells (Fig. 9-11). The *circled area* outlines an extensive junctional complex. Note the discontinuity in the basal lamina, the presence of rough endoplasmic reticulum in the epithelial cells, and the separation of collagen fibrils from the basal lamina. (From Ten Cate AR: *J Anat* 125:183, 1978.)

has not been studied. It must be assumed that the same principles that direct fibroblast movement (Chapter 5) apply, involving fixation of the cell and subsequent contraction. Whatever the situation, the cell, as it migrates, leaves behind a process that comes to occupy a tubule within the mineralized dentin. Thus the dentinal tubule is a permanent record of the track of the odontoblast, which in coronal dentin is S shaped and in root dentin straight. There is an explanation for this configuration: such tracks result from the oscillations of odontoblasts dictated by their crowding as the surface area they occupy decreases during their centripetal movement. This explanation has been tested by a simple model. The outline of the amelodentinal (dentinoenamel) junction in longitudinal section is traced on smoked paper. Beads, representing the odontoblasts, are aligned along the periphery of the drawing and then pushed centripetally following the successive forming fronts of dentin. As they are pushed, they leave behind a record of their movement in the smoked paper that mimics these curvatures of the dentinal tubule in coronal dentin (Fig. 9-22). In root dentin formation, where there is no decrease in surface area, the tubules run a straight course.

PROBLEM OF VON KORFF FIBERS

From the account of dentinogenesis given here it should be appreciated that all the collagen making up the matrix of dentin is formed as a result of odontoblast activity. At one time it was firmly believed that there was a dual origin for dentin matrix collagen, with mantle dentin collagen forming by the activity of cells in the subodontoblast layer and circumpulpal dentin collagen forming as a result of odontoblast activity. In studies of sections stained with silver (once thought to stain only immature collagen) this has certainly seemed to be the case, since such sections generally show what appear to be large collagen fiber bundles arising from the subodontoblast layer and passing spirally between the odontoblasts to fan out against the surface of the basal lamina in the internal dental epithelium and form the fibrillar component of mantle dentin. When such sections are processed for electron microscopic examination, however, no large collagen fiber bundles can be identified between the newly differentiated odontoblasts. Instead, small particles of silver in an extensive extracellular compartment are seen. If similar sections are pretreated with acetic anyhdride (which blocks reducing sugars), this silver staining is abolished; the silver is captured by reducing sugars in the ground substance. Thus it is the extensive extracellular compartment between newly differentiated odontoblasts that captures the silver stain, with the result that when viewed by light microscopy a negative outline of the

odontoblasts appears simulating the outline of fibers (Fig. 9-23). This explanation of the so-called *von Korff fibers* also explains their diminution when circumpulpal dentinogenesis begins. As odontoblasts hypertrophy, they become more closely packed together, develop junctions, and eliminate most of the extracellular compartment between them. Hence there can no longer be capture of silver and therefore no von Korff fibers.

Although this explanation is true for the seeming appearance of interodontoblastic fiber bundles contributing to the formation of mantle dentin in the crown (the electron microscope has consistently failed to show large collagen fiber bundles between odontoblasts in this situation), it is now recognized that intraodontoblastic fiber bundles are sometimes present and can contribute to the dentin matrix in two special circumstances: The first relates to root dentinogenesis in the rat molar, where it has been demonstrated with the electron microscope that large collagen fiber bundles occur among radicular odontoblasts and pass between the distal junctional complexes into the predentin layer to become incorporated in the mineralized dentin. No such fibers have been found associated with coronal dentinogenesis. It should be noted that such fibers do not contribute to the formation of predentin and that the pattern of their occurrence is irregular. The second situation in which interodontoblastic collagen fiber bundles have been described (Fig. 9-24) is during secondary physiologic dentin formation in the root of cat dentin, and again their occurrence is irregular. No information exists as to whether this collagen is the product of the odontoblast, being secreted along its lateral surface, or whether it originates from the activity of pulpal fibroblasts.

Thus it is equivocal whether all dentin collagen is derived from odontoblast activity. Most is, and certainly all that found in coronal dentin is. Should the term von Korff fiber be retained? It is a designation firmly entrenched in the literature and has had a clear connotation with dentinogenesis, indicating that the fibers were the source of mantle dentin collagen; however, this is clearly incorrect, and the designation in this connection should therefore be discontinued.

SECONDARY AND TERTIARY DENTINOGENESIS

As far as is known, secondary dentin formation is achieved in essentially the same way as primary dentin formation, though at a much slower pace. Differences in the staining characteristics between the organic matrices of primary and secondary dentin are such that secondary dentin stains less well for glycosaminoglycans. This characteristic may reflect the minor difference in mineralization between the two dentins, with secondary dentin being less mineralized. Certain stains disclose a well-defined resting line between primary and secondary dentin.

Tertiary, or reparative, dentin is deposited at specific sites in response to injury. The rate of its deposition depends on the degree of injury: the more severe the injury, the more rapid the rate of dentin deposition (with the possibility of as much as 3.5 μm being deposited in a single day). As a result of this rapid de-

position, cells often become trapped in the newly formed matrix and the tubular pattern becomes grossly distorted. At the beginning of this chapter the recruitment of new odontoblasts for reparative dentin production was mentioned, and this issue will be fully discussed in Chapter 20. Here it is necessary only to say that the evidence indicates reparative dentin is produced by odontoblastlike cells and reparative dentin incorporates both type I and type III collagen in its matrix and has a diminished phosphophoryn content.

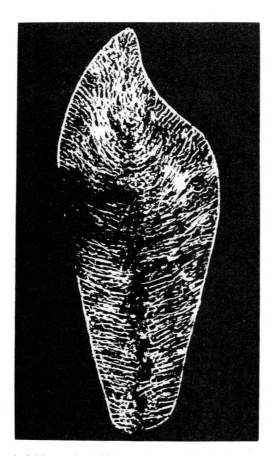

FIG. 9-22 Tracks mimicking odontoblast curvature obtained by crowding of "matchheads" (representing odontoblasts) as they are pushed centrally.(From Osborn JW, Ten Cate AR: *Advanced dental histology,* Bristol UK, 1983, John Wright & Sons.)

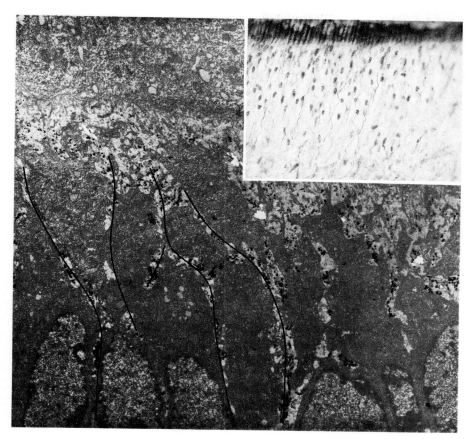

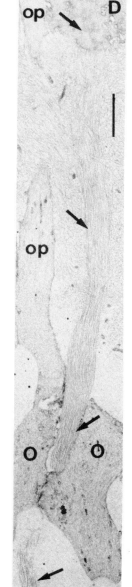

FIG. 9-23 Problem of von Korff's fibers. An electron micrograph shows the fibers after staining with silver. (*Inset:* Light microscope appearance of a similar field also stained with silver.) The silver deposits occupy the extracellular compartment and are captured by reducing sugars in the ground substance. The extracellular compartment *(left)* has been blackened in to indicate how the silver staining would show the presence of fibers in a thick section. (Inset courtesy Dr. S. Bernick.)

FIG. 9-24 Large collagen fiber bundle passing between odontoblasts in the cat secondary to dentinogenesis. Note that it passes through the predentin into mineralized dentin. *O,* Odontoblasts; *op,* odontoblast process; *D,* dentin (From Bishop MA, et al: *Am J Anat* 191:67, 1991.)

BIBLIOGRAPHY

Bishop MA, Malhatra M, Yoshida S: Interodontoblastic collagen (von Korff fibres) and circumpulpal dentin formation: an ultrathin serial section study in the cat, *Am J Anat* 191:67, 1991.

Couve E: Ultrastructural changes during the life cycle of human odontoblasts, *Arch Oral Biol* 31:643, 1986.

Fitzgerald M, Chiego DJ Jr, Heys DR: Autoradiographic analysis of odontoblast replacement following pulp exposure in primate teeth, *Arch Oral Biol* 35:707, 1990.

Fukae M, Kaneko I, Tanabe T, Shimizu M: Metalloproteins in the mineralized compartments of porcine dentine as detected by substrate-gel electrophoresis, *Arch Oral Biol* 36:567, 1991.

Kawasaki K, Tanaka S, Ishikawa T: On the daily incremental lines in human dentine, *Arch Oral Biol* 24:939, 1980.

Linde A: *Dentin and dentinogenesis*, Boca Raton Fla, 1984, CRC Press, vols 1 and 2.

Linde A, Lundgren T: Calcium transport in dentinogenesis, *J Biol Buccale* 18:155, 1990.

Rahima M, Veis A: Two classes of dentin phosphophoryns, from a wide range of species, contain immunologically cross-reactive epitope regions, *Calcif Tiss Intl* 42:104, 1988.

Ruch JV: Odontoblast differentiation and the formation of the odontoblast layer, *J Dent Res* 64:489, 1985.

Salomon JP, Septier D, Goldberg M: Ultrastructure of interodontoblastic fibres in the rat molar, *Arch Oral Biol* 36:171, 1991.

Sandham HJ (ed): The biology of dentin and pulp, *J Dent Res* 64:1, 1985.

Takagi Y, Nagai H, Sasaki,S: Difference in non-collagenous matrix composition between crown and root dentin of bovine incisor, *Calcif Tiss Intl* 42:97, 1988.

Takagi Y, Sasaki S: Histological distribution of phosphophoryn in normal and pathological dentins, *J Oral Pathol* 15:463, 1986.

Thylstrup A, Leach SA, Qvist V: *Dentine and dentine reactions in the oral cavity,* Oxford UK, 1987, IRL Press.

Tominaga H, Sasaki T, Higashi S: Ultrastuctural changes in odontoblasts during early development, *Bull Tokyo Dent Coll* 25:9, 1984.

CHAPTER 10

Dentin-Pulp Complex

DENTIN and pulp are sometimes treated separately in textbooks on dental histology largely because dentin is a hard connective tissue and the pulp is a soft one. However, as explained in Chapter 3, dentin and pulp are embryologically, histologically, and functionally the same tissue and therefore are considered together here.

PHYSICAL PROPERTIES

Dentin is the hard tissue portion of the pulp-dentin complex and forms the bulk of the tooth. Mature dentin is, chemically by weight, approximately 70% inorganic material, 20% organic material, and 10% water (adsorbed on the surface of the mineral or in interstices between crystals), 45%, 33%, and 22% respectively, by volume. Its inorganic component consists mainly of hydroxyapatite, and the organic phase is type I collagen with fractional inclusions of glycoproteins, proteoglycans, phosphoproteins, and some plasma proteins. About 56% of the mineral phase is within the collagen. The inorganic phase makes dentin slightly harder than bone and softer than enamel. This difference can be readily distinguished on radiographs, where the dentin appears more radiolucent (darker) than enamel and more radiopaque (lighter) than pulp.

Dentin is yellowish. Because light can readily pass through thin highly mineralized enamel and be reflected by the underlying dentin, the crown of a tooth has a yellowish appearance. Thicker or hypomineralized enamel does not permit light to pass through as readily, and in such teeth the crown appears whiter. Teeth with pulp disease or without a dental pulp often show discoloration of the dentin, which causes a darkening of the clinical crown.

Physically dentin has an elastic quality (which is important for the proper functioning of the tooth, because it provides flexibility and prevents fracture of the overlying brittle enamel). These two tissues are firmly bound together at the dentinoenamel junction, which is seen microscopically as a well-defined scalloped border. In the root of the tooth the dentin is covered by cementum, and the junction between these two tissues is less distinct.

BASIC ANATOMY

Dentin is characterized by the presence of multiple closely packed dentinal tubules that traverse its entire thickness and contain the cytoplasmic extensions of odontoblasts that once formed the dentin and now maintain it. The cell bodies of odontoblasts are aligned along the inner aspect of the dentin, where they also form the peripheral boundary of the dental pulp.

The dental pulp is the soft connective tissue that occupies the central portion of the tooth. The space it occupies is the pulp space (Fig. 10-1), which is divided into a coronal portion (or pulp chamber) and a radicular portion (the root canal). The pulp chamber conforms to the general shape of the anatomic crown. Under the cusps the chamber extends into pulp horns, which are especially prominent under the buccal cusp of premolar teeth and the mesiobuccal cusp of molar teeth. Their presence is of particular significance in dental restoration, since they must be avoided to prevent exposure of pulp tissue.

The root canal (or root canal system, as it is called in multirooted teeth) terminates at the apical foramen, where the pulp and periodontal ligament (PDL) meet and the main nerves and vessels to the pulp enter and leave the tooth. In the developing tooth the apical foramen is large and centrally located. As the tooth completes its development, the apical foramen becomes smaller in diameter and more eccentric in position. Sizes ranging from 0.3 to 0.6 mm—with the larger diameter occurring in the palatal root of maxillary molars and the distal root of mandibular molars—are typical of the completed foramen. The foramen may be

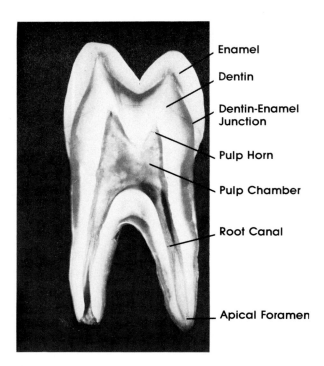

Enamel

Dentin

Dentin-Enamel
Junction

Pulp Horn

Pulp Chamber

Root Canal

Apical Foramen

FIG. 10-1 Halfsection of a young maxillary permanent premolar showing the disposition of dentin in the formed tooth and the anatomy of the pulp space.

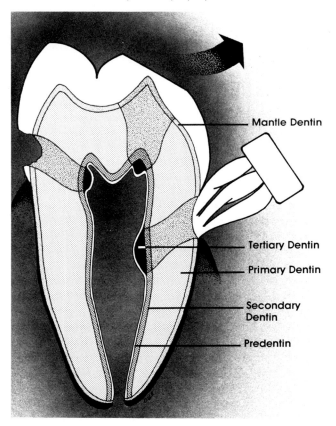

Mantle Dentin

Tertiary Dentin

Primary Dentin

Secondary Dentin

Predentin

FIG. 10-2 Terminology and distribution of dentin.

located at the very end, or anatomic apex, of the root but is usually located slightly more occlusally (0.5 to 0.75 mm) from the apex. If more than one foramen is present, the largest is designated the apical foramen and the others accessory foramina.

Connections between the pulp and periodontal tissues may also occur along the lateral surface of the root through lateral canals. Such canals, which may contain blood vessels, are not present in all teeth and occur with differing frequencies in different types of teeth. The overall incidence in the permanent dentition is approximately 33%, with the highest incidence (55%) occurring in premolar teeth. Occasionally, lateral canals enter the floor of the pulp chamber of multirooted teeth. Since the apical foramen and lateral canals are areas of communication between the pulp space and the periodontium, they can act as avenues for the extension of disease from one tissue to the other. Hence diseases of the dental pulp can produce changes in the periodontal tissues. More rarely do diseases of the periodontium involve the dental pulp.

Primary Dentin

In human teeth three types of dentin can be recognized (Fig. 10-2). Most of the tooth is formed by *primary* dentin, which outlines the pulp chamber. The outer layer of primary dentin, called *mantle* dentin, differs from the rest of the primary dentin. It is the first layer formed by newly differentiated odontoblasts, being approximately 150 μm wide with an organic matrix consisting of ground substance that lacks phosphophoryn and loosely packed coarse collagen fibrils. The matrix is slightly (4%) less mineralized than the rest of the primary dentin, which is referred to as *circumpulpal* dentin.

Secondary Dentin

Secondary dentin develops after root formation has been completed. It was once thought that secondary dentin was formed only in response to functional stimuli, but it has been found in unerupted teeth as well. Thus secondary dentin represents the continuing, but much slower, deposition of dentin by the odontoblasts after root formation has been completed.

Secondary dentin has an incremental pattern and a tubular structure that, though less regular, is for the most part continuous with that of the primary dentin (Fig. 10-3). Although it is deposited around the periphery of the pulp space, it is not deposited evenly, especially in the molar teeth. There a greater deposition of secondary dentin on the roof and floor of the pulp chamber leads to an asymmetric reduction in the size and shape of the chamber and of the pulp horns. These changes in the pulp space, clinically referred to as pulp recession, can be readily detected on radiographs and are important in determining the form of cavity preparation for certain dental restorative procedures. For example, preparation of the tooth for a full crown in a young patient presents a substantial risk of involving the dental pulp by mechanically exposing a pulp horn; in an older patient the pulp horn has receded, presenting less danger. There is also evidence suggesting that secondary dentin scleroses more readily than primary dentin. This tends to reduce the overall permeability of the dentin, thereby protecting the pulp.

Tertiary Dentin

Tertiary dentin (also referred to as reactive, reparative, or irregular secondary dentin) is produced in reaction to noxious stimuli, such as caries or a restorative dental procedure. Unlike primary or secondary dentin, which forms along the entire pulp-dentin border, tertiary dentin is produced only by cells directly affected by the stimulus. The quality (or architecture) and the quantity or degree of tertiary dentin produced are related to the cellullar response initiated, and this depends on the intensity and duration of the stimulus. For example, the stimulus of an active carious lesion causes extensive destruction of dentin and considerable pulp damage. In such instances tertiary dentin is deposited rapidly by odontoblastlike cells that have differentiated from pulpal perivascular cells. Such dentin displays a sparse and irregular tubular pattern with frequent cellular inclusions (Fig. 10-4) and is sometimes called *osteodentin*. It also differs from primary dentin

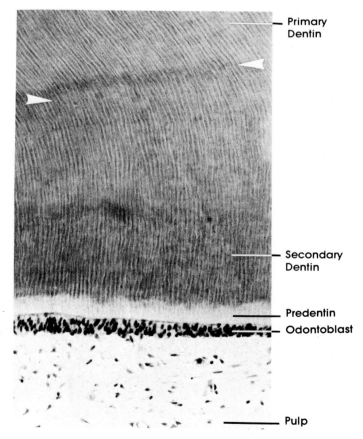

— Primary Dentin

— Secondary Dentin

— Predentin
— Odontoblast

— Pulp

FIG. 10-3 Section of secondary dentin. The darker area between the *arrowheads* marks the junction between primary and secondary dentin.

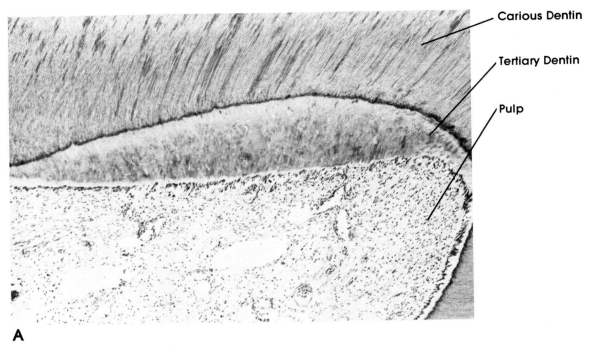

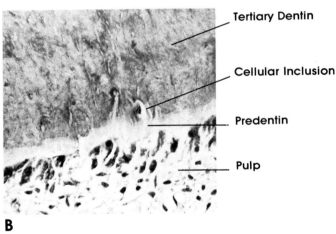

FIG. 10-4 Tertiary (or reparative) dentin. **A,** This form is deposited in response to caries (*dark streaks* in the upper half of the photomicrograph). It contains only a few sparse irregular tubules and some cellular inclusions, **B,** and was most likely laid down very rapidly.

in that it contains both type I and type III collagen expressed by the odontoblastlike cells. If the carious process is less active, however, tertiary dentin is deposited less rapidly, its tubular pattern is more regular, and there are fewer (if any) cellular inclusions (Fig. 10-5). For the most part, there is no continuity between dentinal tubules of tertiary dentin and the overlying primary or secondary dentin. This, in effect, minimizes dentin permeability at the site of deposition and affords protection to the underlying dental pulp.

Although in this text dentin has been categorized into three groups, other classifications recognize only primary and secondary dentin, equating secondary dentin with tertiary dentin.

Predentin

Predentin is a layer of variable thickness (10 to 47 μm) that lines the innermost (pulpal) portion of the dentin. It is unmineralized dentin matrix and consists principally of collagen, glycoproteins, and proteoglycans (other constituents of the dentin matrix are added at the mineralization front). It is similar to osteoid in bone and is easy to identify in hematoxylin and eosin (H&E)–stained sections, because it stains less intensely than mineralized dentin. Predentin is thickest where active dentinogenesis is occurring, and its presence is important in maintaining the integrity of dentin, since when it is absent the mineralized dentin is vulnerable to resorption by odontoclasts.

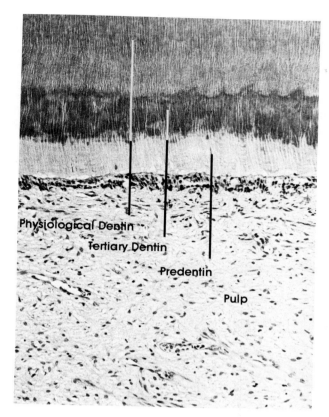

FIG. 10-5 Tertiary dentin. The tubular pattern is more regular, and no cellular inclusions occur. This dentin was probably deposited slowly in response to a mild stimulus.

HISTOLOGY OF PRIMARY DENTIN

When the dentin is viewed microscopically, several structural features can be identified: dentinal tubules, intra- and intertubular dentin, areas of deficient calcification (called interglobular dentin), incremental growth lines, and an area seen solely in the root portion of the tooth known as the *granular layer of Tomes*.

Dentinal Tubules

Dentinal tubules extend through the entire thickness of the dentin from the dentinoenamel junction to the pulp, and their configuration indicates the course taken by the odontoblasts during dentinogenesis. They follow an S-shaped path from the outer surface of the dentin to the perimeter of the pulp in a coronal direction. This S-shaped curvature is less pronounced in root dentin and least pronounced in the cervical third of the root and beneath the incisal edges and cusps (where they may run an almost straight course) (Fig. 10-6). As has been explained (Chapter 9), these curvatures, called

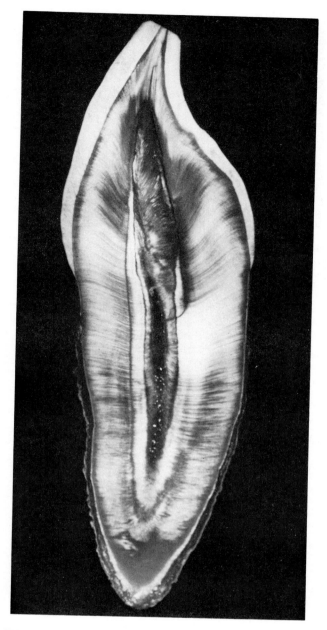

FIG. 10-6 Ground section showing the S-shaped primary curvature of the dentinal tubules in the crown and their straight course in the root. Compare with Figs. 9-22 and 10-7, which are at higher mangifications.

the *primary curvatures*, result from the crowding of odontoblasts as they move toward the center of the pulp. Smaller oscillations within the primary curvatures, called *secondary curvatures*, also occur, but how they are produced has not been established (Fig. 10-7).

The figure 10-5 labels: Physiological Dentin, Tertiary Dentin, Predentin, Pulp.

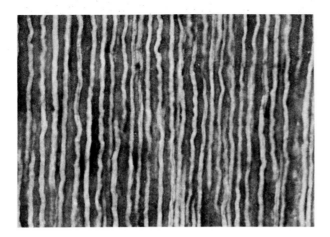

FIG. 10-7 Dentinal tubules. The smaller undulations represent secondary curvatures. Compare this with Figure 10-6.

The dentinal tubules are tapered structures measuring approximately 2.5 μm in diameter near the pulp, 1.2 μm in the midportion of the dentin, and 900 nm near the dentinoenamel junction. In the coronal parts of young premolar and molar teeth their numbers range from 59,000 to 76,000 per square millimeter at the pulpal surface, with approximately half as many per square millimeter near the enamel. This increase per unit voulume is associated with crowding of the odontoblasts as the pulp space becomes smaller. There is also a significant reduction in the average density of tubules in radicular dentin as compared to cervical dentin. Recent studies have shown a higher tubule density on the lingual and buccal walls of the pulp than on the mesial and distal walls. The terminal parts of the tubules branch, resulting in an increased number of tubules per unit length in mantle dentin. This terminal branch-

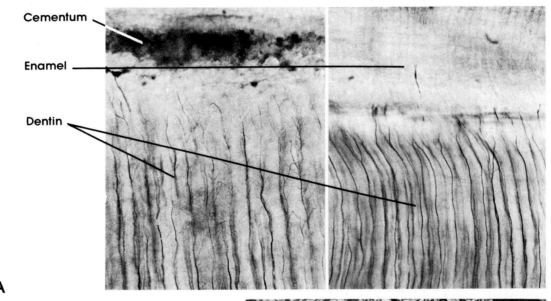

Cementum

Enamel

Dentin

A

B

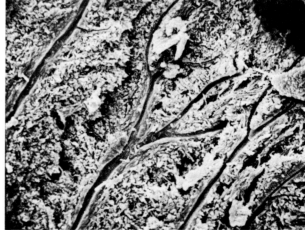

FIG. 10-8 Terminal branching of dentinal tubules. **A,** More profuse in root dentin than in coronal dentin. **B** and **C,** Scanning electron micrograph.

C

ing is especially profuse in root dentin (Fig. 10-8). Dentinal tubules also have lateral extensions that branch from the main lumen at intervals of 1 to 2 μm along its length. A dentinal tubule is generally thought to contain the process of an odontoblast bathed in dentinal fluid and to be lined by an organic sheath, the *lamina lim-* *itans;* but, as will be described, there is much uncertaintity regarding the exact nature of tubule content.

The tubular nature of dentin bestows an unusual degree of permeability on this hard tissue that can enhance a carious process (Fig. 10-9) and accentuate the response of the pulp to dental restorative procedures.

Microorganism in Tubules

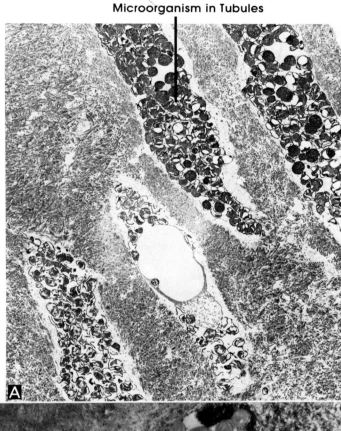

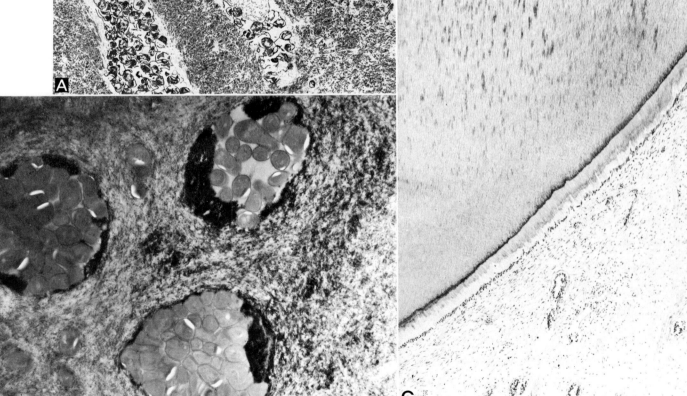

FIG. 10-9 Caries of dentin. Transmission electron micrographs showing the natural pathway created for microorganisms by the dentinal tubules. **A,** In longitudinal section; **B,** in cross section. The microorganisms absorb stain, and in light microscope sections the tubules of carious dentin are seen as dark streaks. **C,** Compare this with Fig. 10-4. (**B,** courtesy Dr. N.W. Johnson.)

Intratubular (Peritubular) Dentin and Sclerotic Dentin

Within the dentinal tubule there is a hypermineralized ring of dentin that is readily apparent when nondemineralized ground sections are cut at right angles to the tubules and examined under the light microscope (Fig. 10-10). This hypermineralized (40% more than intertubular dentin) collar of dentin, which can also be demonstrated by electron microscopy, electron microprobe analysis, and "soft x-ray" radiographs, was originally called *peritubular dentin* at the time of its discovery about 40 years ago, a term that is still widely used. Anatomically, however, the term is incorrect because this dentin forms within the dentinal tubule (not around it), narrowing the tubular lumen; it should therefore be referred to (more accurately) as *intratubular* dentin. Because the intratubular dentin is so highly mineralized, it is lost in decalcified sections. The intratubular dentin is roughly 44 nm wide near the pulpal end and 750 nm wide near the dentinoenamel junction and is sharply demarcated from the intertubular dentin.

The deposition of intratubular dentin causes a progressive reduction in the tubule lumen and, if continued, eventually obliterates the tubule. When this occurs in several tubules in the same area, the dentin assumes a glassy appearance and is brighter than the surrounding dentin in ground sections viewed under transmitted light. The term used to describe this progressive deposition of intratubular dentin and obliteration of the tubule is *sclerosis*, and the dentin so affected is called *sclerotic dentin*. The occlusion of dentinal tubules with mineral to produce sclerotic dentin begins in the root dentin of 18-year-old premolars without any external influence. The assumption therefore is that this is a physiologic response and the occlusion is achieved by continued intratubular dentin deposition. This, of course, begs the question as to how intratubular dentin forms. As mentioned in Chapter 9, this is not understood. Three possibilities exist: (1) there may be passive redistribution of mineral from intertubular dentin into the tubule around the various preexisting components of the tubule; (2) there may be an active response on the part of the odontoblast process, producing an organic matrix that is actively mineralized as a result of odontoblast activity; or (3) the odontoblast may produce an organic matrix that becomes mineralized by redistribution of mineral from intertubular dentin as in the first instance. Whatever the correct explanation, all possibilities involve the deposition of intratubular dentin, which assumes several forms (Fig. 10-11), at the expense of the odontoblast process, which must either retract or be selectively shortened by the loss at its distal extremity. The amount of sclerosed dentin increases with age and is most frequently encountered in the apical third of the root (Fig. 10-12) and in the crown midway between the dentinoenamel junction and the surface of the pulp. Because sclerosis reduces the permeability of dentin, it may help to prolong pulp vitality.

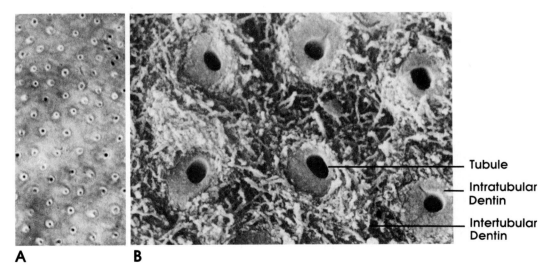

A   B   Tubule

Intratubular Dentin

Intertubular Dentin

FIG. 10-10 Intratubular dentin seen in ground section by light microscopy, **A,** and scanning electron microscopy, **B.** The dark central spots are empty dentinal tubules surrounded by a well-defined collar of intratubular dentin. (**A** from Scott DB, et al: *J Dent Res* 53:54, 1974.)

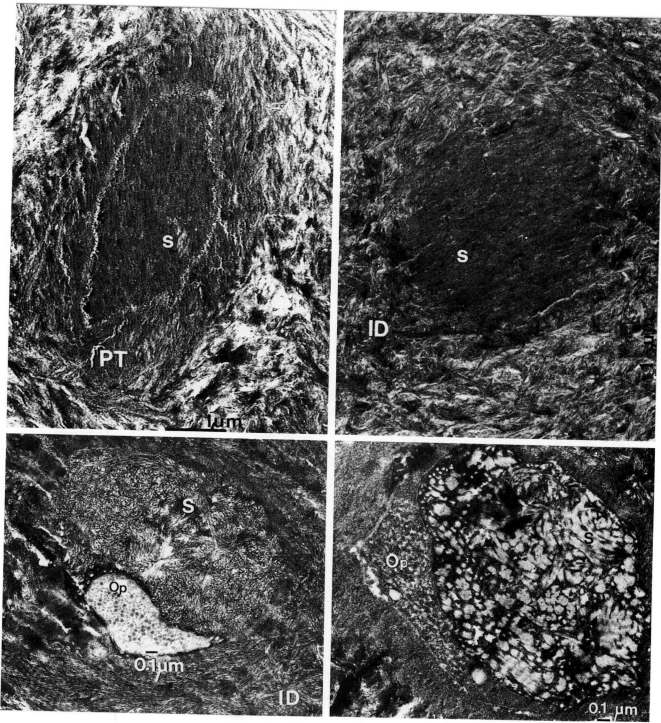

FIG. 10-11 Sclerosis of the dentinal tubule. This occurs in different ways. At *upper left* (from Tsatsas and Frank, *Calcif Tissue Res* 9:238, 1972) the tubule is filled with an even deposition of mineral, which has been interpreted as a spread of intratubular (pertitubular) dentin. However, at *upper right* (from Frank, and Nalbandian, *Handbook of microscopic anatomy,* vol V/6, *Teeth,* 1989) tubular occlusion has occurred in a similar way although no intratubular dentin is present. At *bottom left* (from Frank and Voegel, *Caries Res* 14:367, 1980) diffuse mineralization is occurring with a viable odontoblast process. At *bottom right* (from Tsatsas and Frank, *Calcif Tissue Res* 9:238, 1972) there is mineralization both within the odontoblast process and around the collagen fibrils. *ID,* Intertubular dentin; *Op,* odontoblast process; *S,* sclerotic dentin.

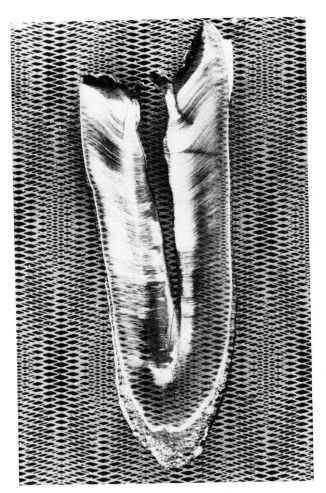

FIG. 10-12 Ground section, approximately 100 μm thick, of an old tooth. The section has been placed over a pattern, which can be seen through the apical translucent sclerotic dentin.

Intertubular Dentin

Dentin located between the dental tubules is called *intertubular dentin*. It represents the primary secretory product of the odontoblasts and consists of a tightly interwoven network of type I collagen fibrils (measuring between 50 and 200 nm in diameter), in which apatite crystals are deposited. The fibrils are randomly arranged in a plane at roughly right angles to the dentinal tubules, and the apatite crystals (averaging 100 nm in length) are generally oriented with their long axes paralleling the fibril. The ground substance consists of phosphoproteins, proteoglycans, γ-carboxyglutamate–containing proteins, glycoproteins, and some plasma proteins.

Interglobular Dentin

Interglobular dentin is the term used to describe areas of unmineralized or hypomineralized dentin where globular zones of mineralization (calcospherites) have failed to fuse into a homogeneous mass within mature dentin (See Fig. 10-14). These areas are especially prevalent in human teeth in which there has been a deficiency in vitamin D or exposure to high levels of fluoride at the time of dentin formation (dentinogenesis). Interglobular dentin is seen most frequently in the circumpulpal dentin just below the mantle dentin, where the pattern of mineralization is largely globular. Because this irregularity of dentin is a defect of mineralization and not of matrix formation, the normal architectural pattern of the tubules remains unchanged, and they run uninterruptedly through the interglobular areas. There is, however, no intratubular dentin where the tubules pass through the globules (Fig. 10-13). These areas are often called interglobular spaces, but this is a misnomer since no true space exists.

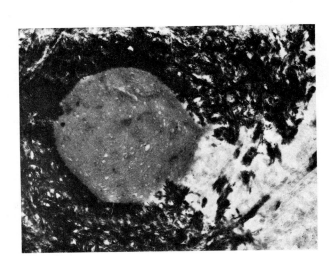

FIG. 10-13 Electron micrograph of interglobular dentin showing the boundary between interglobular and normal intertubular dentin in a human tooth. The mineralized interglobular dentin is at the *bottom left corner*. The tubule contents consist of a dense hyaline material. (From Tsatsas BG, Frank RM: *Calcif Tissue Res* 9:238, 1972.)

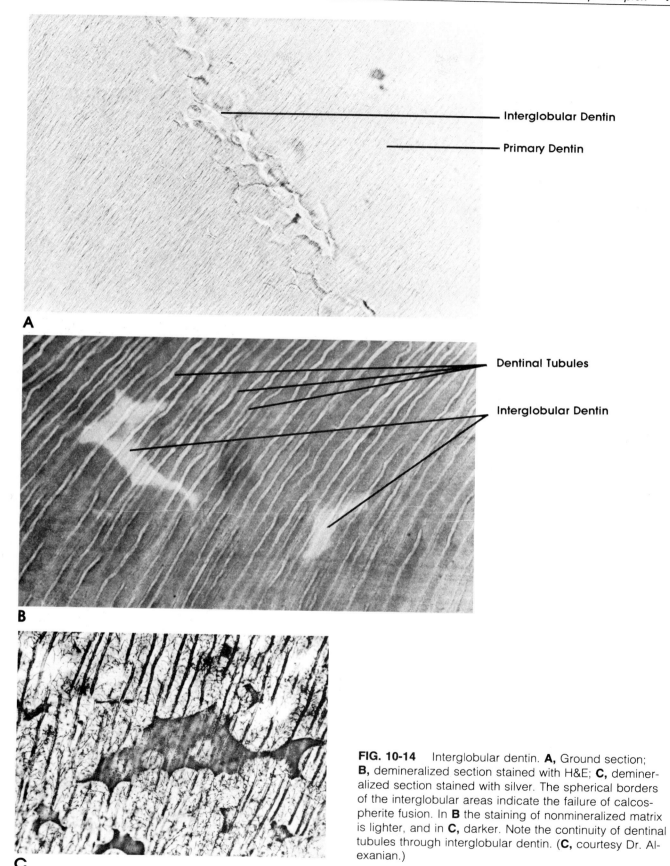

A — Interglobular Dentin

Primary Dentin

B — Dentinal Tubules

Interglobular Dentin

FIG. 10-14 Interglobular dentin. **A,** Ground section; **B,** demineralized section stained with H&E; **C,** demineralized section stained with silver. The spherical borders of the interglobular areas indicate the failure of calcospherite fusion. In **B** the staining of nonmineralized matrix is lighter, and in **C,** darker. Note the continuity of dentinal tubules through interglobular dentin. (**C,** courtesy Dr. Alexanian.)

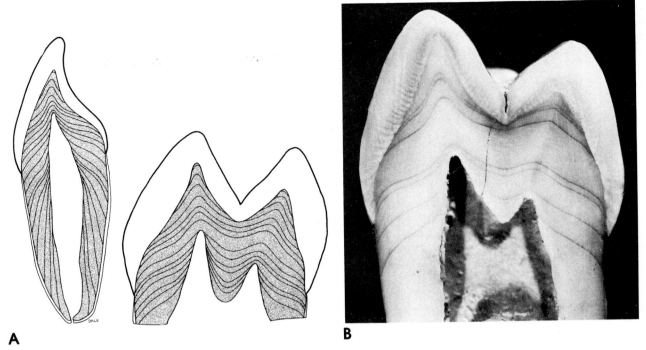

A   **B**

FIG. 10-15   **A,** Pattern of incremental line deposition in dentin. **B,** Tooth section of a person who received tetracycline intermittently. The drug has been incorporated at successive dentin-forming fronts, mimicking incremental line patterns. (**A,** from Kawasaki K: *J Anat* 119:61, 1975.)

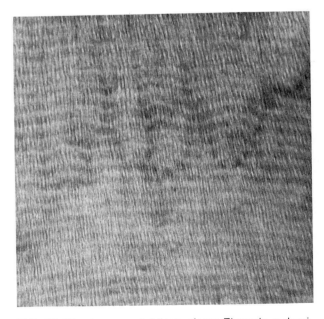

FIG. 10-16   Incremental lines of von Ebner in a demineralized section.

Incremental Growth Lines

Dentinogenesis proceeds rhythmically, with alternating phases of activity and quiescence. These phases are represented in formed dentin as incremental lines that, although often not clearly detectable, can best be seen in longitudinal ground sections of teeth. The incremental lines run at right angles to the dentinal tubules and generally mark the normal rhythmic linear pattern of dentin deposition in an inward and rootward direction (Fig. 10-15). There has been considerable confusion over the nomenclature of incremental lines in dentin. With special staining techniques a daily pattern of dentin deposition can be discerned (Fig. 9-16); no name is given to these incremental lines. There is also a 5-day rhythmic pattern associated with dentin deposition, represented as incremental lines separated by 20 μm intervals. These are the *incremental lines of von Ebner* (Fig. 10-16).

Another type of incremental pattern found in dentin is the *contour lines of Owen*. There is some confusion about the exact connotation of this term. As originally described by Owen, the contour lines result from a coincidence of the secondary curvatures between neighboring dentinal tubules (Fig. 10-17). Other lines, however, having the same disposition but caused by accentuated deficiencies in mineralization, are now more generally known as contour lines of Owen (Fig. 10-18). These are easily recognizable in longitudinal ground sections. An exceptionally wide contour line is the neonatal line found in those teeth mineralizing at birth; it reflects the disturbance in mineralization created by the physiologic trauma of birth. Periods of illness or inadequate nutrition are also marked by accentuated contour lines within the dentin.

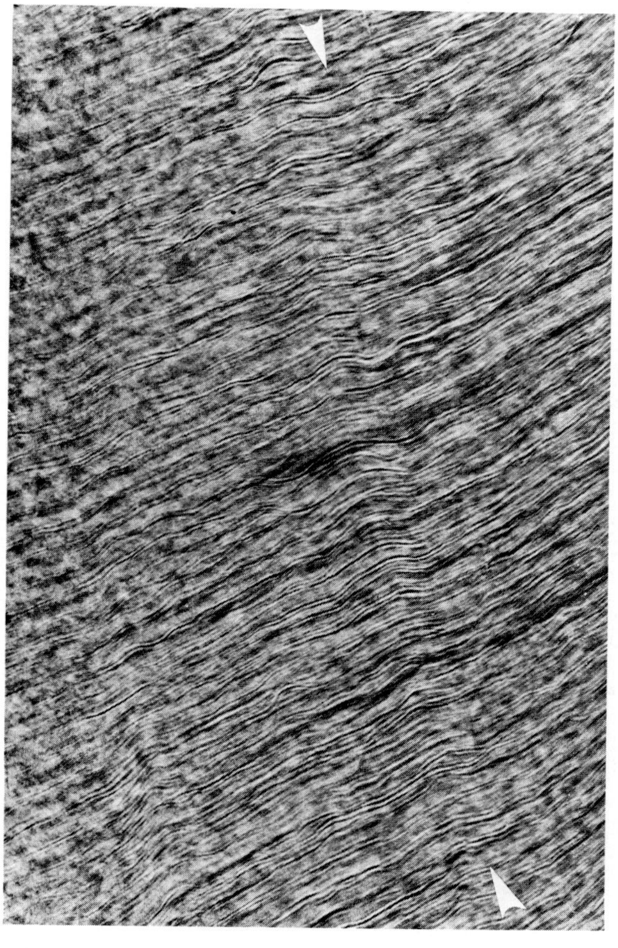

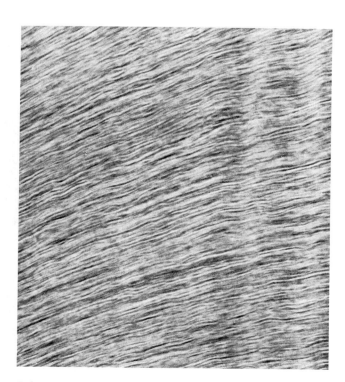

FIG. 10-17 Contour lines of Owen (between *arrowheads*). As originally described, these lines are caused by the coincidence of secondary curvatures in the dentinal tubules.

FIG. 10-18 Contour lines of Owen. As seen here, these are usually considered to be exaggerated incremental lines of von Ebner.

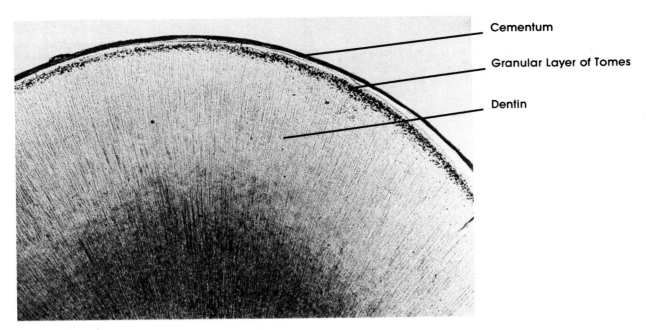

FIG. 10-19 Ground section across the root of a tooth. The granular layer of Tomes is visible just beneath the cementum.

Granular Layer of Tomes

When dentin is viewed under transmitted light in ground sections (and only in ground sections), a granular-appearing area, the granular layer of Tomes, can be seen just below the surface of the dentin where the root is covered by cementum (Fig. 10-19). A progressive increase in so-called granules occurs from the cementoenamel junction to the apex of the tooth (Fig. 10-20). It was once thought that this granular appearance was associated with minute hypomineralized areas of interglobular dentin; but, in fact, they are true spaces. This can be established in a very simple way. When sections are viewed with transmitted light, the granules appear dark, similar to the dead tracts of dentin (see p. 211), which are known to be empty tubules filled with air. The dark coloration results when light is refracted by the microscope lens. If the illumination is changed from transmitted to incident, the dead tracts and the granules of Tomes' layer appear lighter, because the light is refracted by the air within the tubules into the microscope lens. These spaces cannot be seen in H&E–stained sections or on electron micrographs. It has been suggested that the spaces represent sections made through the looped terminal portions of dentinal tubules found only in root dentin and seen only because of light refraction in thick ground sections. This looping has been related to the lower rate of dentin formation in root dentin.

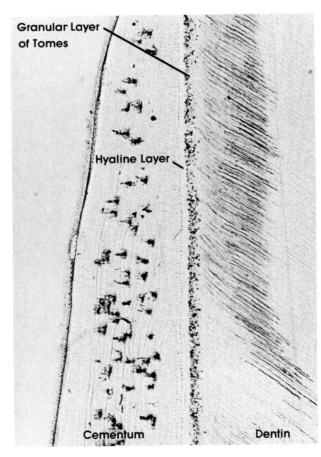

FIG. 10-20 Longitudinal ground section of the granular layer of Tomes. Note the hyaline layer and the increased number of granules as the layer is traced apically.

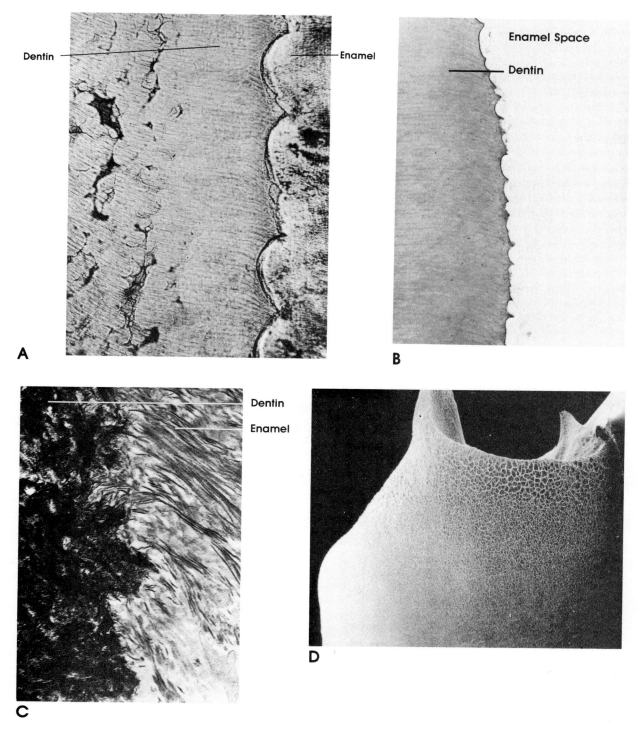

FIG. 10-21 Dentinoenamel junction. **A,** Ground section; **B,** demineralized section after the enamel has been lost. The scalloped nature of the junction when seen in one plane is striking. An electron micrograph, **C,** shows the intermingling of dentin and enamel crystals. A low-power scanning electron micrograph of a premolar from which the enamel has been removed, **D,** which shows that the scalloping is accentuated where the junction is subjected to most functional stress. (**D,** courtesy Dr. W.H. Douglas.)

DENTINOENAMEL JUNCTION

It has already been pointed out that the dentin supports enamel. The junction between the two is the dentinoenamel junction. In ground sections this junction can be easily seen as a series of scallops (Fig. 10-21, *A*) with extensions of odontoblast tubules occasionally crossing the junction and passing into the enamel (the enamel spindles). In a demineralized section where the enamel has been removed, the scalloped nature of the junction can be clearly seen (Fig. 10-21, *B*); and the electron microscope reveals that crystals of dentin and enamel intermix (Fig. 10-21, *C*). The scanning electron microscope reveals the junction to be a series of ridges rather than spikes, which arrangement probably increases the adherence between dentin and enamel; and in this regard it is worth noting that the

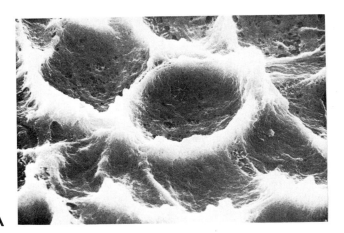

A

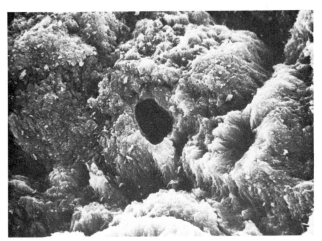

B

10-22 Dentinoenamel junction. **A,** With the scanning electron microscope, the dentinal aspect of the junction is seen. The scallops are a series of ridges, which fit into depressions formed in the enamel face of the junction. **B,** The hole in the center is an enamel spindle. (From Whittaker DK: *J Anat* 125:323, 1978.)

ridging is most pronounced in coronal dentin, where occlusal stresses are the greatest (Figs. 10-21, *D*, and 10-22). The shape and nature of the junction prevent shearing of the enamel during function.

DENTINOCEMENTUM JUNCTION

Peripheral to the granular layer of Tomes, and separating it from the cementum, is a very thin *hyaline layer* that used to be considered a form of dentin. It is now known, however, to be a product of cells of Hertwig's epithelial root sheath with the proposed function of "cementing" cementum to dentin. (See Chapter 13 and Fig. 10-20.)

PULP

The dental pulp is the soft connective tissue that supports the dentin. When its histology is examined, four distinct zones can be distinguished: (1) the odontoblastic zone at the pulp periphery, (2) a cell-free zone (the zone or basal layer of Weil) beneath the odontoblasts, which is prominent in the coronal pulp, (3) a cell-rich zone, where cell density is high, which is again easily seen in coronal pulp adjacent to the cell-free zone, and (4) the pulp core, which is characterized by the major vessels and nerves of the pulp (Fig. 10-23). The principal cells of the pulp are the odontoblasts, fibroblasts, undifferentiated mesenchymal cells, macrophages, and other immunocompetent cells.

Odontoblasts

The most distinctive cells of the dental pulp, and therefore the most easily recognized, are the odontoblasts. They form a single layer lining the periphery of the pulp and have a process extending into the dentin. In the crown portion of the mature tooth, odontoblasts often appear to be arranged in a palisading pattern, seemingly forming a layer three to five cells in depth. This is an artifact caused by crowding of the odontoblasts. The number of odontoblasts corresponds to the number of dentinal tubules and, as mentioned previously, varies with tooth type and location within the pulp space. Although actual cell counts have not been made, the number of dentinal tubules present at the pulp-dentin interface, and therefore the number of odontoblasts, has been estimated to be in the range of 45,000 per square millimeter in coronal dentin, with a lesser number in root dentin. The odontoblasts in the crown are also larger than odontoblasts in the root (Fig. 10-24). In the crown the cell bodies of odontoblasts are columnar and measure approximately 35 μm in length whereas in the midportion of the pulp they are more cuboid and in the apical part more flattened.

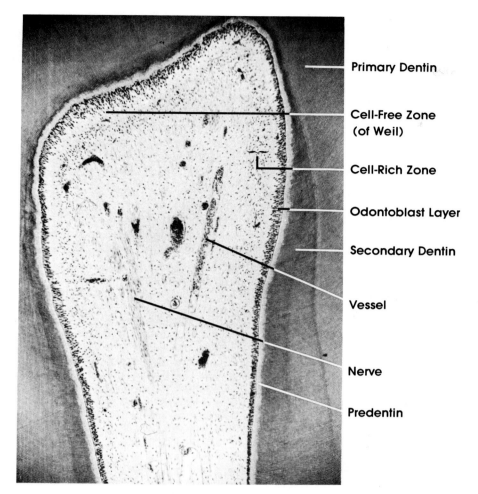

Primary Dentin

Cell-Free Zone (of Weil)

Cell-Rich Zone

Odontoblast Layer

Secondary Dentin

Vessel

Nerve

Predentin

FIG. 10-23 Low-powered photomicrograph of the dentin-pulp complex of a premolar tooth. Primary dentin and secondary physiologic dentin are separated by a hematoxyphilic line. The amount of secondary dentin deposition varies, more having occurred on the right than on the left. The cell-free zone (of Weil) beneath the odontoblast layer is clearly seen, as is the cell-rich zone. Note also the differences in odontoblast layers in the crown and root.

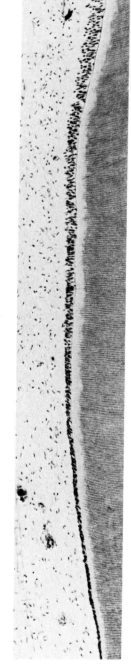

FIG. 10-24 Photomicrograph of the differences in odontoblast morphology in a mature tooth. At *top* the odontoblasts have a palisaded configuration, and they become gradually smaller and more cuboid further down.

The morphology of odontoblasts reflects their functional activity and ranges from an active synthetic phase to a quiesent phase (Fig. 9-5). By light microscopy an active cell can be seen to possess an open-faced nucleus, much basophilic cytoplasm, and a prominent Golgi zone. A resting cell, on the other hand, is flattened, with relatively little cytoplasm, and has a more hematoxophilic (closed) nucleus. By electron microscopy (with its ability to describe more fine detail) a further stage in the life cycle of odontoblasts can be discerned. In addition to the secretory and resting (or aged) states, recognizable by light microscopy, it is possible to define also a transitional stage intermediate between the secretory and resting states. (Secretory odontoblasts were described in Chapter 9 as cells with a basally situated nucleus and a full complement of organelles necessary for synthesis and secretion.) The organelles of an active odontoblast are prominent, consisting of numerous vesicles, much endoplasmic reticulum, a well-developed Golgi complex located on the dentinal side of the nucleus, and numerous mitochondria scattered throughout the cell body. The nucleus contains an abundance of peripherally dispersed chromatin and as many as four nucleoli. The rough endoplasmic reticulum is particularly extensive during dentinogenesis, and its cisternae contain a fine granular material. Arising from the cisternae of the rough endoplasmic reticulum are numerous transport vesicles that pass to, and accumulate at, the immature face of the Golgi complex. At the mature Golgi face many small secretory vesicles are formed that extend to the base of the odontoblast process. Other membrane-bound granules, similar in appearance to lysosomes, are present in the cytoplasm, as are numerous filaments and microtubules. Decreasing amounts of intracellular organelles reflect decreased functional activity of the odontoblast (Fig. 10-25). Thus

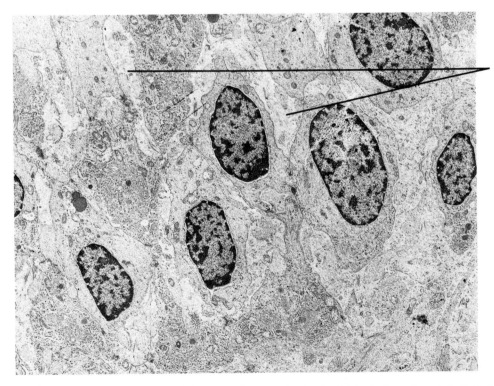

Extracellular Compartment

FIG. 10-25 Electron micrograph of odontoblasts from the mature coronal pulp. This field corresponds to the palisaded appearance visible by light microscopy in Figures 10-23 and 10-24. The cells are not particularly active and therefore do not contain abundant rough endoplasmic reticulum.

A

Predentin ——

Odontoblast —— Process

Odontoblast —— Cell Body

FIG. 10-26 Scanning electron micrograph of the pulp-predentin-dentin interfaces. In **A** the odontoblast process is entering the tubule. In **B** the odontoblast process *(op)* can be seen traversing the predentin *(pd)* into mineralized dentin *(d)*. Note the presence of nerve fibrils *(nf)*. (**A** from Scott DB, et al: *J Dent Res* 53:165, 1974, **B** from Frank RM, Nalbandian J: *Handbook of microscopic anatomy,* New York, 1989, Springer Verlag, vol V/6).

B

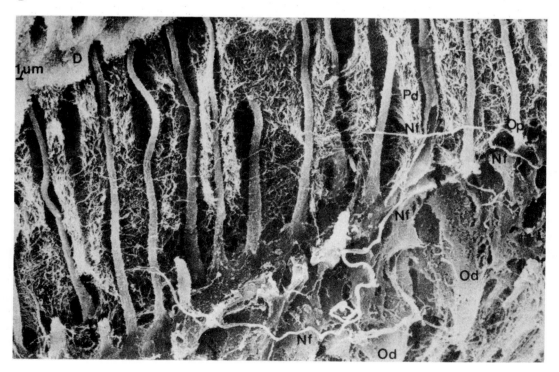

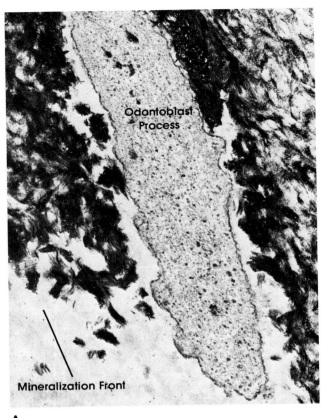

A

Odontoblast Process

Mineralization Front

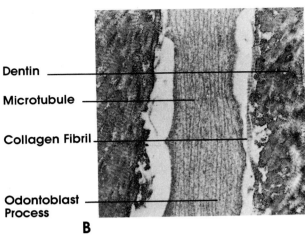

Dentin

Microtubule

Collagen Fibril

Odontoblast Process

B

FIG. 10-27 **A,** Electron micrograph of an odontoblast process as it extends from predentin to dentin. **B,** The microtubular structure within the process.

the transitional odontoblast is a narrower cell, with its nucleus displaced from the basal extremity and exhibiting condensed chromatin. The amount of endoplasmic reticulum is reduced and the reticulum surrounds the nucleus; autophagic vacuoles are present and associated with the reorganization of cytoplasm. Resting, or aged, odontoblasts are smaller cells (about 45 μm tall) crowded together. The nucleus of such a cell is situated more apically, creating a prominent infranuclear region in which fewer cytoplasmic organelles are clustered. The supranuclear region is devoid of organelles, except for large lipid-filled vacuoles in a cytoplasm containing tubular and filamentous structures. Secretory granules are absent.

The odontoblast process begins at the neck of the cells where the cell gradually begins to narrow as it passes through predentin into the mineralized dentin (Fig. 10-26). A major change in the cytology of odontoblasts occurs at the junction between the cell body and the process. The process is devoid of major organelles but does display an abundance of microtubules and filaments arranged in a linear pattern. Coated vesicles are also present that may fuse with the cell membrane. Occasional mitochondria are found in the process, usually where it passes through predentin (Fig. 10-27). The apical cell membrane and the beginning of the cell process exhibit structural specializations related to the exocytosis and endocytosis associated with turnover that occurs within predentin.

Many complex junctions occur between adjacent odontoblasts—gap junctions, zonulae occludentes (tight junctions), and zonulae adherentes (desmo-

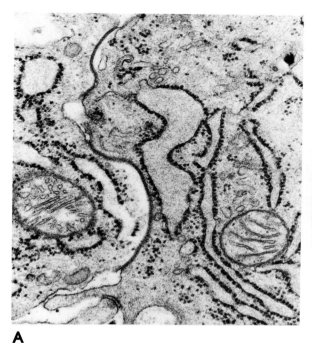

A

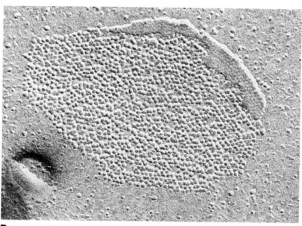

B

FIG. 10-28   Junction between odontoblasts. **A,** Electron microscope view. **B,** Freeze-fractured preparation showing the characteristic blebs of the gap junction. (**A** and **B** courtesy Dr. M. Weinstock.)

somes). The occurrence of gap junctions between adjacent odontoblasts indicates communication between these cells, for it is known that such junctions permit the free interchange of ions and small molecules. The number and location of gap junctions are variable, since they can form, dissolve, and reform rapidly as function dictates (Fig. 10-28).

The life span of odontoblasts is generally believed to equal that of the viable tooth, because odontoblasts are end cells, which means that, once differentiated, they cannot undergo further cell division. This fact poses an interesting problem. It is known that on occasion, when the pulp tissue is exposed, repair can take place by the formation of new dentin. This means that new odontoblasts must have differentiated and migrated to the exposure site from pulp tissue, most likely from the cell-rich subodontoblast zone. Recall that the differentiation of odontoblasts during tooth development requires a cascade of determinants, including cells of the internal dental epithelium or Hertwig's root sheath. Epithelial cells, however, are no longer present in the developed tooth, and the stimulus for differentiation of new odontoblasts under these circumstances is not known. (This problem is discussed at greater length in Chapter 20.)

Contents of the dentinal tubule

At this point it is necessary to discuss further the dentinal tubule and its contents. The account given so far of the tubule and the odontoblast process has been presented in a fairly uncontroversial fashion to help the beginning student understand dentin structure and gain the necessary vocabulary. An appreciation should have been obtained that dentin is tubular, that each tubule is occupied by an odontoblast process (whose presence dictates the formation of the tubule), that the tubule is subsequently constricted by the deposition of intratubular dentin, that it is lined by an organic sheath, and that fluid circulates between this sheath and the process. The foregoing is simplistic, however, and a number of debatable issues exist that require amplification, especially since the dentin-pulp complex is so crucial to the everyday practice of dentistry. Perhaps the most important issue is the extent of the odontoblast process within the dentinal tubule.

The odontoblast process

There is no debate that from the cell body of the odontoblast a single process extends into the dentin housed within the dentinal tubule. The junction of the cell body with the process is characterized by a loss of

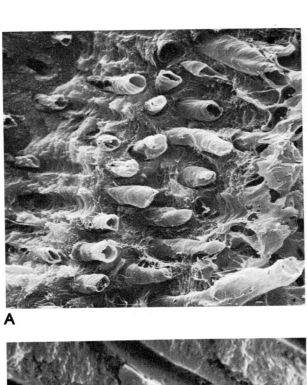

A

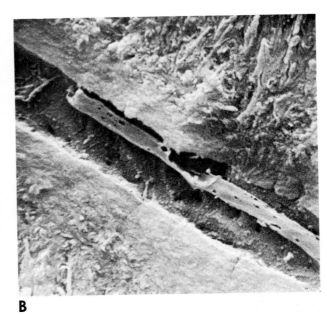

B

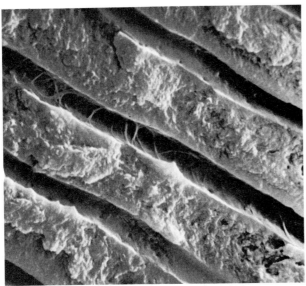

C

FIG. 10-29 Scanning electron micrographs of the tubular configuration from the pulp-dentin border to the dentinoenamel junction. In **A,** at the pulp-dentin interface, the odontoblast process can be seen entering the tubules. In **B,** 0.5 mm into the dentin, the process is within the tubule. In **C,** after 0.07 mm, the tubule contents are empty. These photomicrographs were taken 1.2 mm from the pulp. (**A** to **C** from Brännström M, Garberoglio R.: *Acta Odontol Scand* 30:291, 1972.)

cytoplasmic organelles and the presence of a terminal web. The process itself contains a few secretory vacuoles and an extensive cytoskeletal network (the parallel with a cytoskeleton in osteocyte processes is worth noting). Where there is controversy is whether the odontoblast process extends the full length of the dentinal tubule. The tubule forms only because there is an odontoblast process, and for many years it was assumed that this condition (of a tubule occupied by an odontoblast process) was the norm. There was, however, debate, as to whether the process filled the tubule completely in cross section.

This assumption was challenged some 20 years ago on the basis of simple examination of fractured human dentin with the scanning electron microscope, and it was claimed that the odontoblast process extended only 0.7 mm into dentin, with the remainder of the tubule empty (Fig. 10-29). Understandably, this claim prompted a flurry of further investigation because of its implications with respect to dentin response to various dental clinical procedures; and this important issue, surprisingly, is still not resolved. What follows is a summary of current information.

Light microscope studies. Under an oil immersion lens it is possible to see a structure within dentinal tubules in decalcified sections that can be interpreted as the odontoblast process (Fig. 10-30); and, indeed, early investigators, who dissolved away sections of dentin in hydrochloric acid, published photographs of this structure, which they considered to be the odontoblast process (Fig. 10-31). When such structures are harvested and visualized under the electron microscope, however, they are seen to be not odontoblast processes but the lamina limitans (Fig. 10-32). Many are filled with collagen bundles.

Scanning electron microscope studies. It is these same structures that provide the appearance of processes under the scanning electron microscope. Although such images (Fig. 10-33) are both beautiful and seemingly convincing, the evidence is that they do not show the odontoblast process. Recall that the scanning electron microscope can demonstrate only surfaces and that the tubule (lined by a sheath or membrane known as the lamina limitans) will mimic an odontoblast process unless specific steps are taken to remove the sheath. Thus what appears to be a process is in reality the lamina (Fig. 10-34) and the scanning electron microscope cannot reveal what lies within it.

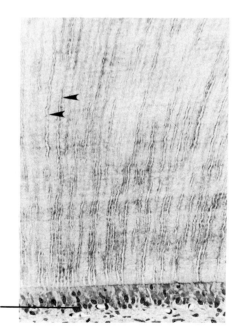

Odontoblasts

FIG. 10-30 Light microscopic appearance of dentin. Odontoblast processes *(arrows)* can be seen within the dentinal tubules.

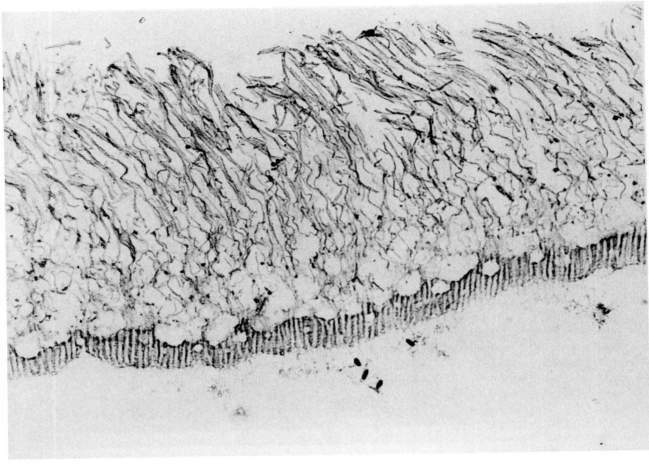

FIG. 10-31 Section of fixed dentin that has been successively demineralized and exposed to collagenase and hyaluronidase to remove all the noncellular elements. Predentin remains because its collagen, unprotected by mineral and therefore exposed to fixative, has become resistant to collagenase digestion. Structures resembling the process appear to be isolated.

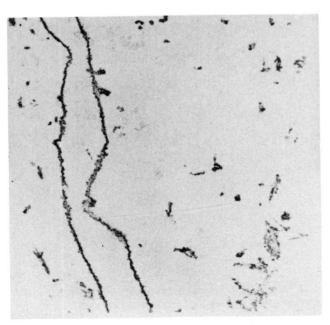
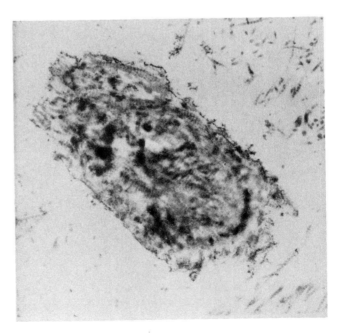

A   B

FIG. 10-32 Electron micrographs of the section illustrated in Fig. 10-31. What resembles a process under the light microscope is seen to be the lamina limitans **(A)** which in some instances close to the predentin encloses a mass of collagen **(B)**.

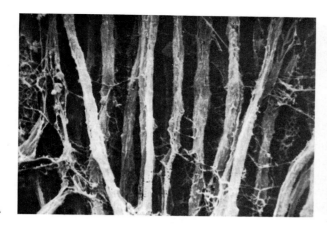

A

FIG. 10-33 Scanning electron micrograph of dentin that has been treated with acid (to remove mineral) and collagenase (to remove collagen). Structures resembling odontoblast processes remain. **A** shows such processes in middentin, and **B** at the dentinoenamel junction *(arrows)*. (Courtesy Dr. M. Sigal.)

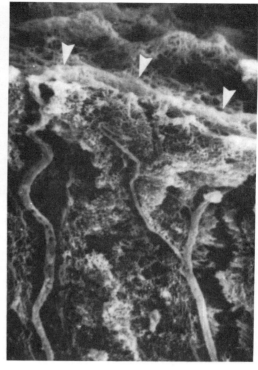

B

A

— Peritubular Dentin

— Odontoblast Process

— Limiting Membrane

B

FIG. 10-34 Electron micrographs of dentinal tubules. **A** is from the inner third of dentin, where the tubule is lined by an electron dense limiting membrane. In **B,** taken from the outer dentin, the odontoblast process is lost and peritubular dentin is demineralized. The limiting membrane remains and under the scanning electron microscope could mimic the structures seen in Figure 10-30. (From Thomas HF: *Arch Oral Biol* 28:465, 1983.)

Immunocytochemical studies. Using labeled antibodies against proteins comprising the cytoskeleton (actin, vimentin, tubulin), researchers have shown that the majority of dentinal tubules exhibit these components along their entire extent (Fig. 10-35). Since these proteins are exclusively intracellular, the presence of a process can be inferred.

Transmission electron microscope studies. Conventional dentin preparatory techniques for electron microscopy fail to demonstrate odontoblast processes in peripheral dentin; yet the demonstration of such processes in inner dentin is easily achieved (Fig. 10-27). Two explanations have been offered to explain this fact: The first is that the demonstration of odontoblast processes in outer dentin is prevented by the difficulty of achieving adequate fixation. This seems a bit hard to understand since it has been shown that fixative can penetrate the entire thickness of dentin. The second argument is that contractile elements within the odontoblast and its process cause its retraction in response to the manipulative procedures involved in preparing a tooth for examination. This argument is not unreasonable when it is remembered that (1) contractile proteins exist within the process, (2) tenascin, a glycprotein associated with motility, has been demonstrated in the dentinal tubule, and (3) when cryofixation is used (which is thought to prevent contraction), the process can be demonstrated in peripheral dentin (Fig. 10-36).

Summary. The extent of odontoblast processes is still an issue not entirely resolved, and it is likely that considerable variation exists.

FIG. 10-35 Photomicrograph of the surface of dentin in a fractured human tooth. An immunofluorescent label for tubulin (found only intracellularly) has been applied to the dentin surface and, as the tubules fluoresce, suggests the presence of odontoblast processes throughout the dentin. (Courtesy Dr. M. Sigal.)

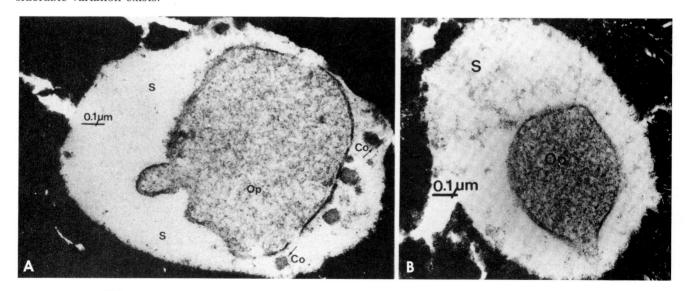

FIG. 10-36 Electron micrographs of coronal dentin just below the dentinoenamel junction demonstrating the presence of a process *(op)* in the tubule following cryofixation. In **A** collagen fibrils *(co)* are also visible in the tubular space *(s)*. (**A** from Frank RM, Nalbandian J: *Handbook of microscopic anatomy,* vol V/6, *Teeth,* New York, 1989, Springer-Verlag; **B** from LaFleche RG, et al: *J Biol Buccale* 13:293, 1985.)

Other contents of the tubule

Recently it has become appreciated that collagen is a significant component of the dentinal tubule. Previous electron microscope studies reported collagen fibrils as occupying the space between the odontoblast process and the tubule wall, with no mention of their extent and distribution (Fig. 10-37). This deficiency has now been corrected, and it has been shown that in human teeth intratubular collagen is a significant feature of dentin, with increasing amounts occurring in the tubules of inner dentin. Indeed, a sizable number of tubules are almost filled with collagen (Figs. 10-32 and 10-38), which would preclude the presence of a process and support the notion that the extent of a process is variable.

Of interest is the observation that this pattern of collagen deposition is common to all tooth families and unrelated to the age of the tooth (Fig. 10-39).

Another question concerns the constituents of the "space" between the odontoblast process and the tubule wall, the so-called dentinal fluid. The assumption has been made that the space is filled with fluid (equivalent to serum), but there is no validity to this. It has also been suggested that a physiologic barrier exits between odontoblasts and that the demonstration of fluid is achieved only after cavity preparation, which involves tissue damage and the production of exudate. What information there is concerning tubule content, in addition to process content (collagen and nerve fibrils), indicates that proteoglycans, tenascin, the serum proteins albumin, α-2 HS, and transferrin (in ratios differing from those found in serum), and type V collagen may all be present—clearly a complex mixture, about which much more needs to be learned. Nerves are also found in some tubules.

Finally, it might be questioned whether the lining membrane (lamina limitans) exists as such or is merely another artifact of tissue preparation. Cryofixed and undemineralized sections show no evidence of this structure (Fig. 10-40). Only after demineralization does the lamina become evident; in fact, it is just possible that this membrane is a chemical condensation of the various components identified in the previous paragraph. Figure 10-41 summarizes tubule contents.

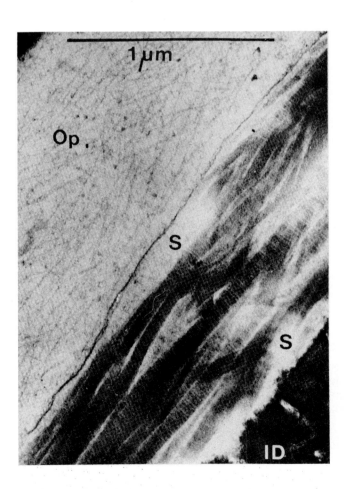

FIG. 10-37 Electron micrograph illustrating collagen fibrils in the dentinal tubule. *ID,* Intertubular dentin; *S,* periodontontoblastic space; *Op,* odontoblast process. (From Frank RM, Nalbandian J: *Handbook of microscopic anatomy,* vol V/6, *Teeth,* New York, 1989, Springer-Verlag.)

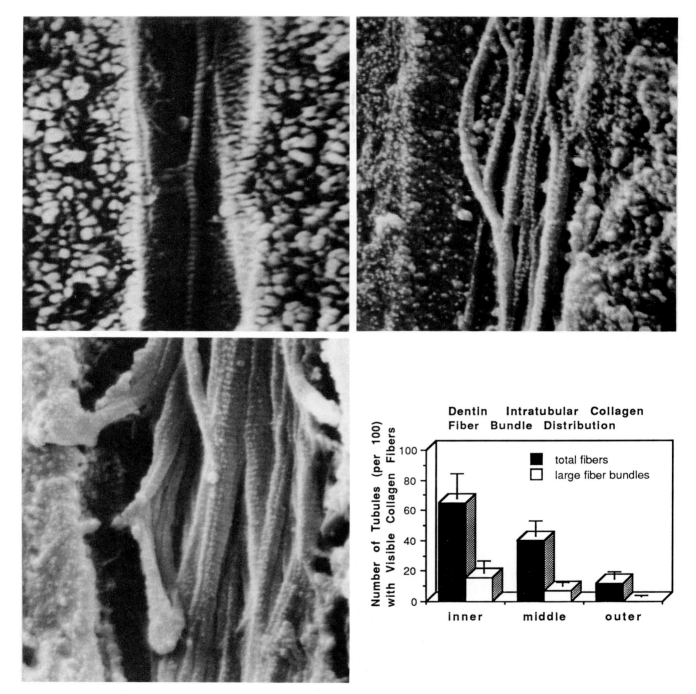

FIG. 10-38   Collagen content of dentinal tubules as seen with the scanning electron microscope. *Upper left,* Sparse in the outer dentin (Fig. 10-36). *Upper right,* increased in the middle dentin. *Bottom left,* Significant in tubules of the inner dentin (Fig.10-32, *B*). *Bottom right* distribution in the dentinal tubules (From Dai XF, et al: *Arch Oral Biol* 36:775, 1991.)

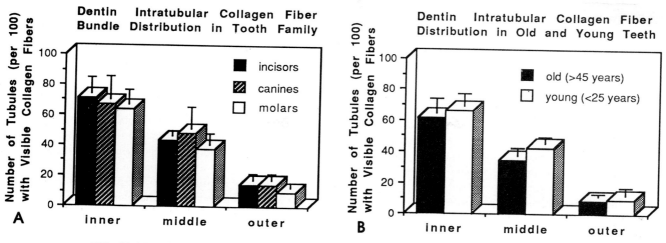

FIG. 10-39 Collagen content of the dentinal tubules in, **A,** tooth families and, **B,** young and old teeth.

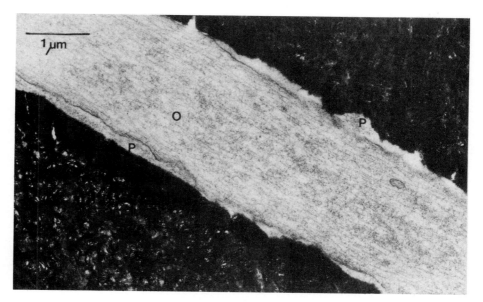

FIG. 10-40 Cryofixation of an odontoblast process in the inner third of root dentin. Note the absence of any structure resembling a lamina limitans. (From Frank RM, Steur P: *Arch Oral Biol* 33:91, 1988.)

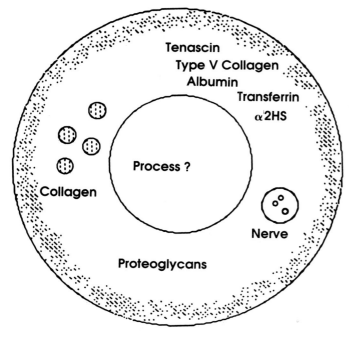

FIG. 10-41 Tubular content.

Fibroblasts

The cells occurring in greatest numbers in the pulp are fibroblasts (Fig. 10-42). They are particularly numerous in the coronal portion of the pulp, where they form the cell-rich zone. The function of fibroblasts in the pulp is to form and maintain the pulp matrix, which consists of collagen and ground substance. The histology of these fibroblasts reflects their functional state. In young pulps the fibroblasts are actively synthesizing matrix and therefore have a plump cytoplasm containing extensive amounts of all the usual organelles associated with synthesis and secretion and an open-face nucleus. With age, the need for synthesis diminishes and the fibroblasts appear as flattened spindle-shaped cells with closed-faced nuclei. Fibroblasts of the pulp also have the capability of ingesting and degrading collagen when appropriately stimulated (Chapter 6). The fine structure of the pulp is shown in Fig. 10-43.

Undifferentiated Mesenchymal Cells

Undifferentiated mesenchymal cells represent the pool from which connective tissue cells of the pulp are derived. Depending on the stimulus, these cells may give rise to odontoblasts and fibroblasts. They are found throughout the cell-rich area and the pulp core and are often related to blood vessels. Under the light microscope they appear as large polyhedral cells possessing a large, lightly staining, centrally placed nucleus. They display abundant cytoplasm and peripheral cytoplasmic extensions. In older pulps the number of undifferentiated mesenchymal cells diminishes, along with the number of other cells in the pulp core. This reduction, in association with other aging factors, reduces the regenerative potential of the pulp.

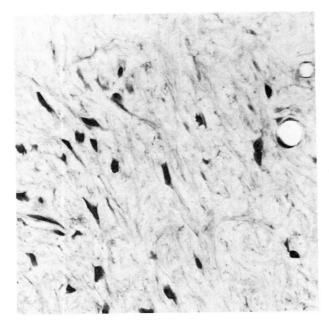

FIG. 10-42 Light microscopic appearance of fibroblasts in the dental pulp. Although in this H&E—stained section the extracellular compartment appears fibrous, the "fibers" are actually fine extensions of the cells. Compare with Figure 10-43.

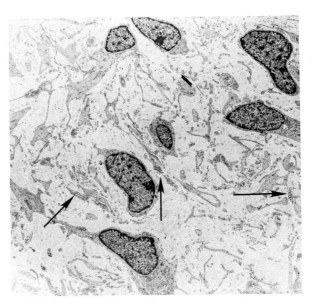

FIG. 10-43 Electron micrograph of the pulp from a mature tooth showing fibroblasts dispersed in an extracellular compartment of ground substance that contains only a few fine collagen fibrils *(arrows)*. Note the many cytoplasmic extensions of the fibroblasts.

Other Immunocompetent Cells

Apart from cells associated with neural and vascular elements, three other types of cells are considered to be normal residents of the dental pulp: the macrophage, a dendritic cell, and the lymphocyte. Monoclonal antibody labeling of normal human dental pulp has indicated that there are various subgroups of T lymphocytes associated with the immune defense system. B lymphocytes, which give rise to antibody-producing plasma cells, are not usually found in normal dental pulp. Monoclonal antibody labeling has also shown the presence of centrally located macrophages (histiocytes) and peripherally located dendritic cells (Fig. 10-44), whose function is similar to that of the Langerhans cell found in the epithelium (Chapter 18) (i.e., the capture and presentation of foreign antigen to the T cells). These cells are nonphagocytitic and participate in pulpal immunosurveillance.

The macrophages appear as large oval or spindle-shaped cells that, under the light microscope, exhibit a dark-staining cytoplasm with darker-staining nucleus. Occasionally, clear areas can be seen in the cytoplasm,

and electron microscopy has shown these to be large lysosomes. Pulp macrophages are involved in the elimination of dead cells, whose existence indicates turnover in the dental pulp. When inflammation occurs, the macrophages remove bacteria and interact with other inflammatory cells. They also present antigens to the lymphocytes. The dendritic and macrophage populations constitute some 8% of the total pulpal cell population, with dendritic cells exceeding macrophages in a 4:1 ratio.

Matrix

The extracellular compartment of the pulp, or matrix, consists of collagen fibers and ground substance.

Fibers

The fibers are principally type I and type III collagen in an approximate ratio of 55:45. This proportion appears to remain constant from the beginning of tooth development to tooth maturity and finding supports the idea that dentin collagen (type I) is an exclusive product of odontoblasts and not a combined product of odontoblasts and pulp fibroblasts.

In young pulps single fibrils of collagen are found scattered between the pulp cells. Whereas the overall collagen content of the pulp increases with age, the ratio between types I and III remains stable, and the increased amount of extracellular collagen is now organized into fiber bundles. The greatest concentration of collagen is generally seen in the most apical portion of the pulp. This fact is of practical significance when a pulpectomy is performed during the course of endodontic treatment. Engaging the pulp with a barbed broach in the region of the apex affords a better opportunity to remove the tissue intact than does engaging the broach more coronally, where the pulp is more gelatinous and liable to tear.

Ground substance

The ground substance of these tissues resembles that of any other loose connective tissue. Composed principally of glycosaminoglycans, glycoproteins, and water, it supports the cells and acts as the medium for transport of nutrients from the vasculature to the cells and of metabolites from the cells to the vasculature. Alterations in composition of the ground substance caused by age or disease interfere with this function, producing metabolic changes, reduced cellular function, and irregularities in mineral deposition.

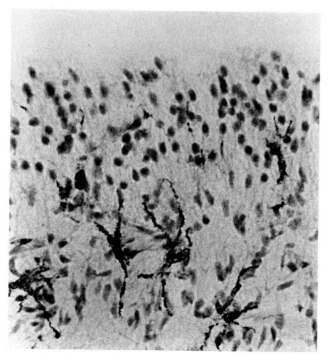

FIG. 10-44 Dendritic cells in the odontoblast layer. (Courtesy Dr. G. Bergenholtz.)

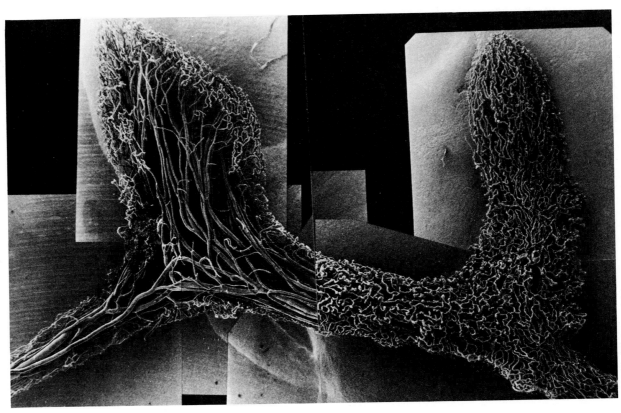

FIG. 10-45 Resin cast of the vasculature of a canine molar. At *right,* the peripheral vasculature can be seen. At *left* this has been removed to show the central pulp vessels and their peripheral ramifications. (Courtesy Dr. K. Takahashi.)

VASCULATURE AND LYMPHATIC SUPPLY

Blood vessels enter and exit the dental pulp by way of the apical and accessory foramina. One or sometimes two vessels of arteriolar size (150 μm) enter the apical foramen with the sensory and sympathetic nerve bundles. Smaller vessels, without any accompanying nerve bundle, enter the pulp through the minor foramina. Vessels leaving the dental pulp are closely associated with the arterioles and nerve bundles entering the apical foramen. Once the arterioles enter the pulp, there is an increase in the caliber of the lumen with a reduction in thickness of the vessel wall musculature. The arterioles occupy a central position within the pulp and, as they pass through the radicular portion of pulp, give off smaller lateral branches that extend toward and branch into the subodontoblastic area. The number of branches given off in this manner increases as the arterioles pass coronally, so that in the coronal region of the pulp they divide and subdivide to form an extensive vascular capillary network. Occasionally U-looping of pulpal arterioles is seen, and this anatomic configuration is thought to be related to the regulation of blood flow.

The extensive vascular network in the coronal portion of pulp can be demonstrated by special scanning electron microscopic techniques, by perfusion, or by microangiography (Fig. 10-45). The capillaries in the subodontoblastic area range from 4 to 8 μm, and the main portion of the capillary bed is located just below the odontoblasts. Some terminal capillary loops may extend upward between the odontoblasts to abut the predentin (Fig. 10-46). Unless dentinogenesis is occurring, the vascular flow in these peripheral capillaries is below their maximum capacity and is not readily seen under the light microscope. Fenestrations are sometimes found in the capillaries that form this bed, appearing as small pores within the wall of the capillary spanned by a thin diaphragm of plasma membrane. Such pores probably permit the rapid transfer of nutrient materials. The basement membrane about a capillary is continuous and intact. Located on the periphery of the capillaries at random intervals are pericytes (or Rouget's cells) whose cytoplasm forms a partial circumferential sheath about the endothelial wall. The function of these cells is controversial, but it is thought that they serve as contractile cells capable of reducing the size of the vessel lumen. Arteriovenous anastomoses have also been identified in the dental pulp. The anastomosis is of arteriolar size, with an endothelium composed of cuboid cells (Fig. 10-47) that project toward the lumen. Anastomoses are points of direct communication between the arterial and venous sides of the circulation and serve to divert blood away from the capillaries.

The efferent, or drainage, side of the circulation is composed of an extensive system of venules whose diameters are comparable to those of arterioles, but their walls are much thinner, making their lumina comparatively larger. The muscle layer in the venule walls is intermittent and thin.

Lymphatic vessels also occur in pulp tissue; they arise as small, blind, thin-walled vessels in the coronal region of the pulp (Fig. 10-48) and pass apically through the middle and radicular regions of the pulp to exit via one or two larger vesels through the apical foramen. The lymphatics are differentiated from small venules by the presence of discontinuities in their vessel walls and basement membranes (Fig. 10-49). Unlike the fenestrations in capillaries, these discontinuities are not covered by plasma membrane but represent actual openings between endothelial cell junctions resulting in communication between the vessel lumen and surrounding connective tissue. The lumen of lymphatic vessels is often wavy and displays multiple cytoplasmic projections that at times interdigitate to form intraparietal channels. The cytoplasm of the endothelial cells is rich in organelles and also contains Weibel-Palade granules. Such granules are found in endothelial cells lining vessels larger than capillaries and contain an agent (von Willebrand factor) that is essential in the hemostatic cascade.

This circulatory pattern establishes the tissue fluid pressure found in the extracellular compartment of the pulp.

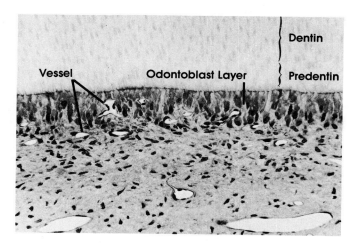

FIG. 10-46 Light photomicrograph of the odontoblast layer. This specimen was fixed by perfusion, which forced the vessels open to show their presence in the layer.

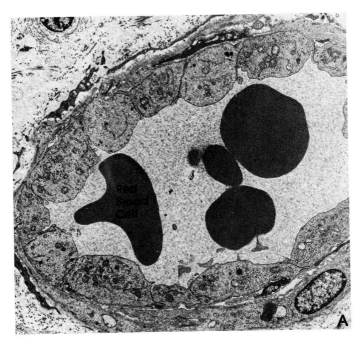

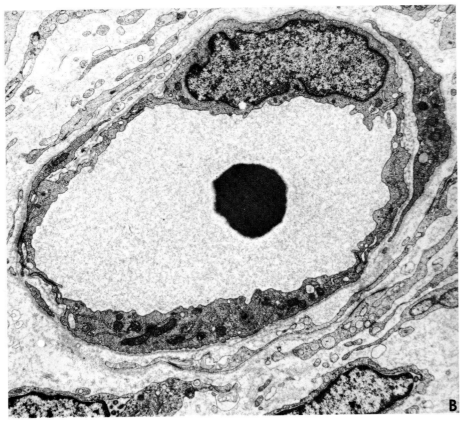

FIG. 10-47 Electron micrographs of an arteriovenous shunt in dental pulp. Such a shunt is characterized by a lining of cuboid endothelial cells, **A,** which contrasts with the flattened endothelial lining cells of venules, **B.**

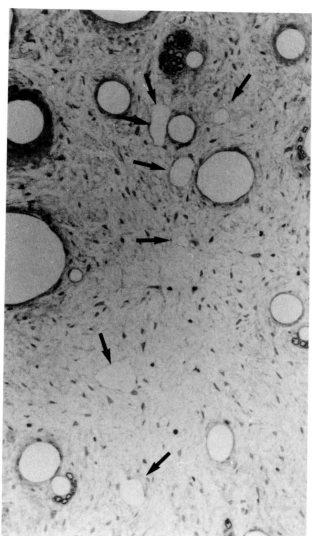

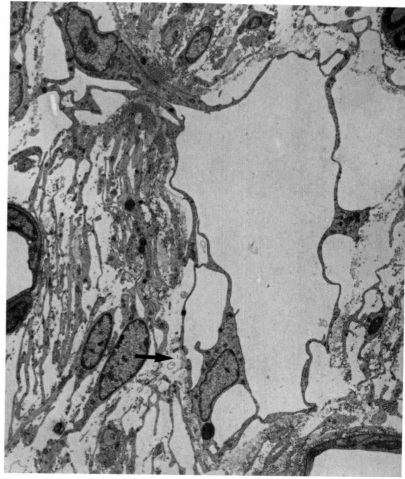

FIG. 10-48 Lymphatic vessels in the dental pulp *(arrow).* (From Bishop MA, Malhotra M: *Am J Anat* 187:247, 1990.)

FIG. 10-49 Higher magnification of pulpal lymphatic vessel. Direct communication to the extracellular space is indicated by the *arrow.* (From Bishop MA, Malhotra M: *Am J Anat* 187:247, 1990.)

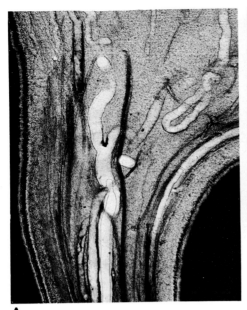

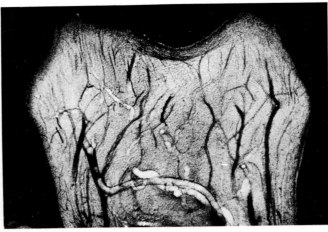

A

B

FIG. 10-50 Photomicrographs of a tooth. The general pattern of distribution of nerves and vessels in the root canal, **A,** and in the pulp chamber, **B,** can be seen. (From Bernick S: *Oral Surg* 33:983, 1972.)

INNERVATION OF THE DENTIN-PULP COMPLEX

The dental pulp is richly innervated (the mean number of fibers entering premolars being over 900). Nerves enter the pulp through the apical foramen, along with afferent blood vessels, and together form the neurovascular bundle. Once in the pulp chamber, the nerves generally follow the same course as the afferent vessels, beginning as large nerve bundles that arborize peripherally as they extend occlusally through the pulp core (Fig. 10-50). It has been estimated that each nerve fiber may provide at least eight terminal branches, which ultimately contribute to an extensive plexus of nerves in the cell-free zone just below the cell bodies of the odontoblasts in the crown portion of the tooth. This plexus of nerves is called the *subodontoblastic plexus of Raschkow* and can be demonstrated in silver-stained sections under the light microscope (Fig. 10-51) or by immunocytochemical techniques to disclose various proteins associated with nerves (e.g., nerve growth factor receptor) (Fig. 10-52).

The nerve bundles entering the tooth pulp consist principally of sensory afferents of the trigeminal (fifth cranial) nerve and sympathetic branches from the superior cervical ganglion. Each bundle contains both myelinated and unmyelinated axons (Fig. 10-53). The myelinated axons are classified according to their diameter and conduction velocities. The majority are Aδ fibers, which are fast conducting and have a diameter

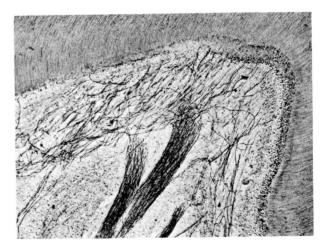

FIG. 10-51 Plexus of Raschkow in a silver-stained demineralized section. The ascending nerve trunks branch to form this plexus, which is situated beneath the odontoblast layer. (From Bernick S: In Finn SB [ed]: *Biology of the dental pulp organ,* Tuscaloosa, 1968, University of Alabama Press.)

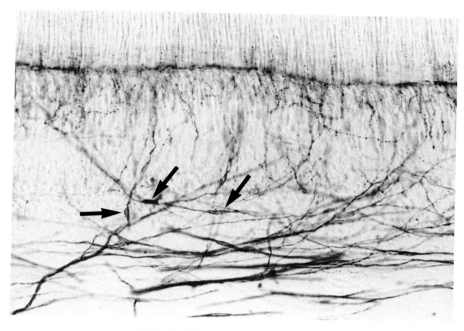

FIG. 10-52 Dentin innervation demonstrated by immunocytochemical staining of nerve growth factor receptor (NGFR). Note the presence of NGRF in some of the dentinal tubules. (From Maeda T, et al: *Proc Finn Dent Soc* 88(Suppl 1):557, 1992.)

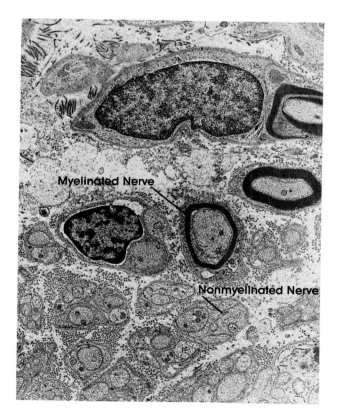

FIG. 10-53 Electron micrograph of a cross section of pulp showing a mixture of myelinated and nonmyelinated nerves.

in the range of 1 to 6 μm, but about 1% have diameters in the 6 to 12 μm range and are identified as Aβ fibers. Nonmyelinated fibers are designated as C fibers and have smaller diameters, in the range of 0.4 to 1.2 μm. In physiologic terms, it is thought that Aδ fibers are associated with the sharp localized pain experienced when dentin is first exposed whereas C fibers are associated with a dull and more diffuse pain. For many years it was thought that stimulation of the dentin-pulp complex initiated only a response appreciated as pain. There is now evidence that pulpal afferents can distinguish among mechanical, thermal, and tactile stimuli as well.

Fine structural investigations of animal tooth pulp have shown increased discontinuities in the investing perineurium as nerves ascend coronally. Furthermore, as the nerve bundles ascend coronally, the myelinated axons gradually lose their myelin coating so that there is a proportional increase in the number of unmyelinated axons in the more coronal aspect of the tooth.

Most of the nerve bundles terminate in the sub-odontoblastic plexus as free nerve endings. A small number of axons lose their Schwann cell coating and pass between the odontoblast cell bodies (sometimes occupying a groove on the surface of the cell) to enter the dentinal tubules (Fig. 10-52) in close approximation (20 nm) to the odontoblast process (Fig. 10-54). No organized junction or synaptic relationship has been noted between axons and the odontoblast process. Intratubular nerves characteristically contain neurofilaments, neurotubules, numerous mitochondria, and many small vesicular structures. These characteristics distinguish them from the odontoblast processes, which, although containing microfilaments and microtubules, do not contain mitochondria and accumulated

vesicles. The close relationship of these nerves to the odontoblast process is of considerable importance and will be discussed more fully in relation to dentin sensitivity. Intratubular nerve fibrils show significant regional differences in distribution. In human premolars it has been shown that in predentin, at the mineralizing front and in mineralized dentin covering the pulpal horns there are nerves in 27%, 11%, and 8% of the tubules respectively, indicating a significant reduction in tubular nerves within mineralized dentin. In coronal dentin not associated with the pulpal horns the figures were 14%, 6%, and 2%; and in root dentin no intratubular nerves were demonstrable although some were found at the pulpal face of predentin (Table 10-1).

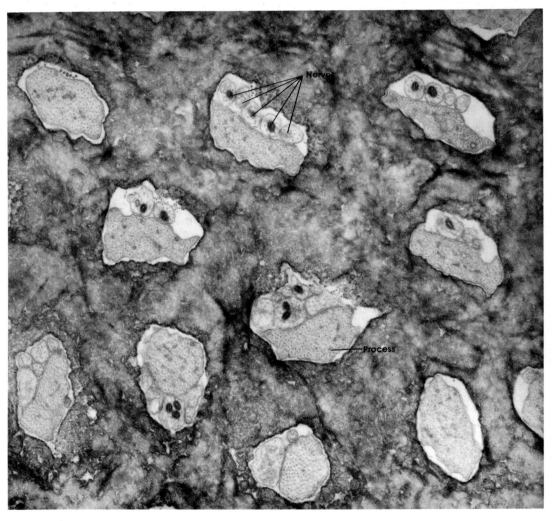

FIG. 10-54   Electron micrograph of pulpal horn dentin seen in cross section. Many of the tubules contain a process and multiple fine neural elements. (Courtesy Dr. R. Holland.)

The density of intratubular nerves also varies and can, in some instances, be as high as one for every two tubules in discrete areas of the coronal dentin (Fig. 10-54). Even so and even if they extend deeper into dentin, the number of tubules containing nerve fibers in relation to the overall number of tubules is small. The literature also contains persistent reports of nerves running within predentin at right angles to the tubules, and it is generally assumed that such loops represent isolated nerve fibrils from the plexus of Rashkow caught up by the advancing process of dentinogenesis (Fig. 10-55). There is a suggestion, however, that this description is too simplified; recent studies examining tangential sections of predentin have indicated that some of these fibers undergo dendritic ramification, which, it has been estimated, permit one nerve fiber entering the predentin to serve an area of 100,000 μm^2 (Fig. 10-56). The functional significance, if any, of this pattern of innervation within the predentin has not been determined. If the pulp is the primary target for pioneer nerve fibers entering the dental papilla, the anatomy of the pulp chamber might explain the pattern of dentin innervation. Growing nerve fibers meeting an obstruction will retract, which would explain the development of the plexus of Raschkow. Nevertheless, some growing nerve fibers approaching the predentin might, by chance, abut against the opening of the dentinal tubule and pass into its lumen between the tubule wall and the odontoblast process. It is then easy to imagine such a growing tip pushing its way along the tubule until it met the surface of the intratubular dentin, at which point further extension would be restricted. This may explain why intratubular nerves are found only for a limited distance within the dentin, why only a portion of tubules contain them (their distribution depending on chance), and why this pattern of neural distribution is not linked to the phenomenon of dentin sensitivity.

TABLE 10-1	Distribution of intratubular nerves		
Location	**Predentin (%)**	**Mineralizing front (%)**	**Dentin to 100 μm (%)**
Pulp horns*	27	11	8
Remaining crown	14	6	2
Root	11	0	0

*Small areas of predentin showed a high density of innervation (as many as every second process could be accompanied by a nerve process).
Data from Lilja J: *Acta Odontol Scand* 37:3346, 1979.

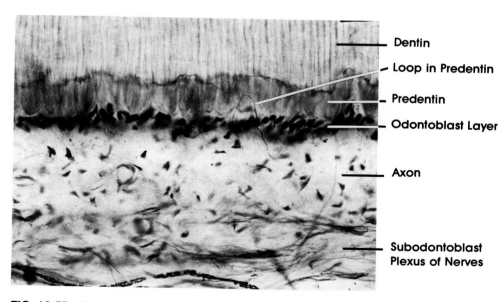

FIG. 10-55 Nerve fibril arising from the plexus of Raschkow. It is shown passing between the odontoblasts and looping within the predentin. (From Bernick S: In Finn SB [ed]: *Biology of the dental pulp organ,* Tuscaloosa, 1968, University of Alabama Press.)

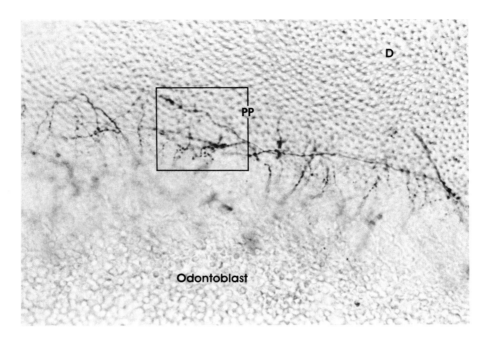

FIG. 10-56 Nerve demonstrated by staining for NGFR in a tangential section of pre-dentin. Note its extensive ramification. (See also Fig. 10-26.) (From Maeda T: *Proc Finn Dent Soc* 88[Suppl 1]:557, 1992.)

DENTIN SENSITIVITY

One of the most unusual features of the pulp-dentin complex is its sensitivity. Why this complex should be so sensitive is difficult to explain, because it provides no apparent evolutionary benefit. The overwhelming sensation appreciated by this complex is pain. Convergence of pulpal afferents with other pulpal afferents and afferents from other orofacial structures often makes pulpal pain difficult to localize.

Numerous stimuli can evoke a painful response when applied to dentin—including many that are related to clinical dental practice—such as thermal change from an air-water spray, mechanical contact by a probe or bur and dehydration with cotton wool or a stream of air.

Dentin is not uniformly sensitive. It is known, for example, to be more sensitive at the dentinoenamel junction, and it is also quite sensitive close to the pulp; overall, its sensitivity is increased when supported by an inflamed pulp.

Three mechanisms might be used to explain dentin sensitivity, all involving an understanding of the structure of dentin and pulp: (1) the dentin contains nerve endings that respond when it is stimulated; (2) the odontoblasts serve as receptors and are coupled to nerves in the pulp; (3) the tubular nature of dentin permits fluid movement to occur within the tubule when a stimulus is applied—a movement registered by pulpal free nerve endings close to the dentin (Fig. 10-57).

There is no debate that the pulp is well innervated, especially below the odontoblasts (the plexus of Raschkow). Nor is there any dispute that some nerves penetrate a short distance into tubules in human teeth. Where there is question, however, is whether these intratubular nerves are involved in dentin sensitivity. No satisfactory evidence has been found that nerves exist in the outer dentin, which is reputedly the most sensitive. Development studies have shown that the plexus of Raschkow and the intratubular nerves do not establish themselves until some time after the tooth has erupted; yet newly erupted teeth are sensitive. In addition, the application of local anesthetics or silver nitrate (a protein precipitant) to exposed dentin does not eliminate dentin sensitivity; and pharmacologic agents that cause pain when applied to skin do not do so when applied to dentin.

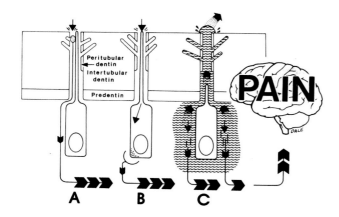

FIG. 10-57 Three theories of dentin sensitivity. **A** suggests that the dentin is directly innervated. **B** suggests that the odontoblast acts as a receptor. **C** suggests that the receptors are in the pulp and are stimulated by fluid movement through the tubules.

The structural features of intratubular nerves, especially their content of mitochondria and numerous microvesicles, might suggest that these nerves in some way control the activity of odontoblasts rather than monitor a change in the environment. The reason for this assumption is that similar features are found in the synapse (i.e., the transmitter half of the synaptic complex), but it has also been reported that some free sensory nerve endings in the buccal mucosa have mitochondria and vesicles in their terminal axoplasm. Cutting the inferior alveolar nerve does not cause all these nerves to degenerate, which means that either there is collateral innervation of the pulp or the nerves are autonomic in origin; however, the effect of these nerves on odontoblast function is not understood, since inferior alveolar nerve resection has also had no effect on dentin formation. At present, all that can be stated is that there are some nerves within some tubules in the inner dentin but dentin sensitivity does not depend solely, if at all, on the stimulation of such nerve endings.

The second mechanism proposed to explain dentin sensitivity, hydrodynamic involves movement of fluid through the dentinal tubules. This theory, which fits much of the experimental and morphologic data, proposes that fluid movement through the tubule distorts the local pulpal environment and is sensed by the free nerve endings in the plexus of Raschkow. Thus, when dentin is first exposed, small blebs of fluid can be seen on the cavity floor. When the cavity is dried with air or cotton wool, a greater loss of fluid is induced, leading to more movement and a further painful experience. The increased sensitivity at the dentinoenamel junction is explained by the profuse branching of the tubules in this region. The hydrodynamic hypothesis also explains why local anesthetics fail to block dentin sensitivity and why pain is produced by thermal change, mechanical probing, hypertonic solutions, and dehydration.

The third possible mechanism to explain dentin sensitivity considers the odontoblast to be a receptor cell. This attractive concept has been considered, abandoned, and reconsidered for many reasons. It was once argued that because the odontoblast is of neural crest origin it retains an ability to transduce and propagate an impulse. What was missing was the demonstration of a synaptic relationship between the odontoblast and pulpal nerves. That the membrane potential of odontoblasts measured in vitro is too low to permit transduction and that local anesthetics and protein precipitants do not abolish sensitivity also militated against this concept. When it was thought that the odontoblast process probably does not extend much further than a third of the way through dentin, this explanation of dentin sensitivity was largely abandoned. The possibility that the odontoblast process extends to the dentinoenamel junction and the demonstration of gap junctions between odontoblasts (and possibly between odontoblasts and pulpal nerves), combined with the knowledge that such junctions permit electronic coupling, have revived interest in the probability that the odontoblast plays a direct role in dentin sensitivity.

Attention must be drawn, however, to the fact that dentin sensitivity bestows no benefit on the organism; also the possibility must be recognized that this sensitivity is secondary to other functional requirements of the innervated dentin-pulp complex. For instance, sensory nerves contain a number of neuropeptides that are released when nerves are stimulated. Most notable are substance P, calcitonin, gene-related peptide, and nerve growth factor. These substances, when released, are thought to play an important role in the vascular and neural responses of pulp tissue following injury and possibly odontoblastic activity.

PULP STONES

Pulp stones, or denticles, are frequently found in pulp tissue (Fig. 10-58). As their name implies, they are discrete calcified masses. They may be singular or multiple in any tooth and are found more frequently at the orifice of the pulp chamber or within the root canal. Histologically they usually consist of concentric layers of mineralized tissue formed by surface accretion around blood thrombi, dying or dead cells, or collagen fibers. Occasionally, a pulp stone may be found that contains tubules and is surrounded by cells resembling odontoblasts. Such stones are rare and, if seen, occur close to the apex of the tooth.

Pulp stones may form in several teeth, and indeed in every tooth in some individuals, an indication that their existence may be genetically controlled. If during the formation of a pulp stone union occurs between it and the dentin wall, or if secondary dentin deposition surrounds the stone, it is termed an attached stone, as distinguished from a free stone (which is completely surrounded by soft tissue). The presence of pulp stones is significant in that they reduce the overall number of cells within the pulp and act as an impediment to debridement and enlargement of the root canal system during endodontic treatment. Attempts have been made to correlate the presence of pulp stones with pulpal pain, but so far no positive results have been achieved. The pain noted clinically when a pulp stone is present can generally be attributed to other factors.

AGE CHANGES

The dentin-pulp complex, as all body tissues, undergoes change with time. The most conspicuous change is decreasing volume of the pulp chamber and root canal brought about by continued dentin deposition (Fig. 10-59). In old teeth the root canal is often no more than a thin channel (Fig. 10-60), and indeed it can on occasion appear to be almost completely obliterated. Such continued restriction in pulp volume probably brings about a reduction in the vascular supply to the pulp and initiates many of the other age changes found in this issue.

From about the age of 20 years cells gradually decrease in number until age 70, when the cell density has decreased by about half. Whereas it was once believed that the collagen content of the pulp increased with age, recent investigations have proven that subsequent to the period of tooth eruption and root formation, when there is a slight decrease in collagen synthesis in the dental pulp, no significant change occurs in pulp collagen content associated with aging. In the absence of disease, stabilization of collagen content is the result of diminished collagen synthesis and a lowered rate of collagen degradation.

With age there is both a loss and a degeneration of myelinated and unmyelinated axons that correlates with an age-related reduction in sensitivity.

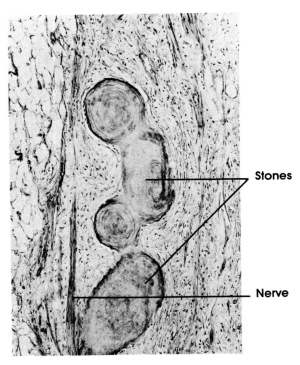

FIG. 10-58 Pulp stones in an aged dental pulp.

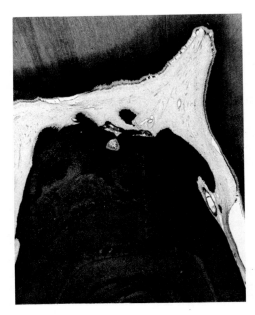

FIG. 10-59 Decreased pulp volume with age. The pulp has been considerably reduced by the continued deposition of dentin on the pulp chamber floor. (From Bernick S, Nedelman CJ: *J Endod* 1:88, 1975; copyright The American Dental Association.)

A further age change is the occurrence of irregular areas of dystrophic calcification, especially in the central pulp. If such areas reach any size, they are known as false pulp stones (Fig. 10-61). Dystrophic calcification may occur in a concentric or linear pattern.

Some histologic changes in the pulp reported to take place with age, however, should be treated cautiously since they may be the result of poor tissue fixation. As the apical foramen decreases in width, adequate fixation of pulpal tissue becomes progressively more difficult to ensure. Thus such changes as vacuolation within the odontoblast layer and clumping (or "wheat sheafing") of the odontoblasts reported in older teeth are probably the result of inadequate fixation.

It has been emphasized that the pulp supports the dentin and that age changes within the pulp are reflected in the dentin. Within dentin there is the continued deposition of intratubular dentin, resulting in a gradual reduction of the tubule diameter. This continued deposition often leads to complete closure of the tubule, as can be readily seen in a ground section of dentin, because the dentin becomes translucent (or sclerotic). Sclerotic dentin is frequently found near the root apex in teeth from middle-aged individuals (Fig. 10-12). Associated with this is an increased brittleness and a decreased permeability of the dentin. Dye introduced into the pulp chamber of a young tooth spreads to reach the dentinoenamel junction. In an older tooth the dye does not spread, indicating that the possibility of bringing about changes within the enamel through the pulp decreases with age.

Another age change found within dentin is the occurrence of dead tracts (Fig. 10-62). Dentinal tubules are, on occasion, emptied either by complete retraction of the odontoblast process from the tubule or through death of the odontoblast. The dentinal tubules then become sealed off so that in a ground section air-filled tubules appear by transmitted light as (black) "dead tracts." Dead tracts occur most often in coronal dentin and are frequently bound by bands of sclerotic dentin.

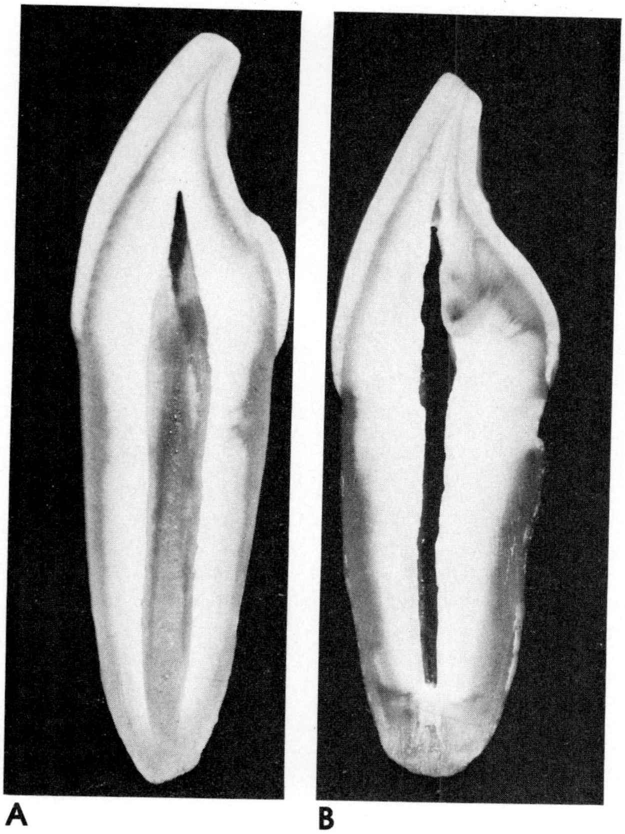

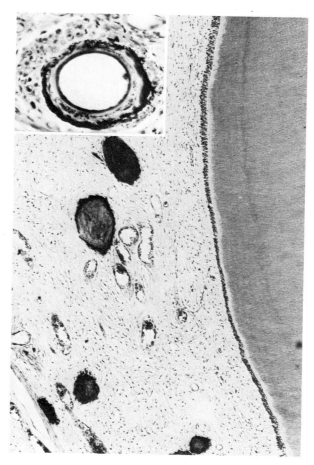

FIG. 10-61 Dystrophic calcification in the center of the pulp chamber. (*Inset:* Dystrophic calcification beginning in a vessel wall.) (From Bernick S: *J Dent Res* 46:544, 1967.)

FIG. 10-60 Difference in pulp volume between halves of a young tooth, **A,** and an old tooth, **B.**

A   B

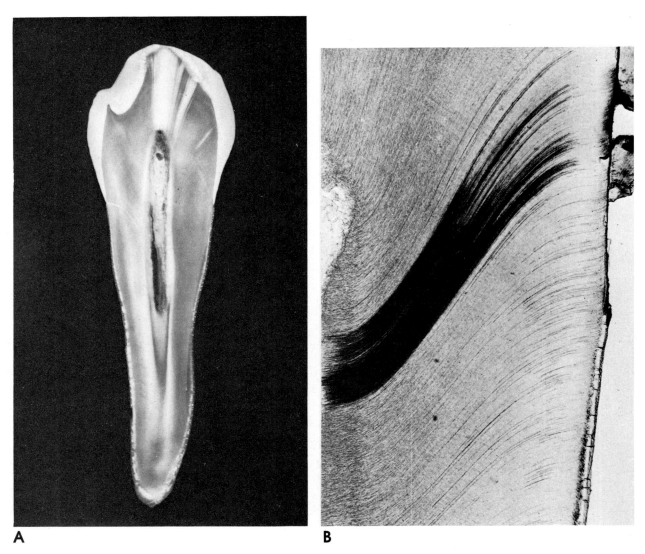

FIG. 10-62   Dead tracts in a ground section of dentin. **A,** Under incident illumination the tracts appear white because light is reflected. **B,** Under transmitted illumination the tracts appear dark because air in them refracts the light.

RESPONSE TO ENVIRONMENTAL STIMULI

Many of the age changes occurring in the pulp-dentin complex render it more resistant to environmental injury. For example, the spread of caries is slowed by tubule occlusion. Age changes are also accelerated in response to environmental stimuli, such as caries or attrition of enamel. The response of the complex to gradual attrition is to produce more sclerotic dentin and deposit secondary dentin at an increased rate. If the stimulus is more severe, tertiary dentin is formed at the ends of the tubules affected by the injury.

Age change, however, also lessens the ability of the pulp-dentin complex to repair itself. Injury has been defined as the interference of a stimulus with cellular metabolism. If pulpal injury occurs, the age of the pulp very much determines its ability to repair the damage. Because cell metabolism is high in young pulps, their cells are prone to injury, which is manifested as altered cell function; but recovery occurs rapidly. An example is the physiologic injury resulting from changes at birth. The odontoblasts are injured and respond by forming, for a brief time, altered dentin, which is seen in sections as the neonatal line. If injury is such that the odontoblasts are destroyed, the possibility exists in young pulps for the differentiation of new odontoblasts from the mesenchymal cells of the pulp and the formation of repair dentin. This potential is considerably reduced with age.

At the beginning of this chapter it was stressed that pulp and dentin should be considered as the same connective tissue. When a clinical procedure on a tooth is undertaken, it must be remembered that cutting enamel and exposing dentin are similar to cutting the skin and exposing the dermis. Only because dental procedures are usually performed with the patient under local anesthesia and because no hemorrhage occurs is cavity preparation regarded by many as a nonsurgical procedure.

BIBLIOGRAPHY

Amerongen JP, van Lemmens IG, Tonino GJM: The concentration, extractibility, and characterization of collagen in human dental pulp, *Arch Oral Biol* 28:339, 1983.

Anderson DJ, Matthews B, Gorretta C: Fluid flow through human dentine, *Arch Oral Biol* 12:209, 1967.

Anderson DJ, Ronning GA: Dye diffusion in human dentine, *Arch Oral Biol* 7:505, 1962.

Anderson DJ, Ronning GA: Osmotic excitants of pain in human dentine, *Arch Oral Biol* 7:513, 1962.

Arwill T: Studies on the ultrastructure of dental tissues. II. The predentine-pulpal border zone, *Odontol Rev* 18:191, 1967.

Arwill T, Edwall L, Lilja J, et al: Ultrastructure of nerves in the dentinal-pulp border zone after sensory and autonomic nerve transection in the cat, *Acta Odontol Scand* 31:273, 1973.

Baume LJ: Dental pulp conditions in relation to carious lesions, *Int Dent J* 20:309, 1970.

Beasley WL, Holland GR: A quantitative analysis of the innervation of the pulp of the cat's canine tooth, *J Comp Neurol* 178:487, 1978.

Bernick S: Innervation of the human tooth, *Anat Rec* 101:81, 1948.

Bernick S: Age changes in the blood supply to human teeth, *J Dent Res* 46:544, 1967.

Bernick S: Effect of aging on the nerve supply to human teeth, *J Dent Res* 46:694, 1967.

Bernick S: Morphological changes in lymphatic vessels in pulpal inflammation, *J Dent Res* 56:841, 1977.

Bernick S, Patek PR: Lymphatic vessels of the dental pulp in dogs, *J Dent Res* 48:959, 1969.

Bevelander G, Nakahara H: The formation and mineralization of dentin, *Anat Rec* 156:303, 1966.

Bhussry BR: Modification of the dental pulp organ during development and aging. In Finn SB (ed): *Biology of the dental pulp organ: a symposium*, Tuscaloosa, 1968, University of Alabama Press.

Bishop MA: A fine-structural investigation of the extent of perineurial investment of the nerve supply to the pulp in rat molar teeth, *Arch Oral Biol* 27:225, 1982.

Bishop MA, Malhotra M: An investigation of lymphatic vessels in the feline dental pulp, *Am J Anat* 187: 247, 1990.

Bishop MA, Yoshida S: A permeability barrier to Lanthanum and the pressure of collagen between odontoblasts in pig molars, *J Anat* 181:29, 1992.

Blake GC: The peritubular translucent zones in human dentine, *Br Dent J* 104:57, 1958.

Boyde A, Lester KS: An electron microscope study of fractured dentinal surfaces, *Calcif Tissue Res* 1:122, 1966.

Bradford EW: The interpretation of decalcified sections of human dentine, *Br Dent J* 98:153, 1955.

Bradford EW: The maturation of the dentine, *Br Dent J* 105:212, 1958.

Bradford EW: The dentine, a barrier to caries, *Br Dent J* 109:387, 1960.

Bradford EW: Microanatomy and histochemistry of dentine. In Miles AEW (ed): *Structural and chemical organization of teeth*, New York, 1967, Academic Press.

Brännström M: Sensitivity of dentine, *Oral Surg* 21:517, 1966.

Brännström M, Aström A: The hydrodynamics of the dentine: its possible relationship to dentinal pain, *Int Dent J* 22:219, 1972.

Brännström M, Garberoglio R: The dentinal tubules and the odontoblast processes: a scanning electron microscopic study, *Acta Odontol Scand* 30:291, 1972.

Brännström M, Johnson G: Movements of the dentine and pulp liquids on application of thermal stimuli: an in vitro study, *Acta Odontol Scand* 28:59, 1970.

Brännström M, Johnson G, Linden LA: Fluid flow and pain response in the dentine produced by hydrostatic pressure, *Odontol Rev* 20:1, 1969.

Brännström M, Lind PO: Pulpal response to early dental caries, *J Dent Res* 44:1045, 1965.

Brännström M, Linden LA, Johnson G: Movement of dentinal and pulpal fluid caused by clinical procedures, *J Dent Res* 47:679, 1968.

Bueltmann KW, Karlsson UL, Edie J: Quantitative ultrastructure of intradental nerve fibres in marmosets, *Arch Oral Biol* 17:645, 1972.

Byers MR: Development of sensory innervation in dentin, *J Comp Neurol* 191:413, 1980.

Byers M, Dong WK: Autoradiographic location of sensory nerve endings in dentin of monkey teeth, *Anat Rec* 205:441, 1983.

Byers MR, Neuhaus SJ, Gehrig JD: Dental sensory receptors structure in human teeth, *Pain* 13:221, 1982.

Calle A: Intercellular junctions between human odonto-b lasts, *Acta Anat* 122:138, 1985.

Chiego DJ, Cox CF, Avery JK: H^{3}HRP analysis of the nerve supply to primate teeth, *J Dent Res* 59:736, 1980.

Coffey CT, Ingram MJ, Bjorndal A: An analysis of human dentinal fluid, *Oral Surg* 30:835, 1970.

Corpron RE, Avery JK: The ultrastructure of intradental nerves in developing mouse molars, *Anat Rec* 175:585, 1973.

Corpron RE, Avery JK, Lee SD: Ultrastructure of terminal pulpal blood vessels in mouse molars, *Anat Rec* 179:527, 1974.

Couve E: Ultrastructural changes during the life cycle of human odontoblasts, *Arch Oral Biol* 31:643, 1986.

Dahl E, Mjör IA: The fine structure of the vessels in the human dental pulp, *Acta Odontol Scand* 31:223, 1973.

Dai XF, Ten Cate AR, Limeback H: The extent and distribution of intratubular collagen fibrils in human dentine, *Arch Oral Biol* 36:775, 1991.

Darvel BW: Effect of dentin thickness on pulpal changes beneath restorative materials, *Aust Dent J* 26:80, 1981.

Diamond RD, Stanley HR, Swerdlow H: Reparative dentin formation resulting from cavity preparation, *J Prosthet Dent* 16:1127, 1966.

Ekblom A, Hansson P: A thin-section and freeze-fracture study of the pulp blood vessels in feline and human teeth, *Arch Oral Biol* 29:413, 1984.

Fearnhead RW: Histological evidence for the innervation of human dentine, *J Anat* 91:267, 1957.

Fearnhead RW: The histological demonstration of nerve fibers in human dentin. In Anderson DJ (ed): *Sensory mechanisms in dentin*, New York, 1963, Pergamon Press.

Finn SB (ed): *Biology of the dental pulp organ: a symposium*, Tuscaloosa, 1968, University of Alabama Press.

Frank RM: Electron microscopy of undecalcified sections of human adult dentine, *Arch Oral Biol* 1:29, 1959.

Frank RM: Étude au microscope électronique de l'odontoblaste et du canalicule dentaire humain, *Arch Oral Biol* 11:179, 1966.

Frank RM: Attachment sites between the odontoblast process and the intradentinal nerve fibre, *Arch Oral Biol* 13:833, 1968.

Frank RM, Steuer P: Transmission electron microscopy of the human odontoblast process in peripheral root dentine, *Arch Oral Biol* 33:91, 1988.

Fried K: Development, degeneration and regeneration of nerve fibres in the feline inferior alveolar nerve and mandibular incisor pulps, *Acta Physiol Scand Suppl* 504:1, 1982.

Fried K, Hildebrand C: Pulpal axons in developing, mature, and aging feline permanent incisors; a study by electron microscopy, *J Comp Neurol* 203:23, 1981.

Furseth R, Mjör I: Electron microscopy of human coronal dentine: a methodological study with emphasis on the "aspiration" of odontoblast nuclei, *Acta Odontol Scand* 27:577, 1969.

Garant PR, Zabo G, Nalbandian J: The fine structure of the mouse odontoblast, *Arch Oral Biol* 13:857, 1968.

Garberoglio R, Brännström M: Scanning electron microscopic investigation of human dentinal tubules, *Arch Oral Biol* 21:355, 1976.

Gotjamanos T: Cellular organization in the subodontoblastic zone of the dental pulp. I. A study of cellfree and cell-rich layers in pulps of adult rat and deciduous monkey teeth, *Arch Oral Biol* 14:1007, 1969.

Gotjamanos T: Cellular organization in the subodontoblastic zone of the dental pulp. II. Period and mode of development of the cell-rich layer in rat molar pulps, *Arch Oral Biol* 14:1011, 1969.

Gotjamanos T, Swedlow D: Scanning electron microscopy of human dental pulp, *Arch Oral Biol* 19:549, 1974.

Graf W, Björlin G: Diameters of nerve fibers in human tooth pulps, *J Am Dent Assoc* 43:186, 1951.

Green DA: Stereoscopic study of the root apices of 400 maxillary and mandibular anterior teeth, *Oral Surg* 9:1224, 1956.

Griffin CJ, Harris R: Ultrastructure of collagen fibrils and fibroblasts of the developing human dental pulp, *Arch Oral Biol* 11:659, 1966.

Griffin CJ, Harris R: The ultrastructure of the blood vessels of the human dental pulp following injury. I to IV, *Aust Dent J* 17:303, 355, 441, 1972; 18:88, 1973.

Grunji T, Kobayashi S: Distribution and organization of odontoblast processes in human dentin, *Arch Histol Jpn* 46:213, 1983.

Gustafson G: Age determinations on teeth, *J Am Dent Assoc* 41:45, 1950.

Gvozdenovic-Sedlecki S, Qvist V, Hansen HP: Histologic variations in the pulp of intact premolars from young individuals, *Scand J Dent Res* 81:433, 1973.

Harcourt JK: Further observations on the peritubular translucent zone in human dentine, *Aust Dent J* 9:387, 1964.

Harris R, Griffin CJ: Histogenesis of fibroblasts in the human dental pulp, *Arch Oral Biol* 12:459, 1967.

Harris R, Griffin CJ: Fine structure of nerve endings in the human dental pulp, *Arch Oral Biol* 13:773, 1968.

Harris R, Griffin CJ: The fine structure of the mature odontoblasts and cell rich zone of the human dental pulp, *Aust Dent J* 14:168, 1969.

Harrop TJ, MacKay B: Electron microscopic observations on healing in the dental pulp in the rat, *Arch Oral Biol* 13:365, 1968.

Hasty DL: Freeze-fracture indices of neonatal mouse incisors, *Anat Rec* 205:405, 1983.

Herold RC, Kaye H: Mitochondria in odontoblastic processes, *Nature* 210:108, 1966.

Herr P, Holz J, Baume LJ: Mantle dentine in man: a quantitative microradiographic study, *J Biol Buccale* 14:139, 1986.

Holland GR: The dentinal tubule and odontoblast process in the cat, *J Anat* 120:169, 1975.

Holland GR: The extent of the odontoblast process in the cat, *J Anat* 121:133, 1976.

Holland GR: Odontoblasts and nerves: just friends, *Proc Finn Dent Soc* 82:179, 1986.

Holland GR, Robinson PP: The number and size of axons at the apex of the cat's canine tooth, *Anat Rec* 205:215, 1983.

Isokawa S, Toda Y, Kubota K: A scanning electron microscopic observation by etched human peritubular dentin, *Arch Oral Biol* 15:1303, 1970.

Isokawa S, Yoshida M, Komura A, Iwatake Y: A preliminary study on the peritubular structure of human dentinal tubules by scanning electron microscopy, *Nihon Univ Sch Dent* 14:122, 1972.

Jacoby BH, et al: An ultrastructural and immunohistochemical study of human dental pulp: identification of Weibel-Palade bodies and von Willebrand factor in pulp endothelial cells, *J Endod* 17:150, 1991.

Johansen E: Ultrastructure of dentine. In Miles AEW (ed) *Structural and chemical organization of teeth*, New York, 1967, Academic Press.

Johansen E, Parks HF: Electron microscopic observations on sound human dentine, *Arch Oral Biol* 7:185, 1962.

Johnsen DC, Harshburger J: Unmyelinated axon networks in most portions of human primary canines, *Neurosci Lett* 6:311, 1977.

Johnsen DC, Harshburger J, Rymer HD: Quantitative assessment of neural development in human premolars, *Anat Rec* 205:421, 1983.

Johnsen D, Johns S: Quantitation of nerve fibres in the primary and permanent canine and incisor teeth in man, *Arch Oral Biol* 23:825-829, 1978.

Johnsen DC, Karlsson UL: Electron microscopic quantitations of feline primary and permanent incisor innervation, *Arch Oral Biol* 19:671, 1974.

Johnsen DC, Karlsson UL: Development of neural elements in apical portions of cat primary and permanent incisor pulps, *Anat Rec* 189:29, 1977.

Johnson, G, Brännström M: Pain reaction to cold stimulus in teeth with experimental fillings, *Acta Odontol Scand* 29:639, 1971.

Johnson G, Brännström M: The sensitivity of dentin changes in relation to conditions at exposed tubule apertures, *Acta Odontol Scand* 32:29, 1974.

Johnson WT, Johnson GK: The effect of inferior alveolar nerve resection on dentin formation, *Oral Surg* 64:212, 1987.

Jontell M, Bergenholtz G, Scheynius A, Ambrose W: Dendritic cells and macrophages expressing class II antigens in the normal rat incisor pulp, *J Dent Res* 67:1263, 1988.

Jontell M, Gunraj MN, Bergenholtz G: Immunocompetent cells in the normal dental pulp, *J Dent Res* 66:1149, 1987.

Kawasaki K: On the configuration of incremental lines in human dentine as revealed by tetracycline labeling, *J Anat* 119:61, 1975.

Kaye H, Herold RC: Structure of human dentine. I. Phase contrast, polarization, interference, and bright field microscopic observations on the lateral branch system, *Arch Oral Biol* 11:355, 1966.

Kelly KW, Bergenholtz F, Cox CF: The extent of the odontoblast process in rhesus monkeys *(Macaca mulatta)* as observed by scanning electron microscopy, *Arch Oral Biol* 26:893, 1981.

Koling A: Freeze-fractured electron microscopy of the nuclear envelope of the human odontoblast, *Arch Oral Biol* 30:691, 1985.

Koling A: Freeze-fracture electron microscopy of simultaneous odontoblast exocytosis and endocytosis in human permanent teeth, *Arch Oral Biol* 32:153, 1987.

Koling A, Rask-Andersen H: Membrane junctions in the subodontoblastic region, *Acta Odontol Scand* 41:99, 1983.

Koling A, Rask-Andersen H: Membrane junctions between odontoblasts and associated cells, *Acta Odontol Scand* 42:13, 1984.

Kramer IRH: The distribution of collagen fibrils in the dentine matrix, *Br Dent J* 91:1, 1951.

Kutter Y: Microscopic investigation of root apexes, *J Am Dent Assoc* 50:544, 1955.

La Fleche RG, Frank RM, Steuer P: The extent of the human odontoblast process, as determined by transmission electron microscopy: the hypothesis of a retractable suspensor system, *J Biol Buccale* 13:293, 1985.

Lechner JH, Kalinsky G: The presence of large amounts of Type III collagen in bovine dental pulp and its significance with regard to the mechanism of dentinogenesis, *Arch Oral Biol* 26:265, 1981.

Lester KS, Boyde A: The surface morphology of some crystalline components of dentine. In Symons NB (ed): *Dentine and pulp: a symposium*, Baltimore, 1968, Williams & Wilkins.

Lilja T: Innervation of different parts of predentin and dentin in young human premolars, *Acta Odontol Scand* 37:339, 1979.

Linde A: *Dentin and dentinogenesis*, Boca Raton Fla, 1984, CRC Press, vols I and II.

Linden LA, Brännström M: Fluid movements in dentine and pulp: an in vitro study of flow produced by chemical solutions on exposed dentine, *Odontol Rev* 18:227, 1967.

Maeda T, Iwanaga T, Fujita T, et al: Immunohistochemical demonstration of nerves in the predentin and dentin of human third molars with the use of an antiserum against neurofilament protein (NFP), *Cell Tissue Res* 243:469, 1986.

Magloire H, Dumont J: Étude ultrastructurale de cellules pulpaires humaines cultivées "in vitro," *J Biol Buccale* 4:3, 1976.

Maniatopoulas C, Smith DC: A scanning electron microscopic study of the odontoblast process in human coronal dentin, *Arch Oral Biol* 28:701, 1983.

Marchetti C, Poggi P, Calligaro A, Casasco A: Lymphatic vessels of the human dental pulp in different conditions, *Anat Rec* 234:27, 1992.

Martens PJ, Bradford EW, Frank RM: Tissue changes in dentine, *Int Dent J* 9:330, 1959.

Matysiak M, Dubois JP, Ducastelle T, et al: Analyse morphométrique des fibres myéliniques pulpaires humaines au cours du vieillissement, *J Biol Buccale* 14:69, 1986.

McWalter GM, El-Kafrany AH, Mitchell DF: Rate of reparative dentinogenesis under a pulp-capping agent in monkeys, *J Dent Res* 56:93, 1977.

Mendis BRRM, Darling AI: Distribution with age and attrition of peritubular dentin in the crowns of human teeth, *Arch Oral Biol* 24:131, 1979.

Miller WA, Eick JD, Neiders ME: Inorganic components of the peritubular dentin in young human permanent teeth, *Caries Res* 5:264, 1971.

Mjör IA: Human coronal dentine: structure and reactions, *Oral Surg* 33:810, 1972.

Mjör IA, Karlsen K: The interface between dentine and irregular secondary dentine, *Acta Odontol Scand* 28:363, 1970.

Nalbandian J, Gonzales F, Sognnaes RF: Sclerotic age changes in root dentin of human teeth as observed by optical, electron, and x-ray microscopy, *J Dent Res* 39:598, 1960.

Narhi MVO: The characteristics of intradental sensory units and their responses to stimulation, *J Dent Res* 64:564, 1985.

Narhi MVO, Hirvouen TJ, Hakumaki MOK: Activation of intradental nerves in the dog to some stimuli applied to dentin, *Arch Oral Biol* 27:1053, 1982.

Närhi M, Jyväsjärvi E, Hirvonen T, et al: Activation of heat-sensitive nerve fibres in the dental pulp of the cat, *Pain* 14:317, 1982.

Nielson CJ, Bentley JP, Marshall FJ: Age-related changes in reducible crosslinks of human dental pulp collagen, *Arch Oral Biol* 28:759, 1983.

Nihei I: A study on the hardness of human teeth, *J Osaka Univ Dent Soc* 4:1, 1959.

Nitzan DW, Michaeli Y, Weinreb M, Azaz B: The effect of aging on tooth morphology: a study on impacted teeth, *Oral Surg* 61:54, 1986.

Okiji T, Kawashima N, Kosaka T, et al: An immunohistochemical study of the distribution of immunocompetent cells, especially macrophages and Ia antigen–expressing cells of heterogeneous populations, in normal rat molar pulp, *J Dent Res* 71:1196, 1992.

Osborn JW: A mechanistic view of dentinogenesis and its relation to the curvatures of the processes of the odontoblasts, *Arch Oral Biol* 12:275, 1967.

Owens PDA: The fine structure of the coronal root region of premolar teeth in dogs, *Arch Oral Biol* 20:705, 1975.

Philippas GA: Influence of occlusal wear and age on formation of dentin and size of pulp chamber, *J Dent Res* 40:1186, 1961.

Philippas GG, Applebaum EA: Age factor in secondary dentin formation, *J Dent Res* 45:778, 1966.

Pimenidis MZ, Hinds JW: An autoradiographic study of the sensory innervation of teeth. II. Dental pulps and periodontium, *J Dent Res* 56:835, 1977.

Pineda F, Kuttler Y: Mesiodistal and buccolingual roentgenographic investigation of 7,275 root canals, *Oral Surg* 33:101, 1972.

Pohto P, Antila R: Acetylcholinesterase and noradrenaline in the nerves of mammalian dental pulps, *Acta Odontol Scand* 26:641, 1968.

Powers MM: The staining of nerve fibers in teeth, *J Dent Res* 31:383, 1952.

Sandham HJ (ed): The biology of dentin and pulp, *J Dent Res* (Special issue) 64:1, 1985.

Sato O, Maeda YT, Kannari K, et al: Immunohistochemical demonstration of nerve growth factor receptor in human teeth, *Biomed Res* 11:353, 1990.

Saunders RL: X-ray microscopy of the periodontal and dental pulp vessels in the monkey and in man, *Oral Surg* 22:503, 1966.

Schellenberg U, Krey G, Bosshardt D, Ramachandran PN: Numerical density of dentinal tubules at the pulpal wall of human permanent premolars and third molars, *J Endod* 18:104, 1992.

Schroder U, Sundstrom B: Transmission electron microscopy of tissue changes following experimental pulpotomy of intact human teeth and capping with calcium hydroxide, *Odontol Rev* 25:1, 1974.

Seltzer S, Soltanoff W, Bender IB, Ziontz M: Biologic aspects of endodontics. 1. Histologic observations of the anatomy and morphology of root apices and surrounding structures, *Oral Surg* 22:375, 1966.

Sessle BJ: The neurobiology of facial and dental pain: present knowledge, future directions, *J Dent Res* 66:692, 1987.

Shovelton DS: Studies of dentine and pulp in deep caries, *Int Dent J* 20:283, 1970.

Sigal MJ, Aubin JE, Ten Cate AR: An immunocytochemical study of the human odontoblast process using antibodies against tubulin, actin, and vimentin, *J Dent Res* 64:1348, 1985.

Sigal MJ, Aubin JE, Ten Cate AR, et al: The odontoblast process extends to the dentinoenamel junction: an immunocytochemical study of rat dentine, *J Histochem Cytochem* 32:872, 1984.

Sigal MJ, Pitaru S, Aubin JE, Ten Cate AR: A combined scanning electron microscopic and immunofluorescence study demonstrating that the odontoblast process extends to the dentinoenamel junction in human teeth, *Anat Rec* 210:443, 1984.

Stanley HR, Ranney RR: Age changes in the human dental pulp, *Oral Surg* 15:1396, 1962.

Stambaugh RV, Wittrock JW: The relationship of the pulp chamber to the external surface of the tooth, *J Prosthet Dent* 37:537, 1977.

Stanley HR, White CL, McCray L: The rate of tertiary (reparative) dentine formation in the human tooth, *Oral Surg* 21:180, 1966.

Stenvik A, Mjör IA: Epithelial remnants and denticle formation in the human dental pulp. *Acta Odontol Scand* 28:721, 1970.

Symons NB (ed): *Dentine and pulp: a symposium,* Baltimore, 1968, Williams & Wilkins.

Takahashi K, Kishi Y, Kim S: A scanning electron microscope study of the blood vessels of dog pulp using corrosion resin carts, *J Endod* 8:132, 1982.

Takuma S: Electron microscopy of the structure around the dentinal tuble, *J Dent Res* 39:973, 1960.

Takuma S: Preliminary report on the mineralization of human dentin, *J Dent Res* 39:964, 1960.

Takuma S, Kurahashi Y: Electron microscopy of various zones in the carious lesion in human dentine, *Arch Oral Biol* 7:439, 1962.

Tanaka T: The origin and localization of dentinal fluid in developing rat molar teeth studied with lanthanum as a tracer, *Arch Oral Biol* 25:153, 1980.

Ten Cate AR: An analysis of Tomes' granular layer, *Anat Rec* 172:137, 1972.

Terrie GG: Identification of lymphocyte antigens in human dental pulp, *J Oral Pathol* 19:246, 1990.

Thomas HF: The effect of various fixatives on the extent of the odontoblast process in human dentin, *Arch Oral Biol* 28:465, 1983.

Thomas HF, Payne RC: The ultrastructure of dentinal tubules from erupted human premolar teeth, *J Dent Res* 65:532, 1983.

Torneck CD: Changes in the fine structure of the dental pulp in human caries pulpitis, blood vessels and nerves, *J Oral Pathol* 3:71, 1974.

Torneck CD: Intracellular destruction of collagen in the human dental pulp, *Arch Oral Biol* 23:745, 1978.

Tronstad L: Scanning electron microscopy of attrited dentinal surfaces and subjacent dentin in human teeth, *Scand J Dent Res* 81:112, 1973.

Tronstad L: Vital staining of coronal dentin in monkey teeth, *Oral Surg* 45:612, 1978.

Tsatsas BG, Frank RM: Ultrastructure of the dentinal tubular substances near the dentino-enamel junction, *Calcif Tissue Res* 9:238, 1972.

Tsukada K: Ultrastructure of the relationship between odontoblast processes and nerve fibres in dentinal tubules of rat molar teeth, *Arch Oral Biol* 32:87, 1987.

Tucker JE, Lemon R, Mackie EJ, et al: Immunohistochemical localization of tenascin and fibronectin in the dentine and gingiva of Canis familiaris, *Arch Oral Biol,* 36:165, 1991.

Turner DF, Marfurt CF, Sattelburg C: Demonstration of physiological barrier between pulpal odontoblasts and its perturbation following routine restorative procedures: a horseradish peroxidase tracing study in the rat, *J Dent Res* 68:1262, 1989.

Vasiliadis L, Darling AI, Levers BGH: The histology of sclerotic human root dentin, *Arch Oral Biol* 28:693, 1983.

Voegel JC, Frank RM: Ultrastructural study of apatite crystal dissolution in human dentine and bone, *J Biol Buccale* 5:181, 1977.

Wang YN, Ashrafi SH, Weber DF: Scanning electron microscopic observations of casts of human dentinal tubules along the interface between primary and secondary dentine, *Anat Rec* 211:149, 1985.

Wasserman F: The innervation of teeth, *J Am Dent Assoc* 26:1097, 1939.

Weber DF: Human dentine sclerosis: a microradiographic survey, *Arch Oral Biol* 19:163, 1974.

Weinberg A, Mjör IA, Heide S: Rate of formation of regular and irregular secondary dentin in monkey teeth, *Oral Surg* 54:232, 1982.

Wysocki GP, Daley TD, Ulan RA: Predentin changes in patients with chronic renal failure, *Oral Surg* 56:167, 1983.

Yamada T, Nakamura K, Hori K, et al: The extent of the odontoblast process in normal and carious human dentin, *J Dent Res* 62:798, 1983.

Zerlotti E: Histochemical study of the connective tissue of the dental pulp, *Arch Oral Biol* 9:149, 1964.

CHAPTER 11

Amelogenesis

AMELOBLAST DIFFERENTIATION

Enamel is an epithelial product whose formation differs significantly from that of other hard tissues of the body, which are all derived from connective tissue. Even so, the principles established in Chapter 7 concerning hard tissue formation apply to enamel formation (or amelogenesis) in that a cell, associated with a good blood supply and alkaline phosphatase activity, produces an organic matrix capable of accepting mineral.

Amelogenesis is a two-step process involving secretion by cells (the ameloblasts) of a distinctive organic matrix, which is almost immediately partially mineralized. All the enamel of a tooth is first formed in this way as a fairly soft hard tissue, and only when this stage of amelogenesis is completed does it become fully mineralized as a result of a maturation activity on the part of ameloblasts, a process that involves not only the addition of further mineral but also the removal of most of the organic matrix.

Ameloblasts differentiate from the cells of the internal dental epithelium beginning first at the tips of the cusp outlines formed in that epithelium and then sweeping down the slopes until all the cells of the epithelium have differentiated into enamel-forming cells. Differentiation requires that dentinogenesis occur first; thus enamel formation always lags behind dentin formation. This dependence on the presence of formed dentin is an example of reciprocal induction, for it will be recalled that cells of the internal dental epithelium were needed to induce odontoblasts and now their product, dentin, becomes the initiator for further differentiation of the internal dental epithelial cells.

Recall also that during dentinogenesis the odontoblasts retreat centrally, leaving behind formed dentin. Ameloblasts also retreat, but in a peripheral direction, leaving newly formed enamel capping the dentin.

When amelogenesis begins, the tooth germ is described as being at the crown stage of tooth development (Fig. 11-1).

Enamel formation is initiated in the presence of a poor nutritive supply, because the ameloblasts are distanced from the blood vessels (which lie outside the dental organ within the dental follicle). Compensation for this distanced vascular supply, however, is achieved by cells of the internal dental epithelium, which accumulate glycogen before beginning their secretory activity and then utilize this stored glycogen during the initial stages of enamel formation until the so-called "collapse" of the dental organ occurs (so-called because much of this collapse is associated with the continued folding of the internal dental epithelium). With the loss of intervening stellate reticulum the ameloblasts are brought much closer to the follicular blood vessels.

The stratum intermedium intimately contacts the ameloblast layer and is functionally associated with amelogenesis. Its cells exhibit intense activity of alkaline phosphatase, with the ameloblasts exhibiting no activity.

ENAMEL MATRIX FORMATION

Thus far we have identified the cellular elements needed to produce enamel, established their nutritive supply, and identified the location of alkaline phosphatase activity. The next step in the process of amelogenesis is synthesis of the organic matrix of enamel. In the case of other hard tissues the term matrix is reserved for the organic component, but during amelogenesis the term matrix is used to designate not only the organic component but also the inorganic component of first formed enamel. This is unfortunate and confusing. To avoid confusion, the first formed (partially

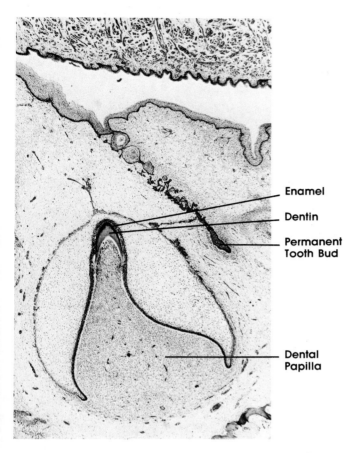

Enamel

Dentin

Permanent Tooth Bud

Dental Papilla

FIG. 11-1 Tooth germ at the early crown stage of development. Enamel formation has just begun at the tip of the cusp.

mineralized) enamel is referred to simply as developing enamel. Its organic component is also referred to as enamel protein, recognizing the fact that there are other minor nonproteinaceous elements associated with the organic content of enamel.

Enamel Protein

The nature and behavior of enamel protein are a long-standing and intriguing problem. Some 30 years ago the term *amelogenin* was coined to describe this protein—which was characterized as having a molecular weight of 22 to 30 kilodaltons (kDa), hydrophobic and rich in proline histidine and glutamine with an ability to flow (thixotropy) under pressure. Amelogenin is now known to constitute approximately 90% of enamel protein in the secretory stage. A second enamel protein, of higher molecular weight (48 to 70 kDa), is also described, called *enamelin;* which is acidic and rich in glutamine acid, aspartic acid, and serine.

It is now known that a single gene on the X chromosome codes for amelogenin. The primary structure of this protein is known for four mammalian species (cow, pig, mouse, and human) and is remarkably similar, indicating a high degree of conservation. In particular, amelogenin contains a 45–amino acid residue sequence known as TRAP (tyrosine-rich amelogenin protein) that may be of considerable functional significance. Almost as soon as the amelogenin is secreted, it undergoes a series of varying and discrete modifications so that a complex of amelogenins exists in the 20 to 25 kDa range. This family of proteins appears to play an important role in crystal growth and organization. For crystal growth to continue, some of the protein must be removed. The following combination of events has been proposed to bring about this removal: Pressure created by crystal growth causes the amelogenin to flow away from between the crystals and back toward the ameloblasts. Some amelogenin, however, becomes trapped between the rapidly growing crystals and is degraded to lower–molecular-weight products through the action of proteolytic enzymes secreted by the ameloblasts. These low–molecular-weight breakdown products are now also squeezed out from between the growing enamel crystals, with the TRAP remaining bound to the hydroxyapatite crystals (Fig. 11-2). There is some question as to whether the higher–molecular-weight family of proteins found in enamel matrix, the so-called enamelins, constitutes a distinct secretory product and what their functions might be. The enamelins (or perhaps, more correctly, nonamelogenins) are thought by some to be aggregations of amelogenin breakdown products, proteolytic enzymes secreted by the ameloblasts, and serum albumin that has leaked into the forming enamel. On the other hand there is good evidence that enamelins are secreted first and are linked to the formation of the hypermineralized layer of enamel first deposited on the dentin surface. They are then retained in mature enamel in the enamel tufts (Chapter 12). It has also been proposed that with progressive and increasing mineralization of the enamel matrix, amelogenin is selectively removed while enamelin remains tightly bound to the mineral.

Whatever the correct situation might be, the point to be grasped is that, unlike other hard tissue proteins (in which the organic matrix, once formed, is static), enamel protein is labile, exhibiting both quantitative and qualitative change during the process of amelogenesis (Fig. 11-3 and Table 11-1).

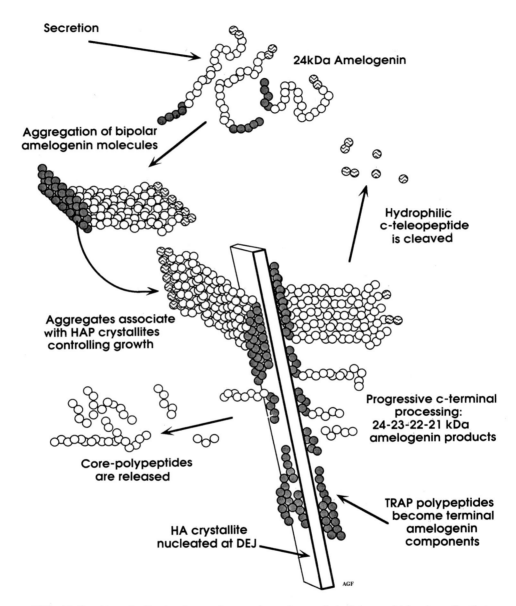

FIG. 11-2 Hypothetical scheme for amelogenin-mediated enamel biomineralization. (Courtesy Dr. A. Fincham.)

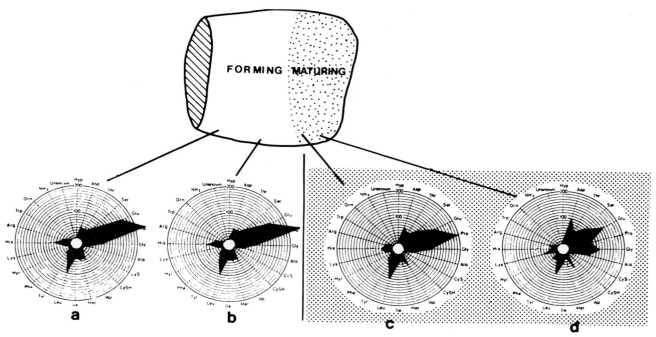

FIG. 11-3 Amino acid composition of enamel samples removed sequentially from a maxillary central incisor of a 9-month human fetus, which contains both forming and maturing enamel. The amino acid values are depicted pictorially in the "rose" diagrams. Actual values are given in Table 11-1. (From Deutsch D, Pe'er F: *J Dent Res* 61:1543, 1982.)

TABLE 11-1	Amino acid composition of two (a and b) enamel samples removed sequentially from a human fetal maxillary first incisor containing both forming and maturing stages*

Amino acid	Forming enamel		Maturing enamel	
	(a)	**(b)**	**(c)**	**(d)**
Aspartic acid	43	39	61	96
Threonine	38	36	42	52
Serine	59	59	74	87
Glutamic acid	150	141	128	142
Proline	241	249	193	80
Glycine	70	74	94	109
Alanine	24	24	35	72
Cystine	1	0	0	3
Valine	41	37	42	55
Methionine	42	41	28	10
Isoleucine	35	34	35	31
Leucine	95	100	96	93
Tyrosine	42	50	46	26
Phenylalanine	24	21	29	36
Histidine	55	53	39	23
Lysine	18	17	29	53
Arginine	24	24	29	33
Tryptophan		Not determined		
Percentage protein	14.7	14.6	5.9	2.5

*Values expressed as residues per 1000.
From Deutsch D, Pe'er F: *J Dent Res* (Special issue) 61:1543, 1971.

Mineralization and Maturation

The way mineral is introduced into this matrix also differs. As soon as enamel protein is secreted by the ameloblast, it almost instantly becomes mineralized; thus no equivalent of predentin or osteoid exists. Enamel protein is deposited directly onto mineralized dentin, and there is strong evidence that its initial mineralization is achieved by nucleation from the apatite crystals located within the dentin (Fig. 11-4). This

method of initial mineralization if correct would also explain why matrix vesicles are absent from the process of amelogenesis. Crystal growth then proceeds rapidly and mi neralizes the entire matrix to approximately 30%. This mineralization process also differs from that found in other hard tissues in that the mineral does not become incorporated within the matrix (as in the collagen molecule) but rather displaces it.

After the formation of partially mineralized enamel

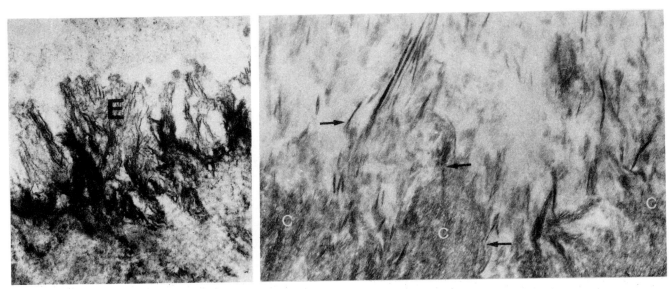

A   **B**

FIG. 11-4   Electron micrographs of initial enamel formation. **A** shows the close intermingling of dentin collagen with the ribbon-like crystals of enamel. **B,** A higher magnification showing the apparent continuity between calcified collagen and enamel crystallites. (From Arsenault AL, Robinson BW: *Calcif Tissue Int* 45(2):111, 1989.)

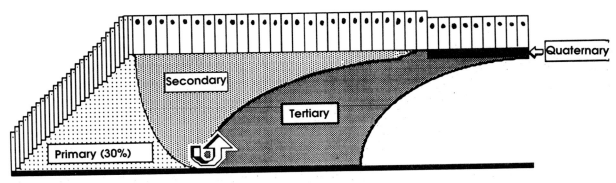

FIG. 11-5   Four phases of enamel mineralization. (Redrawn from Suga S: *Adv Dent Res*, vol 3, p 189, 1989.)

matrix, which involves production of the entire volume of enamel, a process of maturation begins with the continued influx of mineral and removal of protein so that the final consistency of enamel is achieved (with mineralization reaching 96%). It has recently been appreciated that this maturation process is phasic, involving the removal of water and protein, followed by the introduction of additional calcium, followed by the further removal of water and protein, and so on, and that it is dictated by cellular activity.

Although it is correct to describe amelogenesis as a two-step process involving the secretion of an enamel matrix and its subsequent maturation, recent studies involving "soft" x-ray analysis and computer enhancement indicate that the mineralization of enamel involves four stages: The first stage (primary mineralization) is the formation of partially mineralized enamel matrix, during which 30% mineralization is achieved overall (although and perhaps a function of enamelin, a very narrow [8 μm] innermost layer next to the dentin-enamel junction is heavily mineralized as soon as it is formed). The second stage begins with a secondary increase in mineralization that starts at the surface of the enamel and sweeps rapidly into the deeper layers until it reaches the innermost (8 μm) layer. This, in turn, is followed by the third stage, a tertiary increase in mineral rebounding from the innermost layer out toward the enamel surface. A surface layer some 15 μm wide can be distinguished during this phase, and it mineralizes more slowly. However, as the fourth stage commences, this outer layer mineralizes rapidly and heavily (quaternary mineralization), becoming the most mineralized part of the enamel. Thus enamel is most highly mineralized at its surface, with the degree of mineralization decreasing toward the dentinoenamel junction until the innermost layer is reached, where (as has already been noted) there is increased mineralization. These changes are represented diagrammatically in Figure 11-5.

In summary: The process of amelogenesis involves cells with an adequate nutritive supply and associated alkaline phosphatase activity, secreting enamel protein, which is immediately partially mineralized to form enamel matrix, which subsequently becomes further mineralized by a process of maturation. This rather complicated process is under cellular control, and the ameloblast changes significantly with the differing stages of amelogenesis.

LIGHT MICROSCOPY OF AMELOGENESIS

The histology of the dental organ at the bell stage of tooth development has been described (Chapter 4). At the late crown stage most of the light microscopic fea-

tures of amelogenesis can be seen in a single section (Fig. 11-6). Thus in the region of the cervical loop the low columnar cells of the internal dental epithelium are clearly identifiable, supported by a basement membrane that separates them from the acellular zone of the dental papilla. Peripheral to the internal dental epithelium lie the stratum intermedium, stellate reticulum, and external dental epithelium, the last closely associated with the many blood vessels in the dental follicle.

As the internal dental epithelium is traced coronally in a crown-stage tooth germ, its cells become tall columnar and their nuclei become aligned at the proximal ends of the cells adjacent to the stratum intermedium. At this region the acellular zone of the dental papilla is seen to have disappeared as odontoblasts have differentiated and begun dentin secretion. At one time these changes were associated with the inductive function of internal dental epithelial cells in initiating the differentiation of odontoblasts. This is not true; for dental root sheath epithelial cells initiating the differentiation of root odontoblasts do not exhibit such alterations, and therefore these changes must be regarded as entirely preparatory to the cells' assuming a secretive function.

Shortly after dentin formation is initiated, a number of distinct and almost simultaneous morphologic changes associated with the the onset of amelogenesis occur in the dental organ. The cells of the internal dental epithelium, now ameloblasts, begin to secrete the enamel matrix, which immediately becomes partially mineralized. This can be readily identified as a deep-staining layer in demineralized hematoxylin and eosin (H&E)–stained sections (Fig. 11-7). As this first increment of enamel is formed, the ameloblasts begin to move away from the dentin surface; and as they do, each cell forms a conical projection. These projections, called *Tomes processes,* jut into the newly forming enamel, giving the junction between the enamel and the ameloblast a picket-fence or sawtoothed appearance (Fig. 11-8).

At this time the dental organ collapses. The volume of stellate reticulum is reduced by the loss of its intercellular material; this reduction in volume, together with the peripheral migration of ameloblasts, brings the blood vessels in the dental follicle closer to the ameloblasts.

As amelogenesis continues, the cells of the external dental epithelium, stellate reticulum, and stratum intermedium gradually lose their discrete identities and form a stratified epithelial layer adjacent to the ameloblasts. When secretion of the full thickness of enamel is completed, the ameloblasts pass through a brief transitional phase during which significant morpho-

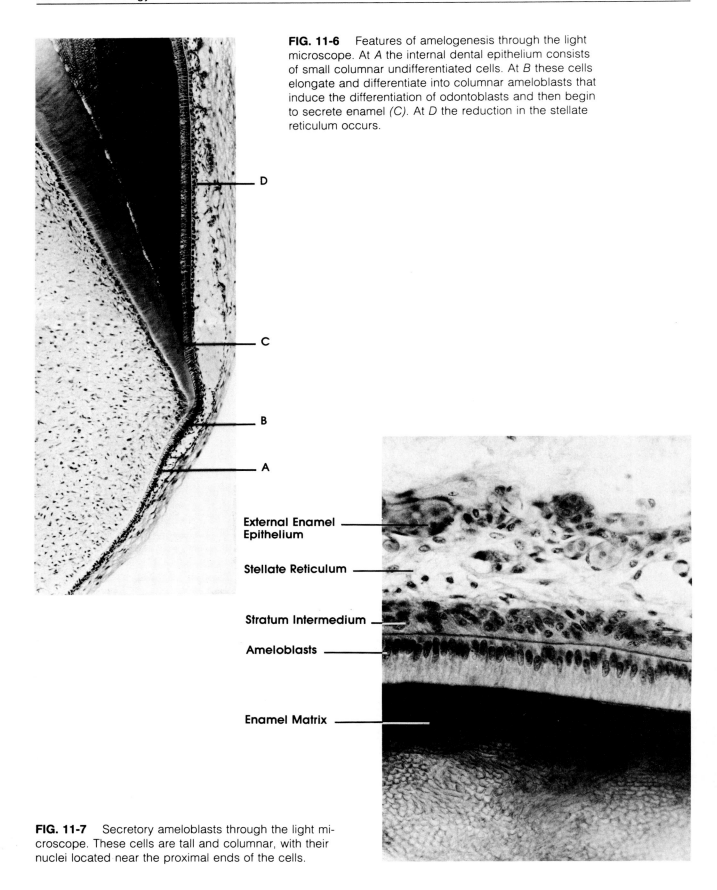

FIG. 11-6 Features of amelogenesis through the light microscope. At *A* the internal dental epithelium consists of small columnar undifferentiated cells. At *B* these cells elongate and differentiate into columnar ameloblasts that induce the differentiation of odontoblasts and then begin to secrete enamel *(C)*. At *D* the reduction in the stellate reticulum occurs.

D

C

B

A

External Enamel Epithelium

Stellate Reticulum

Stratum Intermedium

Ameloblasts

Enamel Matrix

FIG. 11-7 Secretory ameloblasts through the light microscope. These cells are tall and columnar, with their nuclei located near the proximal ends of the cells.

logic changes occur. These postsecretory ameloblasts shorten slightly, lose their Tomes processes, and become involved in enamel maturation.

When enamel maturation is completed, the ameloblast layer and the adjacent stratified epithelium (derived from the stratum intermedium, stellate reticulum, and external dental epithelium) together constitute the reduced dental epithelium (Figs. 13-14 and 13-17). This epithelium, through no longer involved in the secretion and maturation of enamel, continues to cover it and has a protective function. If premature breaks occur in the epithelium, connective tissue cells come into contact with the enamel and deposit cementum on the enamel.

In decalcified sections of developing teeth very little enamel is retained, for its organic component is progressively lost. Only in the most recently formed enamel matrix is sufficient organic material present to reveal some glimpse of the structural organization of this tissue (Fig. 11-9).

Undemineralized or ground sections, however, though providing some information on enamel struc-

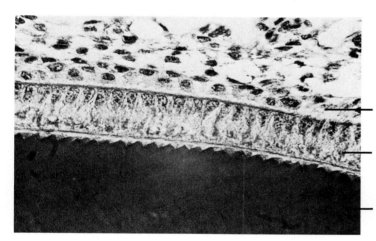

FIG. 11-8 Enamel matrix formation as seen with the light microscope. The Tomes processes of ameloblasts jut into the matrix, creating a picket fence appearance.

— Stratum
Intermedium

— Ameloblasts

— Enamel Matrix

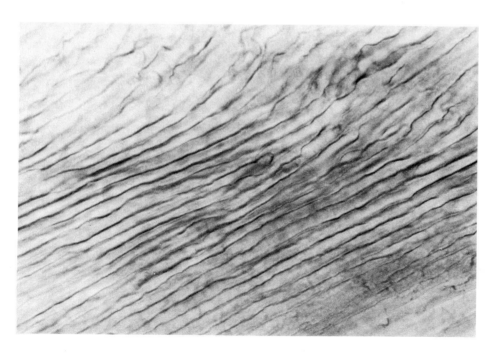

FIG. 11-9 Photomicrograph of mature enamel. Through careful demineralization the organic material has been retained in position. Compare this with Figure 4-18.

ture, are not as informative about the process of amelogenesis because the crucial cellular elements are not retained.

ELECTRON MICROSCOPY OF AMELOGENESIS

Ultrastructural studies by electron microscopy of enamel formation have added greatly to our understanding of this complex process.

Morphogenetic Stage

During the bell and crown stages of tooth development the cells of the dental organ, along with the dental papilla, form the tooth crown. The cells of the internal dental epithelium are cuboidal or low columnar with large centrally located nuclei (Fig. 4-13) and Golgi elements in the proximal portions of the cells (adjacent to the stratum intermedium). Mitochondria and other cytoplasmic components are scattered throughout the cells.

Differentiation Stage

As the cells of the internal dental epithelium begin to differentiate into ameloblasts, they elongate and their nuclei shift proximally toward the stratum intermedium. In each cell the Golgi complex increases its volume and migrates from its proximal position to occupy a major portion of the central core of the cell. The amount of rough endoplasmic reticulum increases significantly, and most of the mitochondria cluster in the proximal region, with only a few scattered through the

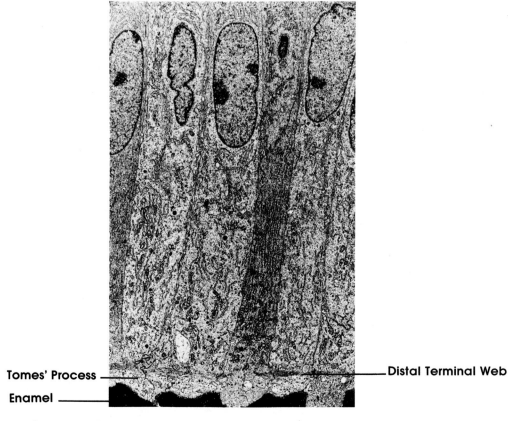

Tomes' Process ———

Enamel ———

———— Distal Terminal Web

FIG. 11-10 Electron micrograph of secretory ameloblasts. The synthetic organelles (Tomes' processes) and the newly formed and mineralized enamel are apparent. Compare with this Figure 11-4. (From Matthiessen ME, Römert P: *Scand J Dent Res* 86:87, 1978.)

rest of the cell. Thus the ameloblast becomes a polarized cell, with the majority of its organelles situated in the cell body distal to the nucleus (Fig. 11-10).

Adjacent ameloblasts are closely aligned to each other, and this alignment is maintained by the development of attachment specializations, or junctional complexes, between them. These complexes encircle the cells at their distal (adjacent to enamel) and proximal (adjacent to the stratum intermedium) extremities. Fine actin-containing filaments radiate from the junctional complexes into the cytoplasm of the ameloblasts and can be distinguished as forming the distal and proximal terminal webs. These junctional complexes play an important role in amelogenesis by determining at different times what may, and what may not, pass between the ameloblasts to enter or leave the enamel. Furthermore, they have the ability to change their functional role, becoming tight or leaky as occasions demand.

The basal lamina supporting the ameloblasts disintegrates after the deposition of predentin and during differentiation of the ameloblast.

Secretory Stage—Synthesis of Enamel

The fine structure of secretory ameloblasts reflects their synthetic and secretory function. The synthesis of enamel protein occurs in the rough endoplasmic reticulum, from where it is passed to the Golgi complex; in the Golgi complex it is condensed and packaged into membrane-bound secretory granules; these granules migrate to the distal extremity of the cell, and their contents are released against the newly formed mantle dentin. Little if any time elapses between the secretion of enamel matrix and its mineralization. Apparently the ameloblasts exert some control over the passage of inorganic ions from capillaries of the dental follicle to the enamel surface. Hydroxyapatite crystals are randomly packed in this first-formed enamel and interdigitate with the crystals of dentin. Some authors consider that the dentin crystals form the nucleation sites for enamel crystals (Fig. 11-4).

After this first structureless enamel layer is formed, the ameloblasts migrate away from the dentin surface, which permits the formation of Tomes processes (already referred to in connection with the light microscopy of amelogenesis). Although the cytoplasm of the ameloblast continues into the Tomes process, the distinction between process and cell body is clearly marked by the distal terminal web and junctional complex. The process contains primarily secretory granules and small vesicles whereas the cell-body cytoplasm contains abundant synthetic organelles (Fig. 11-11).

When the Tomes process is established, the secretion of enamel protein becomes staggered and is confined to two sites. Secretion from the first site (adjacent to the proximal part of the process, close to the junctional complex, around the periphery of the cell), along with that from adjoining ameloblasts, results in the formation of enamel matrix wall. These walls enclose a pit (Fig. 11-12) into which the Tomes process fits. Secretion from the second site (one surface of the Tomes process) later fills this pit with matrix. Crystals in the pit have a different orientation from those in the wall of the pit (Figs. 11-11 and 11-13). This difference (as explained in Chapter 12) gives structure to the enamel, with the walls becoming interrod enamel and the infilling becoming enamel rod. Understand, however, that in both sites the enamel is of identical composition and differs only in the orientation of its crystallites. The Tomes process, which creates structure in the enamel, persists until the final few enamel increments are formed and, as a result, these (like the first few) are structureless.

Enamel proteins are seen throughout the newly forming enamel (Fig. 11-14), but they become much more highly concentrated in the narrow prism sheath areas (to be described in Chapter 12) as enamel matures (Fig. 11-15). Amelogenins have also been localized in lysosomes within secretory ameloblasts. There are two possible interpretations for this observation: First, it has been discovered that the ameloblast begins to synthesize enamel protein well in advance of its secretion and some of this may be destroyed before being secreted. Second, it has been noted that the secretory ameloblast is simultaneously involved with the removal of some enamel protein during the phase of matrix production.

Maturation Stage

After the full thickness of immature enamel has formed, the ameloblasts undergo significant ultrastructural changes in preparation for their next functional role, that of maturing the enamel. There is a brief transitional stage involving a reduction in height of the ameloblasts and a decrease in their volume and organelle content. Excess organelles associated with synthesis are enclosed in autophagic vacuoles and digested by lysosomal enzymes. This development is followed by a shift in many of the remaining organelles to the distal part of the cell.

What happens next is that the ameloblasts become involved in a cyclical process: water and organic material are selectively removed from the enamel while additional inorganic material is introduced by alternate bursts of activity. The cyclical nature of this process is reflected in ameloblast morphology, with the cells alternating between possessing a ruffled border (ruffle ended) and possessing a smooth border (smooth ended)

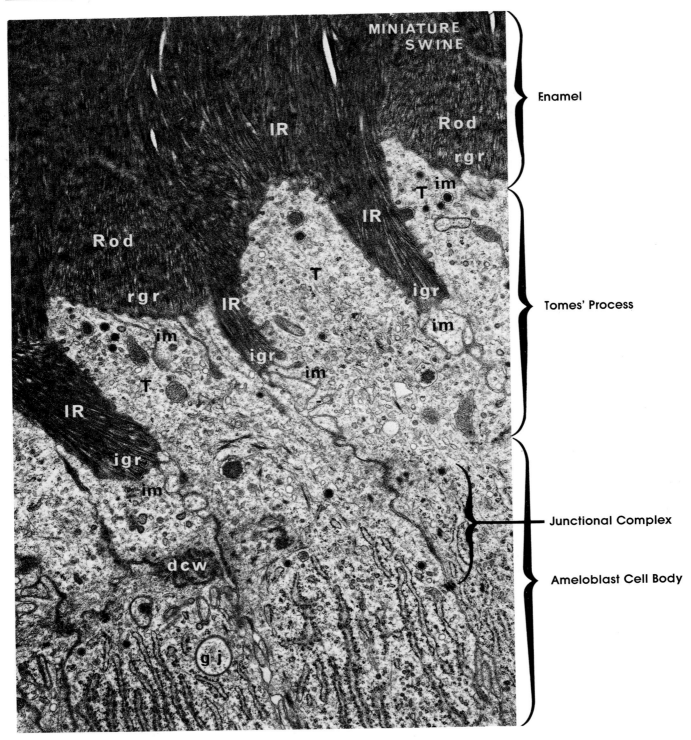

FIG. 11-11 Secretory ameloblast. At bottom are the many profiles of rough endoplasmic reticulum. The transition to Tomes' processes is marked by junctional complexes between the adjacent ameloblasts. Secretory granules are clearly seen in the Tomes processes *(middle)*. Interrod growth regions *(igr)* produce the interrod enamel *(IR)* or pit walls seen in Figure 11-10. At *rgr (top)* the distal portion of a Tomes process fills the base of the pit to form a rod. *gj,* Gap junction; *dcw,* distal cell web; *im,* infolded cell membrane; *igr,* interrod growth region; *IR,* interrod enamel; *rgr,* rod growth region; *T,* Tomes' process. (From Warshawsky H, et al: *Anat Rec* 200:371, 1981.)

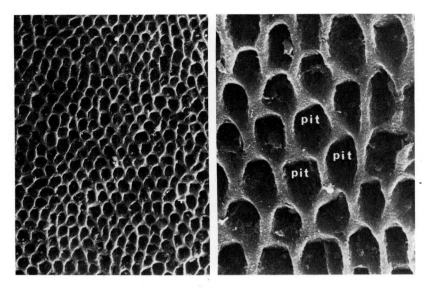

FIG. 11-12 Scanning electron micrograph of the surface of a developing human tooth. The surface consists of a series of pits previously filled by Tomes' processes whose walls are formed by interrod enamel. (From Warshawsky H, et al: *Anat Rec* 200:371, 1981.)

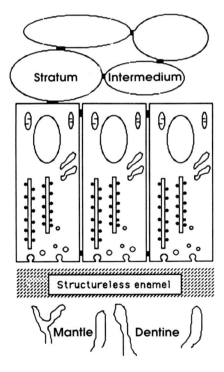

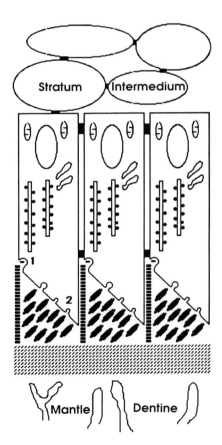

FIG. 11-13 How Tomes' processes create structure. To the left, structureless enamel forms across the straight face of an ameloblast. To the right the two sites of secretion (*1* and *2*) introduce differences in crystallite orientation and hence structure.

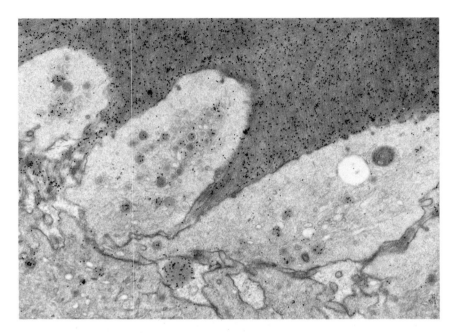

FIG. 11-14 Amelogenesis. Immunocytochemical labeling *(black dots)* of enamel protein in Tomes' processes and in newly formed enamel. (Courtesy Dr. A. Nanci.)

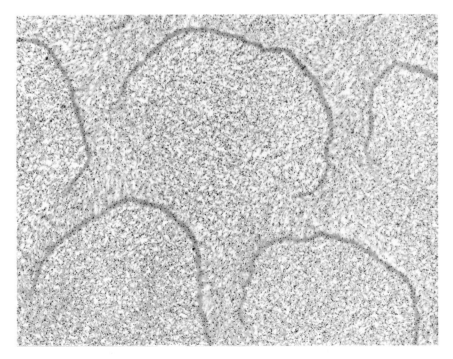

FIG. 11-15 Immunocytochemical labeling of enamel protein. Note the labeling in prism sheaths. (Courtesy Dr. A. Nanci.)

(Fig. 11-16). The ruffle-ended ameloblasts are associated with the introduction of inorganic material, the smooth-ended cells with removal of protein and water. With these changes at the cell surface facing the formed enamel are changes in function of the distal and proximal junctions between adjacent ameloblasts. Thus ruffle-ended ameloblasts possess proximal junctions that are leaky and distal junctions that are tight whereas smooth-ended ameloblasts have distal junctions that are leaky and proximal ones that are tight. These changes indicate that inorganic material must pass through the ruffle-ended ameloblasts (because their distal junctions are tight) and, conversely, larger molecules withdrawn from the developing enamel must pass through the leaky distal junctions between smooth-ended cells (and, because the proxmal junctions are tight, be taken up along the lateral surfaces of these cells). Protein breakdown products may also be absorbed across the ruffled border of ruffle-ended ameloblasts. These functional associations are diagrammed in Figure 11-17.

The above cyclical changes within the ameloblast layer during maturation can also be demonstrated with special stains that reflect the changing nature of the enamel surface (Fig. 11-18)

FIG. 11-16 Ameloblast modulation during maturation. **A** is an electron micrograph of a ruffle-ended ameloblast. Note the developed junctional complex at the distal extremity of the cell. **B** is an electron micrograph of the smooth-ended ameloblast. Note the absence of any well-developed distal junctional complex. (From Nanci A, et al: *Anat Rec* 233:335, 1992.)

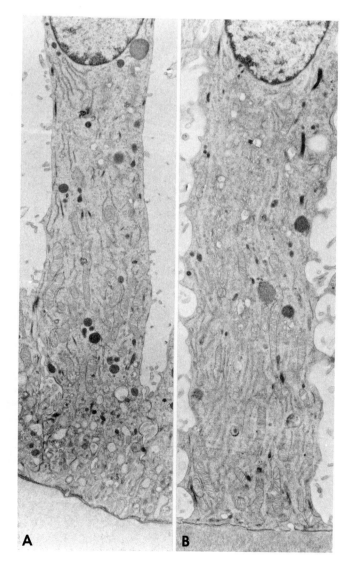

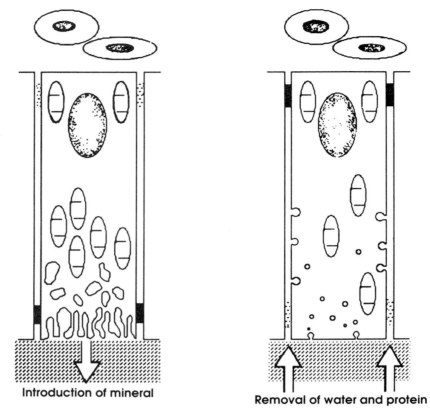

Introduction of mineral

Removal of water and protein

FIG. 11-17   Functional morphology illustrated in Fig. 11-16.

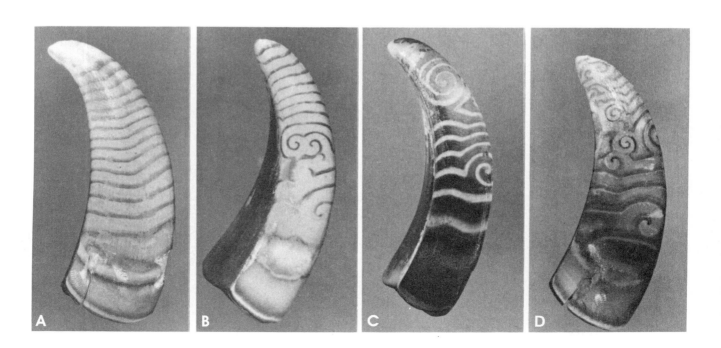

Protective Stage

As enamel maturation nears completion, the ameloblasts secrete a material between the now-flattened distal ends of the cells and the enamel surface. This material appears morphologically identical to a basal lamina. Hemidesmosomes also form along the distal cell membrane, providing a firm attachment for the ameloblasts to the enamel surface, which is especially important in establishment of the dentogingival junction (Fig. 11-19).

The ameloblasts at this stage protect the newly formed enamel surface from the follicular connective tissue. If they fail, for whatever reason, the connective tissue cells differentiate into cementoblasts and deposit cementum on the enamel surface. During this protective phase, however, the cell is still able to modify enamel composition. For instance, fluoride, if available, can still be incorporated into the enamel of an unerupted tooth; and there is evidence that the fluoride content is greatest in those teeth that have the longest interregnum between the completion of enamel formation and tooth eruption (at which time, of course, the ameloblasts are lost).

A few other aspects of enamel formation will be described in Chapter 12 after enamel structure has been discussed.

At this point it is worth recapitulating the many functions that cells of the internal dental epithelium exhibit during their life cycle: Initially they are involved in *determining the crown pattern* of the tooth; at this time they are small and cuboidal (Fig. 4-13) with centrally placed nuclei and they undergo frequent mitoses. Then they are involved in the *differentiation of odontoblasts* within the dental papilla; at this stage morphologic changes occur within them and they become ameloblasts. These changes are preparatory to their entering the next phase, *secretion of the enamel matrix*, wherein they develop a conical extension (called the Tomes process). The secretory phase is followed by the *maturation of enamel* phase, wherein the ameloblasts exhibit cyclical variations with ruffle- and smooth-ended borders against the enamel surface—the ruffle-ended cells allowing the ingress of inorganic material, the smooth-ended cells allowing the removal of protein and water. The final phase is *protection of the newly formed enamel surface* until the time of tooth eruption. Ameloblasts also develop an attachment to the enamel surface during this protective phase that is utilized to form the primary epithelial attachment between the gingiva and the newly erupted tooth (Chapter 13). Figures 4-13, 11-19, and 11-20 summarize the life cycle of ameloblasts.

FIG. 11-18 Developing pig canine stained with various calcium-complexing agents showing the pattern of modulation. In **A** and **B** the stained bands equate with overlying smooth-ended ameloblasts. In **C** the reverse is true, with the stain now demonstrating a surface overlaid by ruffled-ended ameloblasts. **D** illustrates combined staining. (From McKee MD, et al: In Fearnhead RN, [ed]: *Tooth enamel,* Yokohama, 1989, Florence Publishers, Vol 5.)

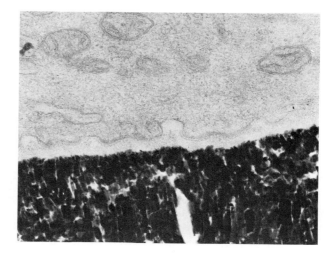

FIG. 11-19 Protective ameloblast. The distal cell membrane is no longer folded and has developed hemidesmosomes as the cell becomes attached to the enamel surface.

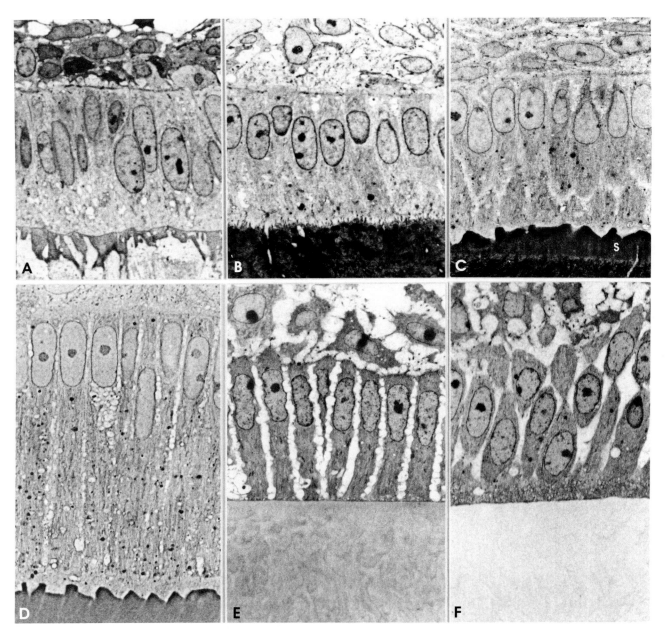

FIG. 11-20   This figure should be studied with Figures 4-13 and 11-19, for together they summarize the entire life-cycle of the ameloblast. In **A** the ameloblasts are depicted overlying the first formed dentin. In **B** the beginning enamel formation is shown. In **C** the formation of Tomes' processes is seen and a distinction between structureless and structured enamel is indicated (*s* denotes structureless enamel). In **D** the active secretory ameloblast is seen, in **E** the smooth-ended ameloblast, and in **F** the ruffled ended ameloblast, the latter two associated with enamel maturation. (From Nanci A, et al: *Anat Rec* 233:335, 1992.)

Mineral Pathway

The way in which mineral ions are introduced into forming enamel is of interest because it spans both the secretory and the maturation phase of enamel formation, with the latter demanding a massive influx of mineral in a relative short time. It also needs to be understood so that some of the defects occurring during amelogenesis can be explained. Although we still do not know for certain how calcium is transported into forming enamel, the following has been suggested based on interpretation of some known facts: (1) The distal intercellular junctions between ruffle-ended ameloblasts are tight and prevent any pericellular transport of mineral to the forming enamel matrix; (2) the calcium–ion concentration in extracellular fluid is 10^{-3} M and in newly secreted enamel 10^{-5} M; (3) calcium–adenosine triphosphatase (Ca-ATPase) is associated with the entire cell membrane of the secretory ameloblast and is more abundant in ruffle-ended than smooth-ended maturation ameloblasts; (4) a calcium-binding protein of 28 kDa has been described that is more abundant in ruffle-ended than smooth-ended ameloblasts; and, finally, (5) the free cytosolic calcium ion concentration has to be within the range of $10^{-6.5}$ to $10^{-7.5}$ M for proper cell function. Recognizing these facts, a number of workers have proposed hypotheses as to how calcium reaches the forming enamel. During the secretory phase of amelogenesis it is thought that Ca-ATPase activity reflects the existence of a pump extruding calcium at a constant rate and thereby pre-

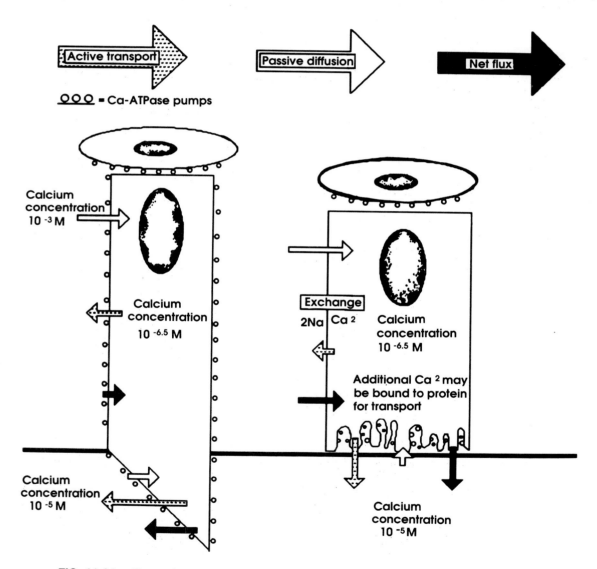

FIG. 11-21 Theoretical pathways of calcium flux during the secretory and maturative phases of amelogenesis. (Redrawn from Bawden JW: *Anat Rec* 224:226, 1988.)

serving the cytosolic free calcium ion concentration in the $10^{-6.5}$ to $10^{-7.5}$ M range. To achieve a flow of calcium ions into the cell, however, there needs to be a net influx of Ca^{2+} into the proximal part of the cell and a net efflux across the distal part beyond the junctional complex. The differences in Ca^{2+} concentration between the extracellular fluid and the enamel matrix are sufficient to cause this without exceeding the range of tolerance for cytosolic free Ca^{2+} (Fig. 11-21). The situation facing the maturation ameloblast is different, and far greater amounts of Ca^{2+} must pass into the enamel. The greater amounts of both Ca-ATPase and 28 kDa calcium-binding proteins in ruffle-ended ameloblasts may indicate an active calcium transport mechanism in these cells. This, coupled with modification of the enamel surface (perhaps related to cycling back and forth between the two cell types,) may allow uptake of transported Ca^{2+} by maturing enamel adjacent to ruffle-ended ameloblasts.

However attractive these hypotheses, a number of flaws exist. There is evidence that the tight junctions between ameloblasts in their secretory phase may permit passage of calcium and phosphorus into the enamel matrix via an intercellular route. Also there is no evidence that the calcium-binding proteins in maturation ameloblasts act in the manner proposed. It is known that cytoskeletal assembly and disassembly are dependent on calcium concentration and, since the formation of a ruffled border is a cytoskeletal phenomenon, could demand an increased Ca^{2+} concentration; and it has been suggested that the appearance of calcium-binding proteins in maturation ameloblasts is related to bringing about this rapid and frequent modulation.

Defects of Amelogenesis

In addition to the genetic dysplasias described in the first chapter, many other conditions produce defects in enamel structure. Such defects occur because ameloblasts are cells that are particularly sensitive to changes in their environment. Even minor physiologic changes affect them and elicit changes in enamel structure that can be seen only histologically. More severe insults either greatly disturb enamel production or produce death of the ameloblasts and the resulting defects are easily seen clinically.

Three conditions affecting enamel formation occur relatively frequently: First, defects in enamel can be caused by febrile diseases. During the course of such a disease, enamel formation is disturbed so that all teeth forming at the time become characterized by distinctive bands of malformed surface enamel. On recovery normal enamel formation is resumed (Fig. 11-22).

Second, defects can be formed by tetracycline-induced disturbances in teeth. Tetracycline antibiotics are incorporated into mineralizing tissues; in the case of enamel, this incorporation may result in a band of brown pigmentation or even total pigmentation. Hypoplasia or absence of enamel may also occur. The degree of damage is determined by the magnitude and duration of tetracycline therapy.

Finally, the fluoride ion can interfere with amelogenesis. Chronic ingestion of F^- concentrations in excess of five parts per million (5 times the amount in fluoridated water supplies) interferes with ameloblast function sufficiently to produce mottled enamel. Mottled enamel is unsightly and is often seen as white patches of hypomineralized and altered enamel. Such enamel, though unsightly, is still resistant to caries.

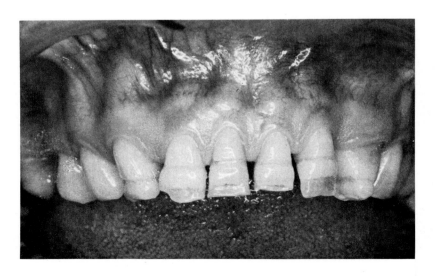

FIG. 11-22 Dentition of a patient who had two illnesses at separate times. The enamel defects, separated by normal enamel, are clearly shown.

In summary: Enamel is an ectodermally derived tissue produced by the dental organ. The cells of the internal dental epithelium differentiate into ameloblasts and have a complex life cycle consisting of five stages: (1) morphogenetic, (2) differentiating, (3) secretory, (4) maturation, and (5) protective. As enamel forms, other cells of the dental organ decrease in prominence. The ameloblasts first produce a partially mineralized enamel and then reorganize their cytology to achieve full maturation of this enamel. Completed enamel is protected by the reduced dental epithelium.

BIBLIOGRAPHY

Bawden JW: Calcium transport during mineralization, *Anat Rec* 224:226, 1989.

Bawden JW, Wennberg A: In vitro study of cellular influence on ⁴⁵Ca uptake in developing rat enamel, *J Dent Res* 56:313, 1977.

Belcourt AB, Fincham AG, Termine JD: Bovine high molecular weight amelogenin proteins, *Calcif Tissue Int* 35:111, 1983.

Boyde A: The development of enamel structure, *Proc R Soc Med* 60:923, 1967.

Burgess RC, Maclaren C: Proteins in developing bovine enamel. In Feanhead RW, Stack MV (eds): *Tooth enamel*, Bristol UK, 1969, John Wright & Sons.

Daculsi G, Kerebel B: High-resolution electron microscope study of human enamel crystallites: size, shape, and growth, *J Ultrastruct Res* 65:163, 1978.

Deakins M: Changes in the ash, water and organic content of pig enamel during calcification, *J Dent Res* 21:429, 1942.

Deutsch D, et al: Rate and timing of enamel development in the deciduous bovine incisor, *Arch Oral Biol* 24:407, 1979.

Deutsch D, Gedalia I: Chemically distinct stages in developing fetal human enamel, *Arch Oral Biol* 25:635, 639, 1980.

Deutsch D, Pe'er E: Development of enamel in human fetal teeth, *J Dent Res* (Special issue), 61:1543, 1982.

Deutsch D, Palmon A, Fisher LW, et al: Sequencing of bovine enamelin ("Tuftalin") a novel acidic enamel protein, *J Biol Chem* 266:16021, 1991.

Eastoe JE: The amino acid composition of proteins from the oral tissues. II. The matrix proteins in dentine and enamel from developing human deciduous teeth, *Arch Oral Biol* 8:633, 1963.

Eisenmann DR, Ashrafi S, Neiman A: Calcium transport and the secretory ameloblast, *Anat Rec* 193:403, 1979.

Fearnhead RW, Stack MV (eds): Tooth enamel: its composition, properties and fundamental structure, vol 2, Bristol UK, 1971, John Wright & Sons.

Fearnhead RW, Suga S (eds): *Tooth enamel*, ed 4, Amsterdam, 1984, Elsevier Science Publishers.

Fincham AG, Hu Y, Lau EC, et al: Amelogenin post–secretory processing during biomineralization in the postnatal mouse tooth, *Arch Oral Biol* 36:305, 1991.

Frank RM, Nalbandian J: Ultrastructure of amelogenesis. In

Miles AEW (ed): Structure and chemical organization of teeth, New York, 1967, Academic Press.

Garant PR, Nalbandian J: Observations on the ultrastructure of ameloblasts with special reference to the Golgi complex and related components, *J Ultrastruct Res* 23:427, 1968.

Glimcher MJ, Brickley-Parsons D, Levine PT: Studies of enamel proteins during maturation, *Calcif Tiss Res* 24:259, 1977.

Hanawa M, Takano Y, Wakita M: An autoradiographic study of calcium movement in the enamel organ of rat molar tooth germs, *Arch Oral Biol* 35: 899, 1990.

Hiller CR, Robinson C, Wetherell JA: Variation in the composition of developing rat incisor enamel, *Calcif Tiss Res* 18:1, 1975.

Josephsen K: Indirect visualization of ameloblast modulation in the rat incisor using calcium-binding compounds, *Scand J Dent Res* 91:76, 1983.

Josephsen K, Fejerskov O: Ameloblast modulation in the maturation zone of the rat incisor enamel organ: a light and electron microscopic study, *J Anat* 124:45, 1977.

Kallenbach E: Electron microscopy of the differentiating rat incisor ameloblast, *J Ultrastruct Res* 35:508, 1971.

Listgarten MA: Phase contrast and electron microscopic study of the junction between reduced enamel epithelium and enamel in unerupted human teeth, *Arch Oral Biol* 11:999, 1966.

Listgarten MA: Structure of surface coatings on teeth: a review, *J Periodontol* 47:139, 1976.

Matthiessen ME, Romert P The secretory ameloblast of the mini pig foetus, *Cell Tiss Res* 169:179, 1976.

Matthiessen ME, von Bulow FA: The ultrastructure of human secretory ameloblasts, *Z Zellforsch Mikroskop Anat* 101:232, 1969.

Nanci A, Bendayan M, Slavkin HC: Enamel protein biosynthesis and secretion in mouse incisor secretory ameloblasts as revealed by high-resolution immunocytochemistry, *J Histochem Cytochem* 33:1153, 1985.

Nanci A, McKee MD, Smith CE: Immunolocalization of enamel proteins during amelogenesis in the cat, *Anat Rec* 233:335, 1992.

Nanci A, Slavkin HC, Smith CE: Immunocytochemical and radioautographic evidence for secretion and intracellular degradation of enamel proteins by ameloblasts during the maturation stage of amelogenesis in rat incisors, *Anat Rec* 217:107, 1987.

Nanci A, Warshawsky H: Characterization of putative secretory sites on ameloblasts of the rat incisor, *Am J Anat* 171:163, 1984.

Nylen MU, Scott DB: Electron microscopic studies of odontogenesis, *J Indiana Dent Assoc* 39:406, 1960.

Pannese E Observations on the ultrastructure of the enamel organ. I. Stellate reticulum and stratum intermedium, *J Ultrastruct Res* 4:372, 1960.

Pannese E: Observations on the ultrastructure of the enamel organ. II. Involution of the stellate reticulum, *J Ultrastruct Res* 5:328, 1961.

Pannese E: Observations on the ultrastructure of the enamel organ. III. Internal and external enamel epithelium, *J Ultrastruct Res* 6:186, 1962.

Reith EJ: The stages of amelogenesis as observed in molar teeth of young rats, *J Ultrastruct Res* 30:111, 1970.

Reith EJ, Cotty VF: Autoradiographic studies on calcification of enamel, *Arch Oral Biol* 7:365, 1962.

Reith EJ, Cotty VF: The absorptive activity of ameloblasts during the maturation of enamel, *Anat Rec* 157:577, 1967.

Robinson C, Briggs HD, Atkinson PJ: Histology of enamel organ and chemical composition of adjacent enamel in rat incisors, *Calcif Tissue Int* 33:513, 1981.

Robinson C, Briggs HD, Atkinson PJ, et al: Matrix and mineral changes in developing enamel, *J Dent Res* 58:871, 1979.

Robinson C, Fuchs P, Deutsch D, et al: Four chemically distinct stages in developing enamel from bovine incisor teeth, *Caries Res* 12:1, 1978.

Robinson C, Kirkham J, Briggs HD, et al: Enamel proteins: from secretion to maturation, *J Dent Res* 61:1490, 1982.

Robinson C, Lowe NR, Weatherell JA: Changes in amino-acid composition of developing rat incisor enamel, *Calcif Tissue Res* 23:19, 1977.

Ronnholm E: An electron microscopic study of the amelogenesis in human teeth. I. The fine structure of the ameloblasts, *J Ultrastruct Res* 6:229, 1962.

Ronnholm E: The amelogenesis of human teeth as revealed by electron microscopy. II. The development of the enamel crystallites, *J Ultrastruct Res* 6:249, 1962.

Ronnholm E: The amelogenesis of human teeth as revealed by electron microscopy. III. The structure of the organic stroma of human enamel during amelogenesis, *J Ultrastruct Res*, 6:368, 1962.

Rosser H, Boyde A, Stewart ADG: Preliminary observations of the calcium concentration in developing enamel assessed by scanning electron probe x-ray emission microanalysis, *Arch Oral Biol* 12:431, 1967.

Salama AH, Zaki AE, Eisenmann DR: Cytochemical localization of Ca^{2+}-Mg^{2+} adenosine triphosphatase in rat incisor ameloblasts during enamel secretion and maturation, *J Histochem Cytochem* 35:471, 1987.

Sasaki S, Takagi T, Susuki M, et al: Amino acid sequence of developing bovine enamel protein. In Fearnhead RW, Suga S (eds): *Tooth enamel*, ed 4, Amsterdam, 1984, Elsevier Science Publishers.

Sasaki T: Endocytotic pathways at the ruffled borders of rat maturation ameloblasts, *Histochemistry* 80:263, 1984.

Schour I, Hoffman MM: Studies in tooth development. I. The 16 microns calcification rhythm in the enamel and dentin from fish to man, *J Dent Res* 18:91, 1939.

Shimizu M, Tanabe T, Fukae M: Proteolytic enzyme in porcine immature enamel, *J Dent Res* 58:782, 1979.

Simmelink JW: Mode of enamel matrix secretion, *J Dent Res* 61:1483, 1982.

Slavkin HC, Grenvlich R (eds): *Extracellular matrix influences on gene expression*, New York, 1975, Academic Press.

Slavkin HC, Mino W, Bringas P Jr: The biosynthesis and secretion of precursor enamel protein by ameloblasts as visualized by autoradiography after trytophan administration, *Anat Rec* 185:289, 1976.

Snead ML, Zeichner-David M, Chandra T, et al: Construction and identification of mouse amelogenin cDNA clones, *Proc Natl Acad Sci USA* 80:7254, 1983.

Takano Y, Crenshaw MA: The penetration of intravascularly perfused lanthanum into the ameloblast layer of developing rat molar teeth, *Arch Oral Biol* 25:505, 1980.

Takano Y, Crenshaw MA, Reith EJ: Correlation of ^{45}Ca incorporation with maturation ameloblast morphology in the rat incisor, *Calcif Tissue Int* 34:211, 1982.

Takano Y, Ozawa H, Crenshaw MA: Ca-ATPase and ATPase activities at the initial calcification sites of dentin and enamel in the rat incisor, *Cell Tissue Res* 243:91, 1986.

Warshawsky H, Smith CE: Morphological classification of rat incisor ameloblasts, *Anat Rec* 179:423, 1976.

Weber DF, Eisenmann DR: Microscopy of the neonatal line in developing human enamel, *Am J Anat* 132:375, 1971.

Weatherell JA, Deutsch D, Robinson C, et al: Fluoride concentration in developing enamel, *Nature* 256:230, 1975.

Weinstock A, LeBlond CP: Elaboration of the matrix glycoprotein of enamel by the secretory ameloblasts of the rat incisor as revealed by radioautography after galactose H^2 injection, *J Cell Biol* 51:26, 1971.

Young RW, Greulich RC: Distinctive autoradiographic patterns of glycine incorporation in rat enamel and dentine matrices, *Arch Oral Biol* 8:509, 1963.

CHAPTER 12

Enamel Structure

ENAMEL is the most highly mineralized tissue known, consisting of 96% mineral and 4% organic material and water. The inorganic content of enamel consists of a crystalline calcium phosphate known as hydroxyapatite, which is also found in bone, calcified cartilage, dentin, and cementum (Fig. 12-1). Various ions—strontium, magnesium, lead, and fluoride—if present during enamel formation, may be incorporated into or adsorbed by the hydroxyapatite crystals. The susceptibility of these crystals to dissolution by acid provides the chemical basis for dental caries.

Although nearly the entire volume of enamel is occupied by the densely packed hydroxyapatite crystals, a fine lacy network of organic material appears between the crystals. The organic material can best be observed in carefully demineralized sections of partially mineralized developing enamel (Fig. 11-9) and is also seen as a lacy network on electron micrographs of mature enamel (Fig. 12-2). The bulk of this organic material consists of the TRAP* peptide sequence tightly bound to the hydroxyapatite crystal as well as nonamelogenin proteins.

*Tyrosine-rich amelogenin protein.

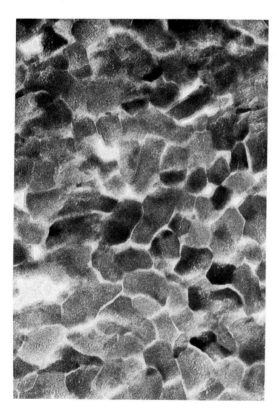

FIG. 12-1   Electron micrograph of enamel crystals. The organic material and water of enamel exist in the spaces between the crystals. (Courtesy Dr. J.W. Simmelink, Dr. V.K. Nygaard, and Dr. D.B. Scott.)

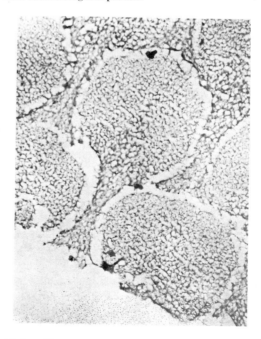

FIG. 12-2   Electron micrograph of demineralized enamel. The rod sheath is greatly widened because of shrinkage of the enamel protein. (Courtesy Dr. A.H. Meckel.)

PHYSICAL CHARACTERISTICS OF ENAMEL

Because of its high mineral content, enamel is extremely hard, a property that enables it to withstand the mechanical forces applied during its functioning. This hardness, which is comparable to that of mild steel, also makes enamel brittle; therefore an underlying layer of more resilient dentin is necessary to maintain its integrity. If this supportive layer of dentin is destroyed by either caries or improper cavity preparation, the unsupported enamel fractures very easily.

Enamel is translucent and varies in color from light yellow to grayish white. It also varies in thickness, from a maximum of approximately 2.5 mm over working surfaces to a featheredge at the cervical line. This variation influences the color of enamel, since the underlying yellow dentin is seen through the thinner regions.

STRUCTURE OF ENAMEL

Because of its highly mineralized nature, the structure of enamel is extremely difficult to study. When conventional demineralized sections are examined, only an empty space can be seen in areas previously occupied by mature enamel, since the mineral has been dissolved and the organic material washed away (Fig. 4-16). Because of its higher organic content, however, sections of decalcified developing human enamel often retain enough organic material to reveal some detail of enamel structure (Figs. 12-3 and 11-7).

Enamel in prepared ground sections can be studied under the light microscope by means of transmitted light. Such sections show it to be composed primarily of elongated structures termed *rods* (Fig. 12-4). The nature of rod structure may be misinterpreted for the crystalline nature of enamel leads to optical interference as the light passes through the section. Because of these factors the basic unit of enamel was at first described as hexagonal and prismlike and the term *enamel prism* was frequently used; but we will not use it here since the basic unit does not have a regular geometry and does not in any way resemble a prism. *Enamel rod* is the more appropriate term.

Another problem met in the study of enamel structure results from the nature and organization of enamel's basic constitutional elements. When the roughly cylindrical enamel rods are sectioned at different angles to their long axes, obliquely cut sections (between 30 and 90 degrees) are easily interpreted as true cross sections, making an assessment of rod direction in any microscopic section extremely difficult (Fig. 12-5). Use of the electron microscope, with much thinner sections and greater resolving power, has overcome some of these interpretative difficulties.

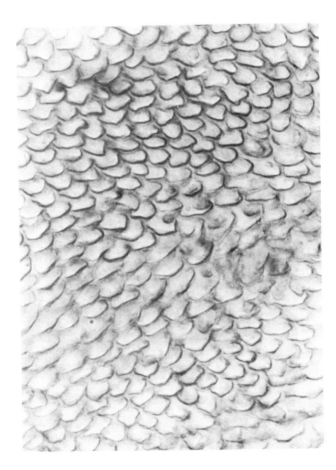

FIG. 12-3 Decalcified section of enamel. Enough organic material has been retained to reveal structure. (Courtesy Dr. K. Katele.)

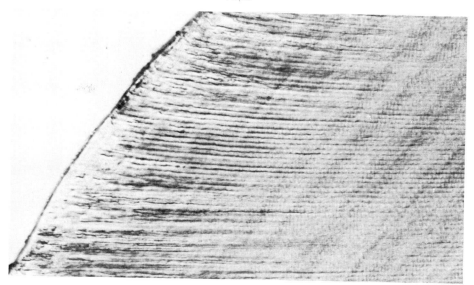

160x

A

FIG. 12-4 Enamel in ground sections. In **A** note the rows of rods running horizontally across the section. In **B** a ground section, the cross sectional appearance of these rods is seen. In **C,** enamel structure has been emphasized by etching (partial demineralization). (Courtesy Dr. D. Weber.)

B

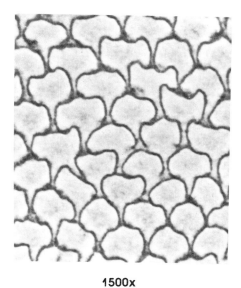

C

1000x

1500x

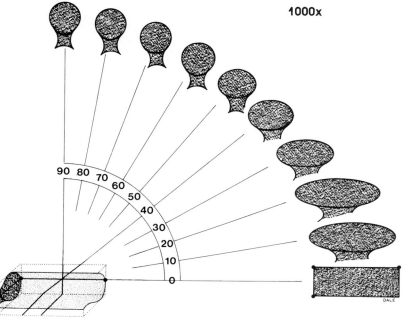

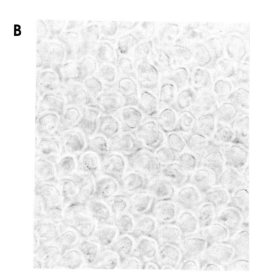

FIG. 12-5 Sections through a rod-shaped structure at different angles. Such sections can sometimes be mistaken for true cross sections. (From Dale AC, Hoard AB: *Ontario Dentist* 55:9, 1978.)

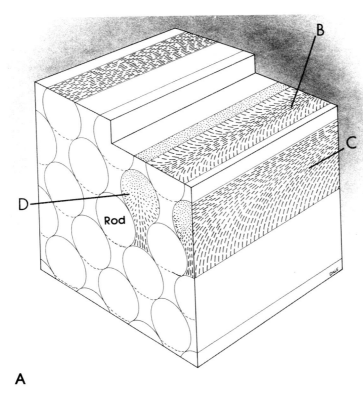

A

FIG. 12-6   Fine structure of enamel. **A,** Crystal orientation of three faces of a block of enamel, showing the rod structure. **B to D,** Electron micrographs of three faces. (Courtesy Dr. A.H. Meckel.)

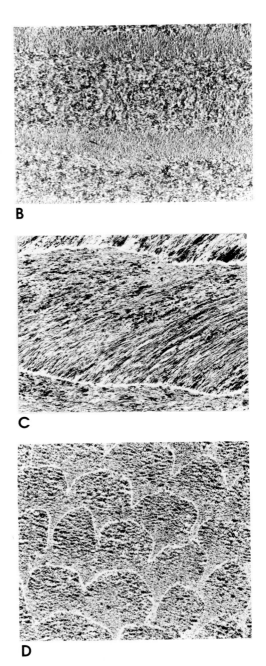

Enamel Rods

Enamel is essentially a tightly packed mass of hydroxyapatite crystals. Indeed, the basic structural unit of enamel—the rod—owes its existence to a highly organized pattern of crystal orientation (Fig. 12-6). The rod is shaped somewhat like a cylinder and is made up of crystals whose long axes run, for the most part, parallel to the longitudinal axis of the rod. This is particularly true for crystals along the central axis of the rod. Crystals more distant from the central axis, however, flare laterally to an increasing degree as they approach the rod periphery. The interrod region is an area surrounding each rod in which crystals are oriented in a different direction from those making up the rod. The degree of difference is significant around approximately three fourths of the circumference of a rod. The boundary where crystals of the rod meet those of the interrod region at sharp angles is known as the *rod sheath* (Figs. 12-6 to 12-9). The rod sheath exists only because of the greater space that occurs between the ends of crystals, which meet at sharp angles.

The complexity of enamel structure is reflected in an intricate pattern of variations in crystal orientation. The portion of the interrod region located directly cervical to a particular rod is not separated from that rod by a sheath, because the crystals there are confluent with those making up the rod. In sections cut along the longitudinal axis of enamel rods, it can be seen that the lateral flaring of rod crystals continues uninterrupted into the cervically located interrod region until they lie nearly perpendicular to the rod (Fig. 12-6). The cross-

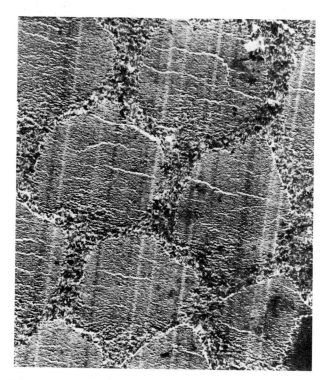

FIG. 12-7 Cross section through enamel rods. The difference in crystal orientation in the enamel rod and in the interrod region is evident. (Courtesy Dr. A.H. Meckel.)

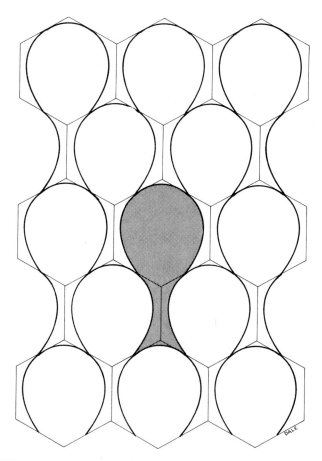

FIG. 12-9 Regions of influence of an ameloblast outlined by the hexagonal profiles. The shaded area indicates the keyhole configuration outlining both a rod and its cervically confluent interrod region.

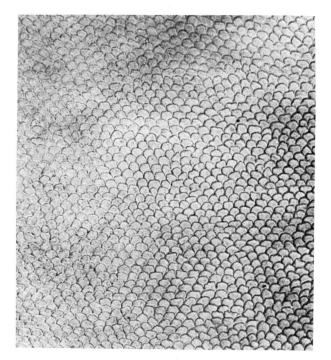

FIG. 12-8 Etched ground section of enamel showing the characteristic fish-scale appearance.

sectional outline of these two related components has been compared to the shape of a keyhole (Fig. 12-9). Since the keyhole analogy does not adequately account for some of the variations in structural arrangement of the enamel components, however, or coordinate with the pattern of secretion by the Tomes processes, this terminology has largely been dropped. The basic unit of enamel is more appropriately described as a cylindrical rod that has a specific spatial relation to the interrod region directly cervical to it.

This configuration of enamel crystals is a property of the ameloblasts and their Tomes processes. The forming surface of enamel consists of pits, each surrounded by a wall made up of newly formed interrod enamel (Fig. 11-13). During active secretion, each of these walled pits is occupied by a Tomes process. The interrod region is formed slightly earlier than the rod enamel, which thus constitutes the walls of the pits. These walls are formed by secretion from proximal sites that completely encircle each Tomes process near its base, where adjacent processes are joined by the distal junctional complexes (Fig. 11-12). Thus each wall (interrod region) is formed as a cooperative effort by adjacent secretory ameloblasts. The rod portion of enamel matrix is subsequently secreted into the pit by the distal secretory site on the Tomes process. Since this distal site is oriented somewhat cervically, the spatial relationship between rods and the adjacent (cervically located) interrod region develops by a confluence of the orientations of these crystals as they form.

Along the remainder of the rod circumference there is a sharp discontinuity between the direction of rod crystals with those of the interrod region, creating the rod sheath. Based on current knowledge of enamel formation, it is apparent that each ameloblast is responsible for the formation of one rod (by its distal secretory site) and a portion of the surrounding interrod region (by its cooperative proximal sites). The region of influence of an ameloblast is indicated in Figure 12-9.

Rod sheaths contain more enamel protein than other regions do because crystals meeting at different angles cannot be packed together tightly. The consistent arrangement of rod sheaths, with their greater protein content, accounts for the fish-scale appearance of enamel matrix seen in sections of demineralized developing enamel or in etched ground sections (Figs. 12-3 and 12-8). The rod sheath can also be visualized in undemineralized light microscope sections because of differences between the refractive indices of the sheath, rod, and interrod regions, so that light is differentially refracted, creating a widened image of the sheath.

Enamel rods have an average width of 5 μm, but they vary somewhat in size and morphology throughout the thickness of enamel. In the first 5 μm, next to the dentin, there is no rod structure (explained by the fact that Tomes' processes have not yet formed when this enamel is laid down). As they traverse the enamel, the rods gradually increase slightly in diameter. At the enamel surface the rod structure is irregular or absent (again explained by the fact that Tomes processes are lost as amelogenesis comes to an end). Rodless enamel occurs in the outermost 30 μm or so of all primary teeth and in the gingival third of the enamel of permanent teeth. Crystals in these regions are aligned perpendicular to the surface of the enamel.

Rod Interrelationships

For two reasons examination of ground sections does not give an accurate indication of rod interrelationships and rod direction: Every rod has an undulating course, and therefore any section contains only short segments of rod. When this factor is combined with the problem of assessing whether a true cross section has been made (Fig. 12-5), the difficulty of seeing the true course of rods in ground sections can be readily appreciated.

In spite of such difficulties, much is known about the complex interrelationships of enamel rods (Fig. 12-10). Rods tend to be maintained in rows arranged circumferentially around the long axis of the tooth. The rods in each row run in a direction generally perpendicular to the surface of the dentin, with a slight inclination toward the cusp as they pass outward. Near the cusp tip the rows have a small radius, and the rods run more vertically. In cervical enamel the rods run mainly horizontally; only a few rows are tilted apically. The arrangement of rod rows has clinical importance, because enamel fractures occur between adjacent rows.

Superimposed on this row arrangement are two other patterns that complicate enamel structure: First, each rod, as it runs to the surface, has an undulating course bending to the right and left in the transverse plane of the tooth (except in cervical enamel, where the rods have a straight course) and up and down in the vertical plane. Second, although the rods in a row run in similar directions, a change in direction of about 2 degrees occurs between successive rows. These complex interrelationships produce some of the structural features seen in enamel and must be remembered when interpreting enamel structure.

FIG. 12-10 Enamel rod orientation. The small diagram *(bottom left)* shows how the enamel rods are arranged circumferentially in rows around the long axis of the tooth. Each row inclines more vertically as the cusp tip is approached so that the final few rows of enamel rods are almost vertical. The larger diagram depicts changes in rod direction as they run from the dentinoenamel junction to the enamel surface. In addition to their S-shaped course in the horizontal plane, successive shifts in rod direction occur in each row. Thus in row *1* the rods run from the dentinoenamel junction to the tooth surface at right angles to the junction. The next vertical row of rods runs to the surface at an angle of 90 + 2 degrees to the junction; the next at 90 + 4 degrees to the junction, and so on until a maximum deviation is reached in row *6*. Rod direction then swings back until row *11*, where the rods change to 90 − 2 degrees, and so on. The result is a wave pattern created in the vertical plane. The scanning electron micrograph depicts successive rows of enamel rods.

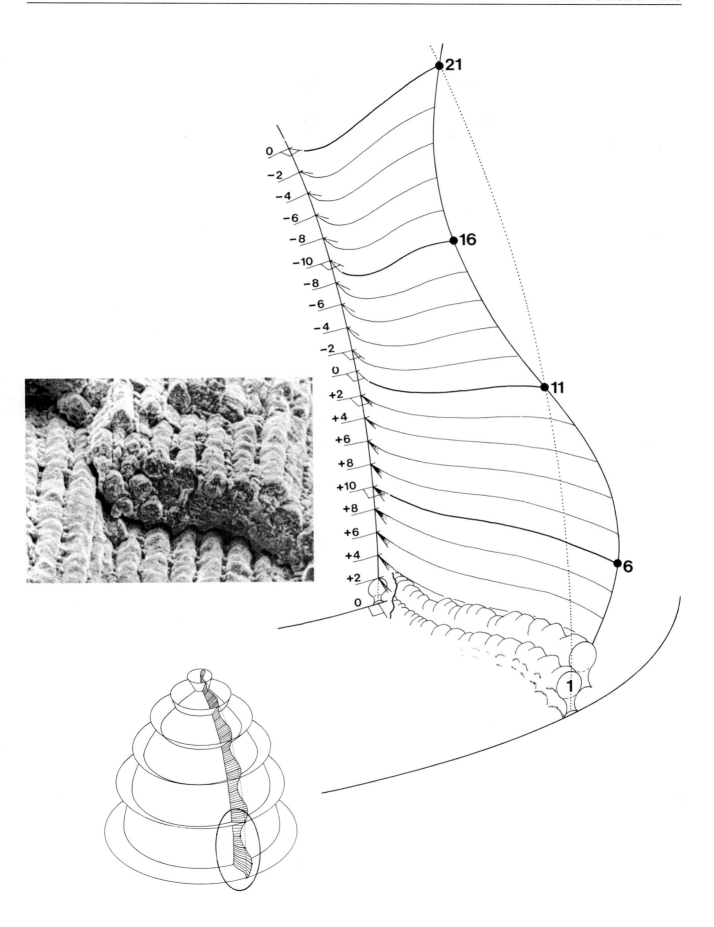

Striae of Retzius

The striae of Retzius are incremental growth lines. In a longitudinal section they are seen as a series of dark bands reflecting successive enamel-forming fronts (Fig. 12-11). In cross section they are seen as concentric rings (Fig. 12-12)—prominent in most human permanent teeth, less prominent in postnatal deciduous enamel, and rare in prenatal enamel. Accentuated incremental lines are produced by systemic disturbances (e.g., fevers) that affect amelogenesis; similar patterns of incremental lines are found in different teeth from the same individual. The structural basis for the production of Retzius lines has recently been examined; it seems that they are formed as the result of a temporary constriction of Tomes processes associated with a corresponding increase in the secretory face forming interrod enamel (Fig. 12-13). As a result enamel structure is altered along the lines. Electron micrographs reveal a possible decrease in the number of crystals in the striae, and there is a suggestion that enamel rods bend as they cross an incremental line (Fig. 12-14). The neonatal line, when present, is an enlarged stria of Retzius that, apparently, reflects the marked physiologic changes occurring at birth.

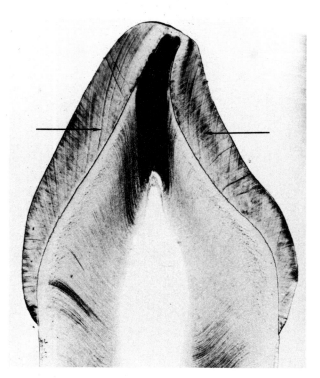

FIG. 12-11 Longitudinal ground section showing disposition of the striae of Reztius (arrows).

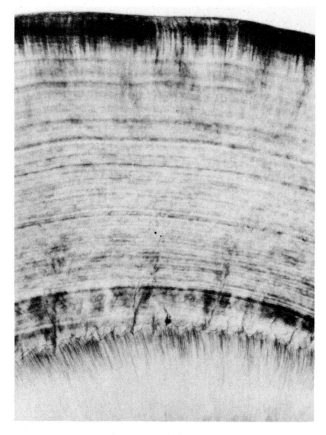

FIG. 12-12 Cross ground section showing disposition of the striae of Retzius. (Courtesy Dr. D. Weber.)

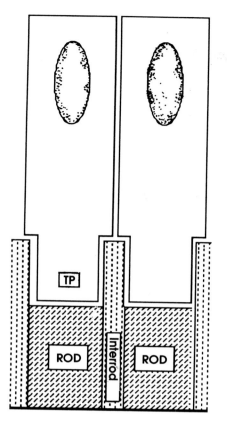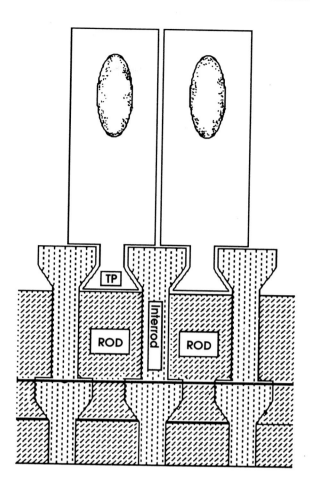

FIG. 12 -13 How the change in diameter of a Tomes process produces a stria of Retzius. (Modified from Risnes, *Anat Rec* 226:135, 1990.)

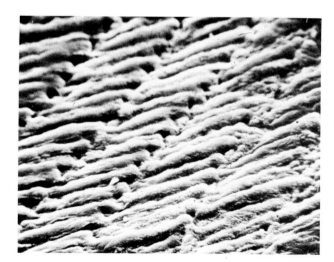

FIG. 12-14 Scanning electron micrograph of partially demineralized enamel. Enamel rods run from left to right. Striae of Retzius, running from bottom left to top right, seem to coincide with a bend in the enamel rod. (Courtesy Dr. D. Weber.)

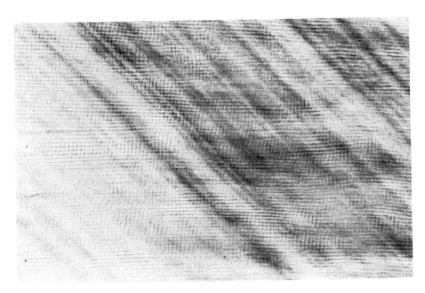

FIG. 12-15 Ground section of enamel. Rods appear to run horizontally and are bisected at regular intervals by cross striations. Oblique lines are striae of Retzius. (Courtesy Dr. D. Weber.)

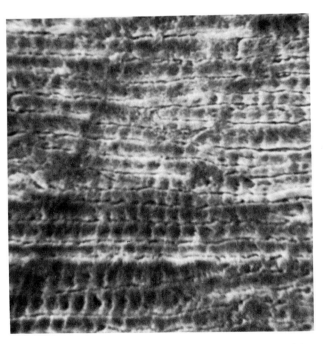

FIG. 12-16 Scanning electron micrograph of an acid-etched ground section. Rods run across the section from left to right. Perpendicular to them, heavily accentuated cross striations can be seen. (Courtesy Dr. D. Weber.)

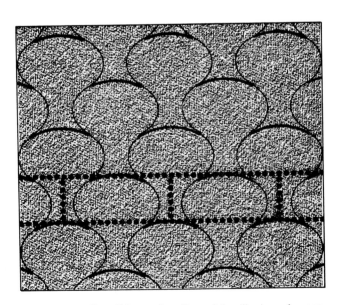

FIG. 12-17 Possible explanation of the illusion of cross striations in oblique sections of enamel. The interrod regions of a series of rods occur about every 4 μm and could create the appearance of cross striations. (From Dale AC, Hoard AB: *Ontario Dentist* 55:9, 1978.)

Cross Striations

Human enamel is known to form at a rate of approximately 4 μm per day. Ground sections of enamel reveal what appear to be periodic bands or cross striations occurring at 4 μm intervals across so-called rods (Fig. 12-15). Scanning electron microscopy reveals alternating constrictions and expansions of the rods in some regions of enamel, which may account for this banded appearance in ground sections (Fig. 12-16). On the other hand, the appearance of cross striations could also result from structural interrelations among groups of rods rather than the modification of a single rod. What may seem to be cross striations of longitudinally sectioned rods are many times obliquely sectioned groups of rods (Fig. 12-17). The rods are aligned in horizontal rows. Situated between the rods at approximately 4 μm intervals are interrod regions. Thus the light microscope may produce an illusion of longitudinally sectioned rods that are really, as demonstrated by electron microscopy, an alignment of obliquely cut rods in horizontal rows. Technical difficulties in achieving true longitudinal planes account for many false observations of cross striations, but do not rule out their existence in some regions of enamel.

In spite of these structural ambiguities it is clear that cross striations indicate a daily (or circadian) variation in the secretory activity of the ameloblasts and that the striae of Retzius represent a weekly (or circaseptimanian) rhythm of the same cells.

Bands of Hunter-Schreger

The bands of Hunter-Schreger are an optical phenomenon produced solely by changes in rod direction. They are seen most clearly in longitudinal ground sections viewed by reflected light and are found in the inner four fifths of the enamel. They appear as dark and light alternating zones that can be reversed by altering the direction of incident illumination (Figs. 12-18 to 12-20).

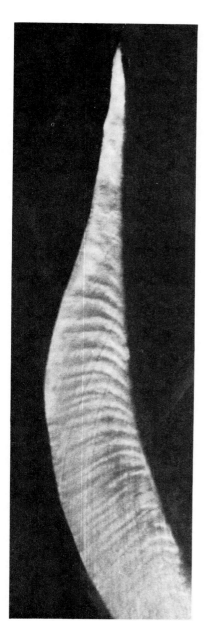

FIG. 12-18 Longitudinal section of enamel viewed by incident light. Note the series of Hunter-Schreger bands (alternating light and dark).

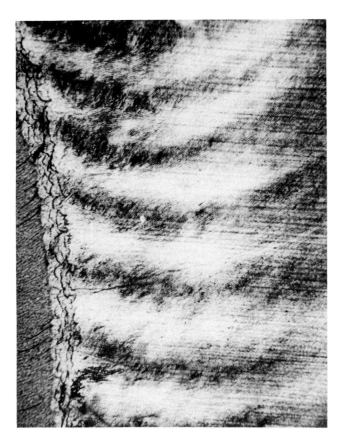

FIG. 12-19 Higher power view of a Hunter-Schreger band as viewed by incident light.

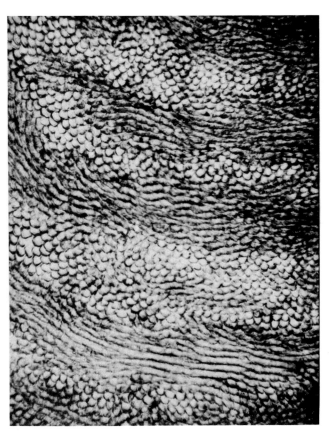

FIG. 12-20 Section corresponding to Fig. 12-19 viewed under transmitted light. The differing orientation of enamel rods is clearly evident.

Gnarled Enamel

Over the cusps of teeth the rods appear twisted around each other in a seemingly complex arrangement known as gnarled enamel. Recall that rods are arranged radially in horizontal rows, each row surrounding the longitudinal axis of the tooth like a washer. The rods undulate back and forth within the rows. This undulation in vertically directed rods around a ring of small circumference readily explains gnarled enamel.

Enamel Tufts and Lamellae

Enamel tufts and lamellae may be likened to geologic faults. They are best seen in transverse sections of enamel (Fig. 12-21). Enamel tufts project from the dentinoenamel junction for a short distance into the enamel, appearing to be branched and containing greater concentrations of enamel protein than the rest of enamel. Lamellae extend for varying depths from the surface of enamel and consist of linear, longitudinally oriented, defects filled with enamel protein or organic debris from the oral cavity.

Tufts and lamellae are usually best demonstrated in ground sections, but they can also be seen in carefully demineralized sections of enamel because of their higher protein content. The protein of tufts is a high-molecular-weight variety similar to enamelin. Tufts are believed to occur developmentally because of abrupt changes in the direction of groups of rods that arise from different regions of the scalloped dentinoenamel junction. A different ratio of interrod and rod enamel in these groups creates less mineralized and weakened planes. Faulting of blocks of enamel occurs to relieve internal strains produced by dimensional changes as the tissue matures. When a fault occurs, it blocks the normal exit for enamel protein, causing the higher organic content of tufts and lamellae. Tufts and lamellae are of no known clinical significance and do not appear to be sites of increased vulnerability to caries attack.

Dentinoenamel Junction and Enamel Spindles

The junction between enamel and dentin is established as these two hard tissues begin to form and is seen as a scalloped profile in cross section (Fig. 10-22). Scanning electron microscopy of the junction shows it to be a series of ridges that increase the surface area and probably enhance the adhesion between enamel and dentin. Before enamel formation occurs, some newly forming odontoblast processes push between adjoining ameloblasts and, when enamel formation begins, become trapped to form enamel spindles (Fig. 12-22). These structures do not follow the direction of enamel rods.

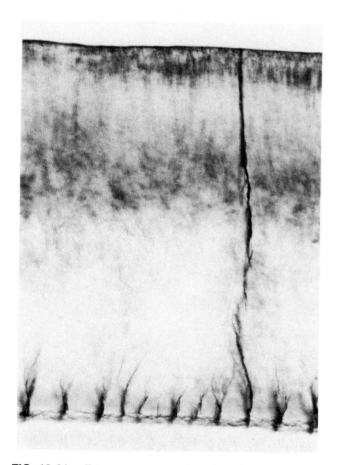

FIG. 12-21 Transverse ground section of enamel. An enamel lamella can be seen running from the outer surface to the dentinoenamel junction. Enamel tufts are the branched structures extending from the junction into the enamel. The junction is seen as a scalloped profile.

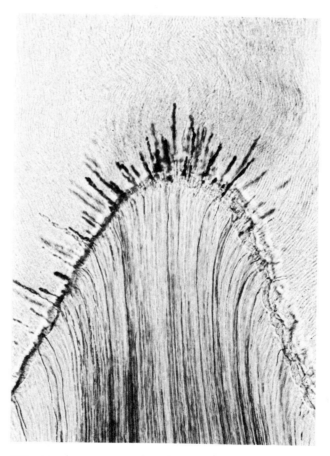

FIG. 12-22 Enamel spindles in ground section. They extend from the dentinoenamel junction into the enamel and are most frequently found at cusp tips. (Courtesy Dr. D. Weber.)

Enamel Surface

The surface of enamel is characterized by several formations. The striae of Retzius often extend from the dentinoenamel junction to the outer surface of enamel, where they end in shallow furrows known as *perikymata* (Figs. 12-23 to 12-25). Perikymata run in circumferentially horizontal lines across the face of the crown. In addition, lamellae or cracks in the enamel appear as jagged lines in various regions of the tooth surface. The electron microscope shows that the surface structure of enamel varies with age. In unerupted teeth the enamel surface consists of a structureless cuticle some 0.5 to 1.5 μm thick. Immediately below this is a layer of small loosely packed crystallites, some 5 nm thick, with cuticular material between them. Interspersed among, in, and on these fine crystallites are randomly distributed large platelike crystals. The fine crystallite layer merges into the subsurface enamel, where crystals are closely packed and approximately 50 nm in size (Fig. 12-26). In erupted teeth the subsurface layer forms the enamel

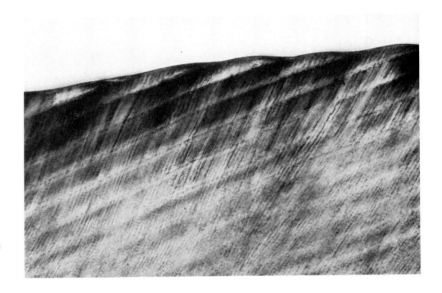

FIG. 12-23 Ground section of enamel showing the relationship between the striae of Retzius and surface perikymata. (Courtesy Dr. D. Weber.)

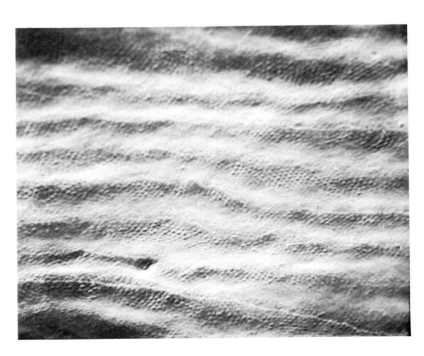

FIG. 12-24 Scanning electron micrograph of the labial surface of a tooth, showing the perikymata. (Courtesy Dr. D. Weber.)

surface, which indicates that the primary cuticle and the surface layer of small crystallites are rapidly lost by abrasion, attrition, and erosion.

Salivary pellicle, a nearly ubiquitous organic deposit on the surface of teeth, always reappears shortly after teeth have been mechanically polished. Dental plaque forms readily on the pellicle, especially in more protected areas of the dentition. The important role of dental plaque in fostering caries as well as other clinical implications of these surface accumulations will be discussed in Chapter 16.

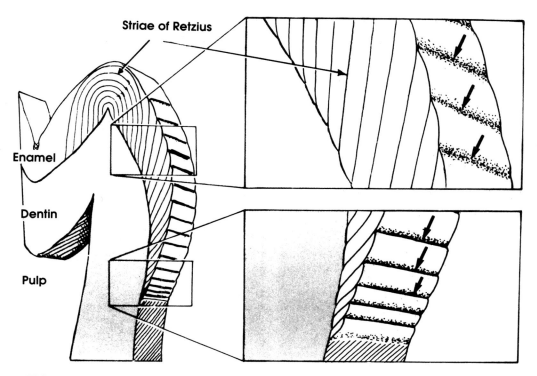

FIG. 12-25 Relationship between the striae of Retzius and surface perikymata as seen in Fig. 12-23 (From Fejerskov O, Thylstruo A: In Mjör I, Fejerskov O. [eds]: *Human oral embryology and histology,* Copenhagen, 1986, Munksgaard.)

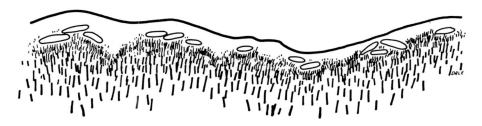

FIG. 12-26 Surface of enamel in an unerupted tooth illustrating the variation in crystal size. (Redrawn from Palmara J, et al: *Arch Oral Biol* 25:715, 1980.)

AGE CHANGES

Enamel is a nonvital tissue and is incapable of regeneration. With age it becomes progressively worn away in regions of masticatory attrition. Wear facets are increasingly pronounced in older people, and in some cases substantial portions of the crown (both enamel and dentin) become eroded. Other characteristics of aging enamel include discoloration, reduced permeability, and modifications in the surface layer. Linked to these changes is an apparent reduction in the incidence of caries.

Teeth darken with age. Whether this is caused by a change in the structure of enamel is debatable. Although it could be due to the addition of organic material to enamel from the environment, it also may be due to a deepening of dentin color seen through the progressively thinning layer of translucent enamel.

There is no doubt that enamel becomes less permeable with age. Young enamel behaves as a semipermeable membrane, permitting the slow passage of water and substances of small molecular size through pores between the crystals. With age the pores diminish as the crystals acquire more ions and increase in size. Because the bulk of the water lies in the pores, it follows that the water content of enamel also decreases with age.

The surface layer of enamel reflects most prominently the changes occurring within this tissue. During aging the composition of the surface layer changes as ionic exchange with the oral environment occurs. In particular, there is a progressive increase in the fluoride content of surface enamel that affects the surface layer (and that, incidentally, can be achieved by topical application).

CLINICAL IMPLICATIONS

An appreciation of the histology of enamel is important for understanding the principles of fluoridation, acid etch techniques, and dental caries.

Fluoridation

It is well known that if the fluoride ion is incorporated into or adsorbed on the hydroxyapatite crystal the crystal becomes more resistant to acid dissolution. This reaction partly explains the role of fluoride in caries prevention, for the caries process is initiated by demineralization of enamel. Obviously, if fluoride is present as enamel is being formed, all the enamel crystals will be more resistant to acid dissolution. The amount of fluoride must be carefully controlled, however, because of the sensitivity of secretory ameloblasts to the fluoride ion and the possibility of producing unsightly mottling. The semipermeable nature of enamel enables topical fluorides, fluoridated toothpastes, and fluoridated drinking water to provide a higher concentration of fluoride in the surface enamel of erupted teeth. Also the fluoride in surface enamel reduces the free energy in this region and thus lessens the adsorption of glycoproteins from the saliva.

It is well established that the presence of fluoride enhances chemical reactions that lead to the precipitation of calcium phosphate. An equilibrium exists in the oral cavity between calcium and phosphate ions in the solution phase (saliva) and in the solid phase (enamel), and fluoride shifts this equilibrium to favor the solid phase. Clinically, when a localized region of enamel has lost mineral (e.g., a white spot lesion), it may be remineralized if the destructive agent (dental plaque) is removed. The remineralization reaction is greatly enhanced by fluoride.

Acid Etching

Acid etching of the enamel surface, or enamel conditioning, has become an important technique in clinical practice. It is involved in the use of fissure sealants, in the bonding of restorative materials to enamel, and in the cementing of orthodontic brackets to tooth surfaces. It achieves the desired effect in two stages: First, it removes plaque and other debris, along with a thin layer of enamel. Second, it increases the porosity of exposed surfaces through selective dissolution of crystals, which provides a better bonding surface for the restorative and adhesive materials.

Several types and concentrations of acid are used to alter the enamel surface; most etch the surface to a depth of only about 10 μm. For example, 30% to 40% phosphoric acid applied to enamel for 60 seconds provides an adequate etch for retention of sealants.

The scanning electron microscope beautifully demonstrates the effects of acid etching on enamel surfaces. Three etching patterns predominate (Fig. 12-27): The most common is *type I*, characterized by preferential removal of the rod core. The reverse, *type II*, also occurs, in which the rod periphery is preferentially removed and the core remains intact. Occurring less frequently is *type III*, which is irregular and indiscriminate. There is still some debate as to why acid etchants produce differing surface patterns. The most commonly held view is that the etching pattern depends on crystal orientation. Ultrastructural studies of crystal dissolution indicate that crystals dissolve more readily at their ends than on their sides. Thus crystals lying perpendicular to the enamel surface are the most vulnerable. The type I etching pattern can easily be explained by noting that crystals reach the enamel surfaces at differing inclinations in the rods as compared to the interrod areas. Regional variations may also play a role, since the same areas on contralateral teeth seem to have almost identical etch patterns. There is, in addition, however, evidence that the type of pattern results from differences in the nature of the etching agent.

In summary: Acid conditioning of enamel surfaces is now an accepted procedure for obtaining improved bonding of resins to enamel. Retention depends mainly on a mechanical interlocking. The conditioning agent removes the organic film from the tooth surface and preferentially etches the enamel surface so that firmer contact is established. In areas where rodless enamel occurs, especially in deciduous teeth, slightly more severe etching is required to obtain adequate mechanical retention.

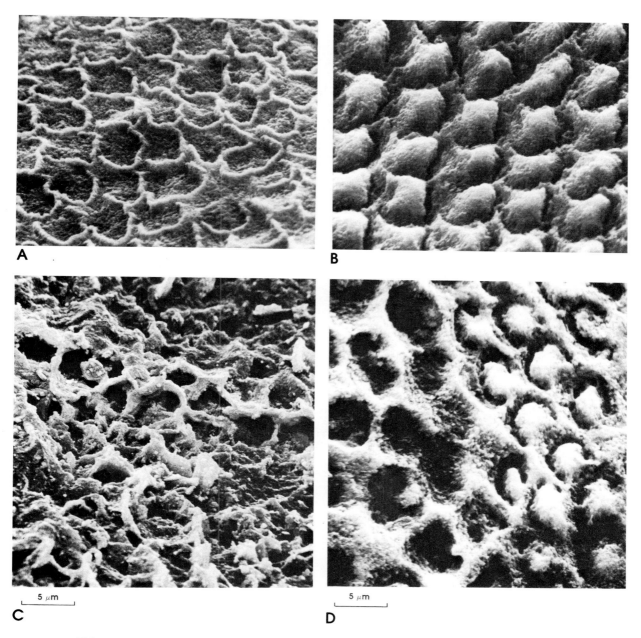

FIG. 12-27 Scanning electron micrographs of etching patterns in enamel. **A,** Type I pattern, rod core preferentially eroded; **B,** type II pattern, rod boundary preferentially eroded; **C,** type III pattern, indiscriminate erosion; **D,** junction between type I and type II etching zones. (Courtesy Dr. L. Silverstone.)

BIBLIOGRAPHY

Boyde A: The development of enamel structure, *Proc R Soc Med* 60:923, 1967.

Dean MC: Growth layers and incremental markings in hard tissues; a review of the literature and some preliminary observations about enamel structure in *Paranthropus boisei, J Hum Evolution* 16:157, 1987.

Fearnhead RW, Suga S (eds): *Tooth enamel,* ed 4, Amsterdam, 1984, Elsevier Science Publishers.

Frank RM: The ultrastructure of the tooth from the point of view of mineralization, demineralization and remineralization, *Int Dent J* 17:661, 1967.

Glantz PO: On wettability and adhesiveness, *Odontol Rev* 20(Suppl 17), 1969.

Glass JE, Nylen MU: A correlated electron microscopic and microradiographic study of human enamel, *Arch Oral Biol* 10:893, 1965.

Gwinnett AM: The ultrastructure of the "prismless" enamel of permanent human teeth, *Arch Oral Biol* 12:381, 1967.

Hinrichsen CFL, Engel MB: Fine structure of partially demineralized enamel, *Arch Oral Biol* 11:65, 1966.

Hirota F: Prism arrangement in human cusp enamel deduced by x-ray diffraction, *Arch Oral Biol* 27:931, 1982.

Johnson NW: Some aspects of the ultrastructure of early human enamel caries seen with the electron microscope, *Arch Oral Biol* 12:1505, 1967.

Kerckaert GA: Electron microscopy of human carious dental enamel, *Arch Oral Biol* 18:751, 1973.

Listgarten MA: Structure of surface coatings on teeth: a review, *J Periodontol* 47:139, 1976.

Meckel AH, Griebstein WS, Neal RJ: Structure of mature human dental enamel as observed by electron microscopy, *Arch Oral Biol* 10:775, 1965.

Miles AEW (ed): *Structural and chemical organization of teeth,* New York, 1967, Academic Press.

Mortimer KV, Tranter TC: A scanning electron microscope study of carious enamel, *Caries Res* 5:240, 1971.

Nylen MU, Eanes ED, Omnell KA: Crystal growth in the rat, *J Cell Biol* 18:109, 1963.

Osborn JW: The cross-sectional outlines of human enamel prisms, *Acta Anat* 70:493, 1968.

Osborn JW: The mechanism of prism formation in teeth: a hypothesis, *Calcif Tiss Res* 5:115, 1970.

Palamara J, Phakey PP, Rachinger WA, et al: Electron microscopy of surface enamel of human unerupted and erupted teeth, *Arch Oral Biol* 25:715, 1980.

Paulsen RB: Scanning electron microscopy of enamel tuft development in human deciduous teeth, *Arch Oral Biol* 26:103, 1981.

Ripa IW, Gwinnett AJ, Buonocore MG: The "prismless" outer layer of deciduous and permanent enamel, *Arch Oral Biol* 11:41, 1966.

Risnes S: Structural characteristics of staircase-type Retzius lines in human dental enamel analyzed by scanning electron microscopy, *Anat Rec* 226:135, 1990.

Robinson C, Kirkham J, Briggs HD, et al: Enamel proteins: from secretion to maturation, *J Dent Res* (Special issue) 61:1490, 1982.

Rolla G, Melsen B: Desorption of protein and bacteria from hydroxyapatite by fluoride and monofluorophosphate, *Caries Res* 9:66, 1975.

Ronnholm E: The structure of the organic stroma of human enamel during amelogenesis, *J Ultrastruct Res* 6:368, 1962.

Silverstone LM: Fissure sealants: laboratory studies, *Caries Res* 8:2, 1974.

Silverstone LM, Poole DFG: Histological and ultrastructural features of remineralized carious enamel. (Proceedings of the Fourth International Conference on Oral Biology, Copenhagen.) *J Dent Res* 48:766, 1969.

Silverstone LM, Saxton CA, Dogon IL, et al: Variation in the pattern of acid etching of human dental enamel examined by scanning electron microscopy, *Caries Res* 9:373, 1975.

Speirs RL: The nature of surface enamel in human teeth, *Calcif Tiss Res* 8:1, 1971.

Stack MV, Fearnhead RW (eds): *Proceedings of the International Symposium on Composition, Properties, and Fundamental Structure of Dental Enamel,* Bristol, 1964, John Wright & Sons.

Swancar JR, Scott DB, Njemirovskij Z: Studies on the structure of human enamel by the replica method, *J Dent Res* 49:1025, 1970.

Warshawsky H: Ultrastructural studies on amelogenesis. In Butler WT (ed): *The chemistry and biology of mineralized tissues,* Birmingham, 1985, Ebsco Media.

Warshawsky H, Josephson K, Thylstrup A, Fejerskov O: The development of enamel structure in rat incisors as compared to the teeth of monkey and man, *Anat Rec* 200:371, 1981.

Weber D, Eisenmann DR, Glick PL: Light and electron microscopic studies of Retzius lines in human cervical enamel, *Am J Anat* 141:91, 1974.

Weber DF, Glick PL: Correlative microscopy of enamel prism orientation, *Am J Anat* 144:407, 1975.

CHAPTER 13

Development of the Periodontium

THE periodontium consists of cementum (Latin *caementum*, quarried stone [i.e., chips of stone used in making mortar]), the periodontal ligament (PDL), bone lining the alveolus (socket), and that part of the gingiva facing the tooth. Recall that very early in tooth development, at the cap stage, three distinct components can be recognized: the dental organ, the dental papilla, and the dental follicle. The dental follicle is that well-defined layer of cells surrounding the tooth germ that is continuous with and derived from the dental papilla at the cervical loop. It gives rise to the supporting tissues of the tooth (i.e., cementum, PDL, and bone). The histologic events leading to formation of these supporting tissues are diagramed in Figure 13-1.

CEMENTOGENESIS

Cementum is deposited on the surface of root dentin. In Chapter 4 it was explained how the Hertwig root sheath was formed and how it differentiates root odontoblasts from the dental papilla. The cells of the root sheath have a further function: they are involved in the formation of a structureless highly mineralized layer some 10 μm thick on the surface of the root dentin (Figs. 10-20, 14-2, 15-7, and 18-8). This layer has variously been described as dentin (the hyaline layer of Hopewell-Smith) and as intermediate cementum, but a study of its development suggests that it is neither and instead may be a form of enamel. As the large collagen fibers of mantle dentin form, they are deposited slightly away from the basement membrane supporting the root sheath (10 to 20 μm in the mouse molar), leaving a gap filled with ground substance and a very fine fibrillar material (Fig. 13-2). The basement membrane supporting the root sheath breaks up; the root sheath cells develop profiles of rough endoplasmic reticulum and actively secrete a distinct class of enamel proteins closely related to the amelogenin family into this gap (Fig. 13-2). The mineralization of mantle dentin does not involve this layer, which mineralizes both later and separately, largely because of its distinct matrix. We now know that this layer contains the product of epithelial cell activity. Whether the connective tissue component is significant needs to be determined; but, because of this admixture, it has been suggested that the layer is a form of enameloid, the hard tissue covering the teeth of many fishes, which has a mesenchymally derived matrix but is mineralized by the epithelial dental organ. Thus the dentin of the root surface is covered by an epithelial product of the root sheath cells (similar to enameloid) that is more mineralized than other dentin. It has been proposed that its function is to "cement" cementum to the dentin as well as provide the initial attachment of ligament fibrils to the tooth (Fig. 13-3).

Primary Cementum Formation

When root dentin formation has been initiated and the hyaline layer formed, the root sheath fragments into a network that allows follicular cells to pass through it and thereby come into apposition with the newly formed root surface. As soon as the follicular cells are in this location, they differentiate into cementoblasts and become larger as well as develop all the cytoplasmic organelles associated with a protein-synthesizing-and-secreting cell. After their differentiation they begin to deposit an organic matrix against the root surface and around the forming ligament fiber bundles or extrinsic fibers (Fig. 13-4). Mineralization of this matrix (cementoid) occurs in a manner similar to that in dentin, with the deposition of apatite crystals initially in matrix vesicles (Fig. 13-5) followed by mineralization of the

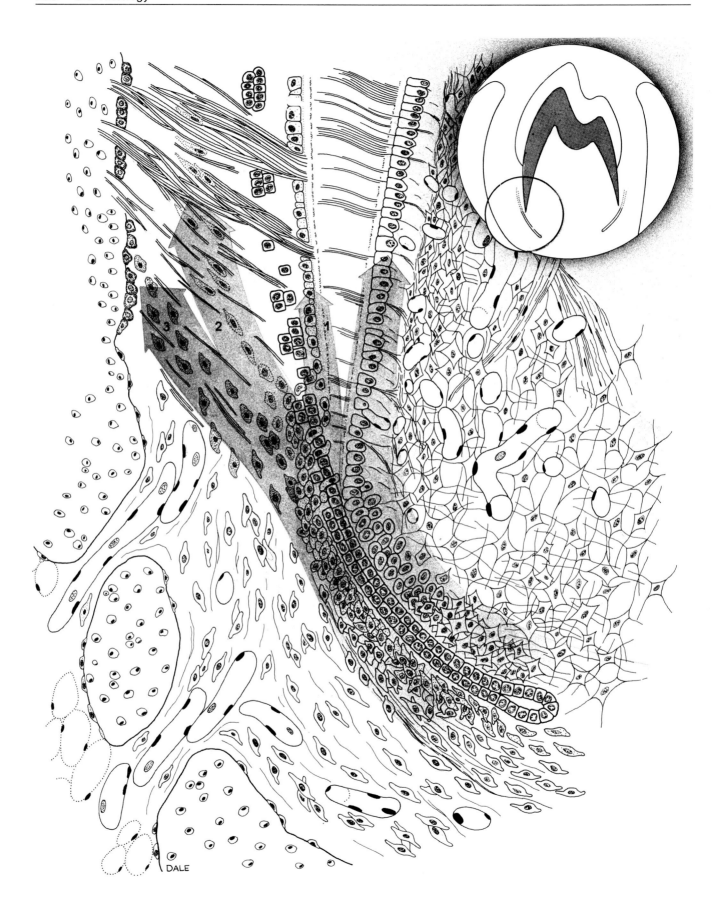

DALE

FIG. 13-1   Events during formation of the periodontium (excluding formation of the dentogingival junction).*1,* Fragmentation of Hertwig's epithelial root sheath and the origin of cementoblasts from follicular cells;
2, follicular contribution to the formation of fiber bundles of the PDL; *3,* formation of bone lining the alveolus. (Inset: site of the activity.)

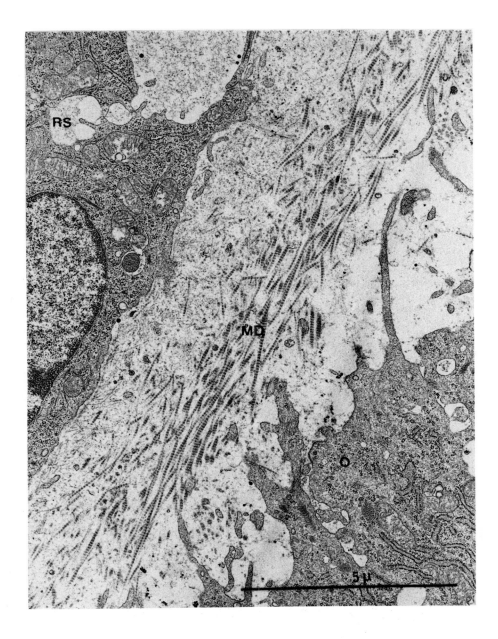

FIG. 13-2   Electron micrograph of early root dentinogenesis. The large collagen fiber bundles of mantle dentin are deposited parallel but not next to the basement membrane that supports the root sheath. *RS,* Root sheath; *MD,* mantle dentin; *O,* odontoblast.

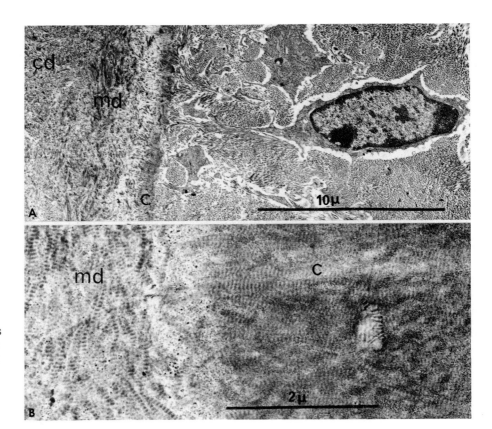

FIG. 13-3 Electron micrographs of early, **A,** and late, **B,** cementogenesis. Note that the cementum is not deposited directly against the mantle dentin. *cd,* Circumpulpal dentin; *md,* mantle dentin; *hl,* hyaline layer; *c,* cementum.

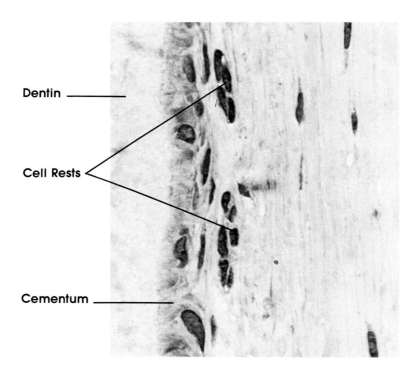

Dentin ————

Cell Rests ◁

Cementum ————

FIG. 13-4 Initial cementum formation. The first increment of cementum is forming against the root dentin surface. Cell rests (remnants of the root sheath) can be seen within the follicular tissue.

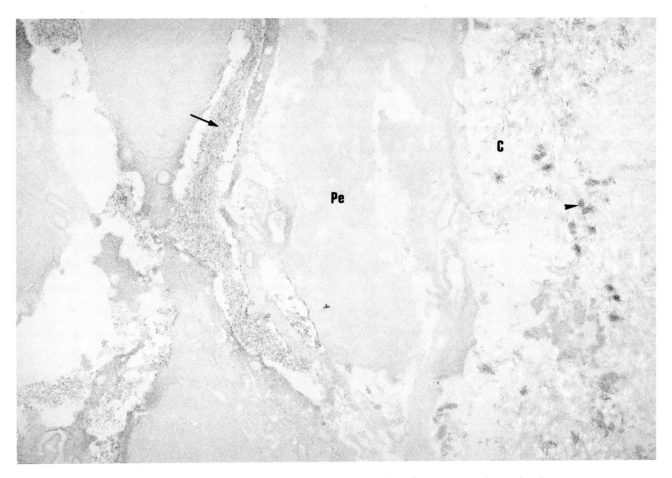

FIG. 13-5 Section through the developing root region of a mouse molar stained to demonstrate type III collagen. Cementum *(c)* is to the right, its collagen (type I) does not stain. The first mineral deposits, associated with matrix vesicles *(arrowhead),* are clearly visible. To the left is dental follicle, where intercellular collagen *(arrow),* which is type III, stains. *Pe,* Periodontal ligament cell. (Courtesy Dr. M.B. Andujar.)

collagen fibrils (Fig. 13-6). This first-formed (or primary) cementum is acellular (Fig. 13-7), develops relatively slowly as the tooth is erupting, and covers at least the coronal two thirds of the root. There is some evidence from the study of mice that, once deposited, the cells forming this primary cementum are lost, to be replaced by cells of a different phenotype, which then form secondary cementum. There is also some debate concerning the nature of the organic matrix: Its collagenous component may be derived entirely from extrinsic fibers of the PDL and the cementoblasts may only form the "glue" around these fibers, or (as seen in Fig. 13-7) some of the collagen of primary cementum between the PDL collagen bundles may derive from cementoblast activity.

Secondary Cementum Formation

After the tooth is in occlusion, more rapidly formed and less mineralized cementum is deposited around the apical two thirds of the root. In this situation the cementoblasts, which could possibly have a different phenotype from those forming primary cementum, usually become trapped in lacunae within the matrix they form so that secondary cementum is generally cellular (Fig. 13-8) (although acellular secondary cementum has also been described). The organic matrix of secondary cementum contains collagen fibers clearly derived from two sources—extrinsic fibers of the PDL and intrinsic fibers formed as the result of cementoblastic activity. The extrinsic fibers are arranged obliquely as they enter the cementum. The intrinsic fibers, arranged parallel to the root surface, weave a lattice around the extrinsic fibers. Secondary cementum formation is a continuous process, with the result that the thickness of cementum on the root surface increases with age, a fact that is used in forensic dentistry to help determine the age of a tooth.

The above account of cementogenesis has been simplified to aid understanding, for there is still much unknown on this subject. It is important to grasp the concept that the hyaline layer provides for the initial attachment of PDL fibers and perhaps also for the attachment of primary cementum to the root surface. Primary cementum appears to be the main tissue attaching the PDL to the tooth, with secondary cementum perhaps forming in response to the functional demands placed on the attachment apparatus (given that cementum is unable to remodel).

FATE OF HERTWIG'S ROOT SHEATH

The fate of cells forming Hertwig's epithelial root sheath should be recounted here. As the sheath frag-

ments and follicular cells migrate through it, the epithelial cells begin to drift away from the root surface and occupy a position within the forming PDL. Fragmentation of the root sheath involves disruption of its basal lamina and possibly some cell loss (transformation into mesenchymal cells has been suggested but not shown); however, most of the cells persist as strands or clusters and reform a basal lamina about themselves. In this process collagen sometimes becomes trapped within the epithelial cluster and is removed by phagocytic activity of the epithelial cells. In conventional histologic sections these remnants of the root sheath appear as seemingly discrete clusters, or islands, of epithelial cells, known as the *epithelial rests of Malassez*. They exhibit dark-staining nuclei and little cytoplasm. In sections cut tangentially to the root they often appear as a network within the PDL close to the cementum surface. Many functions have been proposed for them, but all are speculative. At present there is no known function for these cells. A slight reduction in the number of cell rests occurs with age, although many persist in the PDL for the functional life of the tooth.

Cell rests are the source of epithelial cells that line the walls of a dental cyst, which is an epithelium-lined cavity (and one of the most common cystic lesions) that develops in response to inflammatory changes within the PDL. Epithelium responds characteristically to a change in its supporting connective tissue: it proliferates. Epithelial cell rests are no different; they too proliferate. If cavitation occurs within the resulting mass of epithelium, a dental cyst is formed.

PERIODONTAL LIGAMENT FORMATION

The PDL forms from the dental follicle shortly after root development begins (Fig. 13-9). At its forming front there is a high rate of cell division, which results in an increased number of cells that enlarge and rapidly assume the function of fibrillogenesis, forming collagen fibrils of the PDL. At this early stage the cells already have an oblique orientation, and the fiber bundles they form assume the same orientation.

Before the tooth erupts, the crest of the alveolar bone is above the cementoenamel junction and the developing fiber bundles of the PDL are all directed obliquely. Because the tooth moves during eruption, the level of the alveolar crest comes to coincide with the cementoenamel junction and the oblique fiber bundles just below the free gingival fibers become horizontally aligned. When the tooth finally comes into function, the alveolar crest is positioned nearer the apex. The horizontal fibers, termed *alveolar crest fibers*, again become obliquely oriented, except that now

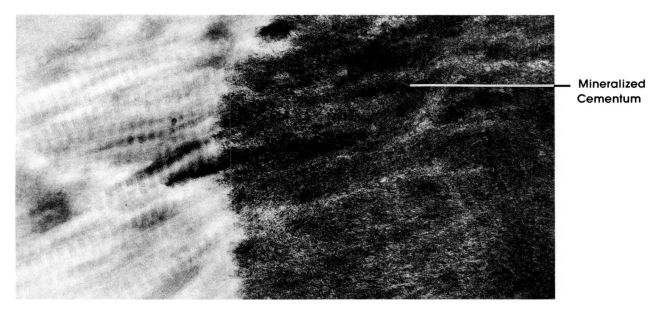

FIG. 13-6 Electron micrograph of the continued mineralization of cementum. Crystals are forming in collagen fibrils of the cementum matrix. (Courtesy Dr. M.A. Listgarten.)

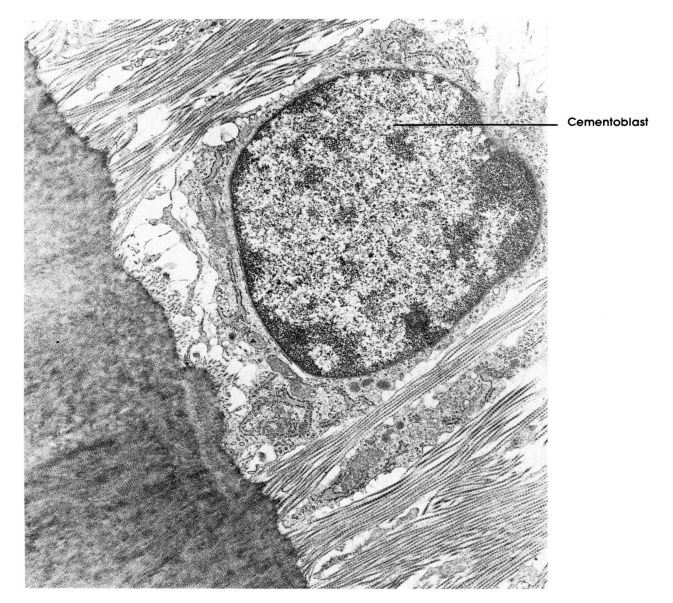

FIG. 13-7 Active acellular cementogenesis. The cementoblast lies between adjacent fiber bundles of the PDL that will form the extrinsic fibers of cementum. The intrinsic fibers can be seen on cementum that lies adjacent to the formative surface of the cell. Note that the cells' organelles are concentrated in this area. A demineralized section, so no electron-dense apatite crystals can be seen.

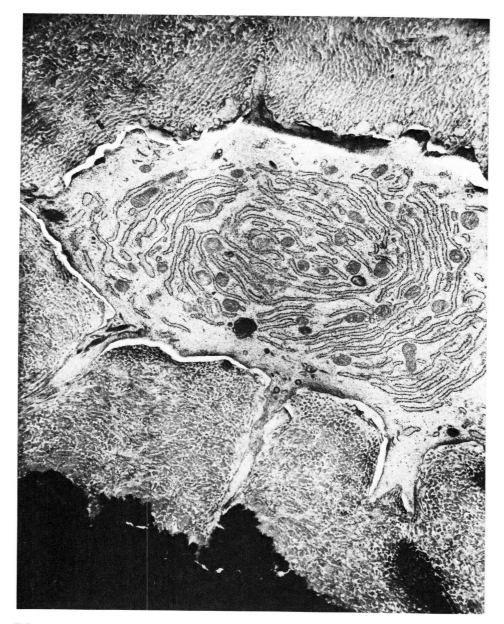

FIG. 13-8 Cellular cementum formation. The cementoblast has embedded itself in the cementum matrix and thus become a cementocyte occupying a lacuna. The mineralization front is at bottom left. (From Furseth R: *Arch Oral Biol* 14:1147, 1969.)

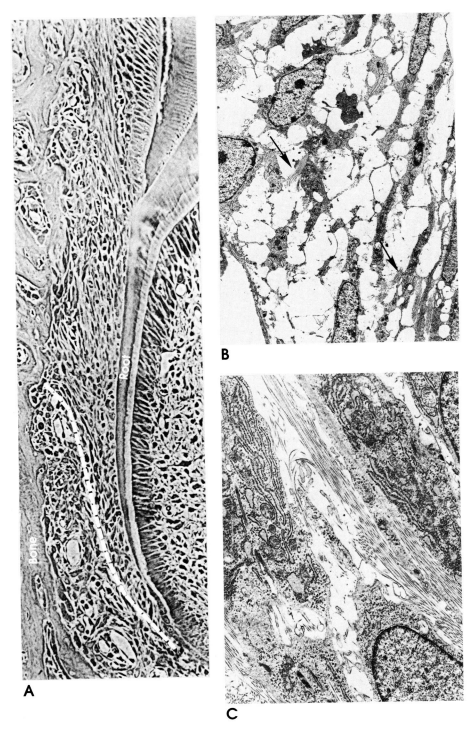

FIG. 13-9 Development of the PDL. **A,** Phase-contrast micrograph. The *white* dotted line indicates how the dental follicle seems to form the ligament by sweeping out toward bone. **B** is an electron micrograph of the follicle. Small undifferentiated fibroblasts exist in an extracellular compartment containing but a few fine collagen fibrils. **C,** The forming ligament. There has been an increase in size of the fibroblasts, which are now actively forming collagen fiber bundles in the ligament. (From Freeman E, Ten Cate AR: *J Periodontol* 42:387, 1971.)

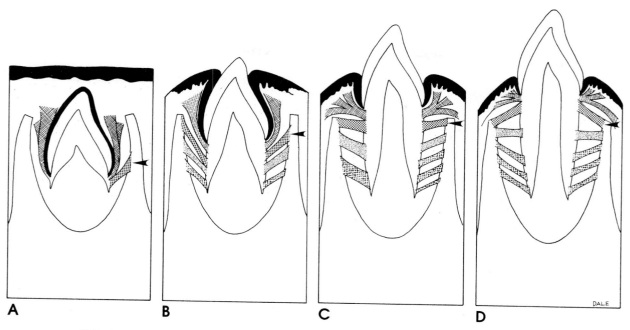

FIG. 13-10 Development of the principal fiber groupings in the PDL. Note how the group of alveolar crest fibers *(arrow)*, first forming in **A,** are initially oblique, **B,** then horizontal, **C,** and then oblique again, **D.**

the cemental attachment has reversed its relation to the alveolar attachment and is more coronal (as opposed to its previous apical orientation) (Fig. 13-10). Only after the teeth have been in function for some time do the fiber bundles of the PDL thicken appreciably, and even then they are constantly being remodeled. (This remodeling of the fiber bundles is achieved by fibroblasts as described in Chapter 6.)

BONE FORMATION

As the PDL is forming, new bone is deposited around the developing ligament fiber bundles against the crypt wall. The deposition of this bone gradually reduces the space between the crypt wall and the tooth to the dimensions of the PDL (Fig. 13-11).

The origin of a tooth's supporting apparatus from the dental follicle has important clinical applications. For example, in the past, when a tooth was avulsed, the practice was to fill the root, clean the root surfaces of all adherent soft tissue, and reimplant the tooth into its socket (with the hope that reattachment might ensue). What sometimes happened, however, was that reattachment occurred by ankylosis (i.e., fusion of the tooth to the jaw by bone, with no intervening PDL) and this did not last long. Nowadays, every effort is made to preserve all the soft tissue still adherent to the root surface of an avulsed tooth before its reimplantation. When this course is followed, regeneration of the tooth's original supporting apparatus is more likely to occur (presumably because the programmed, embryologically specific, cells of the follicle have been retained).

When part of the attachment apparatus is lost because of periodontal disease, it is difficult (if not impossible) to replace the lost tissue. Again, this failing is probably due to the specific origin of the tooth's supporting tissue. Clinical procedures are now being attempted (e.g., guided tissue regeneration) in an effort to influence repair after periodontal surgery by placing

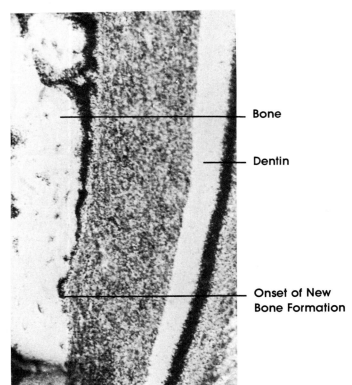

Bone

Dentin

Onset of New
Bone Formation

FIG. 13-11 Photomicrograph of the formation of new bone on the alveolar wall coincident with organization of the PDL. New bone is marked by the dense black precipitate, which indicates where radioactive proline has been incorporated into the collagen of the newly formed bone. (From Ten Cate AR: *Arch Oral Biol* 20:137, 1975.)

a tissue-tolerant barrier between gingival connective tissue and PDL, in the hope that cells from the PDL will repopulate and be responsible for the repair process.

This approach is perhaps simplistic; but it is now appreciated that there is a continuous demand for new cementoblasts, osteoblasts, and ligament fibroblasts as the tooth's supporting apparatus remodels, which means that a source of new cells is constantly required. In animal models there is strong evidence that cells migrate into the PDL from the bone marrow by way of vascular channels, which then come to occupy a perivascular location within the PDL and probably reinforce the resident perivascular population. Cell division of perivascular cells provides the daughter cells, which migrate to the bone and cementum and there differ-

entiate into osteoblasts or cementoblasts. Perivascular cells also are the source of new PDL fibroblasts. What has not been determined is whether there is a single progenitor cell for all three cell types associated with tooth support; the available evidence indicates that a common progenitor for hard tissue–forming cells exists, along with possibly a separate progenitor for PDL fibroblasts. Attempts to "persuade" fibroblasts from other sources such as the gingiva to differentiate into cementoblasts and PDL fibroblasts have been unsuccessful. In summary: The best interpretation of available evidence is that the tooth-supporting tissues have a specific embryologic origin from the dental follicle and that progenitor cells persist in a perivascular location able to replenish the cementoblast, fibroblast, and osteoblast populations. The possibility also exists that perivascular progenitor cells may themselves be replenished by the migration of stromal cells from the marrow.

DEVELOPMENT OF NERVE AND VASCULAR SUPPLIES

Little is known about the development of nerve and vascular supplies to the periodontium. Nerves and vessels ramify around the early tooth germ, but it has not been determined when or how they assume their adult configuration. This is an important omission, especially with respect to the development of innervation, since the PDL plays such an important role in perception.

DENTOGINGIVAL JUNCTION FORMATION

That part of the gingiva facing the tooth also forms part of the periodontium. To understand development of the dentogingival junction, visualize the tissues overlying the tooth before it begins its eruptive movement. At this time the crown is covered by a double layer of epithelial cells (Fig. 13-12). Those cells in contact with the enamel are the ameloblasts, which, having completed their formative function, develop hemidesmosomes, secrete a basal lamina, and become firmly attached to the enamel surface (Fig. 13-13). The outer layer consists of more flattened cells, the remnants of all remaining layers of the dental organ. Together, these two layers of cells are called the reduced dental epithelium. Between the reduced dental epithelium and the overlying oral epithelium is connective tissue that supports both the reduced dental epithelium and the oral epithelium. When tooth eruption begins, this connective tissue breaks down (Figs. 13-14 and 13-15).

In Chapter 6 the relationship between connective tissue and epithelium was discussed and the dependence of epithelium on connective tissue stressed. In

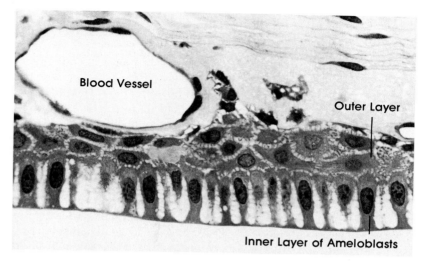

FIG. 13-12 Dental epithelium toward the completion of amelogenesis. Note that it consists of two layers, an inner layer consisting of ameloblasts at the completion of their formative function and an outer layer that has formed from the remaining cells of the dental organ. Together, these layers form the reduced dental epithelium. The white area at bottom is the enamel space.

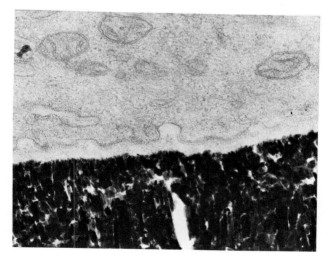

FIG. 13-13 Electron micrograph of the interface between reduced ameloblasts and enamel after the completion of amelogenesis. The ameloblasts have formed a basal lamina, and their plasma membranes are developing hemidesmosomes to provide a firm attachment between the epithelium and the formed enamel. (From Schroeder HE, Listgarten MA: *Fine structure of the developing epithelial attachment of human teeth*, Basel, 1971, S Karger.)

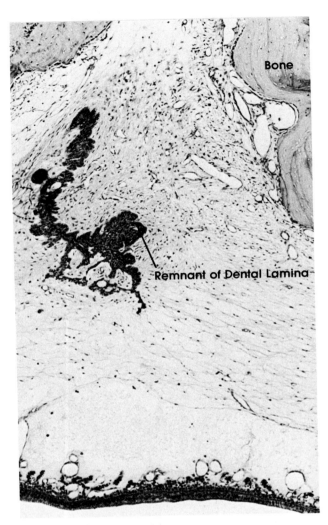

Bone

Remnant of Dental Lamina

FIG. 13-14 Photomicrograph of the tissues in advance of an erupting tooth. At bottom, reduced dental epithelium covers the enamel space. The connective tissue supporting this epithelium is becoming hyalinized. At center, note the mass of epithelium, a remnant of the dental lamina.

response to the degradative changes occurring in connective tissue, epithelial cells of both the reduced dental epithelium and the oral epithelium behave in a manner characteristic of epithelium supported by damaged connective tissue. Thus a widening of the intercellular spaces between the epithelial cells occurs as they proliferate and migrate; and, as a result, cells of the outer layer of reduced dental epithelium and cells of the oral epithelium proliferate and migrate into the degenerating connective tissue, eventually fusing to establish a mass of epithelial cells over the erupting tooth. Cell death in the middle of this epithelial plug leads to the

formation of an epithelium-lined canal through which the tooth erupts without causing hemorrhage (Fig. 13-16).

From this mass of epithelium (also known as the *epithelial cuff*), together with the remaining reduced dental epithelium, an epithelial component of the dentogingival junction is established in relation to the degraded connective tissue. This is an important observation, for it is likely that connective tissue determines the morphology of the dentogingival epithelium. Thus cells of the epithelial cuff proliferate and migrate and become separated by widened intercellular spaces; and it is through these intercellular spaces that antigens from the oral cavity pass as soon as the cusp tip emerges, initiating an acute inflammatory response within the connective tissue (already altered) that supports the epithelium. The clinical manifestation of this inflammatory response is called "teething," and over this inflamed connective tissue further development of the sulcular epithelium of the dentogingival junction occurs.

After the tip of the cusp of the erupting tooth has emerged into the oral cavity, oral epithelial cells begin to migrate over the reduced dental epithelium in an apical direction. At this time the attachment of gingival epithelium to tooth is maintained through the reduced ameloblasts and their hemidesmosomes and basal lamina adjacent to the enamel surface . This is the *primary epithelial attachment* (Fig. 13-17).

A process of transformation then takes place whereby the reduced enamel epithelium gradually becomes *junctional epithelium*. The reduced ameloblasts change their morphology and are transformed into squamous epithelial cells that retain their attachment to the enamel surface. The cells of the outer layer of reduced dental epithelium retain their ability to divide and, because of this, continue to function as basal cells of a forming junctional epithelium. The transformed ameloblasts are eventually displaced by the mitotic activity of these basal cells. As the overgrowing epithelial cells from the cuff stratify, they further separate the cells of the transformed dental epithelium from their nutritive supply, with the consequence that these latter cells degenerate and create a gingival sulcus. Thus, shortly after the tooth has erupted, the epithelium of the dentogingival junction has the characteristics illustrated in Figure 13-18. The final conversion of reduced dental epithelium to junctional epithelium may not occur until 3 to 4 years after the tooth has erupted.

Immediately following the transformation of reduced dental epithelium, the development of a dentogingival junction is considered complete (Fig. 13-19). At this time, it extends to the cementoenamel junction and its epithelial component consists of junctional epithelium

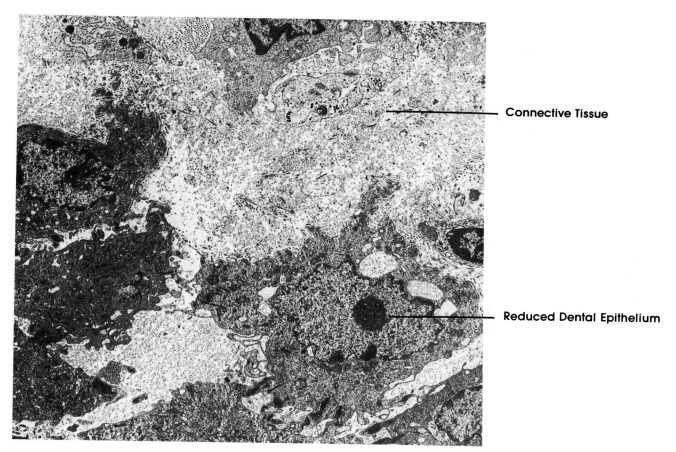

Connective Tissue

Reduced Dental Epithelium

FIG. 13-15 Electron micrograph of the tissues in advance of an erupting tooth. At bottom, epithelial cells of the reduced dental epithelium abut on a disorganized connective tissue.

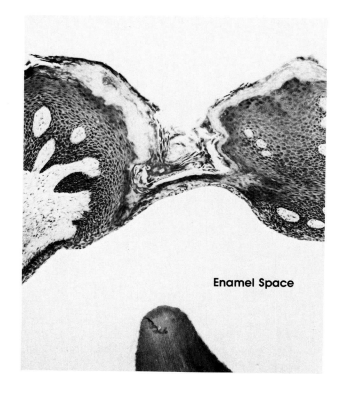

Enamel Space

FIG. 13-16 Preparation for tooth eruption. Fusion of the dental epithelium and oral epithelium has occurred, and the epithelial plug is degenerating to form an epithelium-lined canal through which the tooth will erupt.

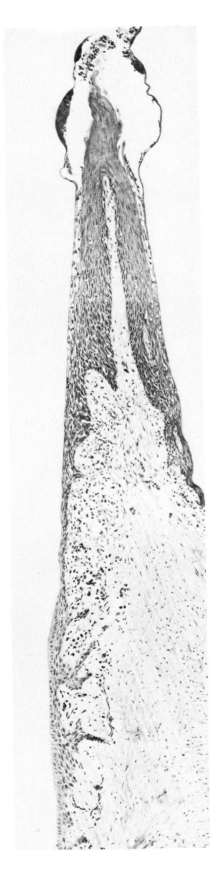

formed largely by the transformation of reduced dental epithelium and sulcular epithelium derived from the epithelial cuff.

Although the dental epithelium contributes specifically to the development of a dentogingival junction, it is not required for the redevelopment of this junction after a gingivectomy. After this surgical procedure, the junction is reestablished at a lower level on the tooth and its epithelial component comes solely from cells of the oral epithelium. That the anatomy of the junction is restored is a property of the connective tissues supporting the epithelium. (See Chapter 14.)

It has already been established that inflammatory changes exist within the connective tissue supporting the junction. This means that with time there is often a gradual loss of the supporting tissue of the tooth and a subsequent apical migration of the dentogingival junction. The junction thus passes on to the cementum surface of the root with advancing age (Fig. 13-20). This apical migration has also been called *passive eruption* because it results in an increased length of the clinical crown (Fig. 13-21). In other words, we become "long in the tooth."

With formation of the dentogingival junction the dental epithelium is finally lost. It is worth recapitulating here the many functions of this epithelium during development of the tooth. First of all, it has a morphogenetic function that helps to determine the crown pattern of the tooth. Second, it has an inductive role in initiating coronal and root dentinogenesis and therefore determines the size, shape, and number of roots of a tooth. Third, it has a formative function in that its cells elaborate enamel. Fourth, it permits tooth eruption without an exposure of connective tissue. Finally, it assists in establishing the dentogingival junction.

FIG. 13-17   Montage photomicrograph of the primary dentogingival junction associated with a recently erupted tooth. At bottom, reduced dental epithelium can be identified by its characteristic inner ameloblast layer. As the epithelium is traced coronally, its morphology changes in becoming junctional epithelium.

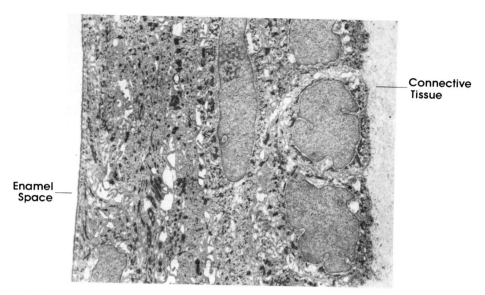

Enamel Space

Connective Tissue

FIG. 13-18 Electron micrograph of the newly formed junctional epithelium. It consists of squamous cells separated by well-marked intercellular spaces. (From Listgarten M: *Oral Sci Rev* 1:3, 1972.)

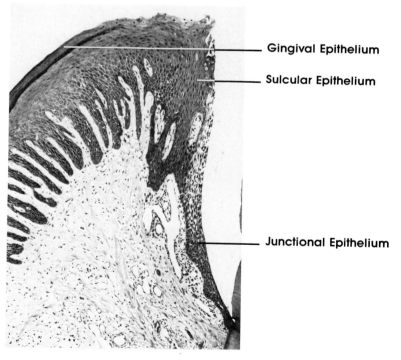

Gingival Epithelium

Sulcular Epithelium

Junctional Epithelium

FIG. 13-19 Light photomicrograph of the completed dentogingival junction. It consists of two components, the junctional epithelium (which is attached to the enamel surface) and the sulcular epithelium (which lines the gingival sulcus). Note that the floor of the sulcus is formed by junctional epithelium.

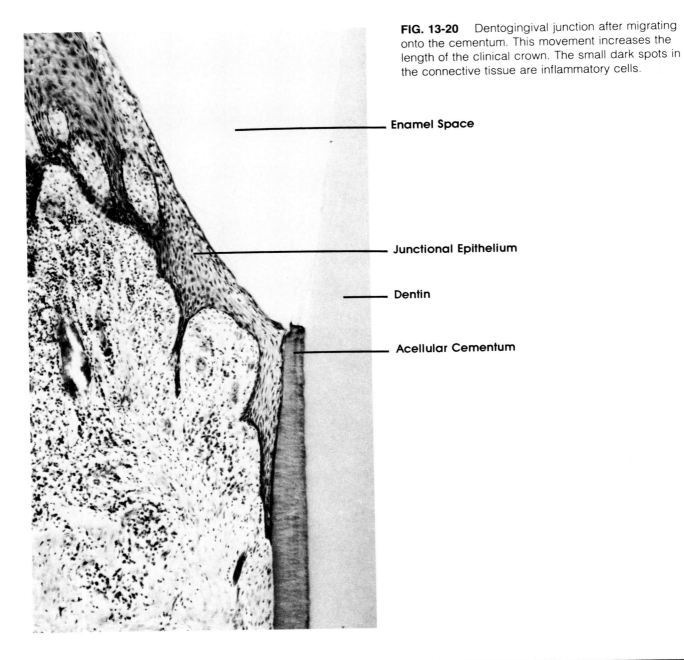

FIG. 13-20 Dentogingival junction after migrating onto the cementum. This movement increases the length of the clinical crown. The small dark spots in the connective tissue are inflammatory cells.

Enamel Space

Junctional Epithelium

Dentin

Acellular Cementum

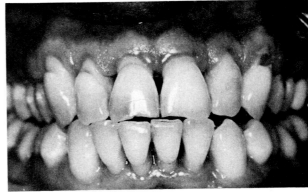

FIG. 13-21 Dentogingival junction after migrating onto cementum. The cementum has become exposed as the attachment migrated apically, thereby lengthening the clinical crown.

BIBLIOGRAPHY

Atkinson ME: The development of the mouse molar periodontium, *J Periodont Res* 7:255, 1972.

Bernick S: The organization of the periodontal membrane fibres of the developing molars of rats, *J Periodont Res* 2:57, 1960.

Cho MI, Garant PR: Radioautographic study of [^{3}H] mannose utilization during cementoblast differentiation, formation of acellular cementum and development of periodontal ligament principal fibres, *Anat Rec* 223:209, 1989.

Diamond M, Applebaum E: The epithelial sheath, *J Dent Res* 21:403, 1942.

Eccles JD: Studies on the development of the periodontal membrane: the principal fibres of the molar teeth, *Dent Pract Dent Rec* 10:31, 1959.

Eccles JD: Studies in the development of the periodontal membrane: the apical region of the erupting tooth, *Dent Pract Dent Rec* 11:153, 1961.

Engler WO, Ramfjord SP, Hiniker JJ: Development of epithelial attachment and gingival sulcus in rhesus monkeys, *J Periodontol* 36:44, 1965.

Freeman E, Ten Cate AR: Development of the periodontium: an electron microscope study, *J Periodontol* 42:387, 1971.

Freeman E, Ten Cate AR, Dickinson J: Development of a gomphosis by tooth germ implants in the parietal bone of the mouse, *Arch Oral Biol* 20:139, 1975.

Furstman L, Bernick S: Early development of the periodontal membrane, *Am J Orthodont* 51:482, 1965.

Glavind L, Zander HA: Dynamics of dental epithelium during tooth eruption, *J Dent Res* 49:549, 1970.

Grant DA, Bernick S: Formation of the periodontal ligament, *J Periodontol* 43:17, 1972.

Grant DA, et al: A comparative study of periodontal ligament development in teeth with and without predecessors in marmosets, *J Periodontol* 43:162, 1972.

Griffin CJ, Harris R: The fine structure of the developing human periodontium, *Arch Oral Biol* 12:971, 1967.

Hayashi Y: Ultrastructural characterization of extracellular matrix vesicles in the mineralizing fronts of apical cementum in cats, *Arch Oral Biol* 30:445, 1985.

Hoffman RL: Formation of periodontal tissues around subcutaneously transplanted hamster molars, *J Dent Res* 39:781, 1960.

Innes PB: The differentiation of cat crevicular epithelium in diffusion chambers in vivo, *Anat Rec* 169:345, 1971.

Kenney EB, Ramfjord SP: Cellular dynamics in root formation of teeth in rhesus monkeys, *J Dent Res* 48:114, 1969.

Lester KS: The incorporation of epithelial cells by cementum, *J Ultrastruct Res* 27:63, 1969.

Lindskog S: Formation of intermediate cementum. I. Early mineralization of aprismatic enamel and intermediate cementum in the monkey, *J Craniofac Genet Develop Biol* 2:147, 1982.

Lindskog S: Formation of intermediate cementum. II. A scanning electron microscopic study of the epithelial root sheath of Hertwig in the monkey, *J Craniofac Genet Develop Biol* 2:161, 1982.

Lindskog S, Hammastrom L: Formation of intermediate cementum. III. ^{3}H-tryptophan and ^{3}H-proline uptake into the epithelial root sheath of Hertwig in vitro, *J Craniofac Genet Develop Biol* 2:171, 1982.

Listgarten MA: Phase-contrast and electron microscopic study of the junction between reduced enamel epithelium and enamel in unerupted human teeth, *Arch Oral Biol* 11:999, 1966.

Luo W, Slavkin HC, Snead ML: Cells from Hertwig's epithelial root sheath do not transcribe amelogenin, *J Periodont Res* 26:42, 1991.

Magnusson B: Tissue changes during molar tooth eruption, *Trans R Sch Dent Stockholm Umea* 13:1, 1968.

Magnusson B: Mucosal changes at erupting molars in germ-free rats, *J Periodont Res* 4:181, 1969.

McHugh WD: The development of the gingival epithelium in the monkey, *Dent Pract Dent Rec* 11:314, 1961.

McHugh WD, Zander HA: Cell division in the periodontium of developing and erupting teeth, *Dent Pract Dent Rec* 15:451, 1965.

Provenza DV, Sisca RF: Fine structure features of monkey (*Macaca mulata*) reduced enamel epithelium, *J Periodontol* 41:313, 1970.

Schroeder HE, Listgarten MA: Fine structure of the developing epithelial attachment of human teeth. In Wolsky A (ed): *Monographs in developmental biology,* vol 2, Basel, 1971, S Karger.

Schonfeld SE, Slavkin HC: Demonstration of enamel matrix proteins on root-analogue surface of rabbit permanent incisor teeth, *Calcif Tiss Int* 24:223, 1977.

Selvig KA: Electron microscopy of Hertwig's epithelial sheath and of dentine and cementum formation in the mouse incisor, *Acta Odontol Scand* 21:175, 1963.

Selvig KA: An ultrastructural study of cementum formation, *Acta Odontol Scand* 22:105, 1964.

Ten Cate AR: The development of the periodontium. In Melcher AH, Bowen WH (eds): *Biology of the periodontium,* New York, 1969, Academic Press.

Ten Cate AR: Physiological resorption of connective tissue associated with tooth eruption, *J Periodont Res* 6:168, 1971.

Ten Cate AR: Cell division and periodontal ligament formation in the mouse, *Arch Oral Biol* 17:1781, 1972.

Ten Cate AR: Developmental aspects of the periodontium. In Slavkin HC, Bavetta LA (eds): *Developmental aspects of oral biology,* New York, 1972, Academic Press.

Ten Cate AR, Mills C: The development of the periodontium: the origin of alveolar bone, *Anat Rec* 173:69, 1972.

Ten Cate AR, Mills C, Solomon, G: The development of the periodontium: a transplantation and autoradiographic study, *Anat Rec* 170:365, 1971.

Thomas HF, Kollar EJ: Tissue interactions in normal murine root development. In Davidovitch Z (ed): *The biological mechanisms of tooth eruption and resorption,* Birmingham Ala, 1988, EBSCO Media.

Tonge CH: The development and arrangement of the dental follicle, *Eur Orthod Soc Trans* 39:118, 1963.

Yamamoto T, Wakita M: Initial attachment of principal fibers to the root dentin surface in rat molars, *J Periodont Res* 25: 113, 1990.

Yamamoto T, Wakita M: The development and structure of principal fibers and cellular cementum in rat molars, *J Periodont Res* 129:266 1991.

CHAPTER 14

Periodontium

THE periodontium is the attachment apparatus of the tooth and consists of cementum, the periodontal ligament (PDL), bone lining the alveolus, and part of the gingiva. The gingiva is discussed in Chapter 18, but the connection of the gingiva to the tooth, the dentogingival junction, is described here because it has a functional relationship to the periodontium. In the previous chapter reference was made to a hyaline layer deposited on the dentin of the root by the root sheath before cementogenesis begins. It is problematic whether this layer should be included as part of the periodontium. What evidence there is suggests that it should, for this layer seems to have the function of "cementing" cementum to root dentin. In studies of ligament repair new cementum may be deposited on denuded dentin, but in histologic section there is always an artifactual split between the newly deposited cementum and the dentin, suggesting a weak union between these two tissues in the absence of this hyaline layer. In addition, it has been shown that collagen fibers of the follicle attach to this layer before cementoblasts deposit further matrix (Fig. 13-3). A further question is how best to name this layer. Because it seems to have a cementation function, is of epithelial origin, and lies between the dentin and primary cementum, the term *intermediate epithelial cement layer* is proposed.

CEMENTUM

Cementum is a hard connective tissue, very much like bone, that covers the roots of teeth, which has as its main function the attachment of fibers of the PDL to those roots. It has an organic matrix consisting largely of collagen (about 90%) and ground substance that is about 50% mineralized with hydroxyapatite. Unlike bone, cementum is not vascularized, nor does it have the ability to remodel, which makes this issue more resistant to resorption. This resistance to resorption is clinically important because, if it were resorbed as readily as bone, the application of orthodontic tech-

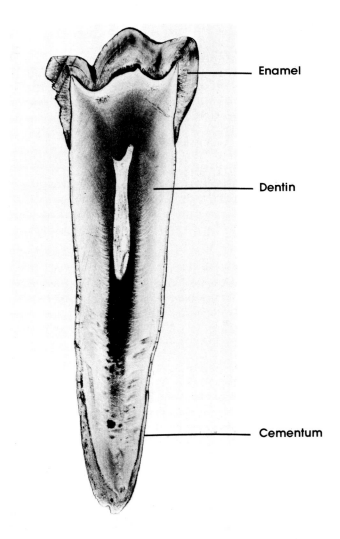

— Enamel

— Dentin

— Cementum

FIG. 14-1 Ground section of a premolar showing the distribution of cementum around the root. Increasing amounts of cementum occur around the apex.

niques would result in the loss of root surface and tooth attachment as the tooth is moved.

At the cementoenamel junction, cementum forms a thin layer (20 to 50 μm) that becomes thicker toward the apex of the root (150 to 200 μm) (Fig. 14-1). Classically, it is stated that in approximately 30% of teeth, the cementum and enamel meet as a butt joint, forming a distinct cementoenamel junction at the cervical margin; in 10% a gap occurs between the cementum and enamel, exposing root dentin; and in approximately 60% the cementum overlaps the enamel. This information was obtained from the study of ground sections (Fig. 14-2), but studies with the scanning electron microscope (Fig. 14-3) indicate that the cementoenamel junction exhibits all of the above forms and shows considerable variation when traced circumferentially. The exposure of root dentin at the cervical margin can lead to sensitivity at this site.

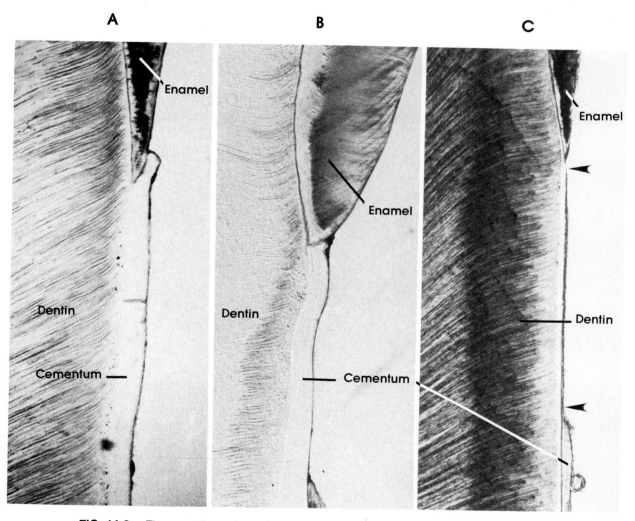

FIG. 14-2 Three configurations of the cementoenamel junction in ground sections. In **A** cementum overlaps the enamel. There is a butt joint in **B,** and in **C** a deficiency of cementum between the *arrows* leaves root dentin exposed. Note the hyaline layer in **B** and **C.**

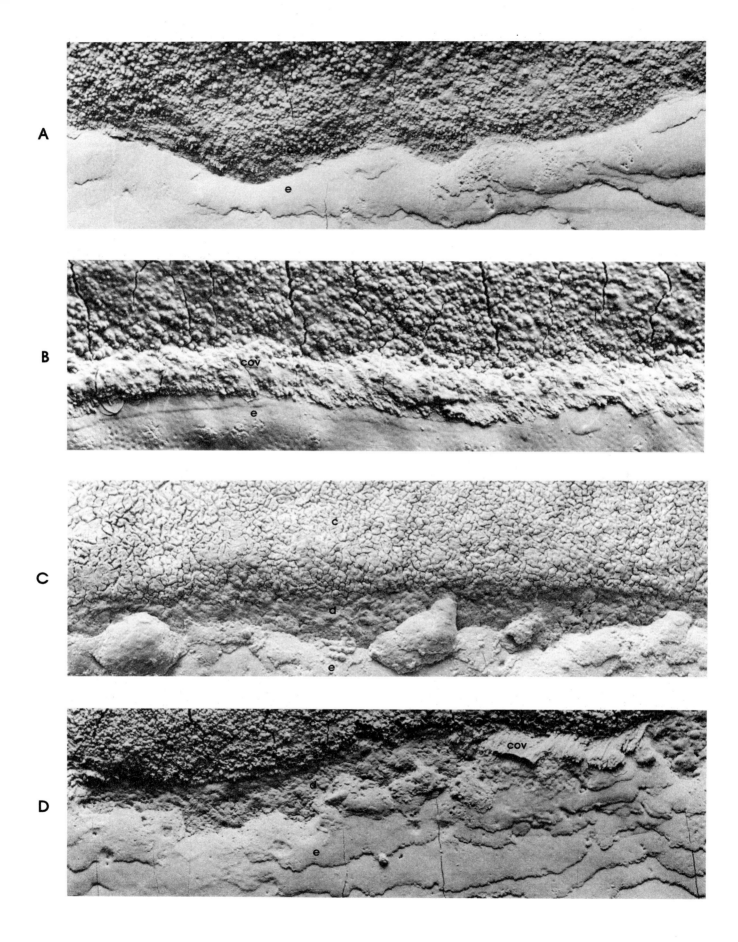

Classification of Cementum

Cementum is classified in three different ways.

There is its distinction as *primary* or *secondary*. Primary cementum is the first formed; it is deposited on the intermediate epithelial cement layer and covers the coronal two thirds of the root. It is acellular, and its matrix consists of noncollagenous proteins elaborated by the cementoblasts and of extrinsic collagen fibers formed by the PDL fibroblasts. Recall (Chapter 13, Fig. 13-7) that there is some evidence that the cementoblast may contribute some collagen to the matrix of primary cementum. Secondary cementum overlies primary cementum and covers at least the apical two thirds of the root. It may be either acellullar (with cementoblast lining its surface) or cellular (with cementoblasts becoming incorporated into its matrix and occupying lacunae). The matrix of secondary cementum consists of intrinsic collagen fibrils (formed by cementoblasts) and extrinsic fibrils (formed by PDL fibroblasts) in roughly equal proportions embedded in a ground substance formed of cementoblasts (Fig. 14-4). Secondary cementum, whether cellular or acellular, covers primary cementum and the pattern of cellular/ acellular secondary cementum deposition is highly variable. If the separation between ligament fiber bundles is sufficient, areas of secondary cementum occur where the organic matrix is formed exclusively by cementoblasts.

Understanding the primary classification of cementum, the secondary classification of cementum as *cellular* and *acellular*, or the tertiary classification as *extrinsic* fiber, *mixed* fiber or *intrinsic* fiber cementum is explained.

Cells

The cells associated with cementum are *cementoblasts* and *cementocytes*.

Cementoblasts form the cementum and are found lining the root surface, interposed between bundles of PDL fibers. Because of their location they are often considered as part of the PDL cell population although there is some evidence that two populations of cement-forming cells exist, one forming primary cementum and

---

FIG. 14-3 Typical scanning electron microscopic appearance of the edge-to-edge contact of cementum *(c)* and enamel *(e)*. **A,** Overlap of enamel by cementum; **B,** exposed dentin *(d)* between the cementum and enamel; **C,** along the cementoenamel junction of a freshly erupted human tooth; **D,** cementum overlap *(cov)* and dentin exposure occurring side by side. (From Schroeder HE, Scherle WF: *J Periodont Res* 23:53, 1988.)

the other secondary cementum. When active, cementoblasts are round plump cells with a basophilic cytoplasm, indicative of an extensive rough endoplasmic reticulum, and have open-faced nuclei (Fig. 13-5). With the electron microscope cementoblasts have been shown to possess collagen-containing phagolysosomes (Fig. 14-5), suggesting that these cells play a role in remodeling the ligament. The phasic deposition of cementum continues throughout life, and resting cementoblasts can often be seen in section. Resting cementoblasts have a closed (or hematoxophilic) nucleus and little cytoplasm. When acellular cementum is being formed, the cementoblasts retreat, leaving behind the cementum matrix. When cellular cementum is being formed, the cementoblasts become trapped in lacunae within their own matrix and are then known as cementocytes.

Cementocytes have sparse amounts of cytoplasm and numerous processes occupying canaliculi in the mineralized cementum matrix. Since the cementum is avascular, the cementocytes depend on diffusion from the PDL for essential nutrients. As a consequence, most cementocyte processes are directed toward the ligament. Another consequence of the avascularity of cementum is that, as more and more cementum is formed, the cementocytes become progressively further removed from the nutritive source, with the result that they degenerate, leaving empty lacunae in the deeper cementum (Fig. 14-6).

Organic Matrix

The collagen fibers of the cementum matrix and their origin have already been described. The noncollagenous components consist of the normal assembly of proteoglycans, glycoproteins, and phosphoproteins.

Because of the continuous but phasic deposition of cementum, resting lines can be clearly seen in section by H&E stain. Another effect of continuous cementum deposition, especially around the root apex, is that the total length of the tooth is maintained despite the loss of enamel from occlusal wear. This accretion of cementum often leads to a constricton of the apical foramen and alteration in the number, size, and shape of such foramina. The overall effect is that in older teeth the complexity of apical foramina is increased, a development that should be borne in mind when considering endodontic treatment.

PERIODONTAL LIGAMENT

The PDL is that soft specialized connective tissue situated between the cementum covering the root of the tooth and the bone forming the socket wall. It

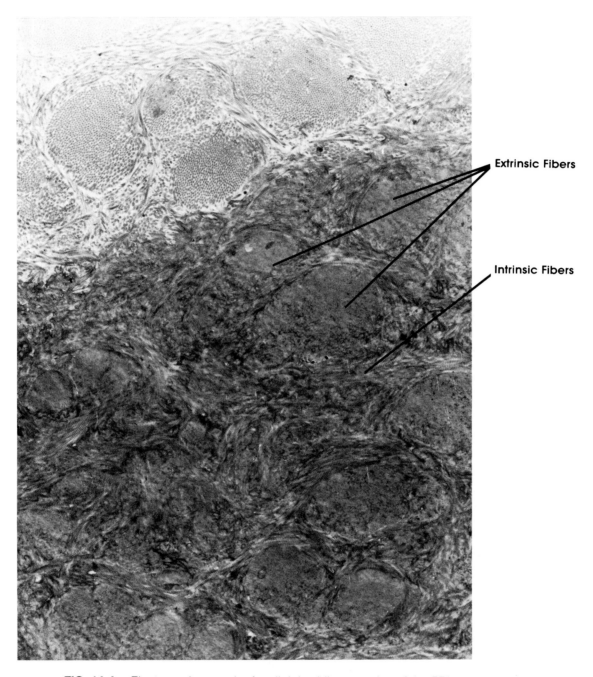

Extrinsic Fibers

Intrinsic Fibers

FIG. 14-4   Electron micrograph of a slightly oblique section of the PDL-cementum interface. The distinction between extrinsic and intrinsic fibers within cementum is apparent. (Courtesy Dr. M.A. Listgarten.)

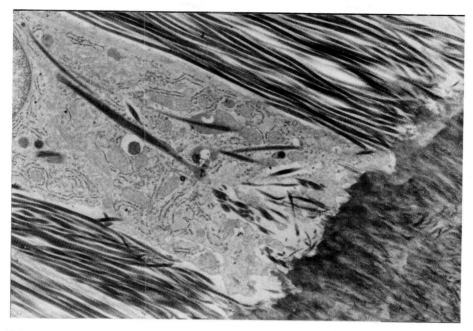

FIG. 14-5   Part of a cementoblast showing the degradation of collagen fibrils. (From Yajima T, et al: *Arch Histol Cytol* 52:521, 1989.)

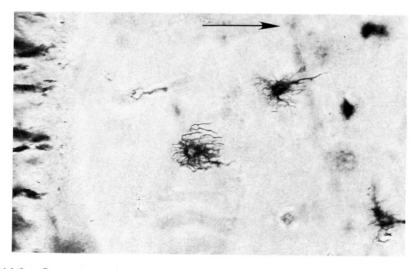

FIG. 14-6   Cementocyte lacunae in ground section. Most of the canaliculi point toward the PDL *(arrow)*. The indistinct dark patches are other cementocyte lacunae deeper within the ground section (and consequently out of focus).

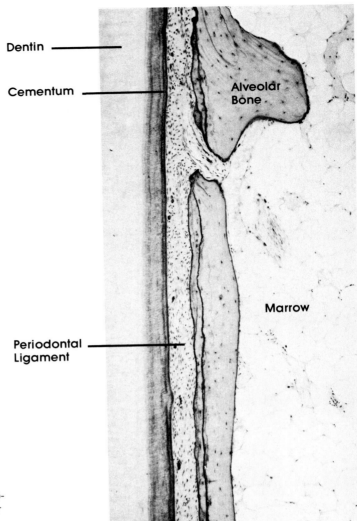

Dentin ————

Cementum ————

Alveolar Bone

Marrow

Periodontal Ligament ————

FIG. 14-7 PDL in longitudinal section. Note the perforation in the alveolar bone that transmits neurovascular bundles. Compare with Figure 14-18.

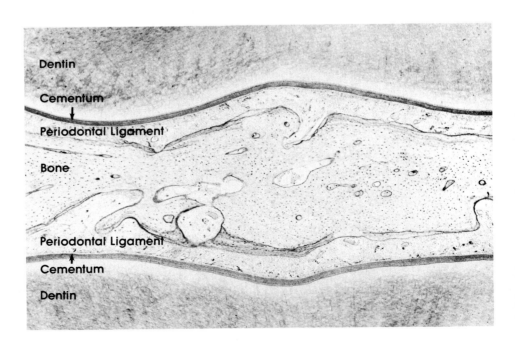

Dentin

Cementum

Periodontal Ligament

Bone

Periodontal Ligament

Cementum

Dentin

FIG. 14-8 PDL in a cross section between two teeth. Note in particular the hyaline layer.

ranges in width from 0.15 to 0.38 mm, with its thinnest portion around the middle third of the root (Figs. 14-7 and 14-8). Its average width is 0.21 mm at 11 to 16 years of age, 0.18 mm at 32 to 52 years, and 0.15 mm at 51 to 67 years, showing a progressive decrease with age. It is a connective tissue particularly well adapted to its principal function, supporting the teeth in their sockets and at the same time permitting them to withstand the considerable forces of mastication. The PDL also has the important function, in addition to attaching teeth to bone, of acting as a sensory receptor—necessary for the proper positioning of the jaws during normal function.

As any other connective tissue, the PDL consists of cells and an extracellular compartment of fibers and ground substance (Fig. 14-9). The cells include osteoblasts and osteoclasts (technically within the ligament but functionally associated with bone), fibroblasts, epithelial cell rests of Malassez, macrophages, undifferentiated mesenchymal cells, and cementoblasts (also technically within the ligament but functionally associated with cementum). The extracellular compartment consists of well-defined collagen fiber bundles embedded in ground substance (Fig. 14-10). Variants of the elastic fiber, eluanin, and oxytalan also occur within the PDL. The ground substance consists largely of glycosaminoglycans, glycoproteins, and glycolipids (Fig. 14-11).

Table 14-1 lists the relative proportions of structural elements in the periodontium of a mouse molar.

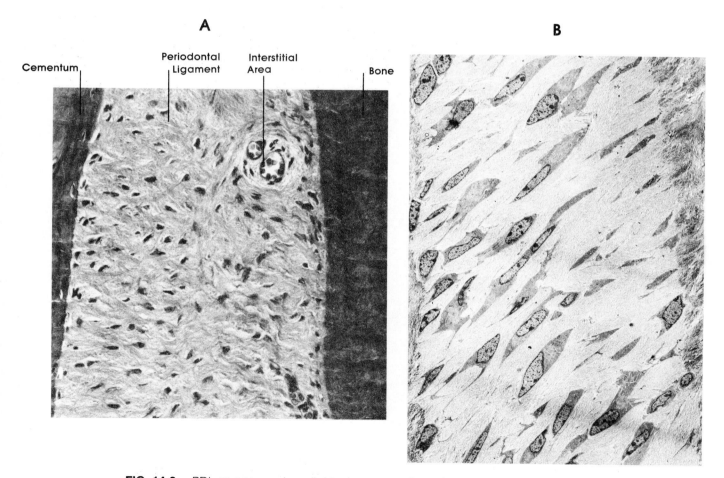

FIG. 14-9 PDL as seen under a light microscope, **A,** and in a low-power electron micrograph, **B. (B** from Beerston W, Everts V: *J Periodont Res.* 15:655, 1980.)

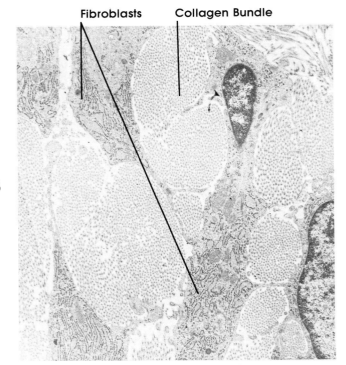

Fibroblasts

Collagen Fiber Bundle

A

Fibroblasts   Collagen Bundle

B

FIG. 14-10 Electron micrograph of the PDL. In **A** elongated fibroblasts can be seen alternating with distinctive fiber bundles. The clear areas are occupied by ground substance. **B,** The fiber bundles have been cut in cross section. Elongated extensions of the fibroblasts encircle the bundles.

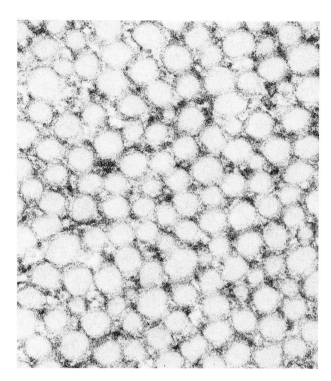

FIG. 14-11 Electron micrograph of ground substance stained in a connective tissue. The collagen fibers have a negative image, and the ground substance appears electron dense. (Courtesy Dr. A.H. Melcher.)

TABLE 14-1	Relative proportions of structural elements found in mouse molar periodontal ligament

Element	Proportion (%)
Fibroblasts	35
Collagen	51
Vessels	10
Nerves	1 (95 unmyelinated)
Oxytalan fibers	0.45
Other cells	2.44

From Freezer SR, Sims MA: *Arch Oral Biol* 32:407, 1987.

Cells of the Periodontal Ligament

Because of the term *ligament*, because of its high collagen content, and because of its function, great importance has always been attached to the anatomy of fiber bundles of the PDL, at the expense of both cellular and nonfibrous components. The fiber bundles are, of course, important, but the cells have an equal or greater role to play in ligament function. Surrounding cells must be viable so there can be tooth movement. If an orthodontic appliance were fitted into the mouth of a cadaver, the force applied to the teeth would not move them.

Fibroblasts

The principal cells of the PDL are fibroblasts. Because of the exceptionally high rate of turnover in the ligament, its constituents are constantly being synthesized, removed, and replaced. This turnover is achieved almost exclusively by the fibroblasts. PDL fibroblasts are large cells with an extensive cytoplasm containing in abundance all the organelles associated with protein synthesis and secretion (e.g., rough endoplasmic reticulum, several Golgi complexes, and many secretory vesicles). Ligament fibroblasts also have a well-developed cytoskeleton (Chapter 5) with a particularly prominent actin network, whose presence is thought to indicate the functional demands placed on the cells, requiring change in shape and migration. Ligament fibroblasts also show frequent cell-to-cell contacts of both the adherens (20 to 30 per cell) and the gap junction types. In addition, associated with PDL fibroblasts are numerous fibronexi (Figs. 5-8 and 14-12). Recall that *fibronexus* is the term used to describe the morphologic relationship between intracellular filaments, the region of dense cell membrane, extracellular filaments, and the sticky attachment glycoprotein fibronectin.

Although fibroblasts look alike microscopically, it is now being recognized that tissues may contain functionally heterogeneous subpopulations of fibroblasts, aligned along the general direction of the fiber bundles and with extensive processes that wrap around the fiber bundles (Fig. 14-10, *B*).

The collagen fibrils of the fiber bundles are continuously being remodeled. It is easy to visualize how a concerted and balanced activity of two cell types, the osteoblast and the osteoclast, achieve the remodeling of a bone. In the PDL, remodeling of collagen is achieved by a single cell, the fibroblast, which is capable of simultaneously synthesizing and degrading collagen (Chapter 5). The remodeling of collagen in the ligament is not confined to any intermediate zone, as previously thought, but occurs across the entire width of the ligament (Figs. 14-5 and 14-13). Because of the exceptionally high rate of turnover of collagen in the ligament, any interference in fibroblast function by disease rapidly produces a loss of the tooth's supporting tissue.

Epithelial cells

The epithelial cells found in the PDL are remnants of Hertwig's epithelial root sheath. They occur as lacy strands close to the cementum surface and are easily

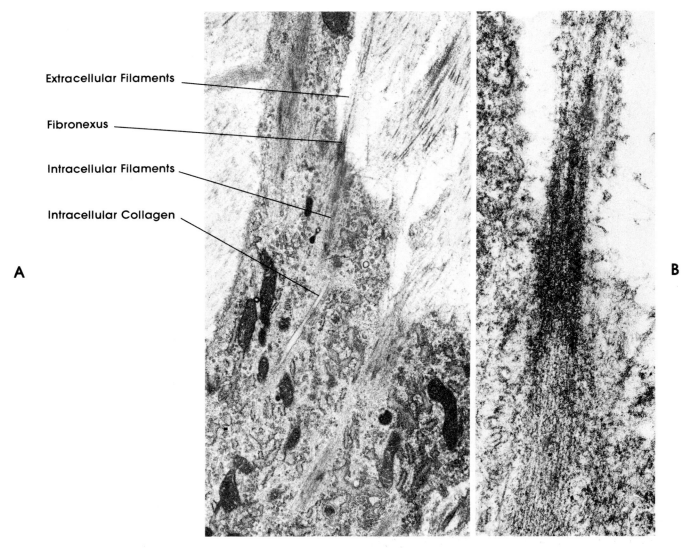

Extracellular Filaments

Fibronexus

Intracellular Filaments

Intracellular Collagen

A

B

FIG. 14-12   Fibronexus. In **A** a PDL fibroblast exhibits a fibronexus whereby intracellular and extracellular filaments are combined. In **B** the fibronexus is shown at higher magnification. (From Garant PR, et al: *J Periodont Res* 17:70, 1982.)

recognized in hematoxylin- and eosin (H&E)–stained sections since their nuclei are closed faced and therefore stain deeply (Fig. 4-22). They are known as the epithelial cell rests of Malassez. As yet, they have no known function; but their presence can lead to the formation of dental cysts if the PDL becomes infected. When infection occurs, the connective tissue supporting these epithelial cells is damaged and the resting cells proliferate to form an epithelial mass that cavitates to form the epithelium-lined cyst.

Undifferentiated mesenchymal cells

Another important cellular constituent of the PDL is the undifferentiated mesenchymal cell or progenitor cell. These cells have a perivascular location within 5 μm of the blood vessels. Although it has been demonstrated that they are a source of new cells for the PDL, it is not known whether a single progenitor cell gives rise to daughter cells that differentiate into fibroblasts, osteoblasts, and cementoblasts, or whether there are separate progenitors for each cell line. The fact that new cells are being produced for the PDL, coupled with the fact that cells of the ligament are in a steady state, means this production of new cells must be balanced by either migration of cells out of the ligament or cell death. Selective deletion of ligament cells occurs by *apoptosis** physiologic cell death (Fig. 15-19), to permit turnover.

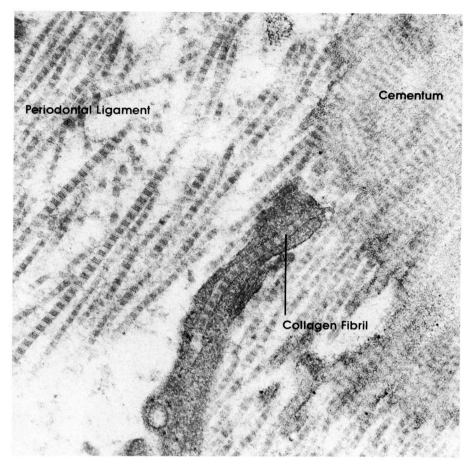

FIG. 14-13 Remodeling within the PDL. A ligament fibroblast is ingesting a collagen fibril immediately adjacent to the cementum surface.

Bone and cementum cells

Although technically situated within the periodontal ligament, bone and cementum cells are properly associated with the hard tissues they form.

Osteoblasts line the bone surface of the ligament and may be either functional or resting depending on the functional state of the ligament. Thus in any light microscope section a mixture of plump osteoblasts and flattened resting cells can usually be found. Osteoclasts may also be found against the bone where resorption is occurring. This variation in the distribution of bone cells along the socket wall reflects the constant state of flux of the alveolus.

Cementoblasts line the ligament surface of the cementum and are most often seen in section in their resting phase. Because cementum does not remodel, cementoclasts (or more properly odontoclasts, for they also destroy dentin and enamel) are not normally found in the ligament. Such cells occur only in certain pathologic conditions, during resorption of the deciduous teeth, and when excessive force is applied during orthodontic tooth movement, particularly with fixed appliances.

---

*Apoptosis describes a form of cell death that results in selective deletion of single cells. This physiological process is characterized by condensation and fragmentation of the cell into membrane-bound particles which are phagocytosed. No inflammatory cells are involved. It is a functionally important mechanism to achieve turnover without architectural disruption of a tissue. In contrast, *necrosis* describes pathological cell death, involves many cells, and is associated with swelling and bursting of cells and involvement of inflammation.

Fibers

Collagen of the PDL is a mixture of type I and III, with individual fibrils having an average diameter of 55 nm. This is a relatively small diameter (tendon collagen fibrils average some 100 to 250 nm in diameter) and is thought to reflect the relatively short half-life of ligament collagen, meaning that there is relatively little time for continuous assembly.

The vast majority of collagen fibrils in the PDL are arranged in definite and distinct fiber bundles. Each bundle resembles a spliced rope; individual strands can be continually remodeled while the overall fiber maintains its architecture and function. In this way the fiber bundles are able to adapt to the continual stresses placed on them. These bundles are arranged in groups that can be easily seen in an appropriately stained light microscope section (Figs. 14-14 and 14-15). They are as follows:

1. The *alveolar crest group*, attached to the cementum just below the cementoenamel junction and running downward and outward to insert into the rim of the alveolus
2. The *horizontal group*, occurring just apical to the alveolar crest group and running at right angles to the long axis of the tooth from cementum to bone just below the alveolar crest
3. The *oblique group*, by far the most numerous in the PDL and running from the cementum in an oblique direction to insert into bone coronally
4. The *apical group*, radiating from the cementum around the apex of the root to the bone, forming the base of the socket
5. The *interradicular group*, found only between the roots of multirooted teeth and running from the cementum into the bone, forming the crest of the interradicular septum (See Fig. 14-15, *A*.)

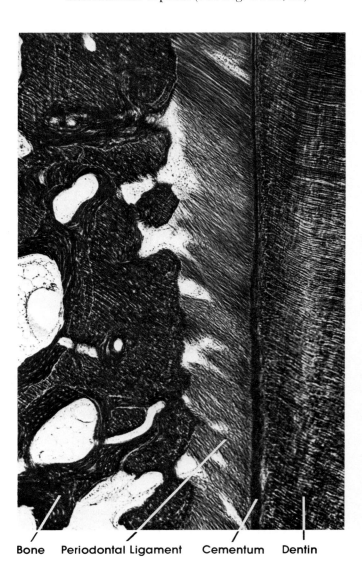

FIG. 14-14 Silver-stained section of the PDL. The disposition of oblique fibers is shown.

Bone   Periodontal Ligament   Cementum   Dentin

A

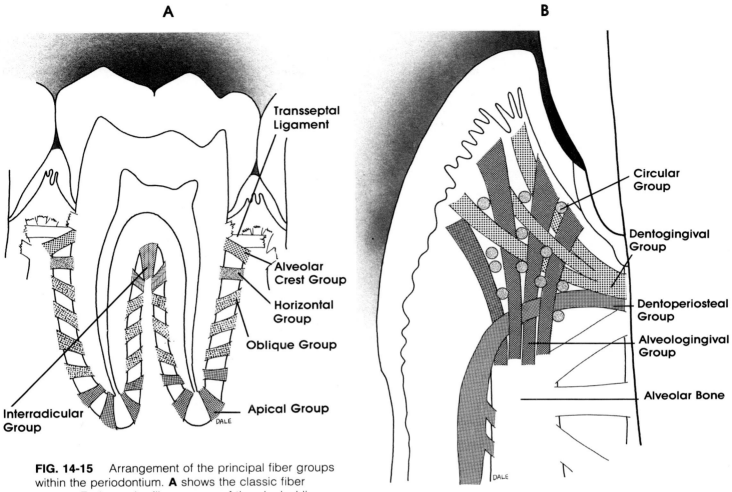

Transseptal Ligament

Alveolar Crest Group

Horizontal Group

Oblique Group

Apical Group

Interradicular Group

B

Circular Group

Dentogingival Group

Dentoperiosteal Group

Alveologingival Group

Alveolar Bone

FIG. 14-15 Arrangement of the principal fiber groups within the periodontium. **A** shows the classic fiber groups; **B** shows the fiber groups of the gingival ligament; **C** shows the gingival ligament fibers as seen interproximally related to the col.

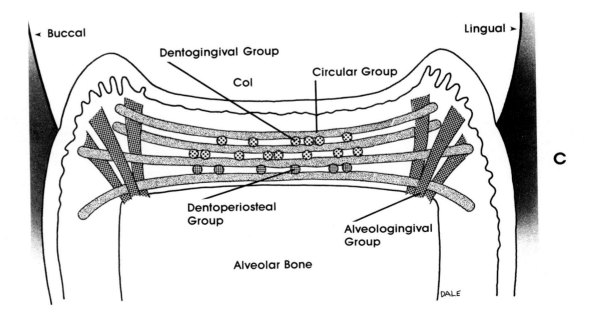

◄ Buccal

Lingual ►

Dentogingival Group

Col

Circular Group

Dentoperiosteal Group

Alveologingival Group

Alveolar Bone

C

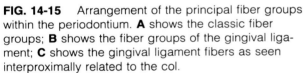

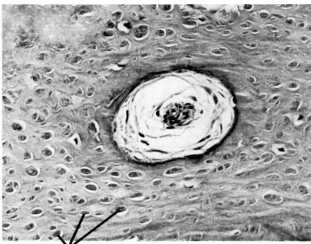

Cross section of Sharpey's fiber insertions

FIG. 14-16 Section through the interface between bundle bone and PDL. The insertion of Sharpey's fibers into the bone is shown. The large hole in the center transmits a vessel from the bone to the ligament.

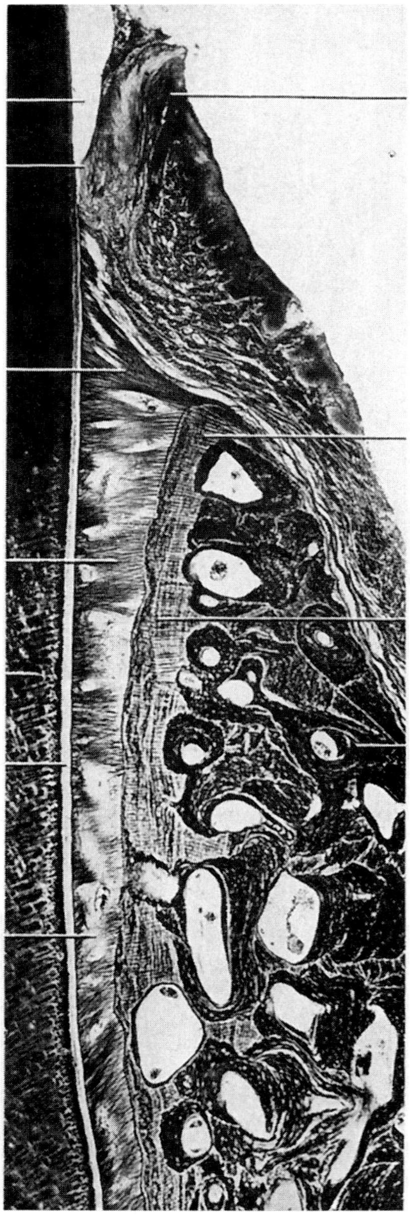

Enamel

Cementoenamel junction

Alveolar crest fibers

Horizontal fibers

Dentin

Cementum

Oblique fibers

Gingiva

Alveolar crest

Alveolar bone

Haversian bone

FIG. 14-17 Silver-stained section of some of the fiber groups of the gingival ligament.

At each end all the principal collagen fiber bundles of the PDL are embedded in cementum or bone (Figs. 13-4 and 14-16). The embedded portion is called a *Sharpey fiber*. Sharpey's fibers in acellular cementum are generally fully mineralized while those in cellular cementum and bone are generally only partially mineralized at their periphery. Occasionally Sharpey's fibers pass uninterruptedly through the bone of the alveolar process to continue as principal fibers of an adjacent periodontal ligament. Or they may mingle buccally and lingually with the fibers of the periosteum covering the outer cortical plates of the alveolar process. Sharpey's fibers pass through the alveolar process only when the process consists entirely of compact bone and contains no Haversian systems. It is not a common occurrence.

Although not strictly part of the periodontal ligament, other groups of collagen fibers in the periodontium are associated with maintaining the functional integrity of the teeth. They are found in the lamina propria of the gingiva and collectively form the gingival ligament (Figs. 14-15, *B*, and 14-17). Five groups of fiber bundles compose this ligament:

1. *Dentogingival group*. These are the most numerous fibers, extending from cervical cementum to lamina propria of both the free and the attached gingiva
2. *Alveologingival group*. These fibers radiate from the bone of the alveolar crest and extend into the lamina propria of the free and attached gingiva
3. *Circular group*. These are a small group of fibers that form a band around the neck of the tooth, interlacing with other groups of fibers in the free gingiva and helping to bind the free gingiva to the tooth (Fig. 14-15, *C*)
4. *Dentoperiosteal group*. Running apically from the cementum over the periosteum of the outer cortical plates of the alveolar process, these fibers insert into either the alveolar process or the vestibular muscle and floor of the mouth. They run interdentally from the cementum of one tooth, over the alveolar crest, to the cementum of the adjacent tooth. Known as transseptal fibers, they constitute the transseptal ligament (Fig. 14-18)
5. *Transseptal fiber system*. These fibers run interdentally from the cementum just apical to the base of the junctional epithelium of one tooth over the alveolar crest and insert into a comparable region of the cementum of the adjacent tooth. Together these fibers constitute the transseptal fiber system, collectively forming an interdental ligament connecting all the teeth of the arch (Fig. 14-18). The supracrestal fibers, and in particular the transseptal fiber system, have been implicated as a major cause of post retention relapse of orthodontically positioned teeth. It is the inability of the transseptal fiber system to undergo physiologic rearrangement that has lead to this conclusion. Recent studies have shown that although the rate of turnover is not as rapid as in the PDL, the transseptal fiber system is capable of protein turnover and/or remodeling under normal physiologic conditions, as well as during therapeutic tooth movement. It would seem reasonable, then, that a sufficiently prolonged retention period following orthodontic tooth movement would allow reorganization of the transseptal fiber system to ensure the clinical stability of tooth position

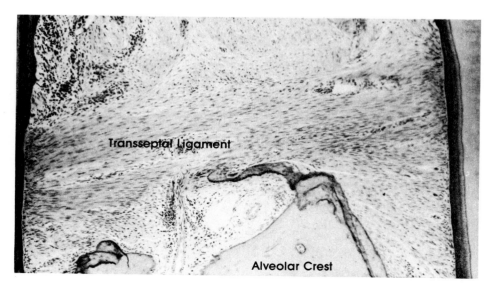

FIG. 14-18 Transseptal ligament. This fiber grouping is identified in sagittal sections running interdentally between adjacent teeth over the alveolar crest.

Elastin Fibers (Oxytalan and Eluanin)

Mature elastin is not found in the PDL but two immature forms of this tissue are, oxytalan and eluanin.

Oxytalan fibers (Fig. 14-19) are bundles of microfibrils (Chapter 5) whose distribution in the PDL is quite extensive when the ligament is examined in sheets rather than in section. They run more or less vertically from the cementum surface of the root apically, forming a three-dimensional branching meshwork that surrounds the root and terminates in the apical complex of arteries, veins, and lymphatics. They are also affiliated with neural elements. Oxytalan fibers are numerous and dense in the cervical region of the ligament, where they run parallel to the gingival group of collagen fibers. Although their function has not been fully determined, it is thought that they act to regulate vascular flow in relation to tooth function. Because they are elastic, they can expand in response to tensional variations, with such variations then registered on the walls of the vascular structures.

Eluanin fibers represent another form of elastic tissue consisting of bundles of microfibrils embedded within a small quantity of elastin (Chapter 5). When steps are taken to remove collagen from the PDL, an extensive

FIG. 14-19 Oxytalan fibers seen through the light microscope, **A,** and the electron microscope, **B.** These fibers run in an oblique direction generally at right angles to the principal collagen fiber bundles, often from the cementum to blood vessels.

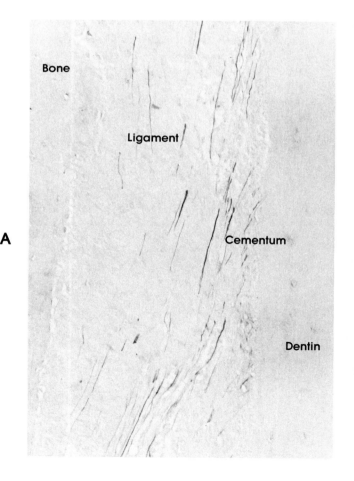

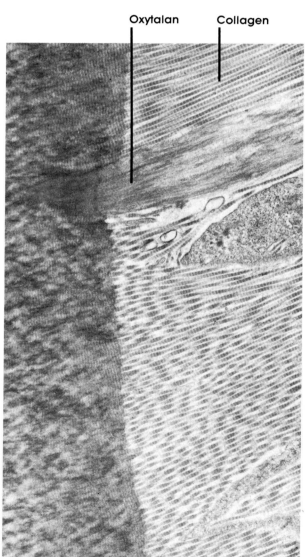

network of eluanin is revealed (Figs. 14-20 and 14-21). This network, together with the oxytalan fibers, forms a meshwork extending from cementum to bone and sheathing the collagen fibre bundles. While it is speculated that the rapid turnover occurring within the PDL prevents the maturation of its elastic component, it is likely that this elastic background of the PDL is of functional significance.

Ground Substance

Although ground substance is a major constituent of the PDL, few studies have been undertaken to determine its exact composition. What information there is indicates a similarity to most other connective tissues in terms of its components, with some variation in ratios, so that in the ligament dermatan sulfate is the principal glycosaminoglycan. It is structureless (Fig. 14-11), and therefore not readily apparent in sections examined with either the light or the electron microscope, but it plays an essential role in ligament function. The PDL ground substance has been estimated to consist of 70% water and is thought to have a significant effect on the tooth's ability to withstand stress loads. This effect will be covered more fully when the total function of the periodontium is discussed.

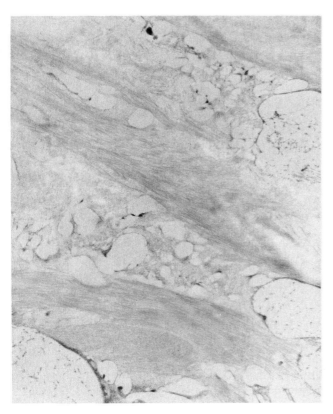

FIG. 14-20 Section of the PDL showing eluanin between partially digested principal collagen fiber bundles. (From Johnson RB, Pylypas SP: *J Periodont Res* 27:239, 1992.)

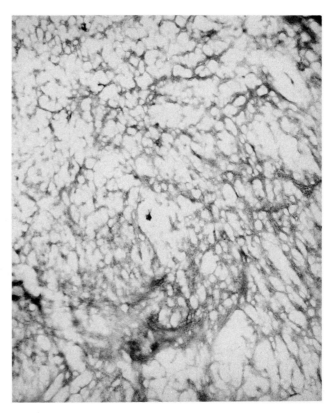

FIG. 14-21 Eluanin network in the PDL following complete digestion of the collagen fiber bundles. (From Johnson RB, Pylypas SP: *J Periodont Res* 27:239, 1992.)

Blood Supply

It has already been mentioned that, for a connective tissue, the PDL is exceptionally well vascularized, which reflects the high rate of turnover of its cellular and extracellular constituents. Its main blood supply is from the superior and inferior alveolar arteries. These arteries pursue an intraosteal course and give off alveolar branches that ascend within the bone as interalveolar arteries. Numerous branches arise from the interalveolar vessels to run horizontally, penetrate the alveolar bone, and enter the PDL space (Figs. 14-7, 14-16, and 14-22). Because they enter the ligament, they are called *perforating* arteries, and they occur more abundantly in the PDL of posterior teeth than that of anterior teeth and in greater numbers in mandibular than in maxillary teeth. In single-rooted teeth they are found most frequently in the gingival third of the ligament, followed by the apical third.

This pattern of distribution has clinical importance: In the healing of extraction wounds, new tissue invades from the perforations and the formation of a blood clot occupying the socket is more rapid in its gingival and apical areas. Once within the ligament, these arteries occupy areas (or bays) of loose connective tissue called *interstitial areas* between the principal fiber bundles and form an arcading pattern closer to the bone surface than to the cementum surface (Fig. 14-9).

Many arteriovenous anastomoses occur within the PDL, and venous drainage is achieved by axially directed vessels that drain into a system of retia (or networks) in the apical portion of the ligament. Lymphatic vessels tend to follow the venous drainage.

Nerve Supply

The use of autoradiographic methods and immunocytochemical labeling of neural proteins has greatly improved our knowledge about the innervation of the PDL over what previously was based on the results of somewhat unpredictable silver staining techniques. Although species differences have been reported, a general pattern of ligament innervation seems to be present (Fig. 14-23). First, there is the general anatomic configuration applicable to all teeth, with nerve fibers running from the apical region toward the gingival margin and being joined by fibers entering laterally through the foramina of the socket wall. These latter vessels divide into two branches, one extending apically and

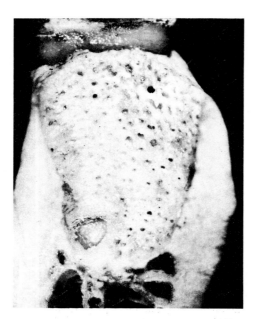

FIG. 14-22 Photomicrograph of the socket wall. The many perforations *(cribriform plate)* that transmit vessels and nerves to and from the PDL ligament are apparent. Compare with Figures 14-7 and 14-16.

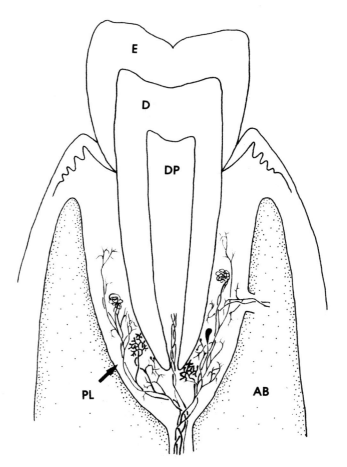

FIG. 14-23 Nerve terminals in a human PDL. (From Maeda T, et al: *Arch Histol Cytol* 53:259, 1990.)

the other gingivally. Second, there is regional variation in the termination of neural elements, with the apical region of the ligament containing more nerve endings than elsewhere (except for the upper incisors, where a particular situation exists in that not only is the innervation generally denser than in molars but further dense distributions of neural elements exist in the coronal half of the labial PDL as well as apically, suggesting that the spatial arrangement of receptors is a factor in determining the response characteristics of the

ligament). Third, the manner in which these nerve fibers terminate is being clarified. Four types of neural terminations have now been described (Fig. 14-24): The first (and most frequent) are free nerve endings that ramify in a treelike configuration. They are located at regular intervals along the length of the root, suggesting that each termination controls its own territory, and extend to the cementoblast layer. They originate largely from unmyelinated fibers but carry with them a Schwann cell envelope with processes that project into

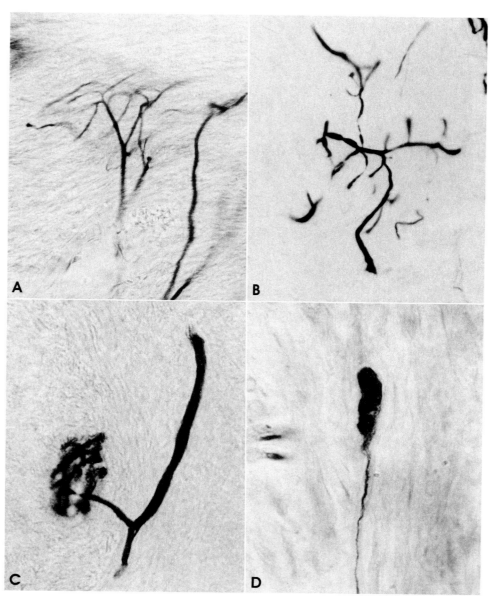

FIG. 14-24 The four types of nerve endings found in a human PDL. **A,** Free endings with treelike ramifications; **B,** Ruffini ending; **C,** coiled ending; **D,** encapsaulated spindle type ending. (From Maeda T, et al: *Arch Histol Cytol* 53:259, 1990.)

the surrounding connective tissue (Fig. 14-25). Such endings are thought to be both nociceptors and mechanoreceptors. The second type of nerve terminal is found around the root apex and resembles Ruffini corpuscles. They appear dendritic and end in terminal expansions among the PDL fiber bundles. By electron microscopy such receptors can be seen to have further subdivided into simple and compound forms, the former consisting of a single neurite and the latter of several terminations following branching. Both have ensheathing Schwann cells that are especially close to collagen fiber bundles (Fig 14-26), which provides morphologic evidence of their known physiologic function as mechanoreceptors. An incomplete fibrous capsule is sometimes found associated with the compound receptors. The third type of nerve terminal is a coiled form found in the midregion of the PDL whose function and ultrastructure have not yet been determined. The final type (with the lowest frequency) is found associated with the root apex and consists of spindlelike endings surrounded by a fibrous capsule.

The autonomic supply of the PDL has not yet been fully worked out, and the few descriptions available concern sympathetic supply. There is no evidence for the existence of a parasympathetic supply. The many free nerve terminals observed in close association with blood vessels are thought to be sympathetic and to affect regional blood flow.

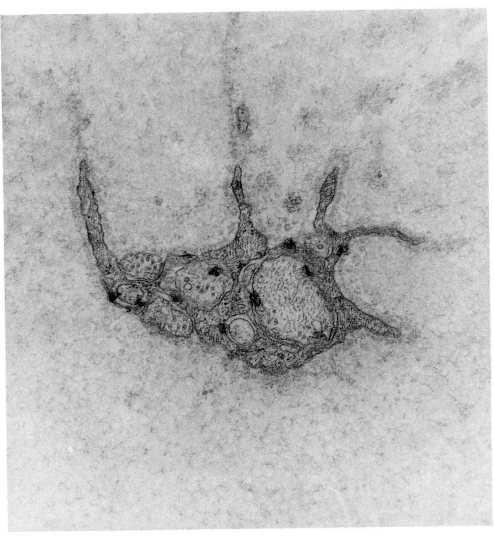

FIG. 14-25 Electron micrograph of free nerve ending *(FNE)* in a human PDL with an associated Schwann cell sending fingerlike projections into the connective tissue. (From Lambrichts I, et al: *J Periodont Res* 27:191, 1992.)

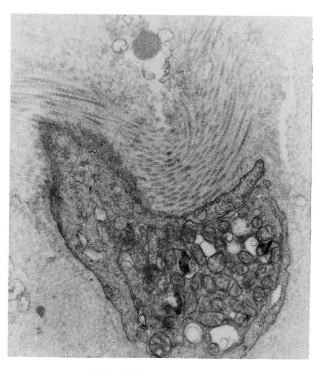

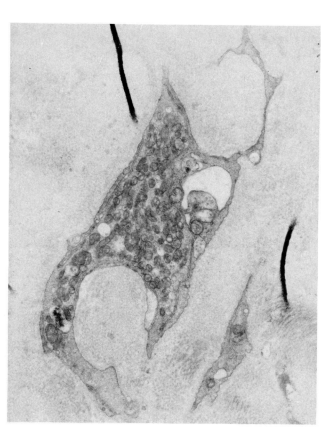

FIG. 14-26 Electron micrographs illustrating the close relationship of Ruffini-like endings with collagen fiber bundles. **A,** insertion of collagen fibrils into the basal lamina of a Schwann cell. **B,** Neurite embracing a bundle of collagen fibrils. (From Lambrichts I, et al: *J Periodont Res* 27:191, 1992.)

Alveolar Process (Bone)

The alveolar process is that bone of the jaws containing the sockets (alveoli) for the teeth. It consists of outer cortical plate, a central spongiosa, and bone lining the alveolus. The cortical plate and bone lining the alveolus meet at the alveolar crest (usually 1.5 to 2 mm below the level of the cementoenamel junction on the tooth it surrounds). The bone lining the socket is specifically referred to as *bundle bone* because it provides attachment for the PDL fiber bundles. Its likely origin is the dental follicle, and it is perforated by many foramina, which transmit nerves and vessels; thus it is sometimes referred to as the *cribriform* plate (Fig. 14-22).

The cortical plate consists of surface layers of fine-fibered lamellar bone supported by compact Haversian system bone of variable thickness. The trabecular (or spongy) bone occupying the central part of the alveolar process also consists of fine-fibered membrane bone disposed in lamellae with Haversian systems occurring in the large trabeculae. The important part of this complex, in terms of tooth support, is the bundle bone.

Bundle bone is that part of the alveolar process into which the fiber bundles of the PDL insert. It is called the *lamina dura* because of an increased radiopacity (Fig. 14-27). This apparent density is due to the thick bone without trabeculations that x rays must penetrate and not to any increased mineral content. The possible specific embryonic origin of bundle bone from the dental follicle has been indicated in Chapter 13. Its histologic structure is generally described as consisting of bundles of coarse-fibered woven bone fibers running

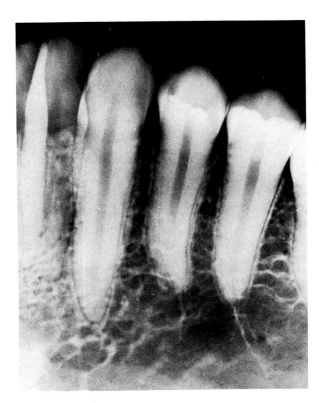

FIG. 14-27 Radiograph of teeth in situ. The white line delineating the socket is the lamina dura. (Courtesy Dr. D.W. Stoneman.)

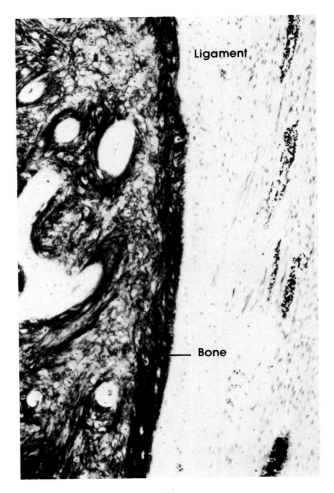

Ligament

Bone

FIG. 14-28 Silver-stained section of alveolar bone showing the intrinsic fiber disposition of the bone lining the alveolus.

parallel to the socket wall and arranged in lamellae (Fig. 14-28). Embedded within this bone are the extrinsic collagen fiber bundles of the PDL (which, as in cellular cementum, are mineralized only at their periphery). This is a simplistic description, however, since (it will be remembered) the tooth is constantly making minor movements and the bone of the socket wall must constantly adapt to many forms of stress. Thus practically all forms of bone histology can be observed lining the alveolus, even in the same field in the same section (Fig. 14-29). This considerable variation reflects the functional plasticity of alveolar bone. In general terms, the lining of the alveolus is fairly smooth in youngsters. With age the socket lining becomes rougher and is seen in histologic section to have a ragged outline.*

The plasticity of bundle bone is reflected in varying forms of Sharpey's fiber attachments. Such variations have only recently been reported, when a high-voltage electron microscope was used to study thick sections of the remodeling interdental septum of mouse alveolar bone, and have been classified as follows:

1. *Severed fibers.* Located within old bone and terminating at the reversal line, marking the junction between old bone and new bone deposited on the surface
2. *Adhesive fibers.* Located entirely within new bone and terminating at the reversal line in a granular material
3. *Arborized fibers.* Located entirely within new bone and terminating in its matrix
4. *Continuous fibers.* Appearing to cross reversal lines as a continuum but, in fact, joining old and new fibrils by nonstriated fibrils (probably link proteins)

---

*It is important to grasp the terminology used here, for many variations exist. The term *alveolar process* is clearly defined and presents no problem. This being so, *alveolar bone* must properly refer to the bone making up the alveolar process. Many dentists, especially periodontists, use the term *alveolar bone* to describe that bone lining the alveolus. Radiologists use *lamina dura* to describe this bone, and others use the term *bundle bone* because the bundles of PDL fibers are embedded in it. (This terminology, too, can be confusing since the bone often consists of coarse-fibered woven bundles of collagen.) In the terminology used here, an alveolar process consists of alveolar bone (which is lost when teeth are lost) containing alveoli (or sockets) lined by bundle bone. *Bundle bone* is chosen because it clearly indicates that such bone incorporates the "bundles" of fibers making up the ligament. The extreme variability of bundle bone (as highlighted in Figure 14-29) indicates the impossibility of ascribing a precise histologic structure to it. Quite likely, as the periodontium first develops, the socket is lined by embryologically distinct coarse-fibered woven bone but it is soon remodeled as the tooth moves during function.

DENTOGINGIVAL JUNCTION

The dentogingival junction represents a unique anatomic feature concerned with attachment of the gingiva to the tooth (Fig. 14-30). It consists of epithelial and connective tissue components, with the epithelium divided into three functional compartments—*gingival, sulcular,* and *junctional*—and the connective tissue into two—*superficial* and *deep*.

Epithelial Component

Three types of anatomically distinct epithelia are associated with the dentogingival junction. The first consists of stratified squamous keratinized gingival epithelium, which is continuous at the crest of the gingiva with the second type, stratified nonkeratinized sulcular epithelium (facing the tooth surface but not attached to it), which in turn is continuous at the base of the sulcus with the junctional epithelium (uniting the gingiva to tooth), which also forms the floor of the sulcus.

Gingival epithelium

Gingival epithelium is a stratified squamous keratinized epithelium (described in Chapter 18) that covers the gingiva and varies in architecture according to location and functional demands.

The *gingival sulcus** is a shallow groove between the tooth and the normal gingiva that extends from the free surface of the junctional epithelium coronally to the level of the free gingival margin. The depth of the sulcus varies from 0.5 to 3 mm, with an average of 1.8 mm. Any depth greater than 3 mm can generally be considered pathologic, a sulcus this deep being known as a periodontal pocket. When the tooth first becomes functional, the bottom of the sulcus is usually found on the cervical half of the anatomic crown; but with age there is a gradual migration of the sulcus bottom, which eventually may pass on to the cementum surface. The sulcus contains fluid that has passed through the junctional epithelium and contains a mixture of both desquamated epithelial cells from the junctional and sulcular epithelia and neutrophils that have also passed through the junctional epithelium.

Sulcular epithelium

Sulcular epithelium is a stratified squamous tissue that in many ways is similar to the stratified gingival epithelium. It differs in one key respect: it is nonkeratinized. The junction between epithelium and connective tissue is straight, and its closely packed cells are characterized by relatively small amounts of cytoplasm, little rough endoplasmic reticulum, and many tonofilaments (Fig. 14-31, *B*). The lack of keratinization

---

*The older term *crevice* is rarely used nowadays.

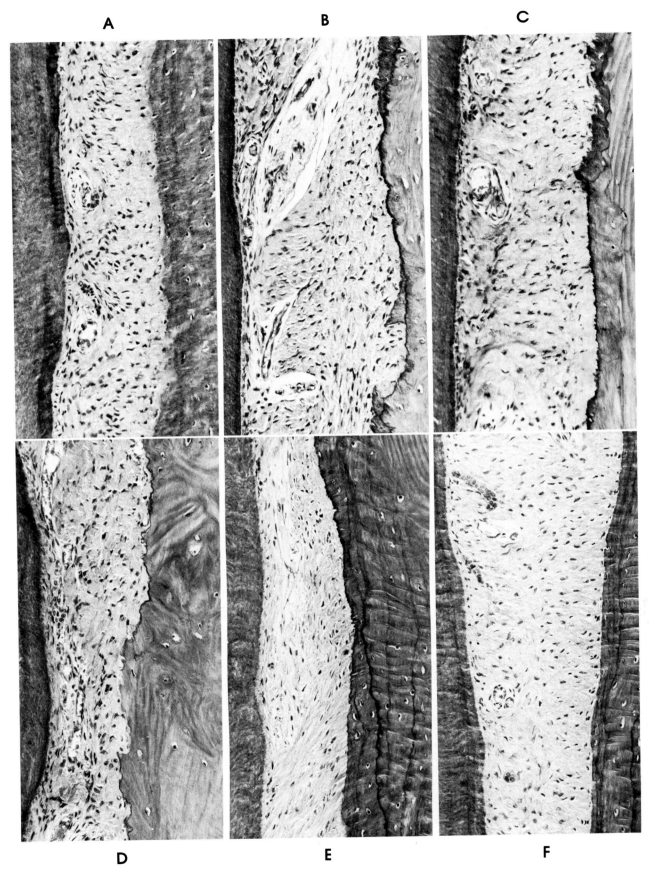

FIG. 14-29 Photomicrographs of the PDL of a single tooth. The considerable variation in morphology of the bone lining this alveolus is produced by the resorption or deposition of bone as it responds to functional demands placed on it. Bone is always to the right.

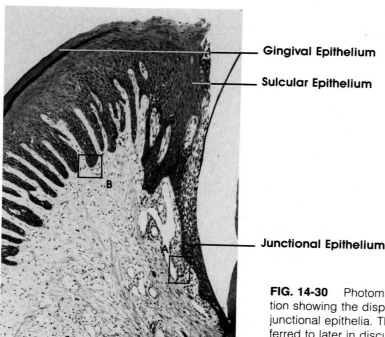

Gingival Epithelium

Sulcular Epithelium

Junctional Epithelium

FIG. 14-30 Photomicrograph of the dentogingival junction showing the disposition of gingival, sulcular, and junctional epithelia. The boxed areas **A** and **B** are referred to later in discussion of the connective tissue component of the junction.

of the sulcular epithelium is the result of inflammation in its supporting connective tissue.

Junctional Epithelium

The junctional epithelium forms a collar around the tooth. It is wider (some 15 to 30 cells thick) at the floor of the gingival sulcus and tapers apically to a final thickness of some 3 to 4 cells. It is made of layers of flattened squamous cells lying parallel to the tooth surface supported by a generally straight basement membrane (Figs. 14-30 and 31, *A* and *C*). The surface cells of the junctional epithelium provide the actual attachment of gingiva to tooth tissue (the epithelium being sometimes referred to as "attachment" epithelium), with the development of hemidesmosomes and a basal lamina that differs from other basal laminae opposed to connective tissue in that type IV collagen is absent.

As in all epithelia, basal cells undergo cell division to replenish the cells sloughed off at the surface. Junctional epithelium presents an unusual circumstance in that its surface cells are specialized for the purpose of attachment and therefore the surface is not available for the elimination of cells. What happens is that the cells stemming from the high turnover of basal cells move to within two or three cell layers of the tooth surface and then join a main migratory route in a coronal direction paralleling the tooth surface to be sloughed off into the gingival sulcus.

The ultrastructural characteristics of junctional epithelial cells are relatively constant throughout the epithelium and differ considerably from those of gingival epithelial cells. The amount of rough endoplasmic reticulum and Golgi complexes is significantly greater, as is the amount of cytoplasm. Conversely, far fewer tonofilaments are present. The extracellular spaces (Fig. 14-31, *C*) between the junctional epithelial cells are also greater (18% of the epithelium is occupied by intercellular space), as reflected by the lower density of desmosomes in junctional epithelium (4 times less) than in gingival epithelium. Within these intercellular spaces, polymorphonuclear leukocytes and monocytes are found passing from the gingival connective tissue to the gingival sulcus. In clinically normal gingiva the relative volume occupied by neutrophils may be as great as 64%. These widened intercellular spaces, besides accommodating the emigration of polymorphonuclear cells, also permit the ingress of antigens.

Such morphologic characteristics are indicative of an immature undifferentiated epithelium, which is confirmed by the analysis of its constituent keratins and surface carbohydrates.

The keratins are a multigene family of proteins (at least 30) (Chapter 18) within which are recognized two subfamilies: the first consisting of relatively large basic proteins (52 to 67 kDa) numbered 1 to 8, and the second of smaller (40 to 56 kDa) and more acidic proteins num-

FIG. 14-31 Photomicrographs of the dentogingival junction. **A,** Thin plastic-embedded section of the junction in the region where junctional and sulcular epithelia meet. The way the junctional epithelium forms the floor of the gingival sulcus is clearly illustrated. **B** and **C,** Ultrastructure of the boxed areas in **A** showing the differences between junctional and sulcular epithelia. **C** also shows the epithelial attachment; the hemidesmosomes, lamina lucida, and lamina densa are readily apparent against the enamel surface. (Courtesy Prof. H.E. Schroeder.)

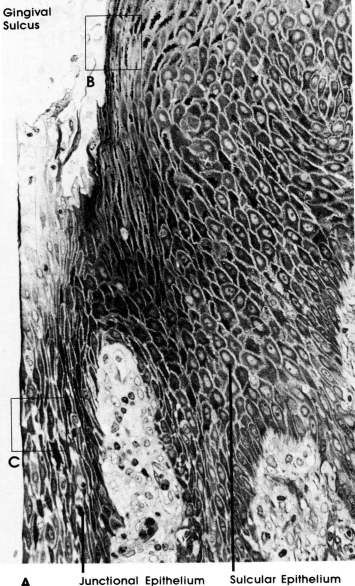

A

Junctional Epithelium   Sulcular Epithelium

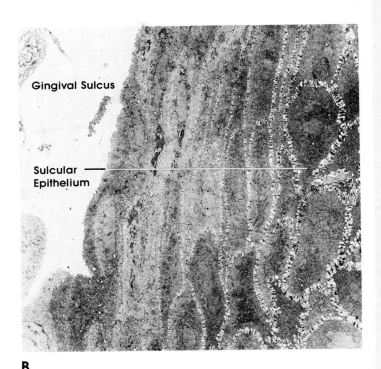

Gingival Sulcus

Sulcular Epithelium

B

C

Intercellular Space

Enamel

Tonofilaments

Lamina Densa

Lamina Lucida

Epithelial Attachment

bered through to 19. Except for no. 19, all keratins occur in linked acid and base pairs in a consistent manner in different types of epithelia. For example, keratins 5 and 14 are found together in all keratinocytes, 1 and 10 in keratinized epithelium, 4 and 13 in stratified squamous epithelium, and 8 and 18 in simple epithelia; keratin 19 occurs alone in simple epithelia. When these various keratins are identified by using immunocytochemistry, their distribution in dentogingival junction epithelium conforms to this pattern (Fig. 14-32) and confirms that junctional epithelium is indeed a simple epithelium. The same conclusion can be derived from an analysis of cell membrane surface carbohydrates, which show elongation correlated to the differentiation and maturity of epithelial cells. Mature cell surface carbohydrate is designated as A, with precursors in descending order labeled H and N. Thus A (indicating the highest level of differentiation) occurs in upper layers of the oral epithelium but in sulcular epithelium is found in only a few cells, where precursor H predominates. Precursor N (indicating the lowest level of cell differentiation) is found in basal cells of the sulcular and gingival epithelia and is the only carbohydrate marker found in junctional epithelium (Fig. 14-32).

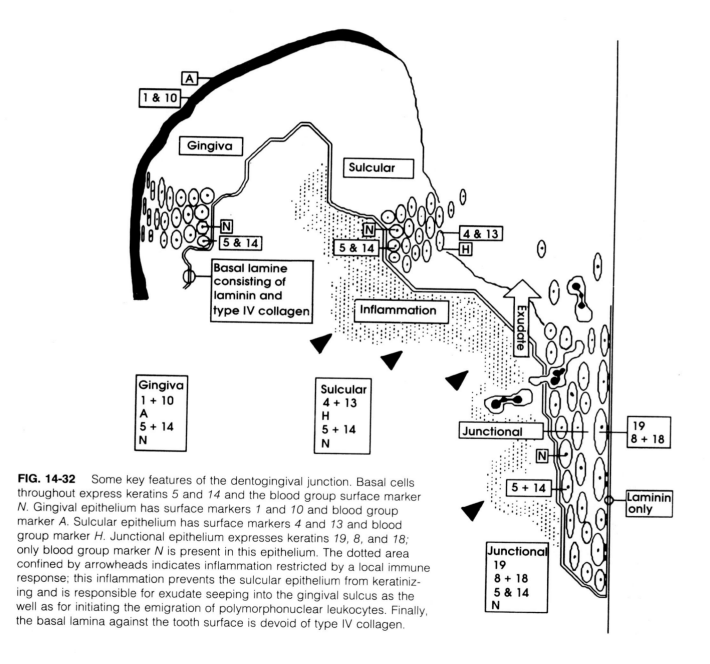

FIG. 14-32 Some key features of the dentogingival junction. Basal cells throughout express keratins 5 and 14 and the blood group surface marker N. Gingival epithelium has surface markers 1 and 10 and blood group marker A. Sulcular epithelium has surface markers 4 and 13 and blood group marker H. Junctional epithelium expresses keratins 19, 8, and 18; only blood group marker N is present in this epithelium. The dotted area confined by arrowheads indicates inflammation restricted by a local immune response; this inflammation prevents the sulcular epithelium from keratinizing and is responsible for exudate seeping into the gingival sulcus as the well as for initiating the emigration of polymorphonuclear leukocytes. Finally, the basal lamina against the tooth surface is devoid of type IV collagen.

Connective Tissue Component

Straightforward microscopic examination of the connective tissue supporting epithelium of the dentogingival junction shows it to be structurally different from connective tissue supporting the oral gingival epithelium (Fig. 14-33) in that, even in clinically normal gingiva, it contains a population of inflammatory cells. This inflammatory lesion is thought to be initiated at the time of tooth eruption (Chapter 13). Cells of the inflammatory series, especially polymorphonuclear leukocytes, continually migrate into both the sulcular and the junctional epithelium and pass between the epithelial cells to appear in the gingival sulcus and eventually in the oral fluid. It has been estimated that some

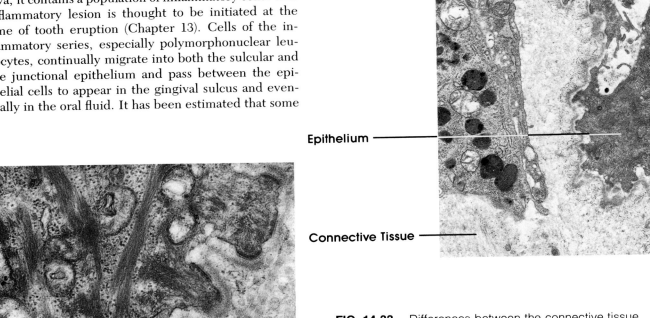

FIG. 14-33 Differences between the connective tissue supporting the junctional epithelium and the gingiva. Ultrastructural appearance. Compare this with Figure 14-30. In **A** the few collagen fibrils supporting junctional epithelium are disorganized. In **B** the fibers are more regularly disposed against the basal lamina supporting gingival epithelium. (**B** from Gelfand HG, et al: *J Periodontol* 49:113, 1978.)

3000 neutrophils migrate every minute into the mouth via this route.

There is evidence that the connective tissue supporting junctional epithelium is also functionally different from the connective tissue supporting sulcular epithelium; and it is worth reviewing this evidence in some detail, because the difference has important connotations for periodontal disease and regeneration of the dentogingival junction after periodontal surgery.

In Chapter 6 epithelial-mesenchymal interactions were discussed; and, on the basis of recombination experiments there described, it has been shown that connective tissue plays a key role in determining epithelial expression. Therefore subepithelial connective tissues (the lamina propria) provide instructive influences for the normal maturation of a stratified squamous epithelium and these influences are absent from deep connective tissue (which posseses only permissive factors required to maintain the epithelium). Thus epithelium combined with deep connective tissue does not mature but instead persists in an immature state closely resembling that of junctional epithelium.

It is believed that gingival and sulcular epithelia (supported by an instructive connective tissue) are able to mature whereas junctional epithelium (supported by a deep connective tissue, the PDL) remains immature (Fig. 14-34). This difference in phenotypic expression is important because, by maintaining a degree of immaturity, the functional epithelium can develop hemidesmosomal attachments where its cells come into contact with the tooth surface.

Mention has been made that the connective tissue associated with the dentogingival junction is inflamed. This inflammation also influences epithelial expression. Thus the sulcular epithelium, in marked distinction to the gingival epithelium, is nonkeratinized, yet both are supported by gingival lamina propria. This difference in epithelial expression is a direct consequence of the inflammatory process, because, if the inflammatory process is removed by implementation of a strict regimen of oral hygiene combined with antibiotic coverage in experimental animals, the sulcular epithelium keratinizes.

The junctional epithelium is also influenced by this inflammatory lesion. Epithelia maintained experimentally in association with deep connective tissue show little capacity to proliferate but can be induced to do so by the introduction of inflammation into the system. Clinically it is recognized that in most people there is a slow apical migration of the attachment level (Fig. 13-21) with age (sometimes referred to as passive eruption) that is probably due to the low-level inflammation in its supporting connective tissue. When this inflammatory process is exacerbated, there is active proliferation with migration of the junctional epithelium, resulting in establishment of a periodontal pocket and the rapid receding of attachment level.

A similar set of biologic events occurs in relation to the proliferation of epithelial cell rests of Malassez and dental cyst formation. Cell rests are supported by the deep connective tissue of the PDL and are proliferative only in the presence of inflammatory changes within that connective tissue.

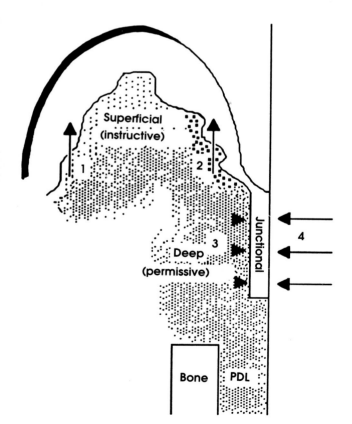

FIG. 14-34 Various influences of connective tissue on the dentogingival junction epithelium: *1,* the instructive influence of superficial connective tissue; *2,* this influence affected by inflammation *(large dots); 3,* the influence of deep connective tissues *(arrowheads); 4,* the influence of surface enamel on epithelial expresson. *(PDL,* Periodontal ligament.)

Col

This description of the dentogingival junction applies to all surfaces of the tooth, even though interdentally the gingiva seems to be different. Interdental gingiva appears to have the outline of a col (or depression), with buccal and lingual peaks guarding it (Fig. 14-35). At one time it was thought that in development of the dentogingival junction the oral epithelium totally replaced enamel epithelium, except in the region of the col, where reduced enamel epithelium persisted. Because of this false assumption, it was suggested that the col area was one of great vulnerability and therefore important in the onset of periodontal disease. In fact, the col is not different in its structure and should be considered to be a duplication of the appearance seen in section through the buccal and lingual surfaces of the tooth (Fig. 14-36).

Col epithelium is identical to junctional epithelium, has the same origin (from dental epithelium), and is gradually replaced by continuing cell division. Thus there is no evidence that the structural elements of the col increases one's vulnerability to periodontal disease. Rather, the incidence of gingivitis interdentally is greater than in other areas because the morphologic relationships of tooth to tooth allow bacteria, food debris, and plaque to accumulate in this location.

Blood Supply

The blood supply to the gingiva is derived from periosteal vessels in the periosteum of the alveolar process. Branches from these vessels run perpendicular to the surface and form loops within the connective tissue papillae of the gingiva. Vessels supplying the dentogingival junction are derived from the continuation of

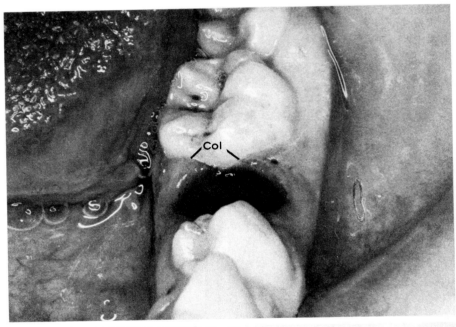

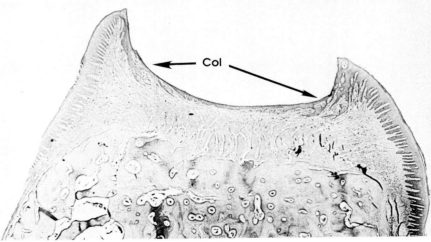

FIG. 14-35 Col. **A** is the clinical appearance, and **B** a histologic section. The distinction between the keratinized gingival epithelium and the epithelium of the col is evident.

interalveolar arteries as they pierce the alveolar crest. These vessels run parallel to the sulcular epithelium, forming a rich network just below the basement membrane (Fig. 14-37). In the presence of inflammation the flat junction between sulcular epithelium and its supporting connective tissue changes as pegs of proliferative epithelium develop. When this occurs, the vessels loop between the pegs.

Thus the blood supply to the periodontium can be divided into three zones for descriptive purposes: (1) that to the PDL, (2) that to the gingiva facing the oral cavity, and (3) that to the gingiva facing the tooth. Connections among the three permit collateral circulation.

Nerve Supply

The gingival component of the periodontium is innervated by terminal branches of periodontal nerve fibers and by branches of the infraorbital and palatine, or lingual, mental, and buccal nerves. In the attached gingiva, most nerves terminate within the lamina propria and only a few endings occur between epithelial cells. In the dentogingival junction, however, there is a rich innervation of the basal layer of epithelium.

Age Changes

With age there is a progressive apical migration of the dentogingival junction. Shortly after the tooth has erupted, the junctional epithelium of the dentogingival junction extends to the cementoenamel junction, which is regarded as its normal anatomic position. When teeth erupt, however, inflammation occurs in the connective tissues. Normally this inflammatory focus is maintained at a very low level and is contained locally by the immune system. Exacerbations of the inflammatory focus (by such factors as poor oral hygiene) lead to gingivitis and a gradual loss of the tooth's supporting tissues. As this happens, the dentogingival junction migrates apically onto the cementum and eventually the cement surface of the tooth is exposed.

Gingival recession has important clinical implications. First, toothbrush abrasion may remove the cervical cementum and expose the dentin, resulting in possible dentin sensitivity in this area. Second, the exposure of cementum to the oral environment usually results in unsightly discoloration and the onset of root caries. Third, gingival recession reflects progressive loss of tooth support and increased tooth mobility.

FUNCTIONS OF THE PERIODONTIUM

All the structural components of the periodontium have now been presented. Together they form a functional system that provides an attachment for the tooth to the bone of the jaw while at the same time permitting the teeth to withstand the considerable forces of mastication.

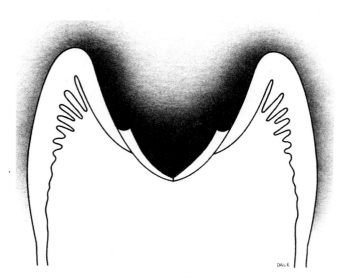

FIG. 14-36   Col. This can be considered a duplication of the appearance of the dentogingival junction as applied to the buccal and lingual surfaces of a tooth. (Modified from McHugh WD: *J Periodont Res* 6:227, 1971.)

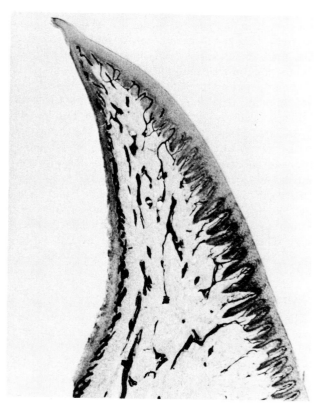

FIG. 14-37   Photomicrograph of the blood supply to the dentogingival junction. Note the differences in shape of vessels related to the gingiva and the dentogingival junction. (From Egleberg J: *J Periodont Res* 1:163, 1966.)

Attachment

There is no dispute that the principal collagen fiber bundles of the PDL attach the tooth to the jaw. And the simple concept of wavy collagen fibers gradually straightening out as force is applied and then acting as inelastic strings or ties transmitting tension to the wall of the alveolus is attractive but incompatible with physiologic findings. For example, if such a concept were true, we might expect the alveolar margins of the sockets to be narrowed when force was applied to the tooth. In fact, the reverse occurs and the margin of the socket is widened. It is now appreciated that all the components of the PDL act together as a hydraulic damper or shock absorber, with the ground substance of the ligament, the tissue fluid, and blood in the blood vessels all acting as a viscoelastic system. Because fluids under pressure are incompressible, it is suggested that when force is applied to the tooth the fluids act as a damper and are then displaced either through the foramina of the cribriform plates or into other regions of the ligament, depending on the direction of the force applied. Thus displacement could cause dilation of the socket margin.

Recently it has been shown that the ground substance of the PDL is not static but that during function alterations occur in its molecular structure. It would appear that these changes in the chemistry and properties of PDL ground substance components account for the changes seen in tooth mobility during function.

When the periodontium is exposed to increased function, as much as a 50% increase in the width of the PDL can occur, with the principal fiber bundles increasing markedly in thickness. Also, the bony trabeculae supporting the alveoli increase number and in thickness, and the alveolar bone itself becomes thicker. Conversely, a reduction in function leads to changes that are the opposite of those described for excess function. The ligament narrows, the fiber bundles decrease in number and thickness, and the trabeculae become fewer. This reduction in width of the PDL is largely due to the deposition of additional cementum (Fig. 14-38).

Sensation

The other major function of the periodontium is sensory, although the nature of this function of the PDL is still being debated. When teeth move in their sockets, undoubtedly they do distort receptors in the PDL and trigger a response. Thus the PDL contributes to the sensations of touch and pressure on the teeth; in addition, the spatial distribution of receptors is significant. It is equally certain, however, that the ligament receptors are not the only organs from which sensations arise. For example, when teeth are tapped, vibrations

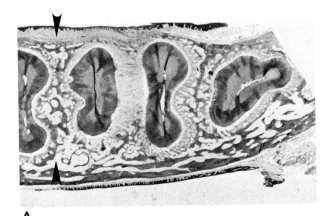

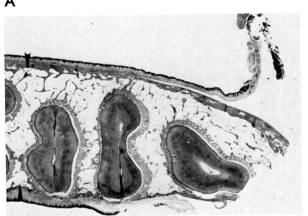

FIG. 14-38 Photomicrographs of the effect of nonfunction on the supporting apparatus of the tooth. **A,** Normal appearance of tissues supporting the teeth. **B,** Effect of nonfunction for 6 months. Note the loss of bone between the *arrows.* The narrowing of the ligament can also be distinguished. (Courtesy Prof. D.C. Picton.)

are passed through the bone and detected in the middle ear. There is also debate as to the exact physiologic function of these receptors. It has been demonstrated that stimulation of the teeth causes a reflex jaw opening and, likewise, that stimulation of periodontal mechanoreceptors initiates this response. Whether such a reflex is required for the normal masticatory process or is a protective mechanism to prevent forces applied to the teeth from reaching potentially damaging levels is not known. (The role of the periodontium in tooth movement is discussed in Chapter 15.)

At this point, all the dental hard tissues have been discussed in detail. As a summary, Table 14-2 presents the similarities and differences among bone, cementum, dentin, and enamel, clearly indicating the distinctive nature of enamel.

TABLE 14-2 Comparison of the dental hard tissues

	Bone	Cementum		Dentin	Enamel
Embryology Tissue Cells in mature tissue	Mesoderm Connective Osteocytes in lacunae	Ectomesenchyme Connective Cementocytes in lacunae in cellular cementum	No cells in acellular cementum	Ectomesenchyme Connective Odontoblasts in pulp with cytoplasmic extensions into dentin (N.B.—correct terminology should be odontocytes)	Ectoderm Epithelial No cells associated with mature enamel
Formative cells	Osteoblasts found on surface of lamellae and incorporated as osteocytes	Cementoblasts found on surface and incorporated as cementocytes	Cementoblasts found only on surface	Odontoblasts in pulp with cytoplasmic extensions	Ameloblasts found only on surface during development
Degradative cells	Osteoclasts	Odontoclasts, characteristics same as osteoclasts; can resorb all three dental hard tissues			
Organic matrix	Collagen and ground substance	Acellular cementum; collagen and ground substance; high proportion of extrinsic fibers; all fibers mineralized	Cellular cementum; collagen and ground substance; many more intrinsic fibers; extrinsic fibers mineralized only at periphery	Collagen and ground substance	Enamel proteins (nonfibrous); trace of carbohydrate; only tissue showing decrease in organic content with maturation
Mineral	Apatite 50% to 60%	Apatite 45% to 50%		Apatite 70%	Apatite 96%
Mineralization matrix vesicles	Present	Present		Present	None present
Viability (ability to repair)	High rate of remodeling; repair potential high; vascularity	No remodeling; repair occurs by new cementum deposition		No remodeling; repair occurs by secondary and tertiary dentin deposition	No remodeling or repair possible (repair of partially demineralized defects by remineralization from salivary ions)
Sensitive	Yes	No		Yes; only pain appreciated	No
Incremental lines	Resting and reversal	Resting		Von Ebner; Owen; neonatal line in deciduous and first lower molar	Retzius; neonatal line in deciduous and first molar
Blood and nutritive supply	Vessels within bone but cells supplied by diffusion	None; cells supplied by diffusion from periodontal ligament		None in dentin; tissue fluid circulates in tubules	Avascular
Age changes (forensic significance)	Lifelong active turnover With age, more resorption and less apposition	Increase in volume of tissue with age especially at the apex		Increase in secondary and sclerotic dentin	Loss of tissue by wear Increase in stains

BIBLIOGRAPHY

Anderson DJ, Hannam AG, Mathews B: Sensory mechanism in mammalian teeth and their supporting structures, *Physiol Rev* 50:171, 1970.

Attström R, Egelberg J: Emigration of blood neutrophil polymorphonuclear leukocytes and monocytes into the gingival crevices, *J Periodont Res* 4:160, 1969.

Bartold PM: Proteoglycans of the periodontium: structure, role and function, *J Periodont Res* 22:431, 1987.

Bartold PM, Miki Y, McAllister B, et al: Glycosaminoglycans of human cementum, *J Periodont Res* 23:13-17, 1988.

Beagrie GS: An autoradiographic study of the gingival epithelium of mice and monkeys with thymidine-H³, *Dent Pract Dent Res* 14:18, 1963.

Becks H: Normal and pathologic pocket formation, *J Am Dent Assoc* 16:2167, 1929.

Berkovitz BKB, et al: *The periodontal ligament in health and disease*, New York, 1982, Pergaman Press.

Bernick S: Innervation of teeth and periodontium after enzymatic removal of collagenous elements, *Oral Surg* 10:323, 1957.

Bevelander G, Nakahara H: The fine structure of the human peridontal ligament, *Anat Rec* 162:313, 1968.

Birn H: The vascular supply of the periodontal membrane, *J Periodont Res* 1:51, 1966.

Blackwood HJJ: Intermediate cementum, *Br Dent J* 102:345, 1957.

Boyde A, Jones SJ: Scanning electron microscope studies of the formation of mineralised tissues. In Slavkin HC, Bavetta LA (eds): *Developmental aspects of oral biology*, New York, 1972, Academic Press.

Breix MC, et al: Variability of histological criteria in clinically healthy human gingiva, *J Periodont Res* 22:468, 1987.

Brill N, Björn H: Passage of tissue fluid into human gingival pockets, *Acta Odontol Scand* 17:11, 1959.

Brill N, Krasse B: The passage of tissue fluid into the clinically healthy gingival pocket, *Acta Odontol Scand* 16:233, 1958.

Carmichael GG: Observations with the light microscope on the distribution and connections of the oxytalan fibre of the lower jaw of the mouse, *Arch Oral Biol* 13:765, 1968.

Carmichael GG, Fullmer HM: The fine structure of the oxytalan fibre, *J Cell Biol* 28:33, 1966.

Carneiro J, Fava De Moraes F: Radioautographic visualization of collagen metabolism in the periodontal tissues of the mouse, *Arch Oral Biol* 10:833, 1965.

Ciancio SC, Neiders ME, Hazen SP: The principal fibres of the periodontal ligament, *Periodontics* 5:76, 1967.

Cohen B: Morphological factors in the pathogenesis of periodontal disease, *Br Dent J* 107:31, 1959.

Cohen B: Study of the periodontal epithelium, *Br Dent J* 112:55, 1962.

Cohn SA: A reexamination of Sharpey's fibres in alveolar bone of the marmoset *(Sanguinus fusciocollis)*, *Arch Oral Biol* 17:261, 1972.

Cohn SA: A reexamination of Sharpey's fibres in alveolar bone of the mouse, *Arch Oral Biol* 17:255, 1972.

Coolidge ED: The thickness of the human periodontal membrane, *J Am Dent Assoc* 24:1260, 1937.

Davidson D, McCulloch CAG: Proliferative behaviour of periodontal ligament cell populations, *J Periodont Res* 21:414, 1986.

Deporter DA, Svoboda EL, Howley TP et al: A quantitative comparison of collagen phagocytosis in periodontal ligament and transseptal ligament of the rat periodontium, *Am J Orthod* 85:519, 1984.

Egelberg J: Diffusion of histamine into the gingival crevice and through the crevicular epithelium, *Acta Odontol Scand* 21:271, 1963.

Egelberg J: The blood vessels of the dentogingival junction, *J Periodont Res* 1:163, 1966.

Eley BM, Harrison JD: Intracellular collagen fibrils in the periodontal ligament of man, *J Periodont Res* 10:168, 1975.

Embery G, Picton DA, Stanbury JB: Biochemical changes in periodontal ligament ground substance associated with short-term intrusive loadings in adult monkeys *(Macaca fascicularis)*, *Arch Oral Biol* 32:545, 1987.

Folke LEA, Stallard RE: Periodontal microcirculation as revealed by plastic microspheres, *J Periodont Res* 2:53, 1967.

Frank RM, Cimasoni G: Ultrastructure de l'épithélium cliniquement normal du sillon et de la jonction gingivo-dentaires. *Z Zellforsch Mikroskop Anat* 43:597, 1972.

Frank R, Fiore-Donno G, Cimasoni G, et al: Gingival reattachment after surgery in man: an electron microscopic study, *J Periodont* 43:597, 1972.

Frank R, Fiore-Donno G, Cimasoni G, et al: Ultrastructural study of epithelial and connective gingival reattachment in man, *Periodontol* 45:626, 1974.

Freezer SR, Sims MR: A transmission electron-microscope stereological study of the blood vessels, oxytalan fibres and nerves of the mouse-molar periodontal ligament, *Arch Oral Biol* 32:407, 1987.

Fullmer HM, Gibson WA: Collagenolytic activity in the gingiva of man, *Nature* 209:728, 1966.

Fullmer HM, Sheetz JH, Narkates AJ: Oxytalan connective tissue fibres: a review, *J Oral Pathol* 3:291, 1974.

Furseth R: A microradiographic and electron microscopic study of the cementum of human deciduous teeth, *Acta Odontol Scand* 25:613, 1967.

Furseth R: The fine structure of the cellular cementum of young human teeth, *Arch Oral Biol* 14:1147, 1969.

Garant PR: Collagen resorption by fibroblasts: a theory of fibroblastic maintenance of periodontal ligament, *J Periodontol* 47:380, 1976.

Garant PR, Mulvihill JE: The ultrastructure of clinically normal sulcular tissues in the beagle dog, *J Periodont Res* 6:252, 1971.

Gargiulo AW, Wentz FM, Orban B: Dimensions and relations of the dentogingival junction in humans, *J Periodontol* 32:261, 1961.

Gathercole LJ: In vitro mechanics of intrusive loading in porcine cheek teeth with intact and perforated root apices, *Arch Oral Biol* 32:249, 1987.

Gavin JB: The ultrastructure of the crevicular epithelium of cat gingiva, *Am J Anat* 123:283, 1968.

Geisenheimer J, Han SS: A quantitative electron microscopic study of desmosomes and hemidesmosomes in human crevicular epithelium, *J Periodontol* 49:113, 1978.

Gould TRL, Melcher AH, Brunette DM: Migration and division of progenitor cell populations in periodontal ligament after wounding, *J Periodont Res* 15:20, 1980.

Gould TRL: Ultrastructural characteristics of progenitor cell populations in the periodontal ligament, *J Dent Res* 62:873, 1983.

Griffin CJ, Harris R: Unmyelinated nerve endings in the periodontal membrane of human teeth, *Arch Oral Biol* 13:1207, 1968.

Hamamoto Y, Nakajima T, Ozawa H: Ultrastructural and histochemical study on the morphogenesis of epthelial rests of Malassez, *Arch Histol Cytol* 52:61, 1989.

Hannam AG: Periodontal mechanoreceptors. In Anderson DJ, Mathews B, (eds): *Mastication*, Bristol UK, 1976, John Wright & Sons.

Hashimoto S, Yamamura T, Shimono M: Morphometric analysis of the intercellular space and desmosomes of rat junctional epithelium, *J Periodont Res* 21:510, 1986.

Hassell TM, Staulk EJ III: Evidence that healthy gingiva contains functionally heterogeneous fibroblast subpopulations, *Arch Oral Biol* 28:617, 1983.

Hill MW, Mackenzie IC: The influence of differing connective tissue substrates on the maintenance of adult stratified squamous epithelia, *Cell Tissue Res* 237:473, 1984.

Johnson RB: A classification of Sharpey's fibres within the alveolar bone of the mouse: a high voltage electron microscope study, *Anat Rec* 217:339, 1987.

Johnson RB, Pylypas SP: A re-evaluation of the distribution of the elastic meshwork within the periodontal ligament of the mouse, *J Periodont Res* 27:239, 1992.

Lambrichts I, Creemers J, van Steenberghe D: Morphology of neural endings in the human periodontal ligament: an electron microscopic study, *J Periodont Res* 27:191, 1992.

Listgarten MA: Normal development, structure, physiology, and repair of gingival epithelium, *Oral Sci Rev* 1:3, 1972.

Listgarten MA: Ultrastructure of the dentogingival junction after gingivectomy, *J Periodont Res* 7:151, 1972.

Löe H: Physiological aspects of the gingival pocket: an experimental study, *Acta Odontol Scand* 19:387, 1961.

Löe H: The structure and physiology of the dentogingival junction. In Miles AEW (ed): *Structural and chemical organization of the teeth*, New York, 1967, Academic Press, Vol 2.

Löe H, Holm-Pedersen P: Absence and presence of fluid from normal and inflamed gingivae, *Periodontics* 3:171, 1965.

Löe H, Karring T: A quantitative analysis of the epithelium-connective tissue interface in relation to assessments of the mitotic index, *J Dent Res* 48:634, 1969.

Mackenzie IC: Nature and mechanisms of regeneration of the junctional epithelium phenotype, *J Periodont Res* 22:243, 1987.

Mackenzie IC, Rittman G, Gao Z, et al: Patterns of cytokeratin expression in human gingival epithelia, *J Periodont Res* 26:468, 1991.

Maeda T, et al: Nerve terminals in human periodontal ligament as demonstrated by immunohistochemistry for neurofilament protein (NFP) and S-100 protein, *Arch Histol Cytol* 53:259, 1990.

Malassez ML: Sur l'existence de masses épithéliales dans le ligament alvéolodentaire (On the existence of epithelial masses in the periodontal membrane), *Comptes Rendus Seances Soc Biol Filiales* 36:241, 1884.

Manson JD: The lamina dura, *Oral Surg Pathol* 16:432, 1963.

Massoth DL, Dale BA: Immunohistochemical study of structural proteins in developing junctional epithelium, *J Periodontol* 57:756, 1986.

McCulloch CAG, Barghava V, Melcher AH: Cell death and the regulation of populations of cells in the periodontal ligament, *Cell Tissue Res* 225:129, 1989.

McCulloch CAG, Bordin S: Role of fibroblast sub-populations in periodontal physiology and pathology, *J Periodont Res* 26:144, 1991.

McDougall WA: Pathways of penetration and effects of horseradish peroxidase in rat molar gingiva, *Arch Oral Biol* 15:621, 1970.

McDougall WA: Penetration pathways of topically applied foreign proteins into rat gingiva, *J Periodont Res* 6:89, 1971.

McHugh WD: The interdental gingivae, *J Periodont Res* 6:227, 1971.

Melcher AH, Bowen WH (eds): *The biology of the periodontium*, New York, 1969, Academic Press.

Melcher AH, Eastoe JE: The connective tissues of the periodontium. In Melcher AH, Bowen WH (eds): *The biology of the periodontium*, New York, 1969, Academic Press.

Minkoff R, Stevens CJ, Karon JM: Autoradiography of protein turnover in subcrestal versus supracrestal fibre tracts of the developing mouse periodontium, *Arch Oral Biol* 26:1069, 1981.

Nakajima T, et al: Fibroblastic cells derived from bovine periodontal ligaments have the phenotypes of osteoblasts, *J Periodont Res* 25:179, 1990.

Nakamura KT, Hanai H, Nakamura MT: Ultrastructure of encapsulated nerve terminalis in human periodontal ligaments, *Jpn J Oral Biol* 24:126, 1982.

Nuki K, Hock J: The organization of the gingival vasculature, *J Periodont Res* 9:305, 1974.

Owings JR: A clinical investigation of the relationship between stippling and surface keratinization of the attached gingiva, *J Periodontol* 40:588, 1969.

Paynter KJ, Pudy G: A study of the structure, chemical nature, and development of cementum in the rat, *Anat Rec* 131:233, 1958.

Picton DCA: On the part played by the socket in tooth support, *Arch Oral Biol* 10:945, 1965.

Picton DCA: Dimensional changes in the periodontal membrane of monkeys, *Arch Oral Biol* 12:1635, 1967.

Pitaru S, Aubin JE, Bhargava U, et al: Immunoelectron microscopic studies on the distribution of fibronectin and actin in a cellular dense connective tissue: the periodontal ligament of the rat, *J Periodont Res* 22:64, 1987.

Quigley MB: Perforating (Sharpey's) fibers of the periodontal ligament and bone, *Alabama J Med Sci* 7:336, 1970.

Ritchey B, Orban B: The crests of the interdental alveolar septa, *J Periodontol* 24:75, 1953.

Romanowski AW, Squier CA, Lesch CA: Permeability of rodent junctional epithelium to exogenous protein, *J Periodont Res*, 23:81, 1988.

Rose GG, Yamasaki A, Pinero GJ, et al: Human periodontal ligament cells in vitro, *J Periodont Res* 22:20, 1987.

Salonen JI, Kautskt MB, Dale BA: Changes in cell phenotype during regeneration of junctional epithelium of human gingiva in vitro, *J Periodont Res,* 24:370, 1980.

Schroeder HE: Extraneous cell surface coat in human inflamed crevicular epithelium, *Helv Odontol Acta* 12:14, April 1968.

Schroeder HE: Ultrastructure of the junctional epithelium of the human gingiva, *Helv Odontol Acta* 13:65, October 1969.

Schroeder HE: Quantitative parameters of early gingival inflammation, *Arch Oral Biol* 15:383, 1970.

Schroeder HE: Transmigration and infiltration of leucocytes in human junctional epithelium, *Helv Odontol Acta* 17:6, April 1973.

Schroeder HE, Listgarten MA: Fine structure of the developing epithelial attachment of human teeth. In Wolsky A (ed): *Monographs in developmental biology,* vol 2, Basel, 1971, S Karger.

Schroeder HE, Münzel-Pedrazzoli S: Morphometric analysis comparing junctional and oral epithelium of normal human gingiva, *Helv Odontol Acta* 14:53, October 1970.

Schroeder HE, Scherle WF: Cemento-enamel junction: revisited, *J Periodont Res* 23:53, 1988.

Schroeder HE, Theilade J: Electron microscopy of normal human gingival epithelium, *J Periodont Res* 1:95, 1966.

Selvig KA: The fine structure of human cementum, *Acta Odontol Scand* 23:423, 1965.

Selvig KA: Current concepts of connective tissue attachment to diseased tooth surfaces, *J Biol Buccale* 11:79, 1983.

Simpson HE: The innervation of the periodontal membrane as observed by the apoxestic technique, *J Periodontol* 37:374, 1966.

Sims MR: Oxytalan fiber system of molars in the mouse mandible, *J Dent Res* 52:797, 1973.

Skougaard M, Beagrie GS: The renewal of gingival epithelium in marmosets *(Calithrix jacchus)* as determined through autoradiography with thymidine-H, *Acta Odontol Scand* 20:467, 1962.

Sodek J: A comparison of the rates of synthesis and turnover of collagen and noncollagen proteins in adult rat periodontal tissues and skin using a microassay, *Arch Oral Biol* 22:655, 1977.

Sodek J, Brunette DM, Feng J, et al: Collagen synthesis as a major component of protein synthesis in the periodontal ligament in various species, *Arch Oral Biol* 22:647, 1977.

Stallard RE, Diab MA, Zander HA: The attaching substance between enamel and epithelium: a product of the epithelial cells, *J Periodontol* 36:130, 1965.

Steffensen B, Lopatin DE, Caffesse RG, Hanks CT: Blood group substances as differentiation markers in human dento-gingival epithelium, *J Periodont Res* 22:451, 1987.

Strahan JD: The relation of the mucogingival junction to the alveolar bone margin, *Dent Pract Dent Rec* 14:72, 1963.

Takata T, Nikai H, Ijuhin N, et al: Ultrastructure of regenerated junctional epithelium after surgery of the rat molar gingiva, *J Periodontol* 57:776, 1986.

Ten Cate AR: The dentogingival junction: an interpretation of the literature, *J Periodontol* 46:475, 1975.

Ten Cate AR, Deporter DA: The role of fibroblast in collagen turnover in the functioning periodontal ligament of the mouse, *Arch Oral Biol* 19:339, 1974.

Valderhaug JP, Nylen MU: Function of epithelial rests as suggested by their ultrastructure, *J Periodont Res* 1:69, 1966.

Van Der Sprenkel H: Microscopical investigation of the innervation of the tooth and its surroundings, *J Anat* 70:233, 1936.

Waerhaug J: The gingival pocket: anatomy, pathology, deepening, and elimination, *Odontol Tidskr* 60(Suppl 1):5, 1952.

Waerhaug J: Effect of C-avitaminosis on the supporting structures of the teeth, *J Periodontol* 29:87, 1958.

Weekes WT, Sims MR: The vasculature of the rat molar gingiva crevice, *J Periodont Res* 21:177, 1986.

Wong RST, Sims M: A scanning electron microscopic, stereo pair study of methacrylate corrosion casts of the mouse palatal and molar periodontal vasculature, *Arch Oral Biol* 32:557, 1987.

Wright DE: The source and rate of entry of leucocytes in the human mouth, *Arch Oral Biol* 9:321, 1964.

Yajima T, Matsuo A, Hirai T: Collagen phagocytosis by cementoblasts at the periodontal ligament-cementum interface, *Arch Histol Cytol* 52:521, 1989.

Yamasaki A, Rose GG, Pinero GJ, et al: Glycogen in human cementoblasts and PDL fibroblasts, *J Periodont Res* 21:128, 1986.

Yamasaki A, et al: Microfilaments in human cementoblasts and periodontal fibroblasts, *J Periodontol* 58:40, 1987.

Zander HA, Hürzeler B: Continuous cementum apposition, *J Dent Res* 37:1035, 1958.

Zwarych PD, Quigley MB: The intermediate plexus of the periodontal ligament: history and further observations, *J Dent Res* 44:383, 1965.

CHAPTER 15

Physiologic Tooth Movement: Eruption and Shedding

THE jaws of an infant can only accommodate a few small teeth. Since teeth, once formed cannot increase in size, the larger jaws of the adult require not only more, but bigger teeth. This accommodation is accomplished in humans by having two dentitions. The first is known as the deciduous or primary dentition, and the second as the permanent or secondary dentition (Figs. 15-1 and 15-2).

The early development of teeth has already been described, and the point has been made that they develop within the tissues of the jaw (Fig. 15-3). Thus for teeth to become functional, considerable movement is required to bring them into the occlusal plane. The movements teeth make are complex and may be described in general terms under the following headings:

1. *Preeruptive tooth movement.* Made by the deciduous and permanent tooth germs within tissues of the jaw before they begin to erupt
2. *Eruptive tooth movement.* Made by a tooth to move from its position within the bone of the jaw to its functional position in occlusion
3. *Posteruptive tooth movement.* Maintaining the position of the erupted tooth in occlusion while the jaws continue to grow and compensate for occlusal and proximal tooth wear

Superimposed on these movements is a progression from primary to permanent dentition, involving the shedding (or exfoliation) of the deciduous dentition.

Although this categorization of tooth movement is convenient for descriptive purposes, it must be recognized that what is being described is a complex series of events occurring in a continuous process. As a result other categorizations exist: for instance, some authors describe tooth movement as having prefunctional and functional phases.

PREERUPTIVE TOOTH MOVEMENT

When the deciduous tooth germs first differentiate, they are extremely small and there is a good deal of space for them in the developing jaw. Because they grow rapidly, however, they become crowded together. This crowding is gradually alleviated by a lengthening of the jaws, which permits the deciduous second molar tooth germs to move backward and the anterior germs to move forward. At the same time the tooth germs are moving bodily outward and upward (or downward, as the case may be) with the increasing length as well as width and height of the jaws.

In Chapter 4 the origin of the successional permanent teeth was described. Recall that those tooth germs develop on the lingual aspect of their deciduous predecessors, in the same bony crypt. From this position they shift considerably as the jaws develop. For example, the incisors and canines eventually come to occupy a position, in their own bony crypts, on the lingual of the roots of their deciduous predecessors, and the premolar tooth germs, also in their own crypts, are finally positioned between the divergent roots of the deciduous molars (Figs. 15-4 and 15-5).

The permanent molar tooth germs, which have no predecessors, develop from the backward extension of the dental lamina (Fig. 4-16). At first there is little room in the jaws to accommodate these tooth germs, so that in the upper jaw the molar tooth germs develop first with their occlusal surfaces facing distally and swing into position only when the maxilla has grown sufficiently to provide room for such movement (Fig. 15-6). In the mandible the permanent molars develop with their axes showing a mesial inclination, which becomes vertical only when sufficient jaw growth has occurred.

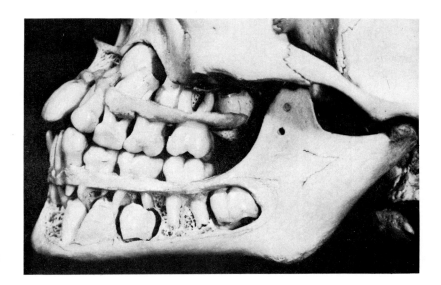

FIG. 15-1 Dried skull of a 7-year-old child. The outer cortical plate has been cut away to show the mixed dentition.

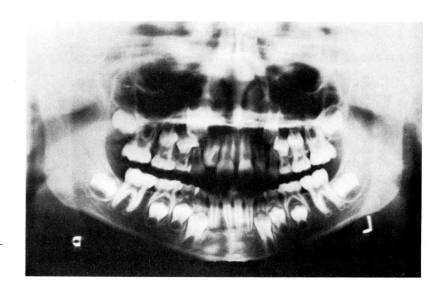

FIG. 15-2 Radiograph of the mixed dentition of a 7-year-old child. (Courtesy Dr. D.W. Stoneman.)

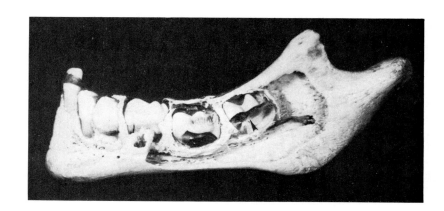

FIG. 15-3 Dried mandible of a 6 month-old child. The teeth occupy most of the body of the mandible. The first deciduous incisor has erupted. Note the amount of crown formation that has occurred in the permanent first molar *(arrow).*

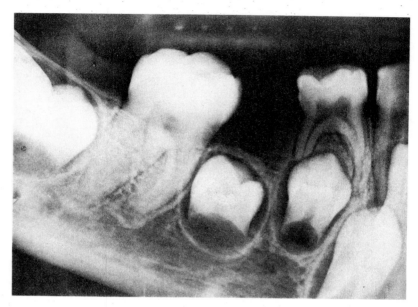

FIG. 15-4 Radiograph of a 7-year-old child. The permanent first premolar is erupting between the divergent roots of the deciduous first molar. The deciduous second molar has been lost early, which could lead to a tipping of the permanent first molar and prevent eruption of the permanent second premolar. (Courtesy Dr. D.W. Stoneman.)

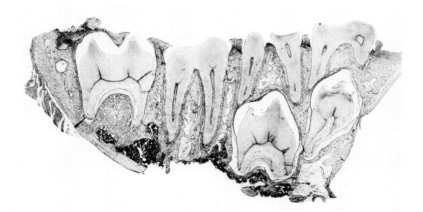

FIG. 15-5 Histologic section through the lower jaw of a monkey at approximately the same dental age as a 7-year-old child. The first premolar has started to erupt, causing resorption of the roots of the deciduous first molar. The second premolar is situated between the roots of the second deciduous molar. The permanent first molar is in function and the permanent second molar is erupting; one cusp tip has pierced the oral mucosa.

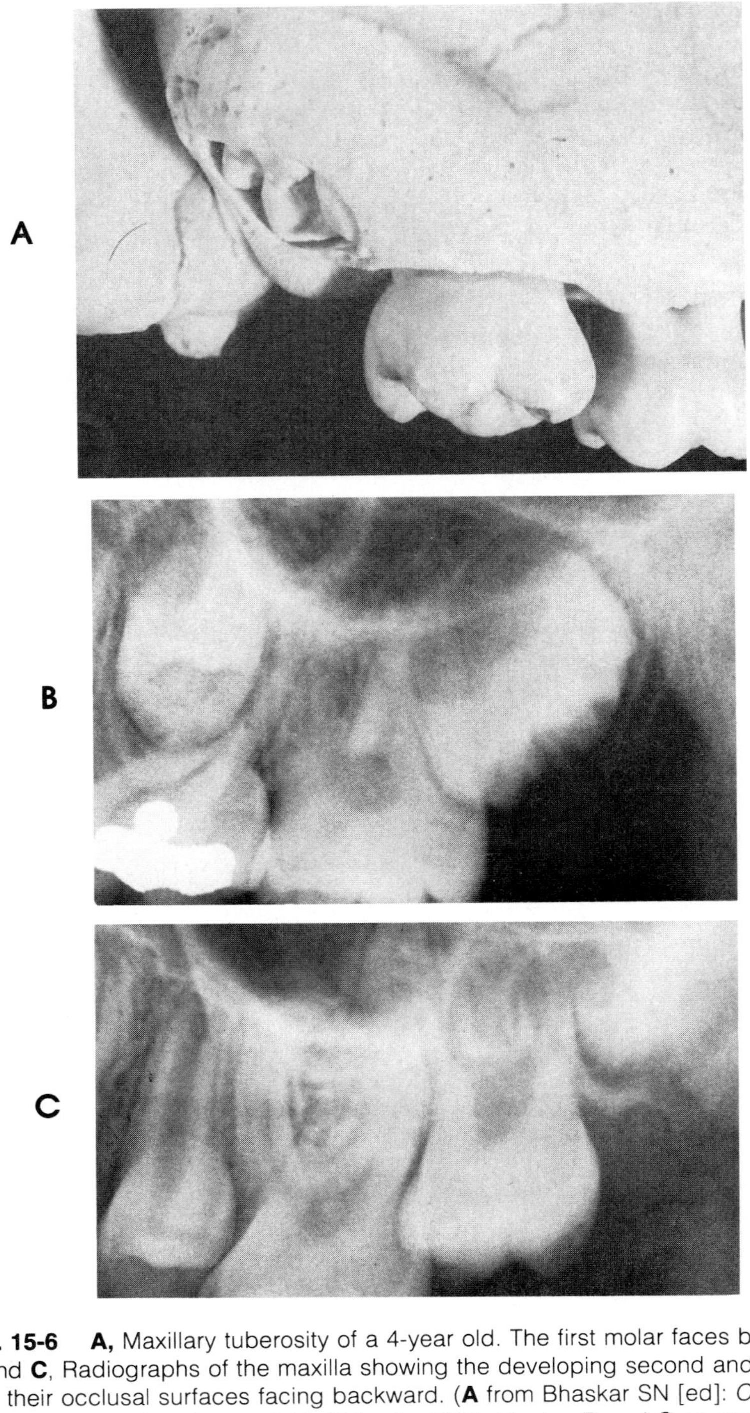

FIG. 15-6 **A,** Maxillary tuberosity of a 4-year old. The first molar faces backward. **B** and **C**, Radiographs of the maxilla showing the developing second and third molars with their occlusal surfaces facing backward. (**A** from Bhaskar SN [ed]: *Orban's Oral histology and embryology,* ed 11, St Louis, 1991, Mosby; **B** and **C** courtesy Dr. D.W. Stoneman.)

These preeruptive movements of both deciduous and permanent tooth germs are best thought of as the means by which the teeth are placed in a position within the jaw for eruptive movement. Analysis has shown that these preeruptive movements of teeth are a combination of two factors. The first is total bodily movement of the tooth germ, and the second is growth in which one part of the tooth germ remains fixed while the rest continues to grow, leading to a change in the center of the tooth germ. This growth explains, for example, how the deciduous incisors maintain their position relative to the oral mucosa as the jaws increase in height.

Preeruptive movements occur in an intraosseous location and are reflected in the patterns of bony remodeling within the crypt wall. For example, during bodily movement in a mesial direction, bone resorption occurs on the mesial surface of the crypt wall and bone deposition occurs on the distal wall as a "filling-in" process (Fig. 15-7). During eccentric growth, only bony resorption occurs, thus altering the shape of the crypt to accommodate the altering shape of the tooth germ. Little if anything is known about the mechanisms that determine preeruptive tooth movements. Whether remodeling of bone to position the bony crypt is important as a mechanism or merely represents an adaptive response is debatable (and will be discussed further when eruptive movement is considered), but the idea that skeletal development determines tooth position has other parallels: thus marrow spaces develop in bones of the appendicular skeleton, and bones grow in length and width by balanced resorption and deposition. As a result, bones can be considered as moving in three-dimensional space.

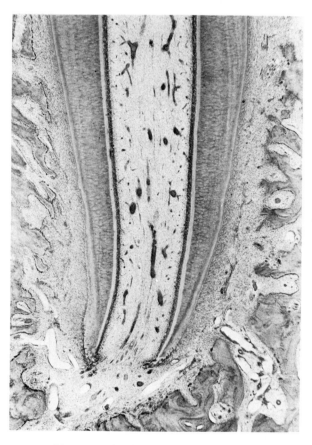

FIG. 15-7 Response of bone to physiologic tooth movement. At left, bone deposition is occurring on the alveolar wall (seen as a continuous row of osteoblasts) whereas on the right resorption is occurring. Resorptive activity is indicated by the many individual osteoclasts (seen as dark spots) on the bone surface. This pattern of bone remodeling is dictated by, and does not cause, tooth movement.

ERUPTIVE TOOTH MOVEMENT

So far as is known, the mechanism of eruption for both deciduous and permanent teeth is similar, bringing about the axial or occlusal movement of the tooth from its developmental position within the jaw to its final functional position in the occlusal plane. The actual eruption of the tooth, when it breaks through the gum, is only one phase of eruption.

Histologic Features

Histologically, many changes occur in association with and for the accommodation of tooth eruption. (Root formation was discussed in Chapter 13, as were the changes occurring in the connective tissues in advance of the erupting tooth.) The periodontal ligament (PDL) develops only after root formation has been initiated; and once established, it must be remodeled to permit continued eruptive tooth movement. The remodeling of PDL fiber bundles is achieved by the fibroblasts, which simultaneously synthesize and degrade the collagen fibrils as required across the entire extent of the ligament (Chapter 5 and Fig. 14-5).

Recall also (from Chapter 6) that the fibroblast has a cytoskeleton, which enables it to contract. This contractility is seen in ligament fibroblasts as well as in fibroblasts of other connective tissues. Ligament fibro-

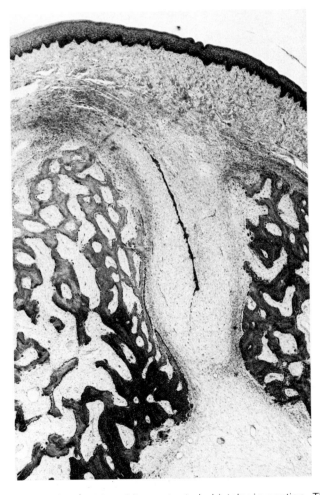

FIG. 15-8 Gubernacular canal and its contents in histologic section. The canal is filled with connective tissue that connects the dental follicle to the lamina propria of the oral epithelium. Strands of epithelial cells, remnants of the dental lamina, often occur.

blasts exhibit numerous (20 to 30 per cell) contacts with each other of the adherens nature and exhibit a close relationship to PDL collagen fiber bundles by means of various transmembrane structures. These combined histologic features provide an explanation for tooth movement (to be discussed later).

The architecture of the tissues in advance of erupting successional teeth differs from that found in advance of deciduous teeth. The fibrocellular follicle surrounding a successional tooth retains its connection with the lamina propria of the oral mucous membrane by means of a strand of fibrous tissue containing remnants of the dental lamina, known as the *gubernacular cord*. In a dried skull holes can be identified in the jaws on the lingual aspects of the deciduous teeth. These holes, which once contained the gubernacular cords, are termed *gubernacular canals* (Figs. 15-8 and 15-9). As the successional tooth erupts, its gubernacular canal is rapidly widened by local osteoclastic activity, delineating the eruptive pathway for the tooth. Interestingly, once the tooth erupts into the oral cavity it continues to erupt at the same rate (about 1 mm every 3 months), slowing only as it meets its antagonist in the opposing arch. This suggests that the resistance to tooth eruption provided by the overlying connective tissue is minimal.

When the erupting tooth appears in the oral cavity, it is subjected to environmental factors that help determine its final position in the dental arch. Muscle forces from the tongue, cheeks, and lips play on the tooth, as do the forces of contact of the erupting tooth with other erupted teeth. A sustained muscular force of only 4 to 5 g is sufficient to move a tooth. The childhood habit of thumb-sucking is an obvious example of environmental determination of tooth position.

Mechanisms of Eruptive Tooth Movement

More is known about the possible mechanisms of eruptive tooth movement than about preeruptive tooth movement. Even so, eruptive mechanisms are not yet fully understood; and most reviews on this subject have concluded that eruption is a multifactorial process in which cause and effect are difficult to separate. Four possible mechanisms are currently favored, although they are not necessarily mutually exclusive: (1) root formation, in which the growing root is accommodated by occlusal movement of the crown; (2) hydrostatic pressure, whereby local increases in tissue fluid pressure in periapical tissues push the tooth occlusally; (3) selective deposition and resorption of bone around the tooth, and (4) a pulling of the tooth into occlusion by the cells or fibers (or both) of the PDL. Others have been proposed but do not warrant serious consideration.

Root formation

Root formation appears to be an obvious cause of tooth eruption, since it undoubtedly causes an overall increase in the length of the tooth that must be accom-

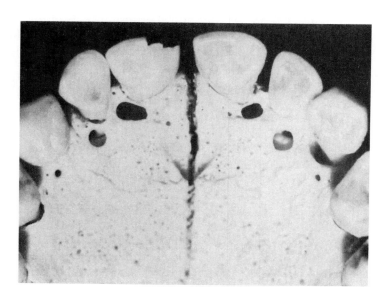

FIG. 15-9   Dried skull. The gubernacular canals are located behind the upper deciduous incisors. (From Bhaskar SN [ed]: *Orban's Oral histology and embryology,* ed 11, St Louis, 1991, Mosby—Year Book.)

modated by the root's growing into the bone of the jaw, by an increase in jaw height, or by the crown's moving occlusally. It is the latter movement, of course, that occurs; but it does not follow that root growth is responsible. Indeed, clinical observation, experimental studies, and histologic analysis argue strongly against such a conclusion. For example, if a continuously erupting tooth (e.g., the rodent incisor or guinea pig molar) is prevented from erupting by being pinned to bone, root growth continues and is accommodated by resorption of some bone at the base of the socket and a buckling of the newly formed root. This experiment yields two conclusions: first, that root growth produces a force; and, second, that this force is sufficient to produce bone resorption. The latter observation is an important aspect of bone biology since it indicates that pressure applied to bone normally results in the removal of bone by osteoclasts. Thus, although it can produce a force, root growth cannot be translated into eruptive tooth movement unless there is some structure at the base of the tooth capable of withstanding this force; and because no such structure exists, some other mechanism must move the tooth to accommodate root growth.

Such a conclusion is further substantiated when it is considered that rootless teeth erupt, that some teeth erupt a greater distance than the total length of their roots, and that teeth will still erupt after the completion of root formation or when the tissues forming the root—the apical papilla, Hertwig's epithelial root sheath, and periapical tissue—are surgically removed.

Hydrostatic pressure

This theory requires a higher pressure system, either within or around the base of the tooth. It is known that teeth move in their sockets in synchrony with the arterial pulse; thus local volume changes can produce limited tooth movement. Ground substance can swell from 30% to 50% by retaining additional water, and the presence of fenestrated capillaries in the PDL suggests a capability for rapid fluid adjustment.

One problem in attempting to link such observations to eruptive tooth movement, however, is to disassociate them from mechanisms required for tooth support. Attempts to establish experimentally a role for vasculature in tooth eruption are further hampered in that such measurements tend to be transient and are made on teeth that have erupted, and often on teeth that erupt continuously. Alterations of the local vascular supply, and in turn tissue fluid pressure, by pharmacologic intervention or by cervical sympathectomy have had far-ranging effects (which could include affecting fibroblast function); but since the surgical excision of a growing root and associated tissues eliminates the periapical vas-

culature without stopping eruption, this means that the local vessels are not absolutely necessary for tooth eruption.

Bony remodeling

Bony remodeling of the jaws has been linked to tooth eruption in that, as in the preeruptive phase, the inherent growth pattern of the mandible or maxilla supposedly moves teeth by the selective deposition and resorption of bone in the immediate neighborhood of the tooth. The strongest evidence in support of bone remodeling as a cause of tooth movement comes from a series of experiments undertaken in dogs: When the developing premolar is removed without disturbing the dental follicle, or if eruption is prevented by wiring the tooth germ down to the lower border of the mandible, an eruptive pathway still forms within the bone overlying the enucleated tooth as osteoclasts widen the gubernacular canal. If the dental follicle is removed, however, no eruptive pathway forms. Furthermore, if the tooth germ is replaced by a metal or silicone replica, and so long as the dental follicle is retained, the replica will erupt, with the formation of an eruptive pathway. These observations need to be analyzed carefully. First, they clearly demonstrate that some "programmed" bony remodeling can and does occur (i.e., an eruptive pathway forms in bone without a developing and growing tooth). Second, they show that the dental follicle is involved but perhaps only indirectly. Osteoclasts are derived from monocytes, and by stripping the follicle they remove the vascular route for these cells to reach the crypt wall. Nor can it be concluded that the demonstration of an eruptive pathway forming within bone means that bony remodeling is responsible for tooth movement, unless it can also be demonstrated that there is coincident bone deposition at the base of the crypt and that the prevention of such bone deposition interferes with tooth eruption. Careful studies using tetracylines as markers of bone deposition have shown that the predominant activity in the fundus of an alveolus in a number of species (including humans) is bone resorption. In humans, for instance, the base of the crypt of the permanent first and third molars continually resorbs as these teeth erupt, although in the second premolar and molar there is some bone deposition on the crypt floor. In the case of the demonstrated eruption of an inert replica, it might be thought that only bony remodeling could bring this about; but, as will be discussed next, there is evidence that follicular tissue is responsible for this movement. The evidence, therefore, sustaining the notion that bone deposition on the crypt floor causes axial tooth movement is insecure and certainly not proven.

What is clear is that the dental follicle is essential to achieving the bony remodeling required to accommodate tooth movement; for it is from this tissue that the osteoblasts differentiate and this is the tissue that permits the conduction of osteoclast precursors, which enable bony remodeling to begin.

Periodontal ligament

Evidence now available strongly indicates that the force for eruptive tooth movement resides in the PDL. It is experimentally possible to disturb the normal architecture of the PDL by interfering with collagen synthesis. This can be done by denying an experimental animal vitamin C, essential for collagen formation (Chapter 5), or by injecting a latharytic agent (which prevents the formation of cross-linkages between aggregating collagen molecules). When either is done, eruptive tooth movement is either slowed or stopped. Furthermore, if a continuously erupting tooth (e.g., the rodent incisor) is cut in half and a barrier placed between the two halves, the distal fragment, which is dissociated from the growing root and the apical vasculature, will still erupt. In this situation the only viable tissue available is the PDL.

Thus the PDL and the dental follicle from which it forms are implicated in the process of tooth eruption; furthermore, there is evidence that the actual force required to move the tooth is linked to the contractility of fibroblasts. In Chapter 5 the structural features associated with the locomotive and contractile properties of fibroblasts were described and it was explained how these properties might be translated into forces acting outside the cell (sailors pulling and climbing ropes). When fibroblasts are plated onto silicone rubber, they crawl about and in so doing create wrinkles or folds in the rubber substrate, indicating that tractional forces are associated with locomotion. A good analogy here is walking in soft sand, where each step demands that the foot dig into the sand, which piles up behind the footprint. Interestingly, when leukocytes, epithelial cells, and fibroblasts are compared in this model system it is the fibroblasts that exert the strongest tractional force. Gingival fibroblasts cultured in this system show relatively little motion, but the degree of wrinkling of the substrate is large, indicating that gingival fibroblasts exert comparatively large and sustained tractional forces. In a similar model system, but using a collagen sheet rather than silicone rubber, PDL fibroblasts have been shown to behave in the same way.

Furthermore, when PDL fibroblasts are embedded in a collagen gel culture they convert the gel into a three-dimensional tissuelike structure in the following way: They adhere to the randomly aligned collagen fibers in the gel and then organize and align the fibers via their cell processes; they then migrate along the aligned fibers, establishing intercellular contacts and junctional complexes with other cells, and then organize themselves into a network exhibiting a three-dimensional tissuelike honeycomb environment. In a model system consisting of a well lined by a perforated mesh (mimicking the cryptal bone) and containing a collagen gel plated with fibroblasts and a slice of root dentin, it has been shown that not only is a three-dimensional network established, with attachment to both the root slice and the mesh, but this network generates sufficient force to raise the root slice from the bottom to the top of the well. Significantly, with this system, it is easy to establish that the cells are responsible for this tractional force since without cells no movement occurs. Furthermore, the use of selective poisons (e.g., colcemid for microtubules, cytochalasin for microfilaments) that disrupt the cell's cytoskeleton and contractility, show a dose-dependent response in relation to the amount of movement achieved. This model system also indicates how the dental follicle can move an inert replica in the experiment referred to earlier.

Thus it is fair to assume that PDL fibroblasts are able to provide a force sufficient to move the tooth, and certainly the proper structural elements exist to translate such force into eruptive tooth movement. The frequent cell-to-cell contacts that occur between PDL fibroblasts permit summation of the contractile forces; a fibronexal connection between the cells and the collagen fiber bundles of the PDL has been demonstrated. For this force to be translated into eruptive tooth movement two further conditions are necessary: (1) the collagen fiber bundles must have an oblique orientation and (2) this orientation must be maintained. Maintenance is achieved by the rapid remodeling of fiber bundles, but how the initial oblique orientation is established is not known. It has been suggested that root formation will create oblique flow lines in a gellike follicle and that the fibroblasts align themselves along these lines.

That the tractional force of fibroblasts is mediated through collagen can be demonstrated by the fact that when the anatomy of the collagen fiber bundles is disrupted experimentally by lathyrogens (which disrupt the formation of cross-linkages between collagen molecules) eruptive movements cease.

In summary: The force moving the tooth is most likely generated by the contractile property of PDL fibroblasts; however, a number of other conditions are needed to translate this contraction into tooth movement—such as root growth and bone and collagen remodeling. Eruption must therefore be considered a multifactorial phenomenon.

POSTERUPTIVE TOOTH MOVEMENT

Posteruptive movements are those made by the tooth after it has reached its functional position in the occlusal plane. They may be divided into three categories: (1) those to accommodate the growing jaws, (2) those to compensate for continued occlusal wear, and (3) those to accommodate interproximal wear.

Accommodation for Growth

Posteruptive movements that accommodate the growth of the jaws are completed toward the end of the second decade, when jaw growth ceases. They are seen histologically as a readjustment of the position of the tooth socket, achieved by the formation of new bone at the alveolar crest and on the socket floor to keep pace with the increasing height of the jaws. Recent studies have shown that this readjustment occurs between the ages of 14 and 18 years, when active movement of the tooth takes place. The apices of the teeth move 2 to 3 mm away from the inferior dental canal (regarded as a relatively fixed reference point). This movement occurs earlier in girls than in boys and is related to the burst of condylar growth that separates the jaws and teeth, permitting further eruptive movement.

Although such movement is seen as remodeling of the socket, it must not be assumed to bring about tooth movement. The same arguments that applied to bony remodeling for preeruptive and eruptive tooth movement apply here.

Compensation for Occlusal Wear

The axial movement that a tooth makes to compensate for occlusal wear is most likely achieved by the same mechanism as eruptive tooth movement. Note that these axial posteruptive movements are made when the apices of the permanent lower molars are fully formed and the apices of the second premolar and molar are almost complete, which indicates again that root growth is not the factor responsible for axial eruptive tooth movement and further emphasizes the role of the PDL. It is often stated that compensation for occlusal wear is achieved by continued cementum deposition around the apex of the tooth; however, the deposition of cementum in this location occurs only after the tooth has moved.

Accommodation for Interproximal Wear

Wear also occurs at the contact points between teeth, on their proximal surfaces; and its extent can be considerable (more than 7 mm in the mandible). This interproximal wear is compensated for by a process known as mesial or approximal drift. Mesial drift and an understanding of its probable causes are important to the practice of orthodontics, since the maintenance of tooth position after treatment depends on the extent of such drift. The forces bringing about mesial drift are multifactorial and include (1) an anterior component of occlusal force, (2) soft tissue pressure, and (3) contraction of the transseptal ligament between teeth.

Anterior component of occlusal force

When teeth are brought into contact (e.g., in clenching the jaws), an anteriorly directed force is generated. That this is so can be easily demonstrated by placing a steel strip between teeth and showing that more force is required to remove it when the jaws are clenched. This anterior force is the result of (1) the mesial inclination of most teeth and (2) the summation of intercuspal planes (producing a forward-directed force). In the case of incisors, which are inclined labially, it would be expected that any anterior component of force would move them in the same direction. In fact, incisors move mesially; but this can be explained by the billiard ball analogy (Fig. 15-10): when cusps are selectively ground, the direction of occlusal force can be either enhanced or reversed. Paradoxically, one experiment designed to demonstrate this anterior component of force also showed that other factors are involved. When opposing teeth were removed, thereby eliminating the biting force, the mesial migration of teeth was slowed but not halted, indicating the presence of some other force; and here the transseptal fibers of the PDL have been implicated.

Contraction of the transseptal ligament

The PDL plays an important role in maintaining tooth position. The suggestion has been made that its transseptal fibers (running between adjacent teeth across the alveolar process) draw neighboring teeth together and maintain them in contact; and there is some evidence to support this. For example, it is known that relapse of orthodontically moved teeth is much reduced if a gingivectomy removing the transseptal ligament is performed. It has also been demonstrated experimentally that in bisected teeth the two halves separate from each other but, if the transseptal ligaments are previously cut, this separation does not occur. Furthermore, remodeling by collagen phagocytosis has been demonstrated in the transseptal ligament, with the rate of turnover increasing during orthodontic tooth movement; however, this only shows that the transseptal ligament is capable of adaptation. A simple and elegant experiment indicates that the cause of mesial drift is multifactorial: by disking away proximal contacts, researchers can provide room for a tooth to move; and when this is done, teeth move to reestablish contact. If teeth are also ground out of occlusion and their proximal surfaces are disked, the rate of drift is slowed. Until the contrary has been demonstrated, it must be assumed that mesial drift is achieved by a contractile mechanism associated with the transseptal ligament fibers and enhanced by occlusal forces.

Soft tissue pressures

The pressures generated by the cheeks and tongue may push teeth mesially. When such pressures are eliminated, however, by constructing an acrylic dome over the teeth, mesial drift still occurs, which suggests that soft tissue pressure does not play a major role (if any) in creating mesial drift. Nevertheless, soft tissue pressure does influence tooth position, even if it does not cause tooth movement.

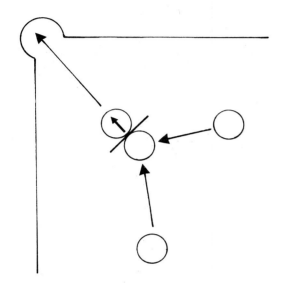

A

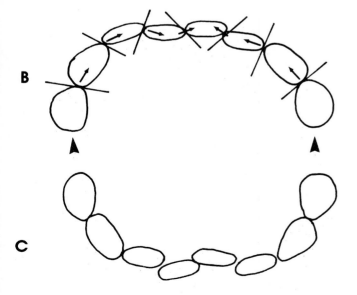

B

C

FIG. 15-10 Billiard ball analogy. **A,** If the two touching balls are in line with the pocket, no matter how the first ball is struck the second will enter the pocket since it travels at right angles to the common tangent between the two balls. **B,** In a young dentition the large arrows indicate the anterior component of force, which drives the first premolars against the canines. Following the example of the billiard balls, the canines and incisors all move in directions at right angles to the common tangents drawn through the contact points. This leads to the imbrication often found in older dentitions, **C.** (From a discussion by J. Osborn. In Poole DFG, Stack MV [eds]: *The eruption and occlusion of teeth. Colston Papers, No. 27,* London, 1976, Butterworths.)

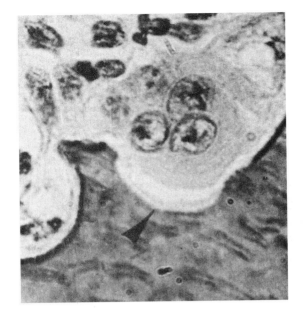

FIG. 15-11 Light microscopic appearance of the odontoclast. Note that it exactly resembles the osteoclast. Its large size, multinucleate appearance, and brush border can all be seen. (From Bhaskar SN [ed]: *Orban's Oral histology and embryology,* ed 11, St Louis, 1991, Mosby.)

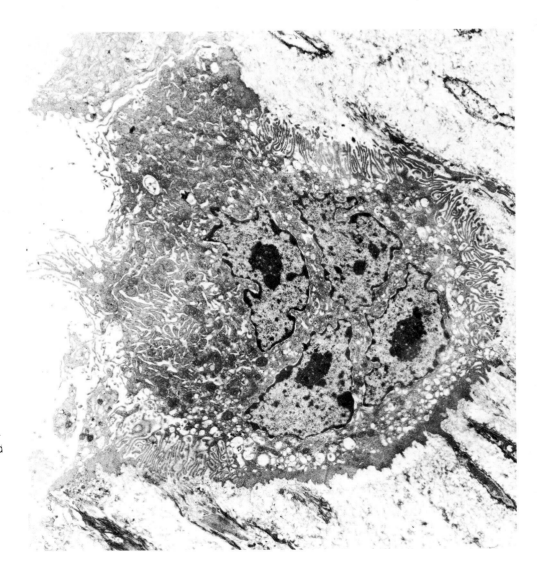

FIG. 15-12 Fine structure of the odontoclast. This cell is resorbing dentin, and extensions extend into the dentinal tubules. The ruffled or brush border can be seen, as can the multinucleated character of the cell. (From Freulich LS: *J Dent Res* 50:1047, 1971.)

SHEDDING OF TEETH

The eruptive pathway of permanent teeth is related to the shedding (or exfoliation) of deciduous teeth as pressure from the erupting successional tooth helps to determine the pattern of deciduous tooth resorption.

Odontoclasts

At all sites where successional teeth contact their deciduous predecessors, local resorption of the deciduous tooth occurs (Figs. 15-4 and 15-5). The resorption of hard tissues of the deciduous tooth is achieved by cells with a histology identical to that of osteoclasts; but because of their involvement in the removal of dental tissue, they are called odontoclasts (Figs. 15-11 and 15-12).

The odontoclast is capable of resorbing all dental hard tissues, including enamel. It is most commonly found on the surface of roots, however, where it resorbs cementum and dentin. It is also found, on occasion, within the pulp chamber, resorbing coronal dentin. This variation depends very much on the position of the successional tooth in relation to the deciduous tooth. Thus since the permanent incisors and canines develop lingually to the deciduous teeth and erupt in an occlusal and vestibular direction, resorption of their roots occurs at the lingual surface of the root and they are shed with much of their pulp chamber intact (Figs. 15-13 and 15-14). Permanent premolars develop between the divergent roots of deciduous molars and erupt in an occlusal

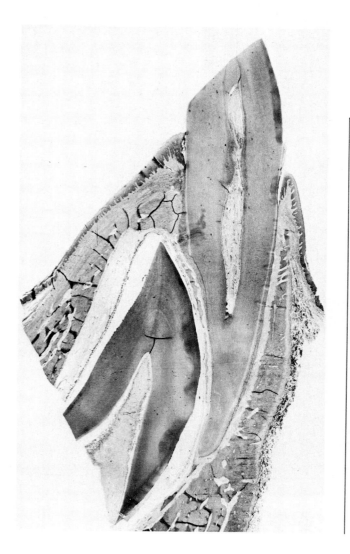

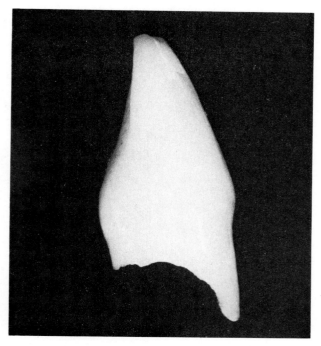

FIG. 15-13 Photomicrograph of the relative positions of deciduous and permanent canines. Resorption occurs on the lingual aspect of the deciduous canine, and the tooth is often shed with much of its lingual root intact.

FIG. 15-14 Exfoliated deciduous canine. This tooth is shed with a considerable portion of its root remaining on the buccal aspect.

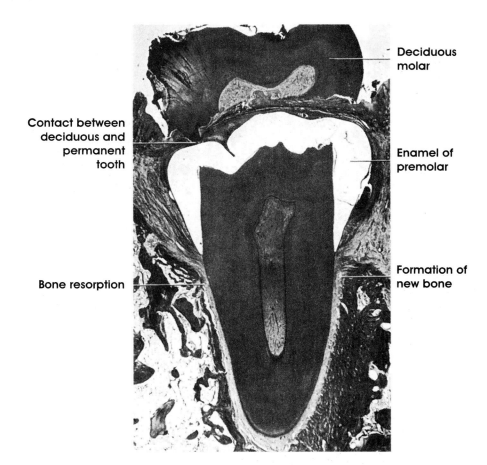

Deciduous molar

Contact between deciduous and permanent tooth

Enamel of premolar

Bone resorption

Formation of new bone

FIG. 15-15 Roots of a primary molar completely resorbed. Dentin is in contact with the premolar enamel. (Courtesy Dr. E.A. Grimmer.)

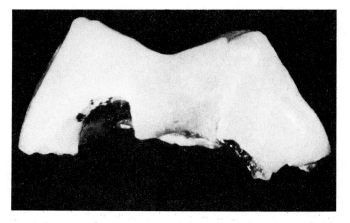

FIG. 15-16 Exfoliated deciduous molar. The roots have been completely lost, and erosion of the enamel has occurred.

direction. Hence the resorption of interradicular dentin occurs with resorption of the pulp chamber and coronal dentin (Figs. 15-15 and 15-16).

Although little is known about the resorption of dental hard tissues, even less is known about resorption of the soft tissues associated with them—the dental pulp and the PDL.

Simple observation of histologic sections shows that the loss of PDL fibers is abrupt (Fig. 15-17). Electron microscopic investigation confirms this finding and also shows that all death in this region occurs without inflammation. Cell death assumes at least two forms. In one instance (Fig. 15-18) the fibroblasts accumulate intracellular collagen, which suggests interference with normal collagen secretory mechanisms. In the other, ligament fibroblasts exhibit morphologic features characteristic of apoptotic cell death (Fig. 15-19). Apoptosis

has been well described and involves "condensation" of the cell with its ultimate phagocytosis by neighboring macrophages or undamaged fibroblasts. It is known to be an important feature of normal embryonic development where cell deletion is important; for example, it is a feature in palatal closure, assisting in the removal of epithelium to permit shelf fusion (Chapter 2). Furthermore, it is now recognized to be programmed; that is, in embryogenesis cells die at specific times during development to permit orderly morphogenesis. The finding of apoptotic cell death in the resorbing PDL suggests that shedding of teeth also is a programmed event. Support for this conclusion is obtained from the study of tooth eruption in monozygotic twins, which indicates that it is mostly determined (80%) by genetic factors (with the remaining determinants local).

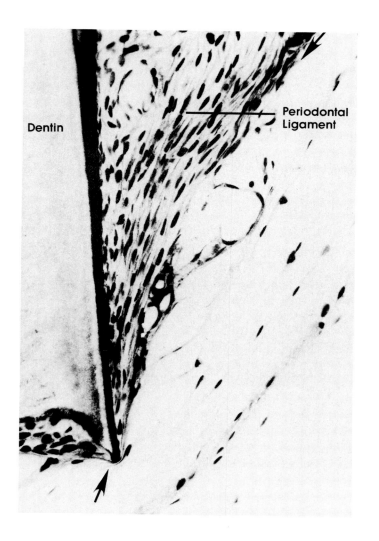

Dentin

Periodontal Ligament

FIG. 15-17 Photomicrograph showing the abrupt loss of periodontal ligament *(between arrows)* in a shedding tooth.

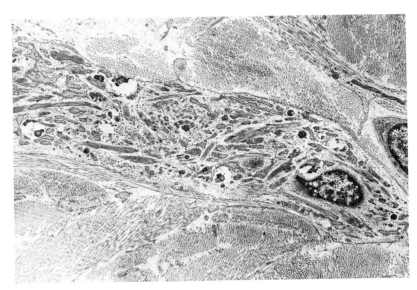

FIG. 15-18 Electron micrograph of a PDL fibroblast just preceding the front shown in Figure 15-16. Its cytoplasm is filled with collagen.

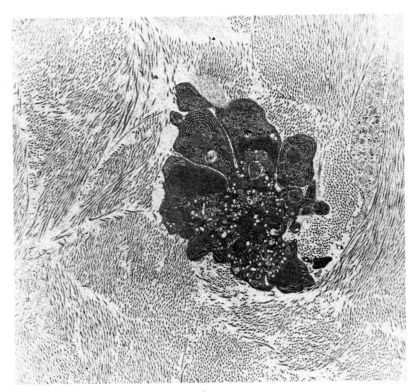

FIG. 15-19 A degenerated fibroblast in the PDL preceding the front illustrated in Figure 15-16. This appearance is characteristic of physiologic cell death.

Pressure

Obviously, pressure from the erupting successional tooth plays a role in shedding of the deciduous dentition. For instance, if a successional tooth germ is congenitally missing or occupies an aberrant position in the jaw, shedding of the deciduous tooth will be delayed. Yet the tooth is eventually shed. The suggestion has also been made that increased force applied to a deciduous tooth can initiate its resorption. Growth of the face and jaws and the corresponding enlargement in size and strength of the muscles of mastication probably increase the forces applied to the deciduous teeth so that the tooth's supporting apparatus is damaged, in particular the PDL, and tooth resorption is initiated (Fig. 15-20).

In fact, the superimposition of both local pressure and masticatory forces on physiologic tooth resorption is likely to determine the pattern and rate of deciduous tooth shedding. Pressure from an erupting permanent tooth results in some root loss, which in turn means that there is a loss of supporting tissue. As the tooth's support diminishes, it is less able to withstand the increasing masticatory forces and thus the process of exfoliation is accelerated.

Pattern of Shedding

In a large population of North American whites it has been shown that the pattern of exfoliation is symmetric for the right and left sides of the mouth. Except for second molars, the mandibular primary teeth are shed before their maxillary counterparts. The exfoliation of all four secondary primary molars is practically simultaneous. Girls exfoliate before boys do. The greatest discrepancy between the sexes is observed for the mandibular canines, the least for the maxillary central incisors. The sequence of shedding in the mandible follows the anterior to posterior order of the teeth in that jaw. In the maxilla this sequence is disrupted by the first molar exfoliating before the canine.

In summary then (Fig. 15-21): Physiologic tooth movement is a complex process. Cells of the PDL can generate forces sufficient to move teeth, but the successful transfer of these to eruption demands that a number of other related events take place involving bone remodeling and connective tissue removal. Failure of such events to proceed properly delays or prevents eruption. Although it might be considered that the force for eruptive tooth movement has been identified, the controlling mechanisms certainly have not. The consistency of eruption dates for the human dentition is really quite remarkable (the so-called 6-year molars as a descriptor for the permanent first molars testifying to this) and surely indicates the involvement of programmed development.

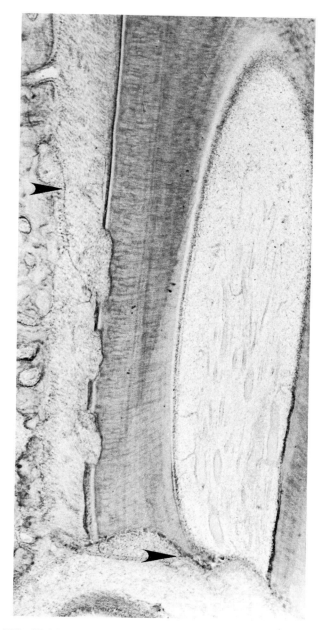

FIG. 15-20 Photomicrograph of the histology of root resorption. At the apex *(arrow)* resorption is occurring, and as a consequence changes are seen in the PDL as this structure becomes less able to cope with the forces applied to it. The downward and oblique orientation of the ligament fibers is progressively lost *(arrow)* and local pockets of cementum resorption occur.

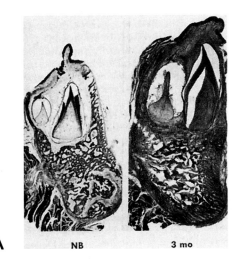

A   NB   3 mo

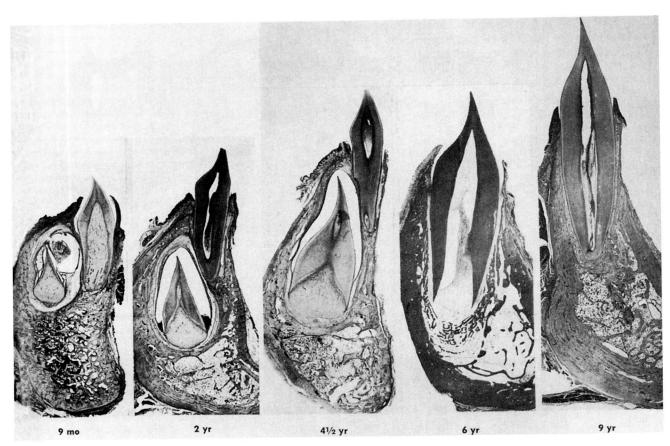

9 mo   2 yr   4½ yr   6 yr   9 yr

FIG. 15-21   Summary of preeruptive and eruptive tooth movement, including the pattern of tooth resorption. **A,** Buccolingual sections through the central incisor region of the mandible at representative stages of development from birth to 9 years of age. At birth both the deciduous and the permanent tooth germ occupy the same bony crypt. Note how, by eccentric growth and eruption of the deciduous tooth, the permanent tooth germ comes to occupy its own bony crypt apical to the erupted incisor. At 4½ years resorption of the deciduous incisor has begun. At 6 years the deciduous incisor has been shed and its successor is erupting. Note the active deposition of new bone at the base of the socket. **B,** Buccolingual sections through the deciduous first molar and permanent first premolar of the mandible at representative stages of development from birth to 14 years. Note how the permanent tooth germ shifts its position. In the section of a 4½- year-old mandible the gubernacular canal is clearly visible. Lack of roots in the 2-, 3-, 4½-, and 11-year sections is the result not of resorption but of the section's having been cut in the midline of a tooth with widely diverging roots. (From Bhaskar SN [ed]: *Orban's Oral histology and embryology,* ed 11, St Louis, 1991, Mosby.)

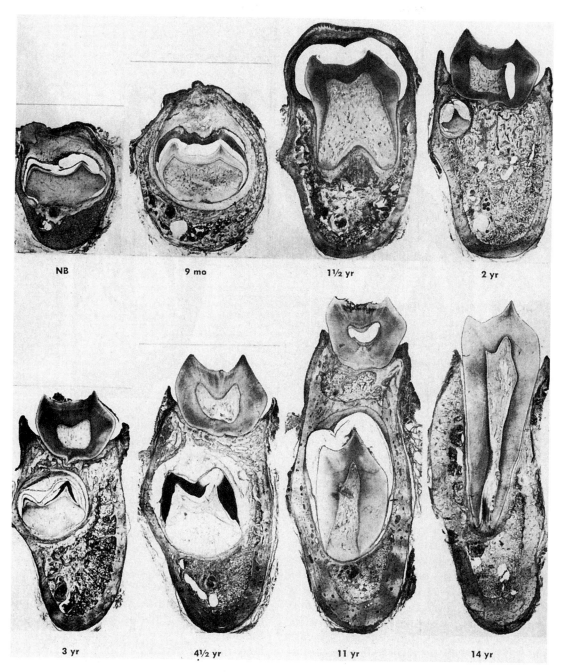

NB   9 mo   1½ yr   2 yr

3 yr   4½ yr   11 yr   14 yr

B

FIG. 15-21 *cont'd.*   For legend, see opposite page.

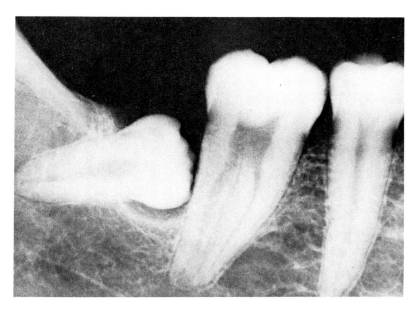

FIG. 15-22 Radiograph of a horizontally impacted mandibular third molar. (Courtesy Dr. D.W. Stoneman.)

ABNORMAL TOOTH MOVEMENT

Obviously, the steps leading to the development of the final permanent dentition are complex, requiring a balance among tooth formation, jaw growth, and the maintenance of function. Not surprisingly, disturbances in this process often indicate some local or systemic abnormality, and thus the pattern of tooth formation and eruption are of considerable diagnostic significance. In fact, the normal pattern is so remarkably consistent that permanent first molars (as just mentioned) often are referred to as 6-year molars because of their predictable time of eruption.

For teeth to erupt earlier than normal is unusual. Sometimes babies are born with a central incisor already erupted, but this represents abnormal dental development and the tooth is extracted to permit suckling. The premature loss of a deciduous tooth will occasionally lead to early eruption of its permanent successor. Delayed eruption of teeth is far more common and may be caused by congenital, systemic, or local factors (with local factors predominating). Congenital absence of teeth most commonly occurs with the permanent third molars. Systemic factors involving delays in tooth eruption may be caused by endocrine deficiencies, nutritional deficiencies, and some genetic factors mentioned in Chapter 1. If teeth have not appeared in an infant during the first year, some underlying cause must be sought. Any systemic lesion delaying eruption of the permanent teeth has usually been identified before the sixth year, when the permanent first molars erupt.

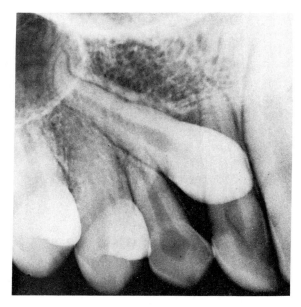

FIG. 15-23 Radiograph of an impacted maxillary canine. (Courtesy Dr. D.W. Stoneman.)

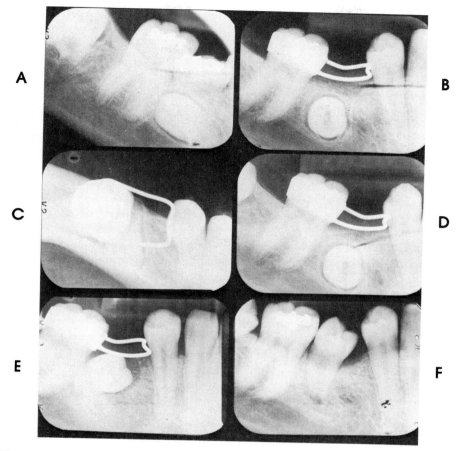

FIG. 15-24   Series of radiographs illustrating an instance of unusual tooth movement. **A,** The permanent second premolar is buried beneath the deciduous second molar. **B,** The deciduous molar has been extracted and a space maintainer inserted to prevent tilting and drift of the permanent first molar. **C** is the same as **B** but seen from above. The premolar has shifted and now occupies a buccolingual position. **E** and **F** show the same tooth erupting and erupted 4 and 5 years later. (Courtesy Dr. F. Pulver.)

Local factors preventing tooth eruption are many. Examples are early loss of a deciduous tooth, with consequent drifting of the adjacent teeth to block the eruptive pathway (Fig. 15-4), and eruption cysts (derived from the dental lamina). Crowding of teeth in small jaws often provides little room for eruption, with consequent impaction of the teeth (Fig. 15-22). The third molars are particularly prone to impaction since they erupt last, when the least room is available. The upper canine is also frequently impacted because of its late eruption (Fig. 15-23). Although much is known about tooth movement and positioning, at times some clinical conditions occur that cannot be explained. Figure 15-24 illustrates just such a case. A tooth has developed in an abnormal location and is lying parallel to the lower border of the mandible. The clinical treatment in this instance was simply to provide room for the tooth to erupt by extraction of the overlying tooth. When this was done, the horizontally inclined tooth righted itself and erupted with no further clinical interference. In this instance the roots of the tooth were fully formed; it is difficult to explain how the periodontal tissues knew the direction in which to move it!

ORTHODONTIC TOOTH MOVEMENT

From this chapter and from Chapter 14, it should be clear that the supporting tissues of the tooth (i.e., the PDL and alveolar bone) have a remarkable plasticity that permits physiologic tooth movement and accommodates to the constant minor movements that the tooth makes during mastication. It is this plasticity of the tooth's supporting tissues that permits orthodontic tooth movement.

Theoretically, it should be possible to bring about tooth movement without any tissue damage by using a light force, equivalent to the physiologic forces determining tooth position, to capitalize on the plasticity of the supporting tissues. It is easy to describe the changes that happen under these circumstances. There will be differentiation of osteoclasts, which will resorb bone of the socket wall on the pressure side. At the same time there will be remodeling of collagen fibers in the PDL to accommodate the new tooth position. On the tension side remodeling of collagen fiber bundles will also occur, but in association with bone deposition on the socket wall. No changes will occur in tooth structure (e. g., in the cementum). Whether current orthodontic techniques duplicate this ideal situation is doubtful; most involve some degree of tissue damage that varies because the forces applied to move the tooth are not equally distributed throughout the PDL.

It is worthwhile to analyze the tissue reactions in terms of a graph illustrating the typical pattern of orthodontic tooth movement (Fig. 15-25). An applied force results in immediate movement of the tooth. This in turn leads to areas of tension and compression within the PDL, resulting in changes within the bone and ligament. Unlike physiologic tooth movement, in which bone resorption of the alveolar wall occurs on its PDL aspect, orthodontic tooth movement causes some in-

ternal or undermining resorption, in which alveolar bone is remodeled from its endosteal face (Fig. 15-26).

This difference in resorption is caused by changes within the PDL resulting from compression. The ligament undergoes *hyalinization*, a light microscopic term describing the loss of cells from an area of ligament because of trauma. Obviously, if no cells are present, no bony remodeling can occur. During the period when hyalinization is present, tooth movement ceases. Only when the hyalinized portion of the ligament is repopulated by new cells, and the bone removed by osteoclasts on the endosteal surface, does tooth movement begin again. This movement coincides with the active remodeling of ligament collagen by the newly arrived fibroblasts and the deposition of new bone. Obviously, heavier forces cause larger areas of hyalinization, a longer period of repair, and slower tooth movement.

In Chapter 14 the point was made that orthodontic tooth movement is possible because of the greater resistance of cementum than bone to resorption. This is certainly true, for if both tissues were resorbed with equal facility root loss would follow orthodontic movement; however, even when radiographs show no visible changes in the root surface, it is now appreciated that most teeth moved orthodontically undergo some minor degree of root resorption (Fig. 15-27) followed by repair. This resorption is seen as small lacunae, created by odontoclasts, that are rapidly repaired by the formation of new cementum (Fig. 15-28). Because cementum is more resistant than bone to resorption, clinically demonstrable resorption usually occurs only after the application of heavy force and the movement of teeth for periods longer than 30 days.

In addition to changes within the periodontium, tooth movement demands remodeling of the adjacent

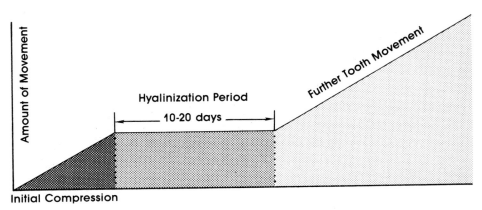

FIG. 15-25 Orthodontic tooth movement over time.

gingival tissues (of which little is known) and some adaptation of pulpal tissue. Too rapid movement can lead to damage of the vessels supplying the pulp, resulting in eventual pulp necrosis, especially when the tooth is tilted too far. It is known that an interrupted force of some magnitude has little effect on the pulp, which is why removable appliances cause little, if any, pulp damage. With a fixed appliance providing a continuous force, some pulp damage usually occurs; but because young pulp is usually involved and the forces are moderate, repair follows.

The development of a functional dentition, from its inception through the deciduous to the permanent dentition, has been fully described. Many of the key events in the process, for both dentitions, are summarized in Figs. 15-29 and 15-30.

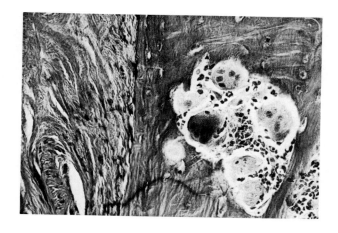

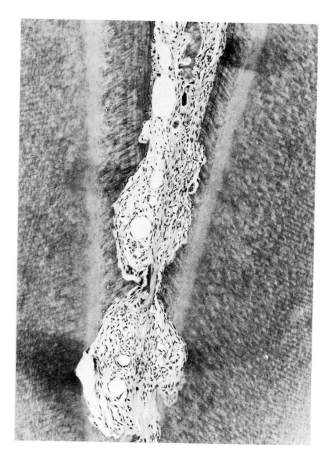

FIG. 15-26 Undermining resorption of alveolar bone 7 days after the beginning of tooth movement with a light tipping force. (From Buck DL, Church DH: *Am J Orthod* 62:507, 1972.)

FIG. 15-27 Photomicrograph of the response of supporting tissues when the roots of teeth come into contact. The two teeth are tipping into contact as a consequence of malocclusion, but the same picture can be created by excessive orthodontic force. The interdental septum has been almost totally lost and the root surfaces are now resorbing. Repair of these resorption bays is possible if the drifting ceases.

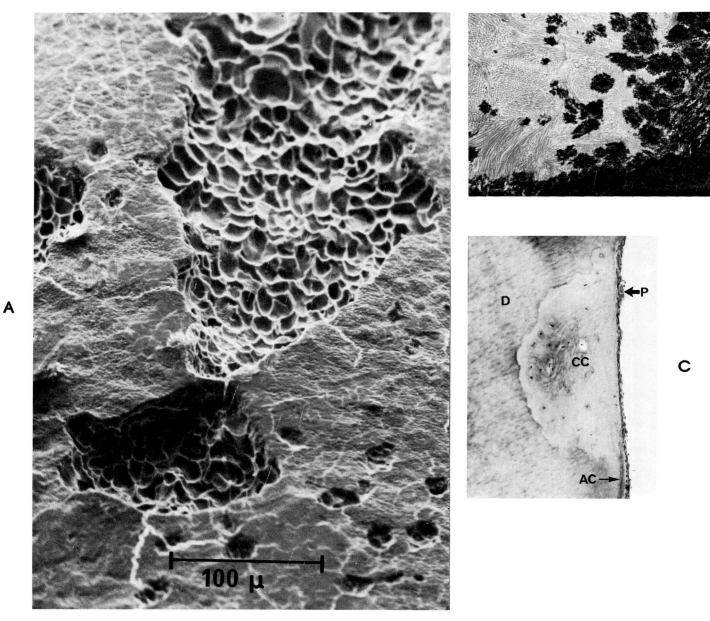

FIG. 15-28 Resorption and repair of the root surface. **A** is a scanning electron micrograph of the root surface of a tooth used as an anchor for rapid maxillary expansion showing resorption bays on the root surface. **B** illustrates repair of a cementum resorption bay seen through the electron microscope. Foci of mineralization occur in the collagenous *(scar)* tissue. **C** is a light microscope picture of completed root surface repair. *D*, dentin; *CC*, cellular cementum; *AC*, acellular cementum; *P*, periodontal ligament. (**A** from Barber AF, Sims MR: *Am J Orthod* 79:630, 1981; **B** from Furseth R: *Arch Oral Biol* 13:417, 1968; **C** from Langford SR, Sims MR: *Am J Orthod* 81:108, 1982.)

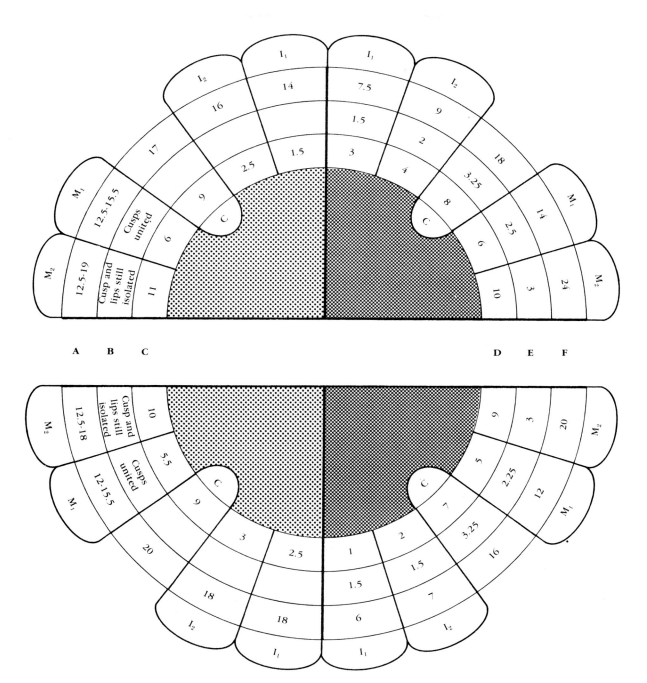

FIG. 15-29 Chronology of the human primary dentition. **A,** Mineralization begins (weeks in utero). **B,** Amount of enamel matrix found at birth. **C,** Enamel complete (months). **D,** Eruption sequence. **E,** Root completed (years). **F,** Emergence into the oral cavity (months).

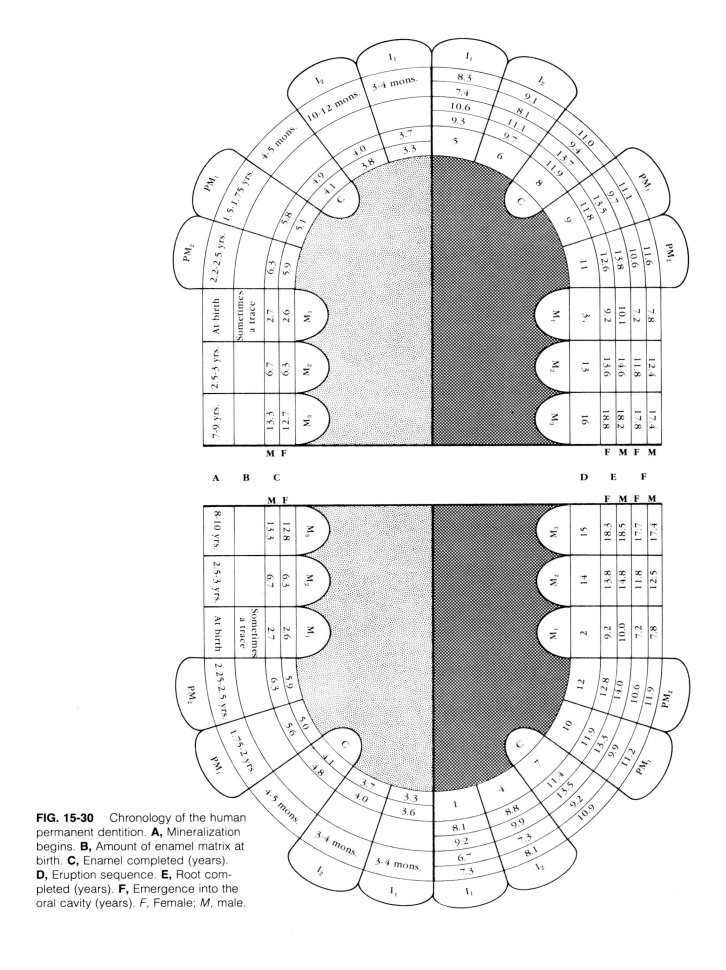

FIG. 15-30 Chronology of the human permanent dentition. **A,** Mineralization begins. **B,** Amount of enamel matrix at birth. **C,** Enamel completed (years). **D,** Eruption sequence. **E,** Root completed (years). **F,** Emergence into the oral cavity (years). *F,* Female; *M,* male.

BIBLIOGRAPHY

Aubin J, Opas M: Cell adhesion and motility. In Davidovitch Z (ed): *The biological mechanisms of tooth eruption and root resorption*, Birmingham Ala, 1988, EBSCO Media.

Beertsen W, Everts V, Van Der Hoff A: Fine structure of fibroblasts in the periodontal ligament of the rat incisor and their role in tooth eruption, *Arch Oral Biol* 16:1033, 1971.

Bellows CG, Melcher AH, Aubin JE: An in-vitro model for tooth eruption utilizing periodontal ligament fibroblasts and collagen lattices, *Arch Oral Biol* 28:715, 1983.

Berkovitz BKB: The effect of root transection and partial root resection on the unimpeded eruption rate of the rat incisor, *Arch Oral Biol* 16:1033, 1971.

Berkovitz BKB: The healing process in the incisor tooth socket of the rat following root resection and exfoliation, *Arch Oral Biol* 16:1045, 1971.

Berkovitz BKB: The effect of preventing eruption on the proliferative basal tissues of the rat lower incisor, *Arch Oral Biol* 17:1279, 1972.

Berkovitz BKB: Mechanisms of tooth eruption. In Lavelle CLB (ed): *Applied physiology of the mouth*, Bristol UK, 1975, John Wright & Sons.

Berkovitz BKB, Thomas NR: Unimpeded eruption in the root resected lower incisor of the rat with a preliminary note on root transection, *Arch Oral Biol* 14:771, 1969.

Bien SM: Fluid dynamic mechanisms which regulate tooth movement. In Staples PH (ed): *Advances in oral biology*, New York, 1966, Academic Press, vol 2.

Björk AE, Skieller V: Facial development and tooth eruption: an implant study at the age of puberty, *Am J Orthod* 62:339, 1972.

Boese LR: Increased stability of orthodontically rotated teeth following gingivectomy in *Macaca nemestrina, Am J Orthod* 56:273, 1969.

Boyde A, Lester KS: Electron microscopy of resorbing surfaces of dental hard tissues, *Z Zellforsch Anat* 83:538, 1967.

Brash JC: The growth of the alveolar bone and its relation to the movements of the teeth, including eruption, *Dent Rec* 46:641, 47:1, 175, 1926.

Brash JC: The growth of the alveolar bone and its relation to the movements of the teeth, including eruption, *Int J Orthod Oral Surg Radiogr* 14:196, 283, 398, 487, 494, 1928.

Brash JC: Comparative anatomy of tooth movement during growth of the jaws, *Dent Rec* 73:460, 1953.

Brodie AG: The growth of alveolar bone and the eruption of the teeth, *Oral Surg* 1:342, 1948.

Bryer LW: An experimental evaluation of physiology of tooth eruption, *Int Dent J* 7:432, 1957.

Burke PH: Eruptive movements of permanent maxillary central incisor teeth in the human, *Proc R Soc Med* 56:513, 1963.

Burn-Murdoch RA: The effect of applied forces on the eruption of rat maxillary incisors, *Arch Oral Biol* 26:939, 1981.

Cahill DR: Eruption pathway formation in the presence of experimental tooth impaction in puppies, *Anat Rec* 164:67-78, 1969.

Cahill DR: The histology and rate of tooth eruption with and without temporary impaction in the dog, *Anat Rec* 166:225, 1970.

Cahill DR: Histological changes in the bony crypt and gubernacular canal of erupting permanent premolars during deciduous premolar exfoliation in beagles, *J Dent Res* 53:786, 1974.

Cahill DR, Marks SC Jr: Tooth eruption: evidence for the central role of the dental follicle, *J Oral Pathol* 189:200, 1982.

Cahill DR, Marks SC Jr, Wise GE, Gorski JP: A review and comparison of tooth eruption systems used in experimentation: a new proposal on tooth eruption. In Davidovitch Z (ed): *Biological mechanisms of tooth eruption and root resorption*, Birmingham Ala, 1988, EBSCO Media.

Carlson H: Studies in the role and amount of eruption in certain human teeth, *Am J Orthod* 30:575, 1944.

Carollo DA, Hoffman RL, Brodie AG: Histology and function of the dental gubernacular cord, *Angle Orthod* 41:300, 1971.

Constant TE: The eruption of the teeth, *Int Dent Congr* 2:180, 1900.

Donohue WB, Perreault JG: The effect of x-ray irradiation on the growth of the teeth and jaws in kittens, *Arch Oral Biol* 9:739, 1964.

Edwards JG: A surgical procedure to eliminate rotational relapse, *Am J Orthod* 57:35, 1970.

Enlow DH, McNamara JA Jr: Varieties of in vivo tooth movements, *Angle Orthod* 43:256, 1973.

Freilich LS: Ultrastructure and acid phosphatase cytochemistry of odontoclasts: effect of parathyroid extract, *J Dent Res* 50:1047, 1971.

Furseth R: The resorption processes of human deciduous teeth studied by light microscopy, microradiography, and electron microscopy, *Arch Oral Biol* 13:417, 1968.

Garant PR, Moon IC, Cullen MR: Attachment of periodontal ligament fibroblasts to the extracellular matrix in the squirrel monkey, *J Periodont Res* 17:70, 1982.

Gowgiel JM: Eruption of irradiation-produced rootless teeth in monkeys, *J Dent Res* 40:538, 1961.

Gowgiel JM: Observations on the phenomena of tooth eruption, *J Dent Res* 46:1325, 1967.

Herzberg F, Schour I: Effects of the removal of pulp and Hertwig's sheath on the eruption of the incisors in the albino rat, *J Dent Res* 20:264, 1941.

Jenkins GN: The physiology of the mouth, ed 3, Oxford, 1966, Blackwell Scientific Publications.

Kenney EB, Ramfjord SP: Patterns of root and alveolar-bone growth associated with development and eruption of teeth in rhesus monkeys, *J Dent Res* 48:251, 1969.

Kronfeld R: The resorption of the roots of deciduous teeth, *Dent Cosmos* 74:103, 1932.

Magnusson B: Tissue changes during molar tooth eruption, *Trans Res Sch Dent Stockholm* 13:1, 1968.

Main JHP: A histological survey of the hammock ligament, *Arch Oral Biol* 10:343, 1965.

Main JHP, Adams D: Experiments on the rat incisor into the cellular proliferation and blood pressure theories of tooth eruption, *Arch Oral Biol* 11:163, 1966.

Manson JD: A study of bone changes associated with tooth eruption, *Proc R Soc Med* 56:515, 1963.

Manson JD: Passive eruption, *Dent Pract Dent Rec* 14:2, 1963.

Manson JD: Bone changes associated with tooth eruption. In Anderson DJ, Eastoe JE, Melcher AH, Picton DCA (eds): *The mechanisms of tooth support*, Bristol UK, 1967, John Wright & Sons.

Marks SC Jr, Cahill DR, Wise GE: The cytology of the dental follicle and adjacent alveolar bone during tooth eruption in the dog, *Am J Anat* 168:277, 1983.

Marks SC Jr, Cahill DR: Experimental study in the dog of the nonactive role of the tooth in the eruptive process, *Arch Oral Biol* 29:311, 1984.

Marks SC Jr, Cahill DR: Ultrastructure of alveolar bone during tooth eruption in the dog, *Am J Anat* 177:427-438, 1986.

Marks SC Jr, Gorski JP, Cahill DR, Wise GE: Tooth eruption: a synthesis of experimental observations. In Davidovitch Z (ed): *The biological mechanisms of tooth eruption and resorption*, Birmingham Ala, 1988, EBSCO Media.

Massler M, Schour I: Studies on tooth development: theories of eruption, *Am J Orthod* 27:552, 1941.

Minkoff R, Stevens CJ, Karon JM: Autoradiography of protein turnover in subcrestal versus supracrestal fiber tracts of the developing mouse periodontium, *Arch Oral Biol* 26:1069, 1981.

Moorrees CF: Dental development: a growth study based on tooth eruption as a measure of physiologic age, *Europ Orthod Soc Rep Congr* 40:92, 1964.

Morita H, Yamishiya H, Shimizu M, et al: The collagenolytic activity during root resorption of bovine deciduous tooth, *Arch Oral Biol* 15:503, 1970.

Moss JP: A review of the theories of approximal migration of teeth. In Poole DFG, Stack MV (eds): *The eruption and occlusion of teeth, Colston papers no. 27*, London, 1976, Butterworth.

Moss JP, Picton DCA: Experimental mesial drift in adult monkeys *(Macaca irus)*, *Arch Oral Biol* 12:1313, 1967.

Moss JP, Picton DCA: Mesial drift of teeth in adult monkeys *(Macaca irus)* when forces from the cheeks and tongue had been eliminated, *Arch Oral Biol* 15:979, 1970.

Moss JP, Picton DCA: The effect on approximal drift of cheek teeth of dividing mandibular molars of adult monkeys *(Macaca irus)*, *Arch Oral Biol* 19:1211, 1974.

Moxham BJ: The effects of section and stimulation of the cervical sympathetic trunk on eruption of the rabbit mandibular incisor, *Arch Oral Biol* 26:887, 1981.

Moxham BJ, Berkovitz BKB: The periodontal ligament and physiological tooth movements. In Berkovitz BKB, Moxham BJ, Newman HN (eds): *The periodontal ligament in health and disease*, New York, 1982, Pergamon Press, Chap 10.

Ness AR: Movement and forces in tooth eruption. In Staple PH (ed): *Advances in oral biology*, New York, 1964, Academic Press, vol 1.

Ness AR: Eruption: a review. In Anderson DJ, Eastoe JE, Melcher AH, Picton DCA (eds): *The mechanisms of tooth support*, Bristol UK, 1967, John Wright & Sons.

Orban B: Growth and movement of the tooth germs and teeth, *J Am Dent Assoc* 15:1004, 1928.

Osborn JW: An investigation into the interdental forces occurring between the teeth of the same arch during clenching the jaws, *Arch Oral Biol* 5:202, 1961.

Parfitt GJ: The physical analysis of the tooth supporting structures. In Anderson DJ, Eastoe JE, Melcher AH, Picton DCA (eds): *The mechanisms of tooth support*, Bristol UK, 1967, John Wright & Sons.

Parker GR: Transseptal fibers and relapse following bodily retraction of teeth: a histologic study, *Am J Orthod* 61:331, 1972.

Picton DCA: The effect of external forces in the periodontium. In Melcher AH, Bowen WH (eds): *Biology of the periodontium*, New York, 1969, Academic Press.

Picton DCA, Moss JP: The part played by the transseptal fibre system in experimental approximal drift of the cheek teeth of monkeys *(Macaca irus)*, *Arch Oral Biol* 18:669, 1973.

Picton DCA, Slater JM: The effect on horizontal tooth mobility of experimental trauma to the periodontal membrane in regions of tension or compression in monkeys, *J Periodont Res* 7:35, 1972.

Reitan K: Tissue rearrangement during retention of orthodontically rotated teeth, *Angle Orthod* 29:105, 1959.

Ripa LW, Leske GS, Sposato AL, et al: Chronology and sequence of exfoliation of primary teeth, *J Am Dent Assoc* 105:641, 1982.

Scott JH: The comparative anatomy of jaw growth and tooth eruption, *Dent Rec* 71:149, 1951.

Scott JH: How teeth erupt, *Dent Pract Dent Rec* 3:345, 1953.

Shore RC, Berkovitz BKB, Moxham BJ: Intercellular contracts between fibroblasts in the periodontal connective tissues of the rat, *J Anat* 133(1):67, 1981.

Sicher H: Tooth eruption: the axial movement of continuously growing teeth, *J Dent Res* 21:201, 1942.

Sicher H: Tooth eruption: the axial movement of teeth with limited growth, *J Dent Res* 21:395, 1942.

Sicher H, Weinmann JP: Bone growth and physiologic tooth movement, *Am J Orthod* 30:109, 1944.

Smith RG: A clinical study into the rate of eruption of some human permanent teeth, *Arch Oral Biol* 25:675, 1980.

Stack MV (ed): *The eruption and occlusion of teeth, The Colston symposium*, London, 1975, Butterworth.

Taylor AC, Butcher EO: The regulation of eruption rate in the incisor teeth of the white rat, *J Exp Zool* 117:165, 1951.

Ten Cate AR: The mechanism of tooth eruption. In Melcher AH, Bowen WH (eds): *Biology of the periodontium*, New York, 1969, Academic Press.

Ten Cate AR: Morphological studies of fibrocytes in connective tissue undergoing rapid remodelling, *J Anat* 112:401, 1972.

Ten Cate AR, Anderson RD: An ultrastructural study of tooth resorption in the kitten, *J Dent Res* 65:1087, 1986.

Ten Cate AR, Deporter DA, Freeman E: The role of fibroblasts in the remodelling of periodontal ligament during physiologic tooth movement, *Am J Orthod* 69:155, 1976.

Thomas NR: The properties of collagen in the periodontium of an erupting tooth. In Anderson DJ, Eastoe JE, Melcher AH, Picton DCA (eds): *The mechanisms of tooth support,* Bristol UK, 1967, John Wright & Sons.

Thomas NR: The effect of inhibition of collagen maturation on eruption in rats, *J Dent Res* 44:1159, 1969.

Van Hassel HJ, McMinn RG Pressure differential favouring tooth eruption in the dog, *Periodontics* 17:183, 1972.

Weatherell JA, Hargreaves JA: Effect of resorption on the fluoride content of human deciduous dentine, *Arch Oral Biol* 11:749, 1966.

Weinmann JP: Bone changes related to eruption of the teeth, *Angle Orthod* 11:83, 1941.

Westin G: Uber Zahndurchbruch und Zahnwechsel, *Z Mikroskop Anatom Forsch* 51:393, 1942.

Wise GE, Marks SC Jr, Cahill DR: Ultrastructural features of the dental follicle associated with formation of the tooth eruption pathway in the dog. *J Oral Pathol* 14:15-26, 1985.

Yaeger JA, Kraucunas E: Fine structure of the resorptive cells in the teeth of frogs, *Anat Rec* 164:1, 1969.

Yilmaz RS, Darling AI, Levers BGH: Mesial drift of human teeth assessed from ankylosed deciduous molars, *Arch Oral Biol* 25:127, 1980.

CHAPTER 16

Surface Coatings of the Teeth

A T differing stages of life the teeth are coated by various structures that can be distinguished as coatings of developmental origin and coatings that are acquired.

COATINGS OF DEVELOPMENTAL ORIGIN

Coatings of developmental origin are formed during the normal development of the tooth and consist of (1) the reduced dental epithelium, (2) coronal cementum, and (3) the dental cuticle.

Reduced Dental Epithelium

The reduced dental epithelium has been described in detail in Chapter 13. It persists until the tooth erupts, when it either is rapidly abraded away on the occlusal surface of the tooth or is involved in formation of the dentogingival junction around the remaining surfaces of the tooth. Remnants may persist, however, in localized protected areas such as occlusal fissures.

Coronal Cementum

In some animals, especially herbivores, the reduced dental epithelium disintegrates as a normal developmental step at the completion of amelogenesis and before tooth eruption. When this occurs, follicular connective tissue cells deposit cementum on the newly formed enamel surface. The end result is an occlusal surface consisting of all three dental hard tissues: enamel, dentin, and cementum. Because these tissues wear differentially, a sharp cutting surface is maintained. In humans thin patches of afibrillar cementum may occasionally be found on the enamel surface in the cervical half of the crown, but it is debatable whether this should be described as a normal surface coating.

Dental Cuticle

In the past the term *cuticle* has been applied erroneously to many different structures. Here it is strictly reserved for the nonmineralized electron-dense structure frequently found between the epithelium of the dentogingival junction and the enamel surface. Dental cuticle is formed by an accumulation of basal lamina material produced by the junctional epithelium of the dentogingival junction (Fig. 16-1).

ACQUIRED COATINGS

Acquired coatings are deposited after tooth eruption and consist of (1) a salivary coating or pellicle, (2) a bacterial coating or plaque, and (3) calculus.

Salivary Pellicle

When a tooth is cleaned in situ, salivary proteins and glycoproteins, as well as traces of some bacterial products, with a strong affinity for enamel very quickly adsorb to the tooth surface and form a very thin layer, usually less than 1.0 μm thick, termed the *salivary pellicle*. In stained transmission electron microscope preparations, this bacteria-free pellicle usually appears as a dark amorphous layer though sometimes it does have a poorly organized lamellar structure (Figs. 16-2 and 16-3).

Bacterial Coating

Dental plaque is the term applied to adherent noncalcified deposits on the tooth surface that are composed of microorganisms embedded in a matrix formed of bacterial products, salivary constituents, and inorganic compounds.

Calculus

Calculus is basically mineralized bacterial plaque. Once mineralized, it is less easily worn away than softer dental plaque by abrasion or salivary washing. Bacteria continue to accumulate on the surface of mineralizing calculus.

FIG. 16-1 Electron micrograph of the dentogingival junction showing the epithelial attachment. An electron-dense cuticle exists between the enamel surface and the lamina lucida of the junctional epithelium. (Courtesy Prof. H.E. Schroeder.)

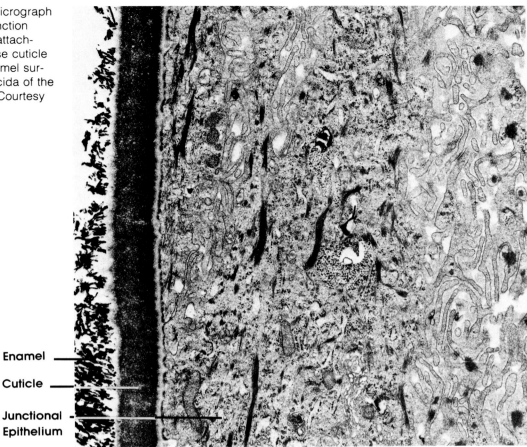

Enamel

Cuticle

Junctional Epithelium

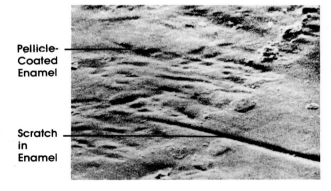

Pellicle-Coated Enamel

Scratch in Enamel

FIG. 16-2 Scanning electron micrograph of salivary pellicle newly formed on a cleaned tooth. The thin film masks scratches on the surface of the enamel *(left)*; enamel scratches are clearly evident in the area where the tooth surface was protected with tape *(right)*. (From Saxton CA: *Caries Res* 7:102, 1973.)

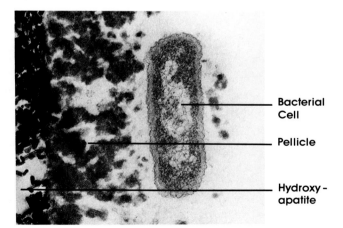

Bacterial Cell

Pellicle

Hydroxy-apatite

FIG. 16-3 Transmission electron micrograph of salivary pellicle freshly formed on a hydroxyapatite surface worn in the mouth. A single rod-shaped bacterial cell is attached to the pellicle. (From Lie T: *J Periodont Res* 13:391, 1978.)

DENTAL PLAQUE

Because dental plaque is present to some extent on all erupted teeth, and because the pathogenic microorganisms within it are involved in the etiology of both dental caries and periodontal disease, a more detailed discussion of its structure than of the structure of other acquired coatings is appropriate.

Dental plaque may be studied by a variety of histologic and histochemical techniques—including light, phase-contrast, darkfield, and electron microscopy. Plaque can be easily prepared in an aqueous suspension and studied by phase-contrast or darkfield microscopy to determine the shape (morphotype) and motility of the bacteria, or it may be fixed, sectioned, and stained for more detailed study by either light or electron microscopy. Because the size of most bacteria is such that they can barely be resolved by the light microscope, electron microscopy has become an indispensable tool for studying the structural details of the complex bacterial cell arrangements in plaque.

Plaque Formation

Plaque formation involves a complex series of physicochemical reactions dependent on the selective ad-sorption of salivary components and bacteria to the teeth and the accumulation of thick bacterial masses through cohesive interactions and growth. Although initial deposition and accumulation probably occur on a temporal continuum, various phases of plaque formation have been designated to facilitate discussion and investigation: (1) acquired pellicle formation, (2) initial attachment of bacteria to the pellicle, and (3) accumulation of bacterial plaque in several layers. These stages can be illustrated by either scanning or transmission electron microscopy. For investigative purposes, most researchers have chosen to study supragingival smooth-surface plaque formed in the mouth on natural teeth or on resin crowns, plastic films, or slabs of enamel and root surfaces worn in removable appliances.

Bacterial cells with a strong affinity for the deposited salivary pellicle proteins attach selectively at the tooth surface to begin the actual formation of bacterial plaque. Bacteria are rarely detected attached directly to the enamel. The specificity of this event should be stressed. The acquired pellicle is formed from only those proteins that bind selectively to the tooth mineral, and not all bacteria available in the bathing saliva can attach well

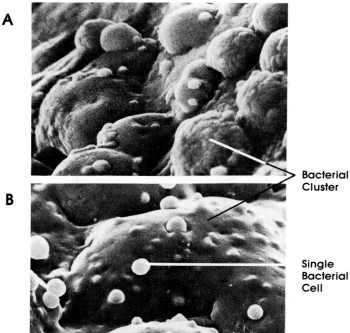

A

B

Bacterial
Cluster

Single
Bacterial
Cell

FIG. 16-4   Scanning electron micrographs of supragingival dental plaque forming close to the orifice of the gingival, sulcus. Aggregates of bacterial cells are seen as large mounds, **A,** whereas individual bacterial cells are seen as smaller prominent spherical structures, **B.** (Courtesy Dr. C.A. Saxton.)

to the pellicle. Only those with a relatively high affinity or multiple binding "adhesins" for pellicle constituents and occurring in sufficient numbers in the saliva are adsorbed. A single layer of cells or single bacterial cells are observed in photomicrographs if samples are taken early enough during plaque formation (Fig. 16-3). The adsorbed bacteria are most often detected in separate clusters or microcolonies superficial to the salivary pellicle (Fig. 16-4).

Plaque mass is increased by the continued deposition of bacteria by selective attachment and especially by the simultaneous growth of the attached bacteria as microcolonies. The bacterial aggregates enlarge and coalesce into deposits. Amorphous intermicrobial matrix is often evident during this accumulation phase (Fig. 16-5). The processes of accumulation, growth, and cohesion continue until the plaque mass, often reaching more than 100 bacterial cells in thickness, is restricted from further growth by abrasion from physiologic oral movements and the bathing action of saliva.

Factors Determining Plaque Morphology

The microbial composition and microscopic structure of dental plaque vary greatly from site to site and from time to time. Bacteria differ in their abilities to attach to the tooth surface, to survive, and to proliferate in the microenvironment of dental plaque. Thus certain species of oral bacteria commonly predominate in newly formed plaque, some become predominant only after plaque has accumulated for several days, and others may not be found routinely in plaque even though they are present in high numbers in saliva and colonize other oral tissues. Also dissimilar areas of the tooth surface (e.g., smooth enamel, occlusal fissures, and subgingival areas) present distinct and selective microenvironments in which different types of bacteria colonize and emerge to predominate in the community. The state of the surrounding tissues—whether inflamed gingiva or carious tooth structure—also affects the microbial population of plaque. Thus the major factors determining the structure of dental plaque include (1) the rate at which an individual forms plaque, (2) the length of time the plaque has accumulated, (3) the populations of bacteria to which the individual has been exposed and that have colonized successfully, (4) the tooth site from which the plaque is collected, and (5) the state of health of the surrounding tissues.

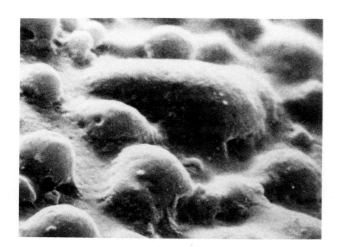

FIG. 16-5 Enlarged and coalesced bacterial aggregates in newly formed plaque. The aggregates appear covered with amorphous material that may be an interbacterial matrix of salivary or bacterial origin. (From Saxton CA: *Caries Res* 7:102, 1973.)

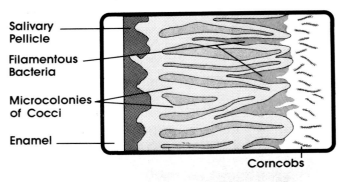

Salivary Pellicle

Filamentous Bacteria

Microcolonies of Cocci

Enamel

Corncobs

Smooth Surface Supragingival Plaque

FIG. 16-6 High magnification of supragingival plaque showing structures common to supragingival smooth-surface plaques. (Inset: Site of the plaque.) Columnar microcolonies of cocci extend outward from the pellicle. Filamentous bacteria are arranged perpendicular to the tooth surface. When these bacteria become coated with cocci, they take on the so-called corncob appearance.

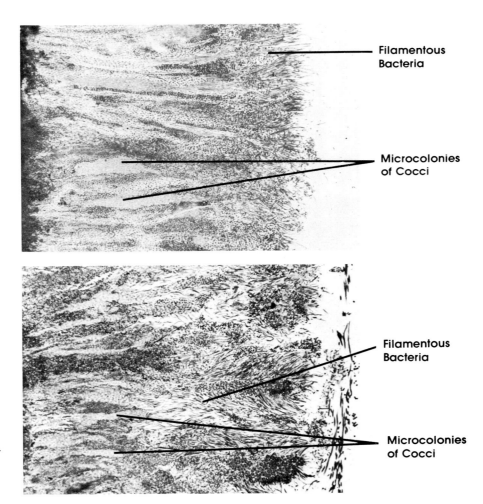

Filamentous Bacteria

Microcolonies of Cocci

Filamentous Bacteria

Microcolonies of Cocci

FIG. 16-7 Photomicrographs of thick supragingival plaques. Filamentous bacteria are numerous near the external surface of the plaque, displacing some of the microcolonies of cocci. (From Listgarten MA, et al: *J Periodontol* 46:10, 1975.)

Morphologic Features

Most investigations into the formation and structure of dental plaque have been concerned with supragingival plaque formed on smooth enamel surfaces. Such smooth-surface plaque may serve to illustrate the structural details common to most plaques (Figs. 16-6 and 16-7). Most of the plaque is composed of densely arranged bacterial cells of coccal (round), bacillary (rod-shaped), and filamentous form. The bacteria are often separated from each other by lightly staining areas that consist of high-molecular weight polysaccharides of bacterial origin, salivary macromolecules, immunoglobulins, simple sugars, and inorganic salts. Occasionally the interbacterial spaces are filled with more darkly staining fibrillar bacterial derivatives or small vesicles likely formed from fragments of bacterial outer membranes. These, along with the other matrix constituents, may foster specific cohesive interactions between bacterial cells.

The bacteria in smooth surface plaque are often arranged in microcolonies that were probably formed by the proliferation of bacteria of a single species in a confined area. Microcolonies of cocci usually form a series of columns perpendicular to the tooth surface (Fig. 16-7). Because distinct bacterial species differ in their abilities to produce various amounts of polysaccharides, the lateral borders of such microcolonies can often be distinguished by observing the amount of intercellular material. Highly specific serologic staining methods have also been used to detect microcolonies of some predominating plaque species. Bacillary and filamentous bacteria are usually aligned with their long axes perpendicular to the tooth surface (Fig. 16-7).

Within long-standing dental plaque, differences in the morphologic features of bacterial cells near the tooth surface (deep) and near the salivary interface (superficial surface) can be detected (Fig. 16-8). Cells closest to the tooth surface, which are probably prevented from easy access to nutrients in the saliva and the host's diet, often exhibit features common to dead cells or cells in a state of unbalanced growth. The most obvious alterations in structure include an increased thickness of cell walls and an increased number of lightly staining intracellular polysaccharide storage granules. By contrast, cells near the salivary interface have morphologic features common to living bacteria growing in laboratory culture. Division planes are more numerous (which, along with the arrangements of cells in columnar microcolonies, suggests that many bacteria in plaque are actively growing). In some long-standing plaques filamentous bacteria predominate at the salivary interface, leaving the impression that they grow into an established plaque from its surface, displacing the cocci that have colonized previously. Filaments at the salivary interface are often coated with cocci, presenting the so-called corncob appearance (Figs. 16-9 and 16-10). Corncob formation is restricted to only those species with mutually attractive surface molecules that can mediate binding or those with a capacity to bind to salivary molecules bridging between them.

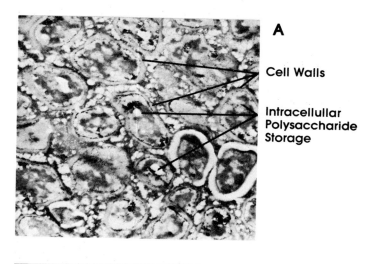

A

Cell Walls

Intracellular Polysaccharide Storage

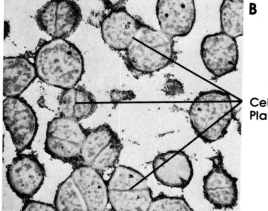

B

Cell Division Planes

FIG. 16-8 Electron micrographs of dental plaque sectioned deep near the tooth surface, **A,** and near the saliva plaque interface, **B.** In **A** densely arranged bacterial cells deep in the plaque contain thickened cell walls and numerous light-staining intracellular polysaccharide storage areas. Bacterial cells near the salivary interface have walls of usual thickness and fewer intercellular polysaccharide storage areas. Cell division planes are numerous. (From van Houte J, Saxton CA: *Caries Res* 5:30, 1971.)

Filaments of
Supragingival
Plaque

Corncobs

Filaments of
Subragingival
Plaque

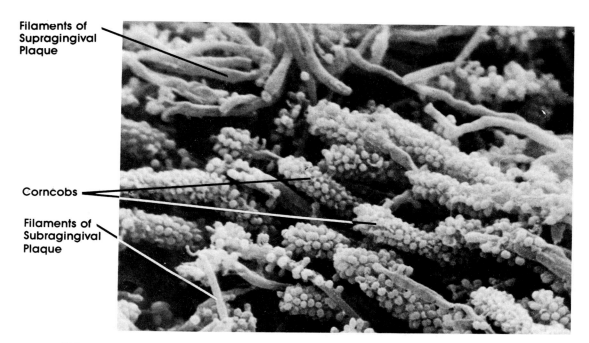

FIG. 16-9 Scanning electron micrograph of cocci-coated filaments of supragingival plaque, the "corncob" formation. Some filamentous bacteria at the plaque surface are not coated with cocci, suggesting a degree of specificity in the mutual affinities between bacterial types forming the corncob. (Courtesy Dr. S. Jones.)

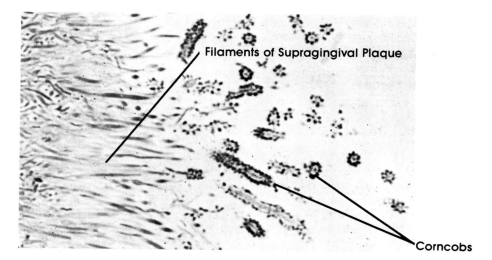

Filaments of Supragingival Plaque

Corncobs

FIG. 16-10 Photomicrograph of supragingival plaque at the saliva-plaque interface demonstrating "corncobs" in both longitudinal and cross section. (From Listgarten MA: *J Periodontol* 47:1, 1976.)

Features of occlusal fissure plaque

Occlusal fissures of teeth are confined retentive sites. The physical and nutrient influences of impacted food in fissures are additional factors contributing to their microbial ecology. These factors have various degrees of influence, depending on the depth, width, and configuration of a fissure.

The morphology of plaque near the orifice of a fissure differs from that in its depth. Plaque near the orifice and that in shallow occlusal grooves are structurally very similar to plaques that form on smooth enamel surfaces (Fig. 16-11). Coccal and short bacillary forms predominate. Columns of cocci are arranged perpendicular to the tooth surface. Occasional filaments are evident. A bacteria-free layer, presumably identical to the salivary pellicle, separates the dense masses of bacteria from the enamel surface.

Deep within fissures, plaque consists mostly of densely arranged cocci among impacted vegetable and food fibers (Fig. 16-12). Filaments and long rods are rarely seen. The cocci are often arranged in clusters or microcolonies. Lightly staining intracellular storage granules are numerous. A thin electron-dense layer of unknown origin, which may be derived from salivary material or remnants of the enamel organ, can usually be seen between the bacterial cells and the enamel fissure wall. Evidence of both intracellular and extracellular mineralization is often noted in long-standing deep fissure plaques.

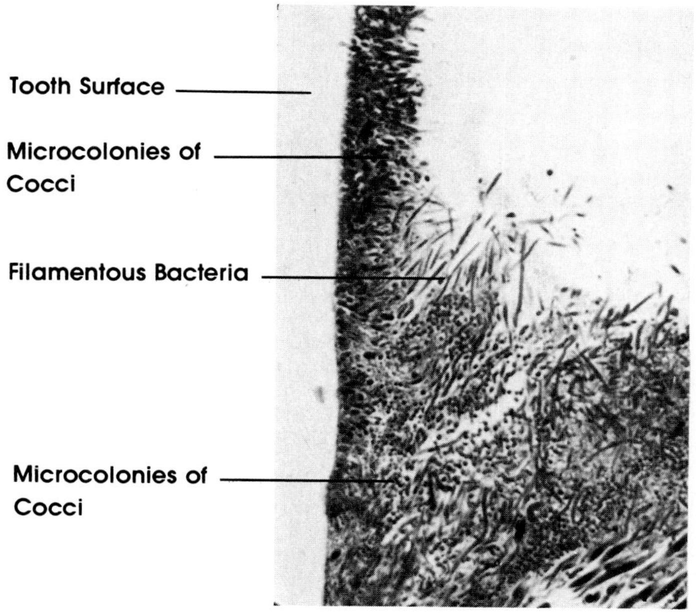

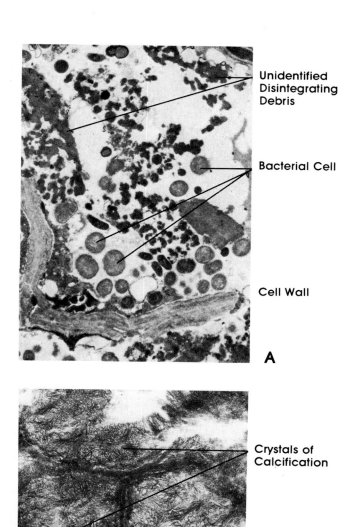

A

B

FIG. 16-11 Low-powered photomicrograph of plaque near the orifice of an occlusal fissure. Note the similarity between its structure and that of smooth-surface plaques. Coccal and filamentous microcolonies radiate from the tooth surface. (From Theilade J, et al: *Arch Oral Biol* 21:587, 1976.)

Tooth Surface

Microcolonies of Cocci

Filamentous Bacteria

Microcolonies of Cocci

Unidentified Disintegrating Debris

Bacterial Cell

Cell Wall

Crystals of Calcification

FIG. 16-12 Electron micrographs of plaque deep within an occlusal fissure. **A,** At low magnification bacterial cells are seen among unidentifiable disintegrating debris and retained plant cell wall material. **B,** At high magnification bacterial cells demonstrate intracellular and extracellular needlelike crystals of calcification. (From Theilade J, et al: *Arch Oral Biol* 21:587, 1976.)

Features of the gingival sulcus microbiota

The gingival sulcus presents a unique environment for the bacterial species that can colonize it. At least four major ecologic conditions account for the differences between supragingival and subgingival plaque: (1) saliva rarely enters the sulcus, so that the composition of pellicle and interbacterial matrix is different; (2) the sulcus is a relatively retentive or stagnant area, which means that less adherent bacteria can accumulate; (3) the oxidation-reduction potential and oxygen tension in the sulcus are relatively low, providing growth conditions for anaerobic bacteria; and (4) serum-derived sulcular fluid or gingival bleeding provides the required nutrients for some fastidious species of bacteria that are unable to colonize the supragingival surfaces of the teeth.

The gingival sulcus thus presents a more hospitable environment than the supragingival tooth surface does for the colonization of strictly anaerobic motile bacteria, with stringent nutrient requirements. The relative

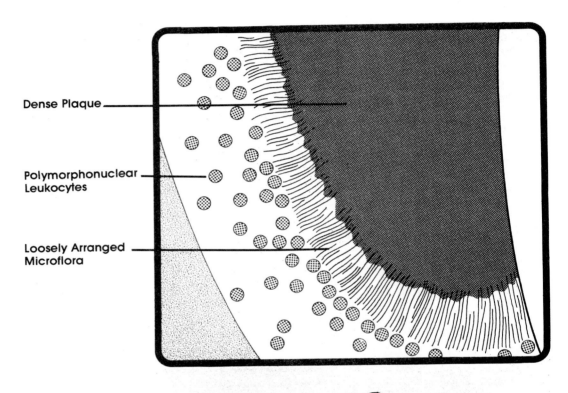

Dense Plaque

Polymorphonuclear Leukocytes

Loosely Arranged Microflora

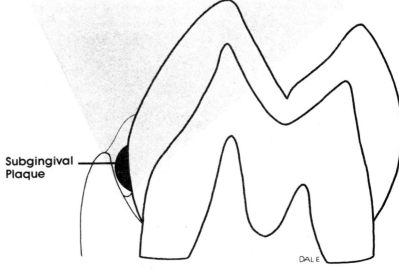

Subgingival Plaque

FIG. 16-13   High magnification of subgingival plaque and microbiota showing features common to subgingival plaques adjacent to areas of peridontal inflammation. (Inset: Site of the plaque). Near the tooth surface dense plaque is covered by a layer of loosely arranged plaque containing many curved and apical bacterial cells. Numerous polymorphonuclear leukocytes that have migrated through the sulcular epithelium line the external surface of the loosely arranged plaque.

abundance of these bacterial types is also greatly influenced by the degree of health of the adjacent periodontal tissues because of increased sulcular depth and increased flow of sulcular fluids during gingival disease. A more diverse microbiota would, in turn, establish a more complex nutrient network for those bacteria dependent on the byproducts of metabolism of other bacteria.

Healthy gingival sulci usually contain sparse formations of plaque similar in morphology to supragingival smooth-surface plaque. Cocci and straight rods predominate. Very few curved or spiral rods are evident, and only a few polymorphonuclear leukocytes (which have passed through the sulcular epithelium) can be seen adjacent to such plaques.

The morphologic features of the subgingival plaque adjacent to tissues affected by inflammatory periodontal disease differ greatly from those found at corresponding healthy sites. There is an increase in the proportion of bacillary and filamentous bacteria, in the number of curved or spiral-shaped rods, and in the number of polymorphonuclear leukocytes lining the surface of the plaque. In some cases bacteria have been detected invading the periodontal tissues.

Subgingival plaque in diseased sites also has a characteristic microscopic arrangement of cells (Figs. 16-13 and 16-14). The area of plaque closest to the tooth surface is often of similar morphology to supragingival plaque, being composed of densely arranged coccal and bacillary forms. External to this area, toward the tissue interface, is a band of more loosely arranged curved and spiral rods as well as so-called bristle brushes and other odd formations of filamentous bacteria with mutual surface affinities (Figs. 16-15 and 16-16). Among the spiral rods, bacteria demonstrating axial filaments characteristic of spirochetes are often found. Numerous polymorphonuclear leukocytes that have migrated from the gingival connective tissue line the external surface of the loosely arranged microbiota. Under some circumstances, subgingival bacteria penetrate the soft tissue wall of the periodontal pocket, through the epithelium and into the connective tissue.

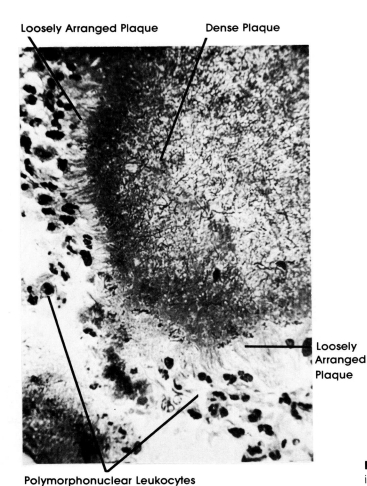

Loosely Arranged Plaque

Dense Plaque

Loosely Arranged Plaque

Polymorphonuclear Leukocytes

FIG. 16-14 Photomicrograph of the features sketched in Figure 16-13. (Courtesy Dr. M.A. Listgarten.)

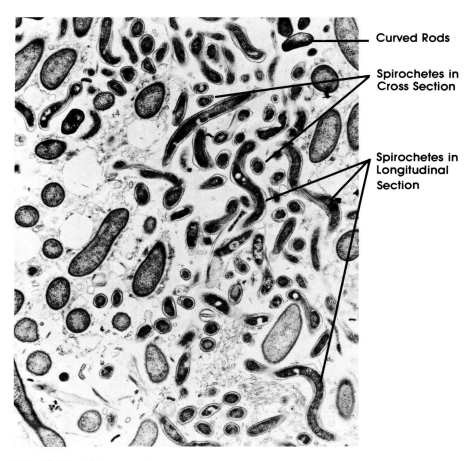

Curved Rods

Spirochetes in
Cross Section

Spirochetes in
Longitudinal
Section

FIG. 16-15 High-magnification electron micrograph of
a loosely arranged area at the surface of subgingival
plaque from an inflamed site. Curved and spiral rods are
very numerous. Most demonstrate axial filaments (in both
longitudinal and cross section) characteristic of spirochetes. (From Listgarten MA, et al: *J Periodontol* 46:10,
1975.)

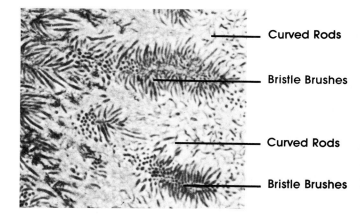

Curved Rods

Bristle Brushes

Curved Rods

Bristle Brushes

FIG. 16-16 Photomicrograph of subgingival plaque.
Many curved rods and filamentous bacterial cell ar-
rangements resembling bristle brushes. (From Listgarten
MA: *J Periodontol* 47:1, 1976.)

CHAIRSIDE MICROSCOPY

Since morphologic features of the microbiota adjacent to healthy and diseased periodontal tissues vary so greatly, it might be possible to use specimens of patients' plaques as adjuncts to diagnosis, prognosis, and patient motivation. For example, subgingival samples can be readily collected with dental instruments, dispersed in saline solution, and examined directly at chairside in a wet preparation by phase-contrast or darkfield microscopy (Figs. 16-17 to 16-19). This technique is ideal for determining microbial shape and motility. It can also detect bacterial morphotypes (e.g., spirochetes) that often are not detected on growth media when samples are cultivated in the laboratory. Samples from healthy gingival sulci usually contain a high percentage of coccal forms but few filamentous, curved rod, or motile organisms. Spirochetes are also rare in preparations from healthy sites. By contrast, samples from inflamed periodontal pockets usually contain high percentages of motile bacteria, many of which resemble curved or spiral rods. Periodontal therapy, by either mechanical debridement or antimicrobial agents, often results in a shift back toward the nonmotile coccal and straight rod morphotypes of health. Astute practitioners can monitor such shifts to assess the effect of therapy or maintenance. Patients who can be made aware of this shift from a highly motile microbiota to one with less activity may benefit from the motivating effect of seeing such positive results of oral hygiene practices and professionally delivered care.

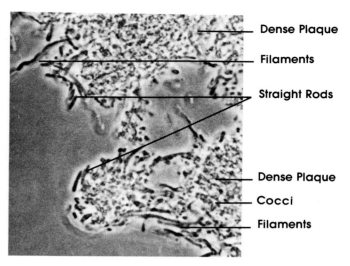

FIG. 16-17 Phase-contrast photomicrograph of an undispersed suspension of subgingival plaque from a healthy gingival sulcus. Cocci, straight rods, and filaments are numerous; but curved motile rods and spirochetes are absent.

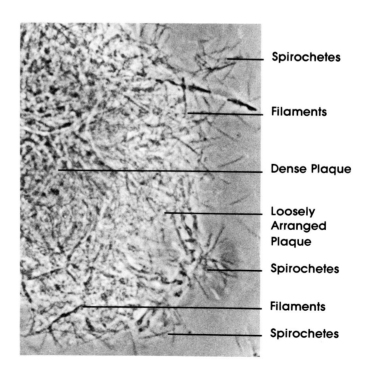

FIG. 16-18 Phase-contrast photomicrograph of suspended subgingival plaque from an inflamed periodontal pocket. This sample was collected at the same time and from the same patient as in Figure 16-17. Spirochetes cover the loosely arranged plaque. The somewhat ill-defined focusing in the photographs is indicative of the high degree of spirochetal motility in aqueous suspensions.

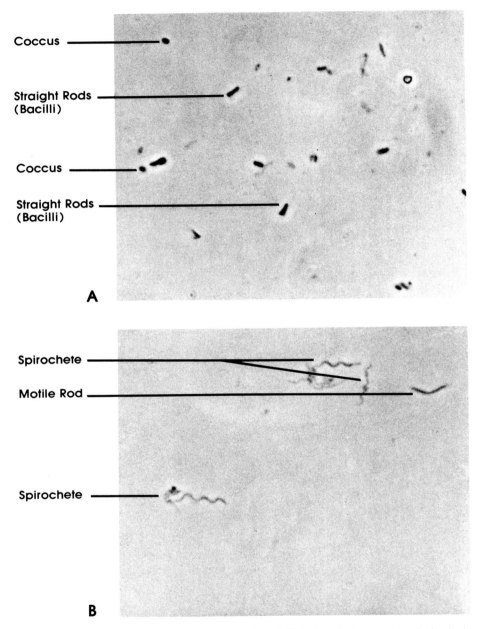

FIG. 16-19 Phase-contrast photomicrographs of diluted and dispersed subgingival plaques from sites of periodontal health and disease in the same patient. **A,** Cocci and short straight rods predominate in health. **B,** Spirochetes and other motile rods are often predominant in inflamed areas.

BIBLIOGRAPHY

Brecx M, Rönström A, Theilade J, et al: Early formation of dental plaque on plastic films. II. Electron microscopic observations, *J Periodont Res* 16:213, 1981.

Critchley P, Saxton CA, Kolendo AB: The histology and histochemistry of dental plaque, *Caries Res* 2:115, 1968.

Dawes C, Jenkins GN, Tongue CH: The nomenclature of the integuments of the enamel surface of teeth, *Br Dent J* 115:65, 1963.

Frank RM, Houver G: An ultrastructural study of human supragingival dental plaque formation. In McHugh WD (ed): *Dental plaque; a symposium at the University of Dundee*, Dundee, 1970, DC Thomson.

Gibbons RJ: Bacterial adhesion to oral tissues: a model for infectious diseases, *J Dent Res* 68:750, 1989.

Hodson JJ: Origin and nature of the cuticula dentis, *Nature* 209:990, 1966.

Jones SJ: A special relationship between spherical and filamentous microorganisms in mature human dental plaque, *Arch Oral Biol* 17:613, 1973.

Kolenbrander PE: Intergeneric coaggregation among human oral bacteria and ecology of dental plaque, *Annu Rev Microbiol* 42:627, 1988.

Lie T: Early dental plaque morphogenesis: a scanning electron microscope study using the hydroxyapatite splint model and a low-sucrose diet, *J Periodont Res* 12:73, 1977.

Listgarten MA: A mineralized cuticular structure with connective tissue characteristics on the crowns of human unerupted teeth in amelogenesis imperfecta: a light and electron microscopic study, *Arch Oral Biol* 12:877, 1967.

Listgarten MA: Structure of the microbial flora associated with periodontal health and disease in man: a light and electron microscopic study, *J Periodontol* 47:1, 1976.

Listgarten MA: Structure of surface coatings on teeth: a review, *J Periodontol* 47:139, 1976.

Listgarten MA, Mayo HE, Tremblay R: Development of dental plaque on epoxy resin crowns in man: a light and electron microscopic study, *J Periodontol* 46:10, 1975.

Marsh PD: Host defenses and microbial homeostasis: role of microbial interactions, *J Dent Res* 68:1567, 1989.

Newman HN: Structure of approximal human dental plaque as observed by scanning electron microscopy, *Arch Oral Biol* 17:1445, 1972.

Newman HN, Britton AB: Dental plaque ultrastructure as revealed by freeze-etching, *J Periodontol* 45:478, 1974.

Nyvad B, Fejerskov O: Scanning electron microscopy of early microbial colonization of human enamel and root surfaces in vivo, *Scand J Dent Res* 95:287, 1987.

Nyvad B, Fejerskov O: Transmission electron microscopy of early microbial colonization of human enamel and root surfaces in vivo, *Scand J Dent Res* 95:297, 1987.

Saglie FR: Bacterial invasion and its role in the pathogenesis of periodontal disease. In Hamada S, Holt SC, McGhee JR (eds): *Periodontal disease: pathogens and host immune responses*, Tokyo, 1991, Quintessence Publishing.

Saxton CA: Scanning electron microscope study of the formation of dental plaque, *Caries Res* 7:102, 1973.

Schroeder HE, de Boever J: The structure of microbial dental plaque. In McHugh WD (ed): *Dental plaque: a symposium at the University of Dundee*, Dundee, 1970, DC Thomson.

Theilade J, Fejerskov O, Horsted M: A transmission electron microscopic study of 7-day-old bacterial plaque in human tooth fissures, *Arch Oral Biol* 21:587, 1976.

Theilade J, Karring T, Ostergaard E, et al: Electron microscopic study of the formation of dental plaque in artificial fissures, *J Biol Buccale* 2:375, 1974.

Van Houte J, Saxton CA: Cell wall thickening and intracellular polysaccharide in microorganisms of the dental plaque, *Caries Res* 5:30, 1971.

CHAPTER 17

Salivary Glands

THE oral cavity is a moist environment; a film of fluid called saliva constantly coats its inner surfaces and occupies the space between the lining oral mucosa and the teeth. Saliva is a complex fluid, produced by the salivary glands, whose important role is maintaining the well-being of the mouth. For example, patients with a deficiency of salivary secretion experience difficulty eating, speaking, and swallowing and become prone to mucosal infections and rampant caries. In humans there are three pairs of major salivary glands—the parotid, submandibular, and sublingual—located outside the oral cavity, encapsulated, and with extended duct systems to discharge their secretions. There are also a multitude of smaller minor salivary glands—the labial, lingual, palatal, buccal, glossopalatine, and retromolar—located just below and within the mucous membranes, unencapsulated, and with short duct systems (Fig. 17-1).

Secretion of each major salivary gland is not the same. The parotid glands secrete a so-called "watery" serous saliva rich in amylase, the submandibular gland produces a more mucinous saliva, and the sublingual gland produces a viscous saliva. Because of these variations saliva found in the mouth is referred to as mixed. The composition of mixed saliva is not the simple additive sum of all salivary secretions as many proteins secreted in saliva are rapidly removed by adhering to hydroxyapatite of teeth and to the oral mucosal surfaces.

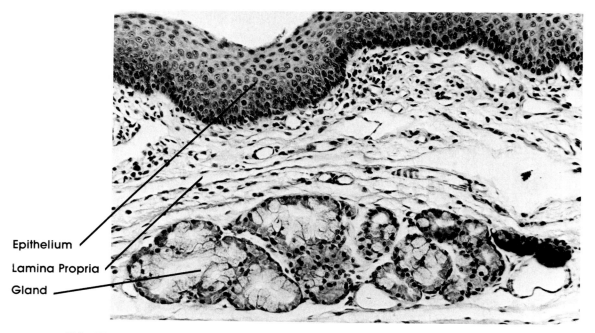

Epithelium

Lamina Propria

Gland

FIG. 17-1 Minor mucous salivary gland. Because it is situated just beneath the surface epithelium, it requires only a short duct.

FUNCTIONS OF SALIVA

Mixed saliva has many functions (Table 17-1), the most obvious being protection of the oral cavity.

Protection

The protective function of saliva is expressed in many ways. Saliva is a lubricant. Its glycoprotein content, which makes it mucinous, protects the lining mucosa by forming a barrier against noxious stimuli, microbial toxins, and minor trauma. Its fluid consistency also provides a mechanical washing action, which flushes away nonadherent bacterial and acellular debris from the mouth. In particular, the clearance of sugars from the mouth by saliva's washing action limits their availability to acidogenic plaque microorganisms. Calcium-binding proteins occur in saliva, and these help form salivary pellicle (Chapter 16), which behaves as a protective membrane.

Buffering

Saliva provides a buffer that protects the oral cavity in two ways. First, many bacteria require a specific pH for maximal growth; the buffering capacity of saliva prevents potential pathogens from colonizing the mouth by denying them optimal environmental conditions. Second, plaque microorganisms can produce acid from sugars, which if not rapidly buffered and cleared by saliva can demineralize enamel. Much of the buffering capacity of saliva resides in its bicarbonate and phosphate ions. Negatively charged residues on salivary proteins are also thought to serve as buffers; a salivary peptide, *sialin*, plays a significant role in raising the pH of dental plaque after exposure to fermentable carbohydrate. The ability of saliva to buffer acid is very important, since saliva and plaque pH are generally lower in caries-active individuals.

Digestion

Saliva is important for digestion. It provides taste acuity, neutralizes esophageal contents, dilutes gastric chyme, forms the food bolus, and, because of its *amylase* contents, breaks down starch.

Taste

Saliva also plays a role in taste. Although it enables the pleasurable sensations of food to be experienced, its primary role is protection in that it permits the recognition of noxious substances. Saliva is required to dissolve substances to be tasted and to carry them to the taste buds. It also contains a protein, called *gustin*, that is thought to be necessary for growth and maturation of the taste buds.

Antimicrobial Action

Saliva has a major ecologic influence on the microorganisms that attempt to colonize oral tissues. In addition to the barrier effect of its mucus content already noted, it contains a spectrum of proteins with antibacterial properties. *Lysozyme* is an enzyme that can hydrolyze the cell walls of some bacteria. *Lactoferrin* binds free iron and in so doing deprives bacteria of this essential element.

Antibodies are present in saliva. The major salivary immunoglobulin, secretory IgA, has the capacity to clump or agglutinate microorganisms. This ability, along with the cleansing action of saliva, serves to remove clumps of bacteria.

Maintenance of Tooth Integrity

Saliva is saturated with calcium and phosphate ions. The high concentration of these ions ensures that ionic exchange with the tooth surface is directed to the tooth. This exchange begins as soon as the tooth erupts, because, although the crown is fully formed morphologically when it erupts, it is crystallographically incomplete. Interaction with saliva results in posteruptive maturation through diffusion of such ions as calcium, phosphorus, magnesium, and chloride into the surface apatite enamel crystals. (See Chapter 7.) This maturation increases surface hardness, decreases perme-

TABLE 17-1 Functions of saliva

	Effect	Active constituent
Protection	Lubrication	Glycoprotein
	Waterproofing	
	Lavage	Water
	Pellicle formation	
Buffering	Maintains pH unsuitable for colonization	Phosphate and bicarbonate
	Neutralizes acid	
Digestion	Bolus formation	Water
	Neutralizes esophageal contents	Phosphate and bicarbonate
	Digests starch	Amylase
Taste	Solution of molecules	Water
	Taste bud growth and maturation	Gustin
Antimicrobial action	Barrier	Glycoprotein
	Antibodies	Immunoglobulin A
	Hostile environment	Lysozyme Lactoferrin
Tooth integrity	Enamel maturation	Calcium and phosphate
	Repair	

ability, and heightens the resistance of enamel to caries. If, however, the carious process intervenes but can be halted before cavitation of enamel occurs (Chapter 12), remineralization of the lesion is possible. Remineralization is achieved largely through the availability of phosphate and calcium ions in the saliva. If the fluoride ion is also available as remineralization occurs, the repaired lesion is less susceptible to future decay.

Tissue Repair

Finally, there is a clinical impression that the bleeding time of oral tissues is shorter than that of other tissues. When saliva is experimentally mixed with blood, the clotting time may be greatly accelerated (although the resulting clot is less solid than normal). Experimental studies in mice have shown that the rate of wound contraction is significantly increased in the presence of saliva, and this is thought due to the presence of epidermal growth factor in the saliva produced by the submandibular glands. The occurrence of growth factor is lower in human saliva, but its effect on repair has yet to be demonstrated.

ANATOMY OF THE SALIVARY GLANDS

The parotid is the largest salivary gland. Situated in front of the ear and behind the ramus of the mandible, it weighs between 14 and 28 g and is intimately associated with peripheral branches of the facial nerve (VII). Its duct runs forward across the masseter muscle and can easily be felt by moving a finger over the cheek when the jaws are clenched. At the anterior border of this muscle, the duct turns inward and opens into the oral cavity in a papilla opposite the maxillary second molar.

Next in size is the submandibular gland. Situated in the posterior part of the floor of the mouth, tucked up against the medial aspect of the mandible, it weighs on average between 10 and 15 g. It has an excretory duct that runs forward and opens into the mouth beneath the tongue by way of a small orifice lateral to the lingual frenum.

The almond-shaped sublingual gland, the smallest of the three paired major salivary glands, weighs about 2 g and is situated in the floor of the mouth between the side of the tongue and the teeth. Its secretions enter the oral cavity through a variable series of small ducts opening into a raised sublingual fold. Often portions of the human sublingual and submandibular glands intermingle to form a gross sublingual-submandibular complex.

Numerous minor salivary glands (estimated to be between 600 and 1000) exists as small discrete masses occupying the submucosa throughout most of the oral

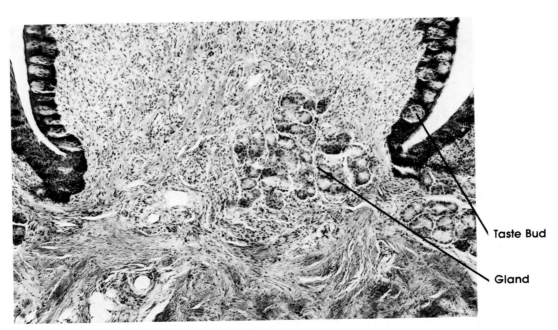

FIG. 17-2 Serous glands of von Ebner. These are situated in the lamina propria at the base of the trough surrounding the circumvallate papillae.

Taste Bud

Gland

cavity. The only places where they do not occur are within the gingiva and in the anterior part of the hard palate. They are mucous glands, except for the serous glands of von Ebner (which exist below the sulci of the circumvallate papillae and in the foliate papillae of the tongue) (Fig. 17-2).

DEVELOPMENT OF THE SALIVARY GLANDS

A salivary gland arises as a focal thickening of the oral epithelium that grows into the underlying ecto-mesenchyme to form a small bud connected to the surface by a trailing cord of epithelium. At the same time ectomesenchymal cells condense around this bud, and to this point the sequence of events is somewhat similar to initial tooth bud formation. The epithelial bulb then clefts to form two or more new buds; and this process continues, producing successive generations, which results in a hierarchical ramification of the gland (Fig. 17-3). As in tooth development, ectomesenchyme plays a significant role in salivary gland development, being required for both morphogenesis and cytodifferentiation of the gland. It has been shown in various recombination experiments that the presence of first arch ectomesenchyme is essential for full salivary gland development. For example, if nonsalivary gland mesenchyme is combined with salivary gland epithelium the epithelium is maintained but does not differentiate into a glandular epithelium. On the other hand, when salivary gland ectomesenchyme is combined with pancreatic epithelium, pancreatic glandular cells differentiate. Such results indicate, again, the delicate interplay between epithelium and mesenchyme during development. In the case of salivary glands, the site of bud clefting is determined by the contraction of microfilaments within the epithelial cells; but the ordered deposition of collagen types I, III, and IV, laminin, and proteoglycan adjacent to the epithelial cells is also needed for further division of the bud to occur.

The development of a lumen within this branched epithelium generally occurs first in the distal end of the main cord and in branch cords, then in the proximal end of the main cord, and finally in the central portion of the main cord (Fig. 17-4). Tubular lumenization is completed throughout the ductal tree before it occurs in the terminal buds. What determines the formation of the lumen is not known; however, it is not due, as has been suggested, to a separation of cells because of a buildup of secretory products from developing end pieces, since the cells have not yet formed; nor is pro-grammed (apoptotic) cell death involved.

As lumina begin to appear in the terminal buds, the buds cleft and further subdivide into a series of units

two cells thick called terminal saccules or *terminal end pieces*. It is within these terminal saccules that the secretory units develop, with the innermost cells differentiating into different types of secretory cells and some of the outer cells forming contractile *myoepithelial* cells. From this brief account of development it can be appreciated why the epithelial component of the salivary gland (the parenchyma) is likened to a bunch of grapes, with the ductal system representing the stalk and stems and the terminal end pieces the grapes. Unlike a bunch of grapes, however, the salivary gland also has a connective tissue component that is rapidly diminished as the parenchyma expands (terminal end pieces alone eventually occupy over 90% of the gland); but even so, every terminal end piece and every duct remain supported by a tenuous connective tissue component carrying blood vessels and nerves. The final

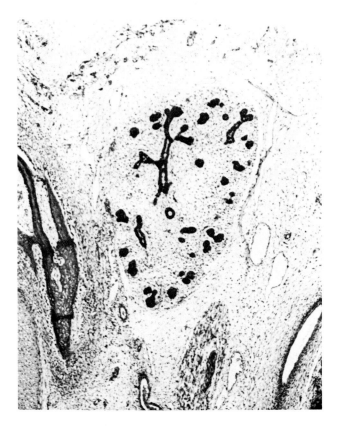

FIG. 17-3 Developing submandibular salivary gland. Epithelium has proliferated into the underlying ectomesenchyme, which has responded with a local proliferative activity.

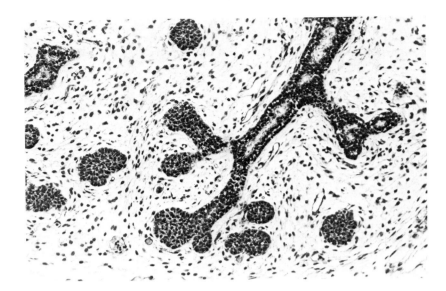

FIG. 17-4 Degeneration of central cells of the epithelial strands. In the ductal branch descending from top the cells are the *white* areas. Their degeneration forms the lumina of the ductal system and terminal secretory end pieces.

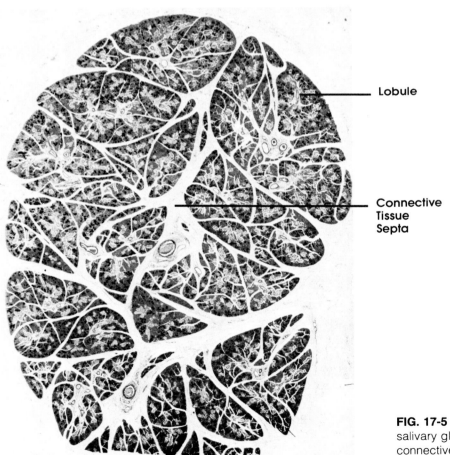

Lobule

Connective Tissue Septa

FIG. 17-5 Low-powered photomicrograph of a salivary gland. The parenchyma is supported by connective tissue septa, which divide the gland into successively smaller lobules.

disposition of connective tissue is in the form of a capsule and septa that divide the gland into lobes and lobules (Fig. 17-5).

There is less understanding of what determines the differentiation of cell types that go to make up a terminal end piece but, again, the presence of ectomesenchyme seems to be an essential requirement.

Little is known about the development of blood supply to the salivary glands. The nerve supply is both sympathetic and parasympathetic, and there is an indication that innervation is necessary if proper functional differentiation of the glands is to occur. Sympathetic innervation is related to acinar differentiation, and parasympathetic innervation to overall growth.

The parotid glands begin to develop at 4 to 6 weeks of embryonic life, the submandibular glands at 6 weeks,

and the sublingual and minor salivary glands at 8 to 12 weeks. Because the capsule of a salivary gland is the last component of the gland to differentiate, it is not uncommon to find misplaced salivary tissue entrapped within facial bones if excessive epithelial proliferation occurs.

STRUCTURE OF THE SALIVARY GLANDS

The description of salivary gland development makes it easy to appreciate that the parenchyma of the glands consists of a series of ducts ending in terminal secretory end pieces. The analogy to a bunch of grapes has already been presented, with the grapes representing the secretory end pieces and the stalks representing the duct system (Fig. 17-6). Thus, following the pattern set by

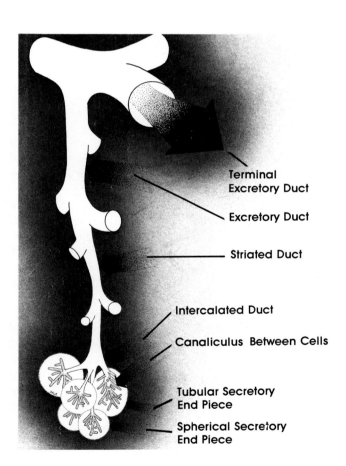

FIG. 17-6   Ductal system of a salivary gland.

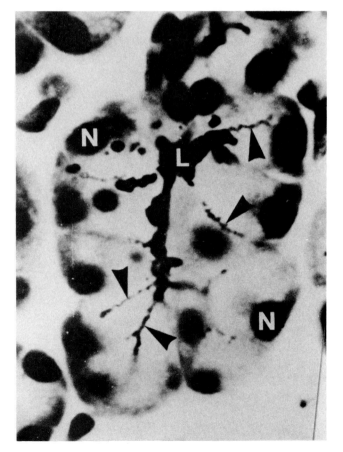

FIG. 17-7   Preparation of an acinus in which the ductal system is displayed. The arrowheads indicate that the system extends between individual cells comprising the acinus.

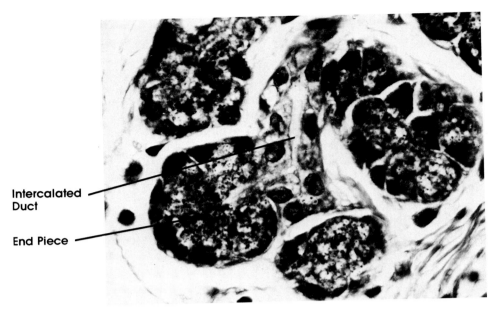

Intercalated
Duct

End Piece

FIG. 17-8 Spherical terminal secretory end piece or spherical acinus. The end pieces are composed of seromucous cells, and their central lumina communicate directly with the intercalated duct.

development, the main secretory duct of the salivary gland breaks up into a series of progressively smaller ducts *(the striated ducts)*, which in turn branch into smaller *intercalated ducts* that open into the blind terminal secretory end pieces, which end as microvillus-lined canaliculi between the parenchymal cells (Figs. 17-7, 17-13, and 17-17). It is also easy to understand how every epithelial cell is supported by connective tissue, even though at times this is tenuous.

Terminal end pieces demonstrate great diversity in size, shape, and cell numbers when seen in section. The shape of end pieces varies from simple circular outlines to tubular outlines to multilobed polygons. They consist of a collection of cells, polygonal in section, supported by a basement membrane that encloses a central space, the lumen. The intercellular spaces between the cells open into the lumina, and technically these spaces constitute the start of the ductal system. In serous glands (e.g., the parotid) the cells in an end piece tend to be arranged in a roughly spherical form around a narrow lumen (Fig. 17-8). In mucinous glands they tend to be arranged in a tubular and/or polygonal configuration with a larger central lumen (Fig. 17-9).

Three cell types may be found in a terminal secretory

end piece: mucous cells, serous cells, and myoepithelial cells. The number and distribution of each type of cell vary from gland to gland and from secretory end piece to secretory end piece.

The basement membrane is continuous around the terminal end piece and the ducts. It forms a complex tubular scaffolding within which the epithelial cells are arranged, and it probably influences the maintenance of normal glandular architecture.

The terminal secretory end piece is also known as an acinus, but the use of this term is confusing. Past practice has been to refer to the spherical serous end piece as an acinus and to the mucus-secreting component end piece as a tubular secretory unit. When a tubular end piece is sectioned obliquely or transversely, however, the appearance of an acinus is created (Fig. 17-9). If the term acinus is to be used to describe the morphology of the gland, it should be qualified as spherical acinus or tubular acinus.

The secretory cells in a salivary gland are described as either serous or mucous. Whereas they exhibit differing histologic features and their secretory products vary, the processes of synthesis and secretion are similar.

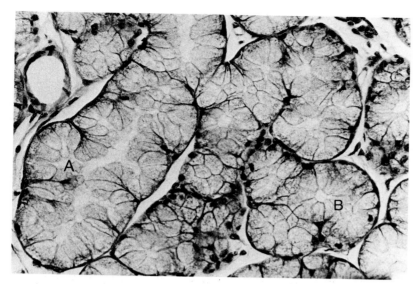

FIG. 17-9 **A,** Tubular polygonal secretory end pieces of mucous cells. **B,** At *right* the end pieces cut in cross section can be seen. Note that they then resemble spherical end pieces. Because mucus does not stain with eosin, the cells appear clear.

Saliva is formed in the secretory end pieces and consists of two components—a macromolecular component derived from the synthetic and secretory activity of the acinar cells and a fluid component derived from the blood. Although the former process is reasonably well understood, the latter is less clear.

Formation of the macromolecular component

The structure of the acinar cells is typical for cells involved in synthesis and secretion: abundant rough endoplasmic reticulum, prominent Golgi complexes, and numerous secretory vesicles. It is clear that the Golgi complex plays a central role in synthesis and secretion—involved as it is in protein transport, concentration, and modification, secretory granule and lysosome formation, and the regulation of membrane traffic throughout the cell.

Proteins, synthesized in the rough endoplasmic reticulum, are shuttled to the Golgi complexes in transport vesicles, where after further modification they are packaged into secretory granules and then transferred to the cell surface where, after fusion of the granulated unit membranes with the surface cell membranes and rupture, they are released to the external environment: a simple enough concept described as *exocytosis*, but one that involves a rather complicated process. As a secretory granule approaches the cell membrane, several events occur: removal of the web of microfilaments beneath the plasma membrane, fusion of the granule and cell membranes, rupture and rearrangement of the lipid layers of both to permit continuity of the granule membrane and cell membrane. Clearly this process, involving the addition of secretory granule membrane to plasma membrane, results in an overall increase in cell surface; thus a compensatory deletion mechanism must exist. Following the pharmacologically stimulated secretion of acinar cells, numerous small vesicles are found in the apical cytoplasm, indicating that endocytosis provides this compensatory mechanism. Indeed, when such vesicles are labeled they can be traced to lysosomes, the Golgi apparatus, or condensing vacuoles. This evidence, combined with biochemical evidence showing that the membrane surrounding the secretory granule derives from the Golgi apparatus and has a much longer halflife than the protein of the granule, provides clear evidence for reutilization.

Formation of the fluid component

This is an active process. Salivary glands are able to secrete their own weight every 15 minutes for up to 1 hour when appropriately stimulated, and such a rate of secretion would simply not be possible if a simple filtration mechanism were responsible for fluid transport.

After appropriate stimulation (discussed later) it is thought that free Ca^{2+} is released from a storage site within the endoplasmic reticulum. Free cytoplasmic Ca^{2+} concentration can increase five- to tenfold in seconds after such stimulation, and this brings about significant compensatory changes that include the opening of two membrane ion channels for passage of K^+ and Cl^-, with the chlorine channel confined to the luminal surface of the cell and the potassium channel to the basolateral surface. When potassium is released from the cell, a compensatory uptake of Na^+ and Cl^- occurs.

Cl^- exits the cell through the channels at the luminal surface; and it is speculated that, to maintain electrical neutrality, Na^+ enters the lumen through the paracellular pathway (Fig. 17-10). The result of these ionic relocations is a flux of water into the lumen via the osmotic coupling of NaCl and H_2O. Although the sodium chloride flux is (as explained) reasonably well understood, the pathway for the flux of water has been debated largely because, for a number of years, it was generally assumed that cell membranes exhibit low permeability to water. Recent studies on gallbladder epithelium, however, have shown that such cells are highly permeable to water and that the smallest changes in osmolarity are sufficient to drive large water fluxes. As a result it is now thought that the production of salivary fluid also is a transcellular event. Given this description of salivary production by the acinus we shall now consider the individual secretory cells.

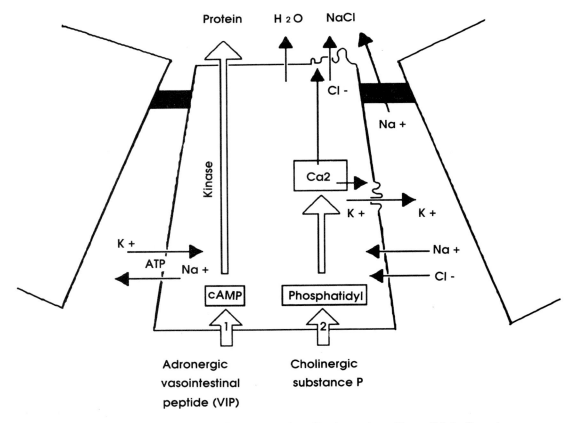

FIG. 17-10 Mechanisms for salivary secretion. (Redrawn from Baum BJ: In Screebny L [ed]: *The salivary system,* Boca Raton, Fla, 1987, CRC Press.)

Serous Cells

The so-called serous cell in human salivary glands also secretes demonstrable amounts of polysaccharide, and therefore these cells are more properly known as seromucous cells. Under the light microscope a seromucous cell is readily identifiable as pyramid shaped with its apex situated toward the central lumen. Its nucleus is spherical and situated in the basal third of the cell. Its cytoplasm stains intensely with hematoxylin and eosin (H&E), giving the cell its characteristic dark color. In some H&E–stained sections, especially after good fixation, the apical cytoplasm can be seen to contain eosinophilic secretory granules about 1 μm in diameter (Fig. 17-11).

With the increased resolution of an electron microscope the seromucous cell is found to have all the features of a cell specialized for the synthesis, storage, and secretion of protein (Fig. 17-12). It has large amounts of rough endoplasmic reticulum arranged in parallel stacks packed basally and laterally to the nucleus. It also has a prominent Golgi complex situated either apically or laterally to the nucleus. Its apical cytoplasm is filled with secretory granules, each surrounded by a unit membrane. In common with most other cells, sero-

mucous cells contain cytoplasmic organelles (e.g., mitochondria, found toward the lateral and basal portions of the cell, lysosomes, free ribosomes, a few microbodies or peroxisomes, microfilaments, and microtubules). It should be appreciated that this secretory process is continuous but cyclical, so that in any end piece seromucous cells at differing stages in the secretory cycle may be found.

In a seromucous end piece the cells are supported by a basement membrane that separates the parenchyma from connective tissue. The relationship between the basement membrane and the seromucous cell that it supports is complicated and shows considerable variation. A straight relationship may exist, with both the basement membrane and the basal plasma membrane in close apposition. On the other hand, the space between the basement membrane and the basal plasma membrane may be increased by complex foldings of the basal plasma membrane, especially when the cell is not distended with secretory material. In the submandibular gland, seromucous cells possess a more complicated basal specialization than in the parotid gland. The plasma membrane is thrown into a series of tall narrow basal folds extending beyond the lateral bor-

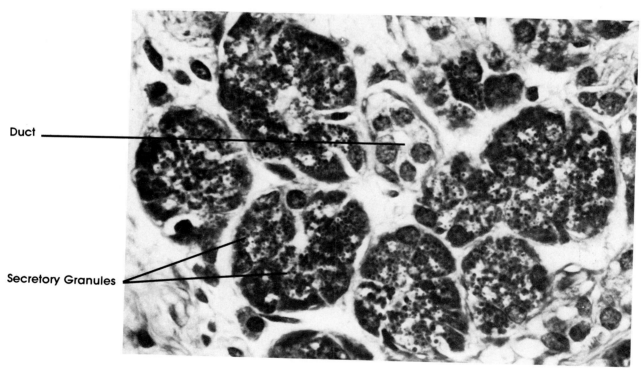

Duct

Secretory Granules

FIG. 17-11 Seromucous cells surrounding an intercalated duct. The cells are roughly pyramidal with basally situated nuclei. Their cytoplasm stains intensely with hematoxylin and is characterized by the presence of many secretory granules. (Compare with Figure 17-12.)

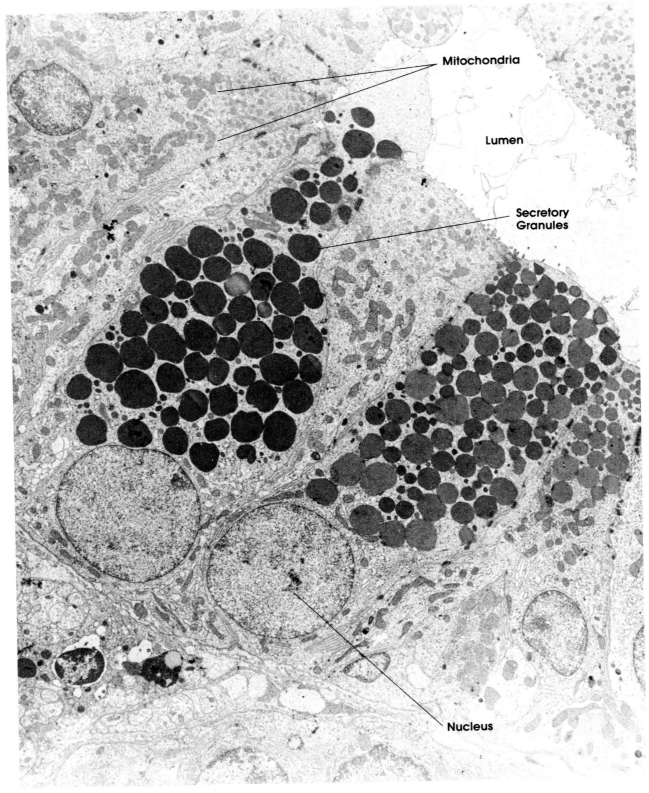

Mitochondria

Lumen

Secretory
Granules

Nucleus

FIG. 17-12   Electron micrograph of seromucous cells at differing stages in ther secretory cycle. Those with dense granules are at the terminal stage. (Courtesy Dr. A. Tamarin.)

ders of the cell as foot processes that penetrate deeply into recesses in the folds of adjoining cells. Thus these cells have the appearance of multipointed stars when viewed from above. This specialization is estimated to increase the basal region of the cell by a factor of 60.

Laterally adjoining seromucous cells also have complex interrelationships. A well-defined intercellular space (or canaliculus) continues from the lumen of the end piece between these cells. The canaliculus terminates in the form of a classic junctional complex consisting of, in order, a tight junction (zonula occludens), an intermediate junction (zonula adherens), and a desmosome (macula adherens). At various points in this canalicular complex apposing cells may contact and join in the form of desmosomal contacts and gap junctions.

The surface of the seromucous cell, lining both the central lumen and the canaliculi, possesses delicate microvilli that extend into the luminal and canalicular spaces.

The complex foldings of these cell surfaces are a reflection of their function of transporting fluid and electrolytes from the serum to saliva (Fig. 17-13). Thus the seromucous cell is structurally adapted to fulfilling its varied purposes.

Although the histology of all seromucous cells is fairly similar, it should be realized that physiologically the secretion of any seromucous cell may vary considerably. In fact, the granules of seromucous cells in the parotid, submandibular, and sublingual glands are morphologically all different, varying in electron density.

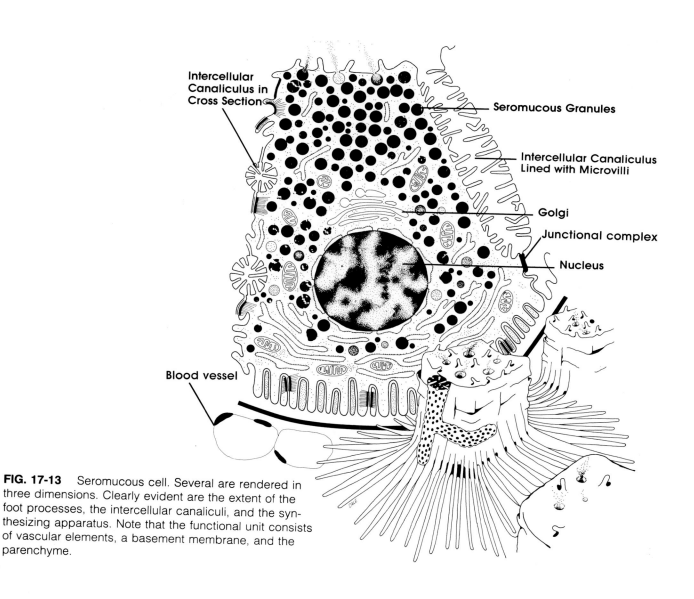

FIG. 17-13 Seromucous cell. Several are rendered in three dimensions. Clearly evident are the extent of the foot processes, the intercellular canaliculi, and the synthesizing apparatus. Note that the functional unit consists of vascular elements, a basement membrane, and the parenchyme.

Mucous Cell

The mucous cell is also well adapted for the production, storage, and secretion of proteinaceous material. Its secretory product differs from that of the seromucous cell in that there is a smaller enzymatic component and the proteins are linked to greater amounts of carbohydrate material—forming mucins. These differences are reflected in the stucture of the cell. Under the light microscope a mucous cell appears as pyramidal with a flattened nucleus situated toward its base. The apical portion of the cell does not stain strongly with H&E (in marked contrast to the seromucous cell) because of its higher carbohydrate content (Fig. 17-14). On the other hand, if a mucous cell is stained specifically for carbohydrates, its apical cytoplasm stains intensely (Fig. 17-15).

Ultrastructurally the mucous cell (Fig. 17-16) differs from the seromucous cell in that it contains more prominent Golgi complexes (which reflect the cell's increased carbohydrate metabolism) and its secretory material is stored in droplets. In resting cells the rough endoplasmic reticulum and other cytoplasmic organelles (e.g., mitochondria) are less conspicuous than in seromucous cells and are mainly confined to the base and lateral aspects of the cell. The interdigitations between adjacent mucous cells tend to be fewer than between seromucous cells. Intercellular canaliculi are found leading to demilunes and also occur between mucous cells (Fig. 17-17). In the submandibular and sublingual glands, mucous cells have a fairly complex system of basal folds; in the labial glands, mucous cells exhibit complex lateral interdigitations.

Secretory granules

Both the seromucous and the mucous cell package their products in secretory granules, and reference has been made to the structural variations of these granules. The variations are described as monopartite for granules containing a dense homogeneous matrix, bipartite for granules with a denser spherical inclusion, and tripartite for granules with a crescent-shaped component adhering to the inner surface of the membrane and enclosing the granule. Despite reports that such structural variations are confined to specific cell types in specific glands, all variations have been found in both serous and mucous cells of all glands. It has been suggested that these variations reflect the stage of maturation of the granule; but evidence is firmer that, because the secretory cells are able to produce a variety of proteins, these structural variations represent the proportional syntheses of different materials.

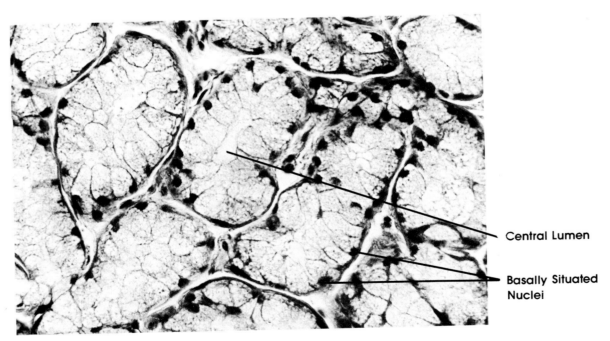

Central Lumen

Basally Situated Nuclei

FIG. 17-14   Mucous cells. Note that they are pyramid shaped with basally situated flattened and condensed nuclei. Their cytoplasm appears empty in this H&E—stained section.

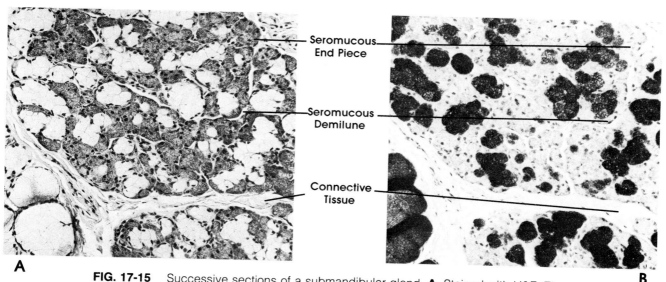

Seromucous End Piece

Seromucous Demilune

Connective Tissue

A

B

FIG. 17-15 Successive sections of a submandibular gland. **A,** Stained with H&E. The mucous units appear unstained. **B,** Stained with periodic—acid Schiff to show mucus; the previously clear cells are now heavily pigmented.

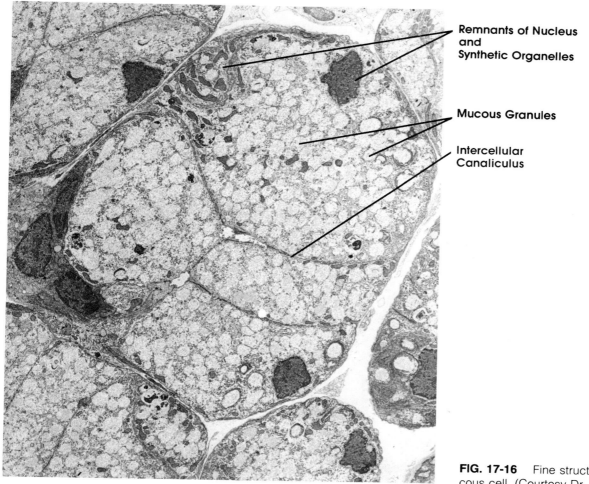

Remnants of Nucleus and Synthetic Organelles

Mucous Granules

Intercellular Canaliculus

FIG. 17-16 Fine structure of a mucous cell. (Courtesy Dr. A. Tamarin.)

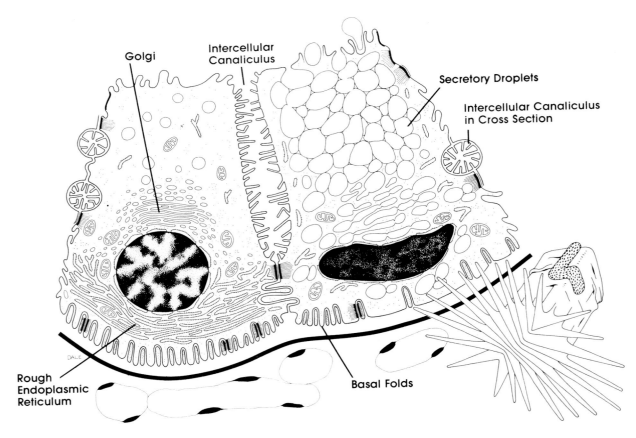

FIG. 17-17 Two mucous cells in section at differing stages of their secretory cycle. The one at right corresponds to that in Figure 17-15.

The identification of a cell as seromucous or mucous by microscopy can be problematic because mucous cells at different stages of the functional cycle have different appearances. Thus a mucous cell at the beginning of its synthetic cycle may stain well with hematoxylin and closely resemble a seromucous cell. Recent studies taking this similarity into account have shown that the labial glands (previously regarded as mixed glands) are in fact mucous glands. It could be that some of the mixed secretory end pieces in submandibular and sublingual glands are also entirely mucous cells, but this has not been established.

Myoepithelial Cells

The myoepithelial cell is found close to the terminal secretory end piece and the intercalated duct, occupying the space between basement membrane and basal plasma membrane of the secretory epithelial cells. There is usually one myoepithelial cell per secretory end piece, but two or three are not uncommon. Only their nuclei are visible in ordinary H&E–stained light microscope sections.

The morphology of a myoepithelial cell depends on its location. Cells associated with the secretory end pieces have been likened to an octopus sitting on a rock (Figs. 17-18 and 17-19). Each cell consists of a central body (where the nucleus is situated) from which four to eight processes radiate and embrace the long axis of the secretory unit (from which other processes branch). The net effect is that the secretory end pieces are encompassed by processes of the myoepithelial cells running between the basement membrane and plasma membrane of the secretory cells in depressions on their surface. Desmosomal attachments are present between the myoepithelial cells and the underlying secretory cells to provide structural stability and prevent the processes from sliding over the acinar or duct cells during contraction. These processes contain many microfilaments (myofilaments) that frequently aggregate to form dark bodies along the course of the process. The microfilaments can be demonstrated by using immunofluorescence techniques to provide precise identification of myoepithelial cells in section (Fig. 17-20). The normal cytoplasmic organelles found in any cell are mainly

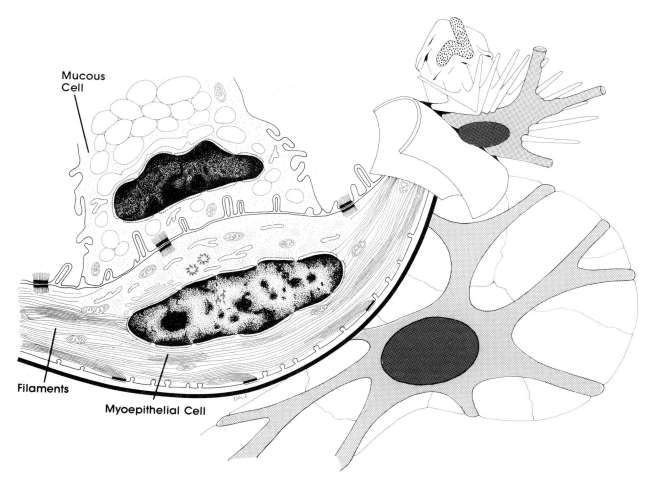

Mucous
Cell

Filaments

Myoepithelial Cell

FIG. 17-18   Myoepithelial cell from two aspects.

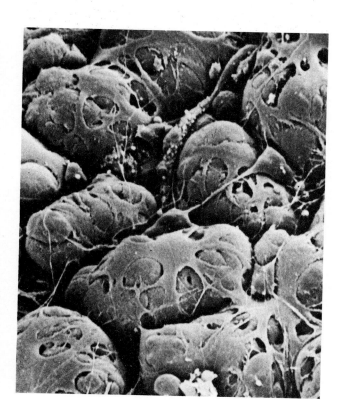

FIG. 17-19   Scanning electron micrograph of myoepithelial cells "clasping" terminal end pieces in an exocrine gland. (From Nagato T, et al: *Cell Tissue Res* 209:1, 1980.)

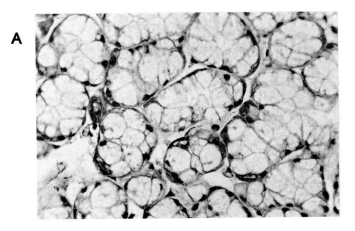

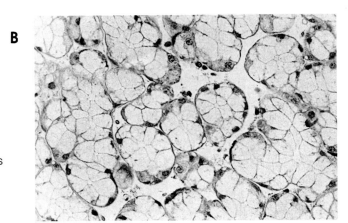

FIG. 17-20 Shows the distribution of myoepithelial cells in a rat sublingual gland stained using immunocyto-chemical techniques. **A** indicates actin filaments, and **B** myosin filaments. (Courtesy Drs. M. Shimino, T. Tsuji, T. Yamamura, O. Watanabe, and T. Ikeno.)

located in the perinuclear region of the cell. The cytoplasm has been described as being sequestered into filamentous and nonfilamentous portions. The stromal surface of the cell has many invaginations containing neural elements that influence the cell's function.

Myoepithelial cells related to the intercalated ducts are more spindle shaped and have fewer processes. On occasion some are found with the cell body situated in the intercalcated duct region with processes extending backward onto parts of the secretory end piece.

The ultrastructural features of myoepithelial cells are very similar to those of smooth muscle cells (Fig. 17-21). The microfilaments, desmosomal attachments, and dark bodies are each found in myoepithelial cells as well as in smooth muscle cells. Because of this similarity, myoepithelial cells are thought to have several possible functions, all related to the ability to contract. One function may be to act as a support for the secretory cells, preventing overdistention as secretory products accumulate within the cytoplasm. Another may be to contract and widen the diameter of the intercalated ducts, thus lowering or raising their resistance to out-

flow. Finally, a third may be to aid in the rupture of acinar cells packed with mucus secretion. The origin of myoepithelial cells has not yet been determined. They are generally considered to be of epithelial origin because of being situated between the parenchyma cell and its basement membrane.

The histology of a terminal secretory end piece having thus far been described, it is worth recapitulating how the constituent cells are assembled to form end pieces of different morphology and function in any salivary gland. First is the spherical end piece consisting usually of seromucous cells (Fig. 17-8). Second is the tubular end piece consisting of mucous cells intermixed with some seromucous cells and often capped by a crescent of seromucous cells, known as a demilune (Fig. 17-22), that discharge their secretion into the tubular lumen via intercellular canaliculi running between the mucous cells. Third is the tubular end piece consisting solely of mucous cells (Fig. 17-9). A salivary gland can therefore consist of a varied mixture of acinar and tubular secretory end pieces. Often whole lobes tend to consist of similar morphologic units (Fig. 17-23).

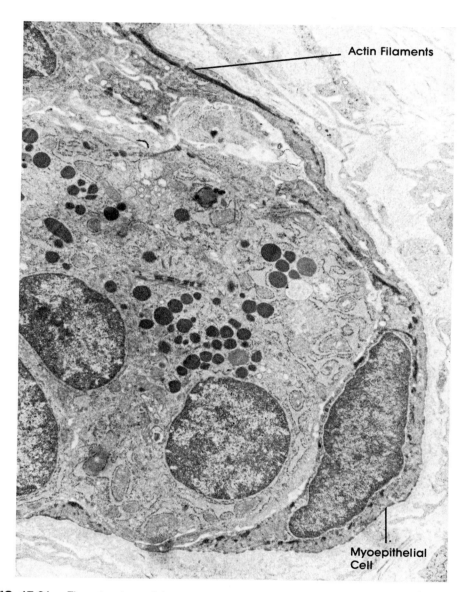

Actin Filaments

Myoepithelial Cell

FIG. 17-21 Fine structure of the myoepithelial cell. Note the actin filaments. (Courtesy Dr. A. Tamarin.)

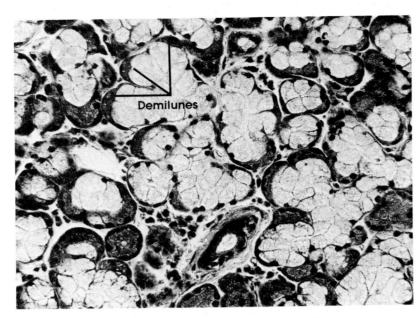

FIG. 17-22 Photomicrograph of a human sublingual gland. The tubular end piece is "capped" by a demilune of seromucous cells.

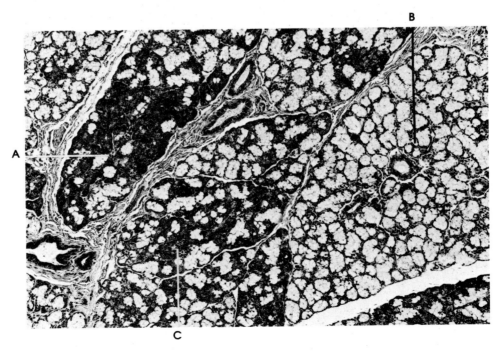

FIG. 17-23 Salivary gland. One lobule *(A)* consists predominantly of serous cells, another *(B)* of mucous cells, and a third *(C)* of both.

DUCTAL SYSTEM

The ductal system of salivary glands comprises a varied network of ducts characterized by progressively smaller membranes. The network contains three classes of ducts: intercalated, striated, and terminal. The system is not a simple conduit, for it actively participates in the production and modulation of saliva.

Intercalated Ducts

The secretion of the terminal end pieces passes first through the intercalated ducts (Fig. 17-24). These ducts are of small diameter and lined by short cuboidal cells with centrally placed nuclei and little cytoplasm containing some rough endoplasmic reticulum situated basally and some Golgi complexes apically. Secretory granules are occasionally found in these cells, especially in cells closest to the secretory end piece. These cuboidal cells have a few microvilli projecting into the lumen of the duct, and their lateral borders interdigitate with each other and interconnect by means of junctional complexes situated apically as well as by scattered desmosomal attachments below the junctional complexes. Myoepithelial cells, or their processes, are usually present between the basement membrane and the ductal cells. A high degree of structural pleomorphism has been described in the intercalated ducts of human labial and soft palate glands with respect to arrangement, location, length, diameter, and epithelial thickness within individual lobules. The simplest form of duct is lined by simple cuboidal epithelium. In human soft palate salivary glands the intercalated ducts are usually relegated to connective tissue septa, are long and highly convoluted, and consist of mucus-secreting cells, simple cuboidal epithelial cells, and myoepithelial cells. The functional activity of intercalated duct cells is not properly understood. Intercalated ducts are especially prominent in salivary glands having a watery secretion and therefore occur frequently in the parotid gland. They may be difficult to distinguish if embedded in a mass of secretory units.

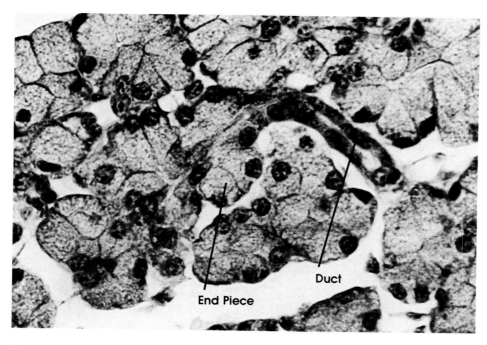

FIG. 17-24   Intercalated duct stemming from a seromucous end piece. Note the short cuboidal cells making up the duct.

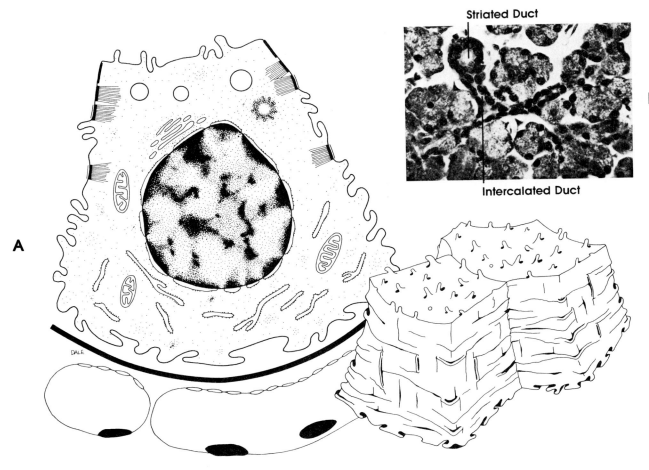

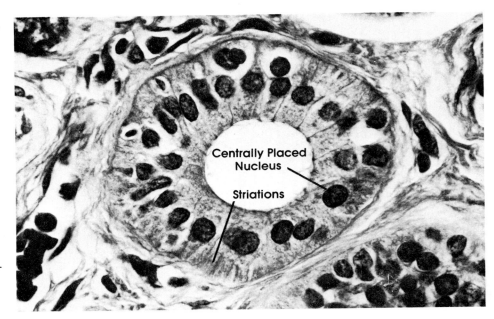

FIG. 17-25 Intercalated duct. In **A** note that the functional unit consists of vascular elements, a basement membrane, and the parenchyme. In **B** it is seen passing into a striated duct.

FIG. 17-26 Higher magnification photomicrograph of a striated duct. Note the associated clear cells.

Striated Ducts

The intercalated duct passes into the striated duct (Fig. 17-25). Striated ducts are lined by columnar cells, which have centrally placed nuclei and intensely eosinophilic cytoplasm, making the ducts clearly recognizable in H&E—stained sections. The most characteristic feature of such cells, however, is their prominent striations at the basal ends of the cells, giving the ducts their name (Fig. 17-26). These striations are seen by electron microscopy as particularly deep indentations of the basal plasma membrane into the cell (Fig. 17-27). They also extend beyond the lateral boundaries of the cell as a series of foot processes that, in turn, possess complex secondary extensions. The lateral processes interlock in a highly complex fashion with adjacent cells and at the same time provide a large increase in the surface area of the basal plasma membrane. Many elongated mitochondria following the long axis of the folds occur in the cytoplasm between the folds. Around the nucleus a few profiles of rough endoplasmic reticulum

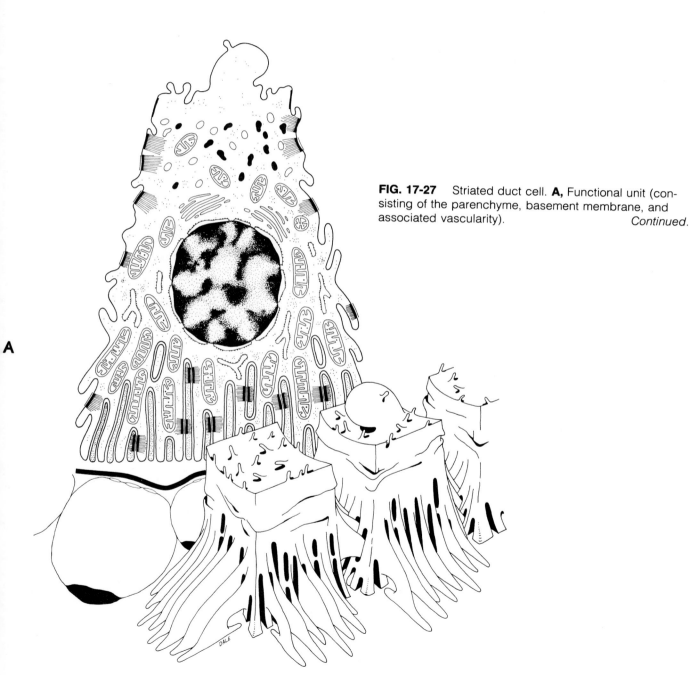

A

FIG. 17-27 Striated duct cell. **A,** Functional unit (consisting of the parenchyme, basement membrane, and associated vascularity). *Continued.*

FIG. 17-27, cont'd.   B, Electron micrograph in which the many mitochondria and basal foldings can be identified.

are found, along with some Golgi complexes. The apical cytoplasm often contains a few scattered vesicles, smooth endoplasmic reticulum, free ribosomes, and lysosomes. The luminal surface of the striated cell is characterized by short stubby microvilli, and again adjacent cells are united by junctional complexes and desmosomal attachments (Fig. 17-27). Occasional dark cells containing numerous mitochondria and scattered small basal cells are usually also present. Striated ducts are always surrounded by a number of longitudinally oriented small blood vessels (Fig. 17-28).

Interspersed between cells of the ductal epithelium of both intercalated and striated ducts are cells described simply as clear cells (Fig. 17-26). They are thought to be of two types, one macrophagelike and the other lymphocytic, and both are involved in immune surveillance.

The specialized structure of the striated ducts implies a particular function: they modify the secretions passing through them. Recall that this fluid is characterized by an isotonic protein content, a high sodium content (hypertonic), and a low potassium content (hypotonic). As it passes along the striated duct, it changes to a generally hypotonic state (low and concentrations). The massive infoldings of the basal plasma membrane, associated with the elongated mitochondria, are thought to reflect the sodium-pumping capacity of the cell wall in this location. Thus sodium, extracted from the cell, passes into the tissue fluid and establishes a concentration gradient between the cell and the luminar fluid. Sodium therefore diffuses into the cells from the luminal fluid; at the same time active transport of potassium occurs in the opposite direction. Bicarbonate ions are also actively secreted. Because under normal conditions of flow the striated duct cells do not absorb water, these ionic changes result in the formation of a hypotonic solution.

Terminal Excretory Ducts

After passing through the striated ducts, salivary fluid is secreted into the oral cavity through the terminal excretory ducts. The histology of these ducts varies as they pass from the striated ducts to the oral cavity. Near the striated ducts they are lined by a pseudostratified epithelium consisting of tall columnar cells (much like striated cells) admixed with small basal cells; goblet cells also occur (Fig. 17-29). As the terminal secretory ducts approach the oral cavity, their epithelium changes to a true stratified epithelium merging with that of the oral cavity at the ductal orifice. The main excretory ducts modify the final saliva by altering its electrolyte concentration and perhaps also adding a mucoid component. Special eosinophilic cells, loaded with mitochondria, tend to be found in the ducts, particularly in mucosal glands. These cells, known as oncocytes, probably represent an age change. The structure of a typical gland is illustrated in Figure 17-30.

This completes the formal description of salivary gland parenchyma. There is, however, one further observation that needs to be made. It is now recognized that, once development is completed, turnover of the parenchyma occurs, with continued replacement of acinar cells following their apoptotic deletion. This replacement is achieved by cell division at all sites within the parenchyma. That this is so has only recently been worked out; and as a result a number of theories to explain turnover exist, all linked to provide a satisfactory classification for salivary gland tumors.

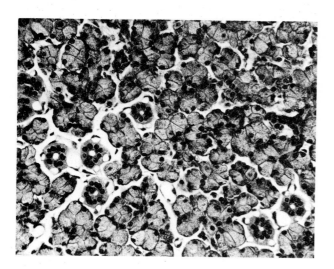

FIG. 17-28 Section of striated ducts. Each is surrounded by a number of blood vessels.

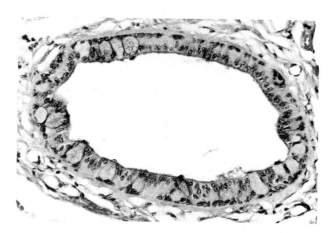

FIG. 17-29 Terminal secretory duct. The pseudostratified nature of the epithelium and the numerous goblet cells can be seen. Note the associated blood vessels.

FIG. 17-30 Typical salivary gland. **A,** Seromucous end piece; **A'**, cross section. **B,** Seromucous demilune; **B'**, cross section. **C,** Mucous end piece; **C'**, cross section. **D,** Intercalated duct; **D'**, cross section. **E,** Striated duct; **E'**, cross section. **F,** Terminal excretory duct.

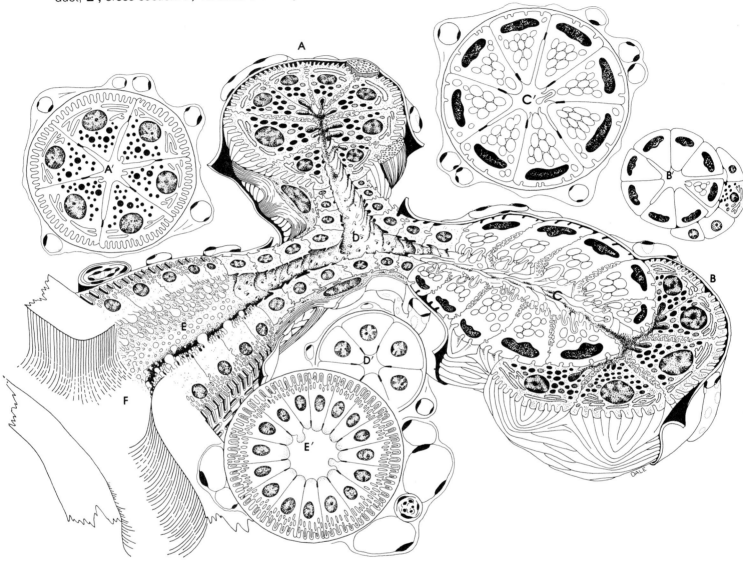

CONNECTIVE TISSUE

The connective tissue component of the salivary glands is the same as connective tissue elsewhere and comprises fibroblasts, macrophages, mast cells, adipose cells, and plasma cells all embedded in an extracellular matrix of collagen fibers and a ground substance of glycoproteins and proteoglycans. Oxytalan fibers are found in the submandibular and minor salivary glands. They are located in connective tissue supporting the mucous end pieces and around the smaller intralobular ducts and are thought to substitute for the elastic fibers that surround the larger extralobular ducts. The connective tissue stroma of the salivary glands serves to carry the nerves and blood vessels (which are both highly specialized).

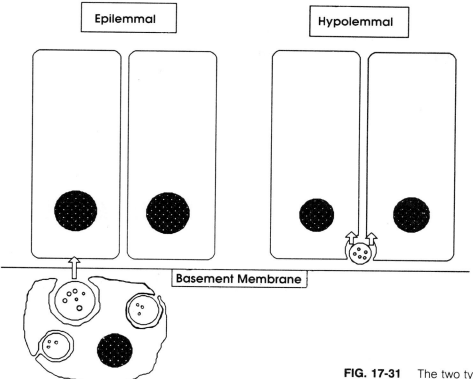

FIG. 17-31 The two types of innervation found in salivary glands.

NERVE SUPPLY

In most glands secretory activity is controlled by impulses reaching the cells via secretomotor nerves. In some glands, especially the smaller mucosal glands, a slow background of spontaneous secretion may occur independently of neural control. Salivary gland innervation is especially complicated; currently available information, obtained from the study of glands from many species, indicates that the glands receive postganglionic secretomotor nerves from both sympathetic and parasympathetic sources but there are wide variations among species, among the glands, and among cell types in the same gland. Despite these complexities in innervation patterns, it is possible to recognize (morphologically at least) two patterns of innervation.

Nerves entering the salivary glands follow the blood vessels and break up into progressively smaller bundles until they form a final plexus adjacent to the terminal parenchyma. In this plexus the nerves consist of unmyelinated axons embedded in Schwann cell cytoplasm. From here they are distributed to muscle arterioles, to secretory cells of the terminal end pieces, to myoepithelial cells, and to cells of the intercalated and striated ducts. It is now that the two patterns of innervation are established (Fig. 17-31).

In the first (described as *epilemmal*) axons remain in the connective tissue separated from the secretory cells by the basement membrane. Where such axons come close to a secretory cell, they lose their Schwann cell covering, and in the adjacent exoplasm many vesicles containing transmitter substances exist. Presumably, some of the neurotransmitter substance is released when a nerve impulse passes and diffuses some 100 to 200 nm across the basement membrane before influencing the secretory cell. In the second *(hypolemmal)* axons penetrate the basement membrane, losing their Schwann cell covering in the process, and run between the secretory cells, separated from them by a gap of only 10 to 20 nm. Small beadings occur along the course of these "bare" axons at sites where small vesicles and many mitochondria are often accumulated and where transmitter substance is considered to be principally released. With this type of innervation a single axon may quickly affect several secretory cells or the small cell several times.

In the ductal system, innervation is usually confined the connective tissue.

The flow of saliva is controlled entirely by nervous stimulation (Fig. 17-32). Generally it is considered that β-adrenergic (sympathetic) stimulation particularly induces protein secretory mechanisms whereas L-adrenergic and cholinergic stimulation regulates water and electrolyte release.

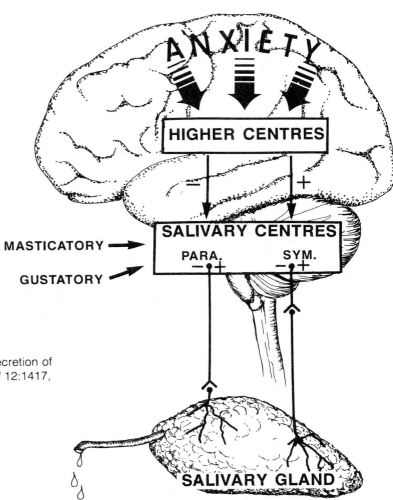

FIG. 17-32 Nerve pathways involved in the secretion of saliva. (Modified from Garrett JR: *Arch Oral Biol* 12:1417, 1967.)

It is important to recognize here that there is no direct inhibitory innervation of the salivary glands. The nervous "dry mouth," long thought to be the result of sympathetic inhibition as part of the fight and flight response, is explained by the direct inhibitory influence of higher centers on medullary centers.

In summary then: normal active reflex secretion of saliva involves the centrally coordinated formation of

1. Parasympathetic impulses, which tend to be more prevalent and
   a. May occur in isolation
   b. Usually evoke most of the fluid secreted
   c. Cause variable degrees of exocytosis from some cells
   d. Induce contraction of myoepithelial cells
   e. Cause vasodilation as part of the secretory process
   f. May have a direct influence on resynthesis

2. Sympathetic impulses, which are likely to occur more intermittently and
   a. Act essentially on cells receiving parasympathetic impulses (and thus produce synergistic effects)
   b. Often do not cause much mobilization of fluid
   c. Tend to modulate the composition of saliva by increasing exocytosis from certain cells

Neurotransmitters

Stimulation of cellular activity is achieved by the release of neurotransmitters, principally norepinephrine and acetylcholine. These substances, found in small vesicular structures of approximately 40 nm diameter, appear agranular in cholinergic axons and granular in adrenergic axons. Scattered larger (80 to 120 nm) dense-cored granular vesicles also occur in axons and are thought to be the site of various other neurotransmitter peptides such as substance P and VIP (vasoactive intestinal peptide).

Although there is some evidence that the conventional transmitters are released in subminimal amounts without any stimulation, when stimulated neurons appear capable of releasing inexhaustable amounts of acetylcholine and norepinephrine. On the other hand, the release of any neuropeptide requires high-frequency stimulation and its supply is soon exhausted.

Regardless, when the neurotransmitter is released it affects the parenchymal cell by binding with cell surface receptors and initiating further signaling mechanisms within the cell. Two such mechanisms occur (Fig. 17-10): one involves the generation of cyclic adenosine monophosphate (AMP), and the other a breakdown of phosphatidylinositol-4,5-biphosphate (with the breakdown products serving as intracellular messengers). Cyclic AMP generation results from adrenergic stimulation, which activates protein kinase to stimulate the secretion of protein, whereas cholinergic transmitters stimulate the second system, ultimately releasing free calcium (whose effect has already been described).

It is also known that a salivary reflex exists involving periodontal receptors.

Finally, in addition to neurotransmitter regulation, hormones exert varying levels of salivary gland regulation. The hormones include estrogens, androgens, glucocorticoids, and peptide hormones. Although they can cause modification of salivary constituents, hormones cannot themselves initiate the flow of saliva. Myoepithelial cells contract because of impulses from both sympathetic and parasympathetic systems.

BLOOD SUPPLY

An extensive blood supply to the salivary glands is required for the rapid secretion of saliva (which is 99% water). One or more arteries enter the gland and give rise to numerous arterioles, which tend to run in a countercurrent direction around the ducts. These vessels branch into a dense distribution of capillaries, particularly around the striated ducts. The distribution of capillaries around the secretory end pieces is not as dense and takes the form of arterial arcades as the capillaries arise from the ends of the vessels supplying the intralobular ducts. Venous return is accomplished by venae comitantes as well as by larger veins that drain directly to the periphery of the gland. Arteriovenous anastomoses are found, related particularly to the acinar circulation. Definitive information concerning the lymphatic drainage is lacking. The pattern of microcirculation reflects the different functional components of a gland: a major concentration of capillaries is found around the striated ducts, where ionic exchange occurs,

whereas a lesser density occurs around the terminal secretory systems. A profound increase in blood flow normally accompanies salivary secretion.

AGE CHANGES

Whether the salivary glands become less active with age is problematic, because such a great variation exists in the secretion of saliva. No longitudinal studies of salivary secretion on a single individual have thus far been reported. Even so, histologic changes associated with age have been reported within the salivary glands. Fatty degenerative changes, fibrosis, and the progressive accumulation of lymphocytes in the salivary glands are thought to occur.

Oncocytes, epithelial cells that can be identified by their marked granularity and acidophilia under the light microscope, are thought to represent an age change, although their significance has not been established. Ultrastructurally, they exhibit an accumulation of structurally altered mitochondria. Oncocytes are found in acini and in the intercalated and striated ducts of salivary glands and may give rise to neoplasms.

CLINICAL CONSIDERATIONS

The rate of saliva production varies throughout the day. Of the 640 ml secreted daily, only about 10 ml is produced at night. This nocturnal reduction in salivary secretion, along with the concomitant loss of its cleansing effect, is one reason why people should brush their teeth before retiring to bed.

Developmental defects of salivary tissue are rare. Diagnostic techniques are now successfully applied to the readily available saliva, and saliva has also become a commonly used source of information regarding the metabolism and clearance of many drugs. In addition, biopsy of the labial gland is easily performed in the diagnosis of some systemic lesions. The most common conditions affecting the salivary glands are inflammatory disorders resulting from bacterial or viral infection (e.g., mumps). Painful swelling is then the usual symptom.

Disease of the salivary glands usually brings about changes in the rate of salivary secretion and composition. These changes have a secondary effect, in that they lead to the formation of plaque and calculus, which in turn has a direct bearing on the initiation of caries and periodontal disease. These diseases may become severe after therapeutic irradiation in and around the mouth.

Obstructions to salivary flow may occur as a result of the formation of salivary calculi (stones) in the ducts, which tend to cause atrophy of the gland with an accompanying loss of function. The submandibular acinar cells often seem more resistant to such atrophic changes than the parotid glands; and the more mucinous glands (e.g., sublingual) are the most resistant. On the other hand, calculi occur most frequently in submandibular glands. Thus the type of gland determines the outcome of ductal obstruction.

MINOR SALIVARY GLANDS

The minor salivary glands—lingual, buccal, and palatal—are small mucosal glands with short ducts that produce a primarily mucoprotein-rich secretion with a high secretory IgA concentration.. The exception is the serous glands of von Ebner. The mucins from these glands come into close contact with the tooth and mucosal surfaces and as a result are important contributors to the protective mechanism of saliva. Since the minor salivary gland secretions are especially rich in mucosubstances, they are assumed to play an important role in the formation of acquired pellicle.

An interesting feature of the minor salivary glands is the occurrence of focal accumulations of lymphocytes around the duct walls (Fig. 17-33), which are thought to have a role to play in the immune surveillance of the mouth.

SUMMARY OF MAJOR SALIVARY GLANDS

The above description of saliva and the glands that produce it has indicated that great differences exist in the composition of saliva from different glands and this composition can vary for each gland at different times. It was stated that considerable variation in salivary gland structure exists, not only from species to species but also within the same species and even within the same gland. Thus an exact description of any one gland at any one time is difficult. It is worthwhile, therefore, to summarize the primary features of the main salivary glands as seen under the light microscope in H&E–stained sections, to aid in their histologic identification.

Parotid Gland

In the parotid gland the terminal secretory end pieces are seromucous (Fig. 17-34). Pyramidal cells, which have a spherical basally situated nucleus, surround a small central lumen. The basal cytoplasm stains blue (basophilic), and in well-fixed sections secretory granules can be seen. In older glands fat cells are readily observable.

Intercalated ducts in the parotid gland are numerous and elongated. In cross and oblique sections they can be found interposed between seromucous acini. They

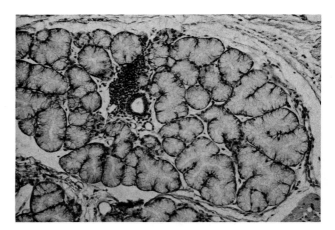

FIG. 17-33 Human retromolar mucous salivary gland showing lymphocytes accumulated around the duct.

have a narrow lumen surrounded by cuboidal cells with a round central nucleus and sparse basophilic cytoplasm.

The striated ducts are easy to recognize and have been described as "pink necklaces" permeating the gland. The cells are columnar and stain intensely pink (acidophilic) with eosin. The nucleus is centrally located; and at higher magnifications the striations can be recognized adjacent to the basement membrane, not the lumen.

Submandibular Gland

Approximately 80% of secretory end pieces in the submandibular gland are seromucous and have the same features as those described in the parotid gland (Fig. 17-35). The remaining secretory units are usually a mixture of mucous and seromucous cells. The mucous secretory cells can be identified by a larger lumen than that of the seromucous unit surrounded by pyramidal cells whose nuclei are flattened and situated basally and by cytoplasm that does not stain very strongly. The mixed units are easy to recognize because of the crescent-shaped caps, or demilunes, of seromucous cells at the terminal ends of the mucus-secreting tubules. Intercalated ducts are shorter in the submandibular gland, and therefore fewer can be found in section. The striated ducts are well developed and longer in the submandibular gland, have the characteristics already described, and pose little difficulty recognizing.

Sublingual Gland

The most variable of the major salivary glands is the small almond-shaped sublingual gland. In H&E–stained preparations the sublingual glands appear to

Seromucous End Piece Striated Duct

Fat Cells

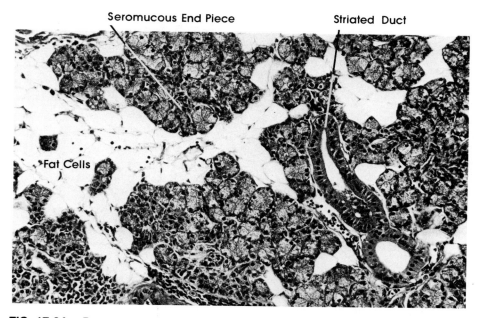

FIG. 17-34　Parotid gland. Seromucous units and striated ducts are clearly seen. The clear areas are fat cells, which accumulate in the gland with age.

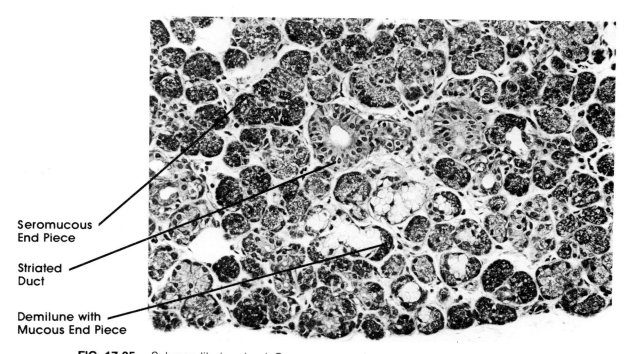

Seromucous End Piece

Striated Duct

Demilune with Mucous End Piece

FIG. 17-35　Submandibular gland. Seromucous and mucous units are present, with seromucous units predominating. Again the striated ducts are easily identified.

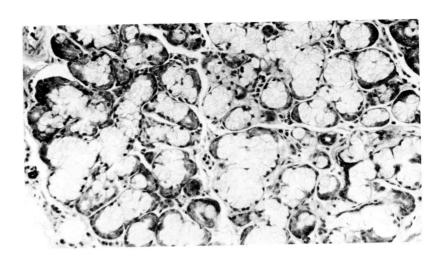

FIG. 17-36 Sublingual gland. Mucus-secreting cells predominate. There are no seromucous end pieces. Instead, seromucous-like units exist in the form of demilunes, capping the mucous end pieces.

have a mixed complement of cells, with individual acini varying according to the cell type. Some end pieces contain large mucus-filled cells, and other end pieces are composed of cells with few secretory granules. All gradations between these two types can be found. Seromucous end pieces are rarely found, but seromucous demilunes capping the mucous tubules exist (Fig. 17-36). Morphologically, then, the sublingual gland is a mixed gland. Intercalated ducts are either extremely short or absent and are difficult to find. Striated ducts also are short and difficult to find and may even be absent. In spite of these morphologic distinctions, histochemical studies indicate that the gland is purely a mucus-secreting gland.

The morphologic heterogeneity of the human sublingual gland appears to be related to the differing stages of maturation exhibited by mucus-producing cells.

BIBLIOGRAPHY

Anderson DJ, Hector MP: Periodontal mechanoreceptors and parotid secretion in animals and man, *J Dent Res* 66:578, 1987.

Ball WD: Development of the rat salivary glands. III. Mesenchymal specificity in the morphogenesis of the embryonic submaxillary and sublingual glands of the rat, *J Exp Zool* 188:277, 1974.

Baum BJ: Regulation of salivary Secretion. In Screebny LM (ed): *The salivary system*, Boca Raton Fla, 1987, CRC Press.

Bellis CJ, Scott FH: Saliva and coagulation of blood, *Proc Soc Exp Biol Med* 30:1373, 1933.

Black JB: The structure of the salivary glands of the human soft palate, *J Morphol* 153:107, 1977.

Bogart BI: The effect of aging on the rat submandibular gland: an ultrastructural, cytochemical and biochemical study, *J Morphol* 130:337, 1970.

Brandtzaeg P: Mucosal and glandular distribution of immunoglobulin components: differential localization of free and bound SC in secretory epithelial cells, *J Immunol* 112:1553, 1974.

Castle JD, Jamieson JD, Palade GE: Radioautographic analysis of the secretory process in the parotid acinar cell of the rabbit, *J Cell Biol* 53:290, 1972.

Cutler LS: Functional differentiation of salivary glands. In Forte J (ed): Salivary, pancreatic, gastric, and hepatobiliary secretion, New York, 1989, American Physiological Society Press, vol 3.

Cutler LS: The role of extracellular matrix in the morphogenesis and differentiation of a salivary gland, *Develop Biol* 4:27, 1990.

Cutler LS, Chaudhry AP: Differentiation of the myoepithelial cells of the rat submandibular gland in vivo and in vitro: an ultrastructural study, *J Morphol* 140:343, 1973.

Dawes C, Wood CM: The contribution of the oral minor mucous gland secretions to the volume of whole saliva in man, *Arch Oral Biol* 18:337, 1973.

Dawes C, Wood CM: The composition of human lip mucous gland secretion, *Arch Oral Biol* 18:343, 1973.

Drummond JR, Chisholm DM: A quantitative and qualitative study of the aging human labial salivary glands, *Arch Oral Biol* 29:151, 1984.

Emmelin N: Nerve interactions in salivary glands, *J Dent Res* 66(2):509, 1987.

Emmelin N, Gjörstrup P: On the function of myoepithelial cells in salivary glands, *J Physiol* 230:185, 1973.

Ferguson DB: Salivary glands and saliva. In Lavell CLB (ed): *Applied physiology of the mouth*, ed 2, Bristol UK, 1975, John Wright & Sons.

Ferguson DB: Current diagnostic uses of saliva, *J Dent Res* 66(2):420, 1987.

Garrett JR: The innervation of normal human submandibular and parotid salivary glands: demonstrated by cholinesterase histochemistry, catecholamine fluorescence and electron microscopy, *Arch Oral Biol* 12:1417, 1967.

Garrett JR: Neuro-effector sites in salivary glands. In Emmelin N, Zotterman Y (eds): *Oral physiology,* New York, 1972, Pergamon Press.

Garrett JR: Structure and innervation of salivary glands. In Cohen B, Kramer I (eds): *Scientific foundations of dentistry,* London, 1976, William Heineman Medical Books.

Garrett JR: The proper role of nerves in salivary secretion, *J Dent Res* 66(2):387, 1987.

Garrett JR: Innervation of salivary glands: neurohistological and functional aspects. In Screebny LM (ed): *The salivary system,* Boca Raton Fla, 1987, CRC Press.

Ham SS, Sreebny L, Suddick R (eds): *Symposium on the mechanism of exocrine secretion,* Ann Arbor, 1973, University of Michigan Press.

Hand AR: The fine structure of von Ebner's gland of the rat, *J Cell Biol* 44:340, 1970.

Hand AR: Morphology and cytochemistry of the Golgi apparatus of rat salivary gland acinar cells, *Am J Anat* 130:141, 1971.

Hand AR: Adrenergic and cholinergic nerve terminals in the rat parotid gland: electron microscopic observations on permanganate-fixed glands, *Anat Rec* 173:131, 1972.

Hand AR: Functional ultrastructure of the salivary glands. In Screeby LM (ed): *The salivary system,* Boca Raton Fla, 1987, CRC Press.

Hensten-Pettersen A: Biological activities in human labial and palatine secretions, *Arch Oral Biol* 20:107, 1975.

Hensten-Pettersen A, Kornstad L: The contribution of the minor mucous glands to the concentrations of blood group specific substances, carbohydrates and proteins in human mixed saliva, *Arch Oral Biol* 21:485, 1976.

Jamieson JD: Biology of the secretory process in exocrine cells. In Rowe NH (ed): *Salivary glands and their secretion. Proceedings of a symposium,* Ann Arbor, 1972, University of Michigan Press.

Kagayama M: The fine structure of the monkey submandibular gland with a special reference to the intra-acinar nerve endings, *Am J Anat* 131:185, 1971.

Kim SK, Nasjleti CE, Han SS: The secretion processes in mucous and serous secretory cells of the rat's sublingual gland, *J Ultrastruct Res* 38:371, 1972.

Kraus FW, Mestecky J: Immunohistochemical localization of amylase, lysozyme and immunoglobulins in the human parotid gland, *Arch Oral Biol* 16:781, 1971.

Levine MJ, Reddy MS, Tabak LA, et al: Structural aspects of salivary glycoproteins, *J Dent Res* 66:436, 1987.

MacFarlane TW: Salivary glands and saliva. In Lavelle CLB (ed): *Applied physiology of the mouth,* ed 2, Bristol UK, 1975, John Wright & Sons.

Mandel L: The labial accessory salivary glands in the diagnosis of systemic disease. In Walker RV (ed): *Oral Surgery,* Edinburgh, 1970, E & S Livingstone.

Mason DK, Chisholm DM (eds): *Salivary glands in health and disease,* Philadelphia, 1975, WB Saunders.

Munger BL: Histochemical studies on seromucous and mucus-secreting cells of human salivary glands, *Am J Anat* 115:411, 1964.

Nagato T, Yoshida H, Yoshida A, Vehara Y: A scanning electron microscope study of myoepithelial cells in exocrine glands, *Cell Tissue Res* 209:1, 1980.

Nair PNR, Schroeder HE: Retrograde access of antigens to the minor salivary glands in the monkey *macaca fascicularis, Arch Oral Biol* 28:145, 1983.

Nair PNR, Zimmerli I, Schroeder HE: Age-related changes of simian duct associated lymphoia tissue (DALT), *J Dent Res* 66(2):407, 1987.

National Institute of Dental Research: *Challenges for the eighties—salivary glands and secretions. Long range research plans, 1985-89,* Publ no. 111, Bethesda, December 1983, NIH.

Newbrun E: What is the relationship of saliva to dental caries activity? In Rowe NH (ed): *Salivary glands and their secretion. Proceedings of a symposium,* Ann Arbor, 1972, University of Michigan Press.

Nour-Eldin F, Wilkinson JH: The blood clotting factors in human saliva, *J Physiol* 136:324, 1957.

Redman RS: Development of the salivary glands. In Screebny LM (ed): *The salivary system,* Boca Raton Fla, 1987, CRC Press.

Riva A, Riva-Testa F: Fine structure of acinar cells of human parotid gland, *Anat Rec* 176:149, 1973.

Riva A, Motta G, Riva-Testa F: Ultrastructural diversity in secretory granules of human major salivary glands, *Am J Anat* 139:293, 1974.

Riva A, Tandler B, Riva-Testa F: Ultrastructure observations on human submandibular gland, *Am J Anat* 181:385, 1988.

Rowe NH (ed): *Salivary glands and their secretion. Proceedings of a symposium,* Ann Arbor, 1972, University of Michigan Press.

Sato Y, Okamoto N, Ikeda T: Observations by electron microscope of the submaxillary glands of human fetuses and newborns, *Hiroshima J Med Sci* 18:233, 1969.

Schneyer LA, Young JA, Schneyer CA: Salivary secretion of electrolytes, *Physiol Rev* 52:720, 1972.

Schroeder HE, Moreillon MC, Nair PNR: Architecture of minor salivary gland duct–lymphoid follicle associations: a possible antigen recognition site in the monkey *macaca fascicularis, Arch Oral Biol* 28:133, 1983.

Schulte W: Saliva and blood coagulation. In Walker RV (ed): *Oral surgery,* Edinburgh, 1970, E & S Livingstone.

Shackleford JM, Schneyer LH: Ultrastructural aspects of the main excretory duct of rat submandibular gland, *Anat Rec* 169:679, 1971.

Shimono M, Yamamura T: Ultrastructure of the oncocyte in normal human palatine salivary glands, *J Electron Microsc* 24:119, 1975.

Spiers RL: Saliva and dental health, *Dent Update* 11(10):605, 1984.

Spiers RL: Secretion of saliva by human lip mucous glands and parotid glands in response to gustatory stimuli and chewing, *Arch Oral Biol* 29(11):945, 1984.

Spooner BS, Wessells NK: An analysis of salivary glands morphogenesis: role of cytoplasmic microfilaments and microtubules, *Develop Biol* 27:38, 1972.

Suddick RP, Dowd FJ: The microvascular architecture of the rat submaxillary gland: possible relationship to secretory mechanisms, *Arch Oral Biol* 14:567, 1969.

Tamarin A, Sreebny LM: The rat submaxillary salivary gland: a correlative study by light and electron microscopy, *J Morphol* 117:295, 1965.

Tandler B: Ultrastructure of the human submaxillary gland. I. Architecture and histological relationships of the secretory cells, *Am J Anat* 111:287, 1962.

Tandler B: Ultrastructure of the human submaxillary gland. II. The base of the striated duct cells, *Am J Ultrastruct Res* 9:65, 1963.

Tandler B: Ultrastructure of the human submaxillary gland. III. Myoepithelium, *Z Zellforsch Microskop Anat* 68:852, 1965.

Tandler B: Fine structure of oncocytes in human salivary glands, *Arch Pathol Anat* 341:317, 1966.

Tandler B: Microstructure of salivary glands. In Rowe NH (ed): *Salivary glands and their secretion. Proceedings of a symposium*, Ann Arbor, 1972, University of Michigan Press.

Tandler B: Salivary gland changes in disease, *J Dent Res* 66(2):398, 1987.

Tandler B: Structure of the human parotid and submandibular glands. In Screebny LM (ed): *The salivary system*, Boca Raton Fla, 1987, CRC Press.

Tandler B, Denning CR, Mandel ID, et al: Ultrastructure of human labial salivary glands. I. Acinar secretory cells, *J Morphol* 127:383, 1969.

Tandler B, Denning CR, Mandel ID, et al: Ultrastructure of human labial salivary glands. III. Myoepithelium and ducts, *J Morphol* 130:227, 1970.

Tandler B, Paulsen JH: Fusion of the envelope of mucous droplets with the luminal plasma membrane in acinar cells of the cat submandibular gland, *J Cell Biol* 68:775, 1976.

Tandler B, Paulsen JH: Ultrastructure of the main excretory duct of the cat submandibular gland, *J Morphol* 149:183, 1976.

Tandler B, Paulsen JH: Ultrastructure of the cat sublingual gland, *Anat Rec* 187:153, 1977.

Taubman MA, Smith DJ: Secretory immunoglobulins and dental disease. In Hans SS, Sreebny L, Suddick R (eds): *Symposium on the mechanism of exocrine secretion*, Ann Arbor, 1973, University of Michigan Press.

Thoma KH: A contribution to the knowledge of the development of the submaxillary and sublingual salivary glands in human embryos, *J Dent Res* 1:95, 1919.

Wheatcroft MG: Saliva and plaque interrelationships. In Rowe NH (ed): *Salivary glands and their secretion. Proceedings of a symposium*, Ann Arbor, 1972, University of Michigan Press.

Yakeda Y, Komori A: Focal lymphocytic infiltrations in the human labial salivary glands: a post mortem study, *J Oral Pathol* 15:83, 1986.

Young JA, Van Lennep EW: Morphology and physiology of salivary myoepithelial cells, *Int Rev Physiol* 12:105, 1977.

Zajicek G, Yagil C, Michaeli Y: The streaming submandibular gland, *Anat Rec* 213:150, 1985.

CHAPTER 18

Oral Mucosa

THE term *mucous membrane* is used to describe the moist lining of the intestinal tract, nasal passages, and other body cavities that communicate with the exterior. In the oral cavity this lining is called the oral mucous membrane, or oral mucosa. At the lips the oral mucosa is continuous with the skin, a dry covering layer whose structure resembles that of the oral lining in some respects; at the pharynx it is continuous with the moist mucosa lining the rest of the intestine. Thus the oral mucosa is situated anatomically between skin and intestinal mucosa and shows some of the properties of each.

The skin, oral mucosa, and intestinal lining each consist of two separate tissue components: a covering epithelium and an underlying connective tissue. Because these tissues together perform a common function, the oral mucosa (like the skin and the intestinal lining) should be considered an organ. It is often easier to understand the complex structure of a tissue or organ when its function is known. This is particularly true of the oral mucosa, whose structure reflects a variety of functional adaptations. The major adaptations are a result of evolutionary changes in the species that have taken place over a very long time. Although small and usually reversible changes in structure may be seen in response to function during the lifetime of an individual, these are not heritable.

FUNCTIONS OF THE ORAL MUCOSA

The oral mucosa serves several functions. The major one is protection of the deeper tissues of the oral cavity. Among its other functions are acting as a sensory organ and serving as the site of some glandular activity.

Protection

As a surface lining the oral mucosa separates and protects deeper tissues and organs in the oral region from the environment of the oral cavity. The normal activities of seizing food and biting and chewing it expose the oral soft tissues to mechanical forces (compression, stretching, shearing) and surface abrasions (from hard particles in the diet). The oral mucosa shows a number of adaptations of both the epithelium and the connective tissue to withstand these insults. Furthermore, there is normally a resident population of microorganisms within the oral cavity that would cause infection if they gained access to the tissues. Many of these organisms also produce substances that have a toxic effect on tissues. The epithelium of the oral mucosa acts as the major barrier to these threats.

Sensation

The sensory function of the oral mucosa is important because it provides considerable information about events within the oral cavity whereas the lips and tongue perceive stimuli outside the mouth. In the mouth there are receptors that respond to temperature, touch, and pain; there also are the taste buds, which are not found anywhere else in the body. Certain receptors in the oral mucosa probably respond to the "taste" of water and signal the satisfaction of thirst. Reflexes such as swallowing, gagging, retching, and salivation are also initiated by receptors in the oral mucosa.

Secretion

The major secretion associated with the oral mucosa is saliva, produced by the salivary glands, which contributes to the maintenance of a moist surface. The major salivary glands are situated far from the mucosa, and their secretions pass through the mucosa via long ducts; however, many minor salivary glands are associated with the oral mucosa. (The salivary glands are fully described in Chapter 17.) There are frequently sebaceous glands present in the oral mucosa, but their secretions are probably insignificant.

Thermal Regulation

In some animals (such as the dog) considerable body heat is dissipated through the oral mucosa by panting;

for these animals the mucosa plays a major role in the regulation of body temperature. The human oral mucosa, however, plays practically no role in regulating body temperature; there are no obvious specializations of the blood vessels for controlling heat transfer.

ORGANIZATION OF THE ORAL MUCOSA

The oral cavity consists of two parts (see also p. 45): an outer vestibule, bounded by the lips and cheeks, and the oral cavity proper, separated from the vestibule by the alveolus bearing the teeth and gingiva. The superior zone of the oral cavity proper is formed by the hard and soft palates, and the floor of the mouth and base of the tongue form the inferior border. Posteriorly the oral cavity is bounded by the pillars of the fauces and the tonsils. The oral mucosa shows considerable structural variation in different regions of the oral cavity, but three main types of mucosa can be recognized, identified according to their primary function: masticatory mucosa, lining mucosa, and specialized mucosa. The anatomic location of each type is shown diagrammatically in Figure 18-1, and the types are fully described later in the chapter.

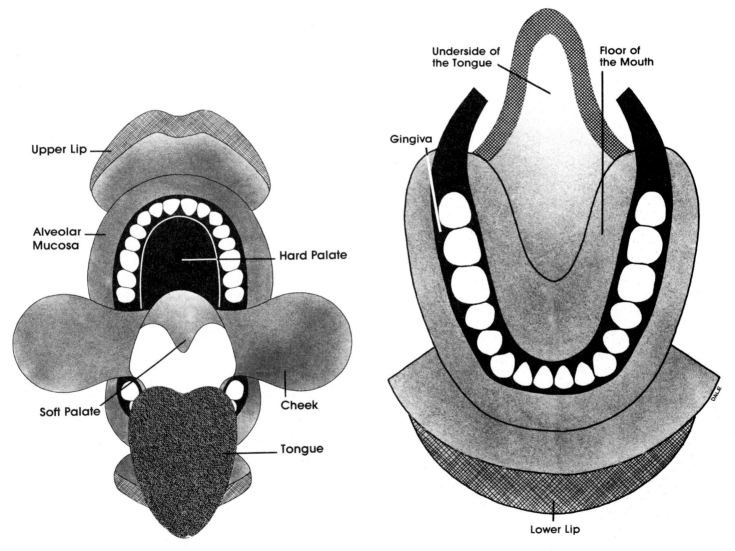

FIG. 18-1 Anatomic locations occupied by the three main types of mucosa in the oral cavity. Masticatory mucosa is shown by black shading; lining mucosa by gray shading; specialized mucosa by the dotted area. (Modified from Roed-Petersen B, Renstrup G: *Acta Odontol Scand* 27:681, 1969.)

Clinical Features

Although the oral mucosa is continuous with the skin, it differs considerably in appearance. Generally it is more deeply colored, most obviously at the lips (where the bright vermilion border contrasts with the skin tone). This coloration represents the combined effect of a number of factors—the concentration and state of dilation of small blood vessels in the underlying connective tissue, the thickness of the epithelium, the degree of keratinization, and the amount of melanin in the epithelium. Color gives an indication as to the clinical condition of the mucosa; inflamed tissues are red, because of dilation of the blood vessels, whereas normal healthy tissues are a paler pink.

Other features that distinguish the oral mucosa from skin are its moist surface and the absence of appendages. Skin contains numerous hair follicles, sebaceous glands, and sweat glands, whereas the glandular component of oral mucosa is represented primarily by the minor salivary glands. These are concentrated in various regions of the oral cavity, and the openings of their ducts at the mucosal surface are sometimes evident on clinical examination (Fig. 18-2, *B*). Sebaceous glands are present in the upper lip and buccal mucosa in about three quarters of adults and have been described occasionally in the alveolar mucosa and dorsum of the tongue (Fig. 18-3). They appear as pale yellow spots and are sometimes called *Fordyce's spots* or Fordyce's disease, although they do not represent a pathologic condition.

The surface of the oral mucosa tends to be smoother and have fewer folds or wrinkles than the skin, but a number of topographic features are readily apparent on clinical examination. The most obvious are the different papillae on the dorsum of the tongue and the transverse ridges (or rugae) of the hard palate. The healthy gingiva

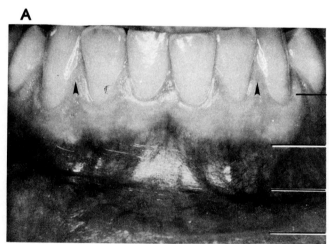

A

Gingiva

Mucogingival junction

Alveolar mucosa

Labial mucosa

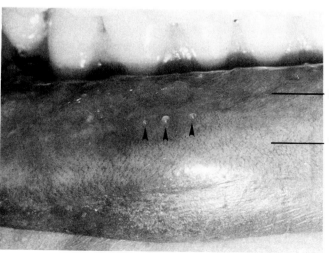

B

Labial mucosa

Vermilion zone

FIG. 18-2 Healthy oral mucosa. **A,** Attached gingiva and the alveolar and and labial mucosae. Gingival stippling is most evident in the interproximal regions *(arrows)*. The mucogingival junction between keratinized gingiva and nonkeratinized alveolar mucosa is clearly evident. **B,** Vermilion zone adjoining the labial mucosa. Several small globules on the mucosa *(arrows)* represent sites of secretion, where minor salivary gland ducts open to the surface.

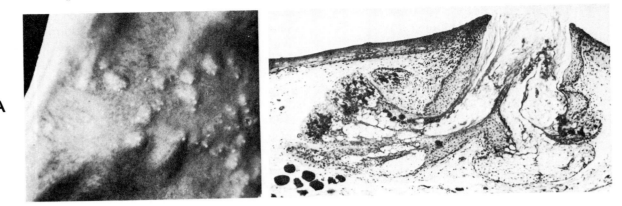

FIG. 18-3 Sebaceous glands in oral mucosa. **A** is a photomicrograph of a large, rosette-shaped gland in the buccal mucosa of a 43-year-old individual. **B** is a histologic section through such a gland. The dilated duct orifice is filled with desquamated cells. (From Miles AEW: In Montagna W, et al [eds]: *Advances in biology of skin,* New York, 1963, Pergamon Press, vol 4.)

shows a pattern of fine surface stippling, consisting of small indentations of the mucosal surface (Fig. 18-2, *B*). In many people a slight whitish ridge occurs along the buccal mucosa in the occlusal plane of the teeth. This line, sometimes called the linea alba (white line), is a keratinized region and may represent the effect of abrasion from rough tooth restorations or cheek biting.

The oral mucosa varies considerably in its firmness and texture. The lining mucosa of the lips and cheeks, for example, is soft and pliable whereas the gingiva and hard palate are covered by a firm immobile layer. These differences have important clinical implications when it comes to giving local injections of anesthetics or taking biopsies of oral mucosa. Fluid can be easily introduced into loose lining mucosa, but injection into the masticatory mucosa is difficult and painful. On the other hand, lining mucosa gapes when incised and may require suturing but masticatory mucosa does not. Similarly, the accumulation of fluid with inflammation is obvious and painful in masticatory mucosa but in lining mucosa the fluid disperses and inflammation may not be so evident.

COMPONENT TISSUES AND GLANDS

The two main tissue components of the oral mucosa are a stratified squamous epithelium, called the *oral epithelium,* and an underlying connective tissue layer, called the *lamina propria* or corium (Fig. 18-4). In the skin these two tissues are known by slightly different terminology: epidermis and dermis. The interface between epithelium and connective tissue is usually irregular, and upward projections of connective tissue, called the connective tissue papillae, interdigitate with epithelial ridges or pegs, sometimes called the rete ridges or pegs (Fig. 18-21). In a typical hematoxylin-and-eosin (H&E)–stained section the interface between epithelium and connective tissue appears as a structureless layer about 1 to 2 μm thick, called the basement membrane (Fig. 18-21, *A*). At the ultrastructural level this region has a complex structure that will be described later.

Although the junction between oral epithelium and lamina propria is obvious, that between the oral mucosa and underlying tissue, or submucosa, is less easy to recognize. In the gastrointestinal tract the lining mucosa is separated from underlying tissues by a layer of smooth muscle and elastic fibers called the muscularis mucosae (literally, "muscle of the mucosa") (Fig. 18-5, *A*). This clearly delineates the mucosa from the submucosa beneath and in functional terms may allow for some isolation of the internal lining from movements of the outer muscular layers of the intestine.

The oral mucosa has no muscularis mucosae, and clearly identifying the boundary between it and the underlying tissues is difficult. In many regions (e.g., cheeks, lips, parts of the hard palate) a layer of loose fatty or glandular connective tissue containing the major blood vessels and nerves that supply the mucosa separates the oral mucosa from underlying bone or muscle. This represents the submucosa in the oral cavity (Fig. 18-5, *B*), and its composition determines the flexibility of the attachment of oral mucosa to the underlying structures. In regions such as the gingiva and parts

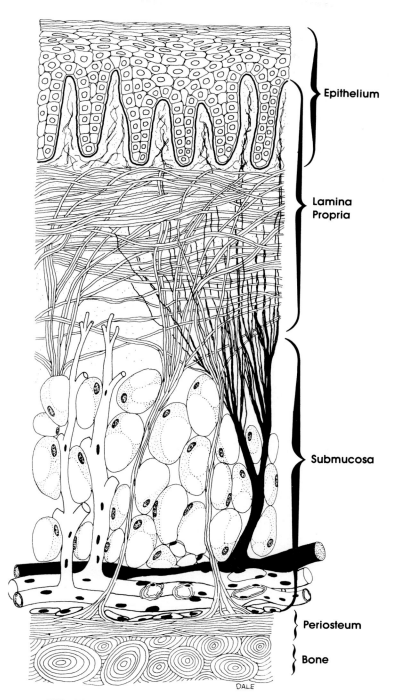

FIG. 18-4 Main tissue components of the oral mucosa.

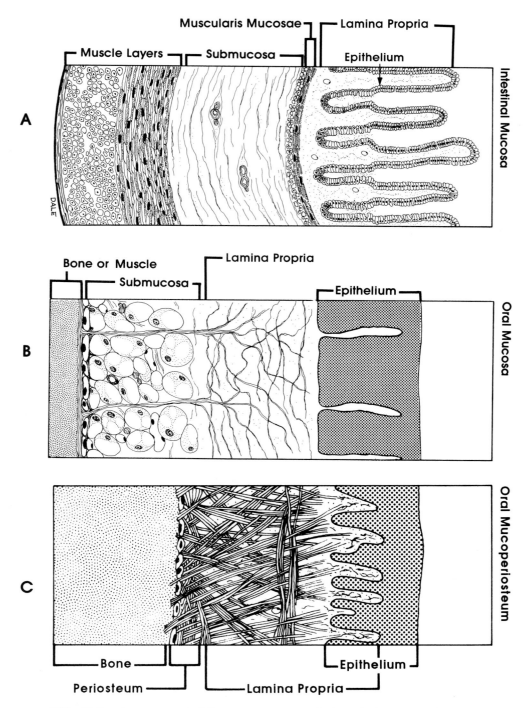

FIG. 18-5 Arrangement of tissue components: **A,** intestinal mucosa; **B,** oral mucosa; **C,** oral mucoperiosteum.

of the hard palate, oral mucosa is attached directly to the periosteum of underlying bone, with no intervening submucosa (Fig. 18-5, C). This arrangement is called a *mucoperiosteum* and provides a firm inelastic attachment.

The minor salivary glands are situated in or just beneath the lamina propria of the mucosa. Sebaceous glands are less frequent than salivary glands; they lie in the lamina propria and have the same structure as those present in the skin. Sebaceous glands produce a fatty secretion, called sebum, whose function in the oral cavity is unclear. The presence of sebaceous glands in oral mucosa may actually be an accident of embryologic development, by which some of the potential of skin ectoderm is retained in the ectoderm that invaginates to form the lining of the oral cavity.

In several regions of the oral cavity there are nodules of lymphoid tissue consisting of crypts formed by invaginations of the epithelium into the lamina propria. These areas are extensively infiltrated by lymphocytes and plasma cells. Because of their ability to mount immunologic reactions, such cells play an important role in combating infections of the oral tissues. The largest accumulations of lymphoid tissue are found in the posterior part of the oral cavity, where they form the lingual, palatine, and pharyngeal tonsils, often known collectively as *Waldeyer's ring*. Small lymphoid nodules also occur in the mucosa of the soft palate, the ventral surface of the tongue, and the floor of the mouth.

ORAL EPITHELIUM

As the tissue that forms the surface of the oral mucosa, the oral epithelium constitutes the primary barrier between the oral environment and deeper tissues. It is a stratified squamous epithelium consisting of cells tightly attached to each other and arranged in a number of distinct layers or strata. As the epidermis and the lining of the gastrointestinal tract, the oral epithelium maintains its structural integrity by a system of continuous cell renewal in which cells produced by mitotic divisions in the deepest layers migrate to the surface

to replace those that are shed. The cells of the epithelium can thus be considered to consist of two functional populations: a *progenitor population* (whose function is to divide and provide new cells) and a *maturing population* (whose cells are continually undergoing a process of differentiation or maturation to form a protective surface layer). These two important processes, proliferation and maturation, will now be considered in more detail.

Epithelial Proliferation

The progenitor cells are situated in the basal layer in thin epithelia (e.g., the floor of the mouth) and in the lower two to three cell layers in thicker epithelia (cheeks and palate). Dividing cells tend to occur in clusters that are seen more frequently at the bottom of epithelial ridges than at the top. Recent studies on both the epidermis and the oral epithelium indicate that the progenitor compartment is not homogeneous but consists of two functionally distinct subpopulations of cells. A small population of progenitor cells cycles very slowly and is considered to represent stem cells, whose function is to produce basal cells and retain the proliferative potential of the tissue. The larger portion of the progenitor compartment is composed of amplifying cells, whose function is to increase the number of cells available for subsequent maturation. Despite their functional differences, these proliferative cells cannot be distinguished by appearance. Because it divides infrequently, the epithelial stem cell may be important in protecting the genetic information of the tissue, for DNA is most vulnerable to damage during mitosis.

Regardless of whether the cells are of the stem or amplifying type, cell division is a cyclic activity and is commonly divided into four distinct phases (Fig. 18-6). The only phase that can be distinguished histologically is mitosis, which can be further subdivided into the recognizable stages of prophase, metaphase, anaphase, and telophase. After cell division, each daughter cell "makes the decision" either to recycle in the progenitor population or to enter the maturing compartment. This decision-making period is known as the *dichophase*.

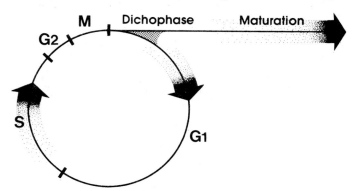

FIG. 18-6   Phases of the cell cycle. Cells in the progenitor compartment preparing to divide initially double their DNA content during the synthetic phase. After a short rest period *(G2)* they enter the visible phases of mitosis to produce two daughter cells. On average, one daughter cell enters the maturation compartment for each one entering the postmitotic presynthetic period *(G1)*. During periods of increased proliferative activity, however, both cells may "decide" at dichophase to remain in the cell cycle.

The rate at which new cells are produced in the progenitor population can be determined by a number of methods (Fig. 18-7). Certain substances, such as the plant alkaloid colchicine, can arrest dividing cells as they enter metaphase. By counting the number of dividing cells arrested over a known period of time, a mitotic index can be determined. An alternative method involves the administration of radioactively labeled thymidine which is incorporated into the DNA of cells preparing for division. Such cells can subsequently be recognized in histologic sections by autoradiography and the result expressed as a labeling index (Fig. 18-7, *B*). Proliferating cells can also be identified by immunocytochemistry following the administration of bromodeoxyuridine (BdU), which is selectively incorporated into DNA. Apart from measuring the number of cells in division, it is also possible to estimate the time necessary to replace all the cells in the epithelium. This is known as the *turnover time* of the epithelium and is derived from a knowledge of the time it takes for a cell to divide and pass through the entire epithelium.

The use of different techniques has led to a wide range of estimates of the rate of cell proliferation in the various epithelia; but, in general, the turnover time is 52 to 75 days in the skin, 4 to 14 days in the gut, 41 to 57 days in the gingiva, and 25 days in the cheek. Although only limited data are available, regional differences in the patterns of epithelial maturation appear to be associated with different turnover rates; for example, nonkeratinized buccal epithelium turns over faster than keratinized gingival epithelium.

The control of epithelial proliferation and maturation has been extensively researched, and there are many biologically active substances produced by different cell types that appear to have an effect on cell division. These compounds are collectively termed cytokines (see Chapter 6); those that may influence epithelial cell proliferation include epidermal growth factor, transforming growth factor alpha, and interleukin 1.

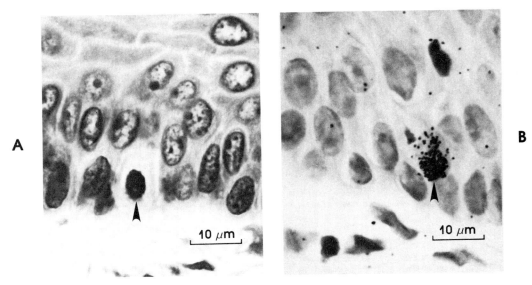

FIG. 18-7 Two methods of identifying proliferating cells in histologic sections. In **A** the arrowhead points to a dividing basal epithelial cell arrested at metaphase by the systemic administration of colchicine. It can be identified by the darkly staining mass of clumped chromatin characteristically surrounded by a clear halo. **B** is an autoradiograph of the deeper layers of palatal epithelium. The arrowhead indicates an epithelial cell nucleus that has incorporated radioactive thymidine into its DNA during the synthesizing phase of its cell cycle. This label produces an accumulation of small black silver grains over the nucleus; the single grains randomly scattered over the rest of the tissue represent nonspecific background.

Mitotic activity can also be affected by factors such as the time of the day, stress, and inflammation. For example, the presence of slight subepithelial inflammatory cell infiltrates stimulates mitosis whereas severe inflammation causes a marked reduction in proliferative activity. The mechanism of such action is not known, but the effect may be important in oral epithelium and especially in relation to determining turnover of the epithelium in regions that are frequently inflamed such as the dentogingival junction (Chapter 14).

Our views on the mechanisms that control the proliferation and differentiation of oral mucosa, skin, and many other tissues have been dramatically influenced in recent years by the discovery of biologically active substances called cytokines (see also Chapter 6). A cytokine is a soluble glycoprotein or protein secreted by living cells that acts in minute concentrations to regulate functions including cell division, growth, and differentiation. Cytokines are produced by epithelial cells, fibroblasts, and inflammatory cells and can promote cell adhesion, influence proliferation, and induce cells to interact with matrix. Examples of cytokines are interleukins such as interleukins 1, 2, and 3 (IL-1, IL-2, and IL-3) and tumor necrosis factor alpha (TNF-α); colony-stimulating factors (CSF); peptide growth factors such as epidermal growth factor (EGF) and fibroblast growth factor (FGF); and suppressor factors such as transforming growth factor beta (TGF-β).

It is becoming evident that the association between nonkeratinocytes and keratinocytes in skin and oral mucosa represents a subtle and finely balanced interrelationship in which cytokines are the controlling factors. Thus keratinocytes produce IL-1, CSF, and TNF-α, which modulate the function of Langerhans cells. In turn, the Langerhans cells produce IL-1, which can activate T lymphocytes, which secrete IL-2 and thus bring about the proliferation of T cells capable of responding to antigenic challenge. IL-1 also increases the number of receptors to melanocyte-stimulating hormone in melanocytes and so can affect pigmentation. The influence of keratinocytes extends to the adjacent connective tissue, where cytokines produced in the epithelium can influence fibroblast growth and the formation of fibrils and matrix proteins.

Epithelial Maturation

As indicated in the previous section, the cells arising by division in the basal or parabasal layers of the epithelium either remain in the progenitor cell population or undergo a process of maturation as they move to the surface. In general, maturation in the oral cavity follows two main patterns: keratinization and nonkeratinization. The histologic appearance of these patterns will now be described (Table 18-1).

TABLE 18-1 Major features of maturation in keratinized and nonkeratinized epithelium

Keratinized epithelium		Nonkeratinized epithelium	
Features	Cell layer	Features	Cell layer
Cuboidal or columnar cells containing bundles of tonofibrils and other cell organelles; site of most cell divisions	Basal	Cuboidal or columnar cells containing separate tonofilaments and other cell organelles; site of most cell divisions	Basal
Larger ovoid cells containing conspicuous tonofibril bundles; membrane-coating granules appear in upper part of this layer	Prickle-cell	Larger ovoid cells containing dispersed tonofilaments; membrane-coating granules appear in upper part of layer; filaments become numerous	Prickle-cell
Flattened cells containing conspicuous keratohyaline granules associated with tonofibrils; membrane-coating granules fuse with cell membrane in upper part; there is also internal membrane thickening	Granular	Slightly flattened cells containing many dispersed tonofilaments and glycogen	Intermediate
Extremely flattened and dehydrated cells in which all organelles have been lost; cells filled only with packed fibrillar material; when pyknotic nuclei are retained, there is parakeratinization	Keratinized	Slightly flattened cells with dispersed filaments and glycogen; fewer organelles present, but nuclei persist	Superficial

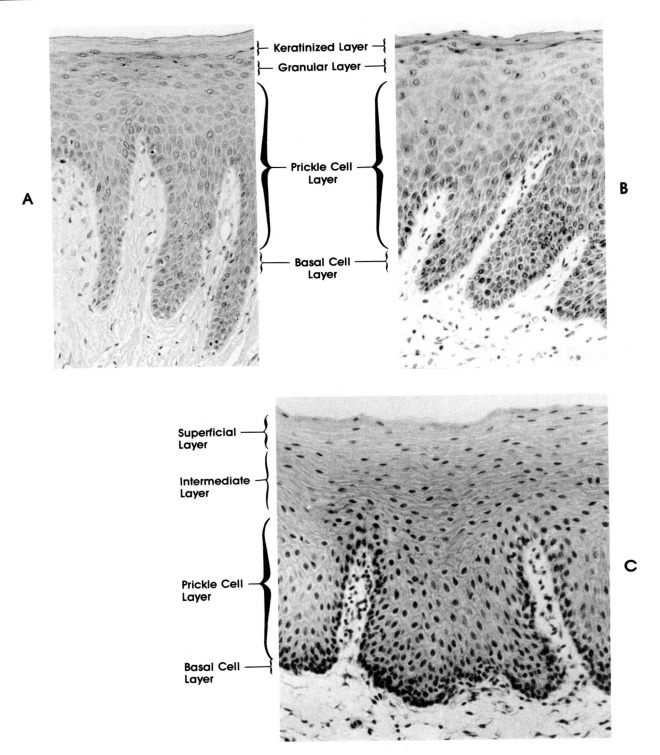

FIG. 18-8   Histologic sections of the main types of maturation in human oral epithelium (at the same magnification). **A** illustrates orthokeratinization in gingiva. Note the narrow darkly staining granular layer. **B** shows parakeratinization in gingiva. The keratin squames retain their pyknotic nuclei, and the granular layer contains only a few scattered granules. **C** shows nonkeratinization in buccal epithelium. There is no clear division into strata, and nuclei are apparent in the surface layer. Note the differences in thickness and epithelial ridge pattern as well as in the patterns of maturation.

Keratinization

The epithelial surface of the masticatory mucosa (e.g., that of the hard palate and gingiva and in some regions of specialized mucosa on the dorsum of the tongue) is inflexible, tough, and resistant to abrasion. This results from the formation of a surface layer of keratin, and the process of maturation is called keratinization or cornification. In routine histologic sections a keratinized epithelium shows a number of distinct layers or strata (Fig. 18-8, *A*). The basal layer (frequently given the Latin name stratum basale) is a layer of cuboidal or columnar cells adjacent to the basement membrane. Occasionally, the term *proliferative* or *germinative* layer (stratum germinativum) is used to describe the cells in the basal region that are capable of division, but this is a functional classification not discernible from appearances in normal histologic sections and should be avoided. Above the basal layer are several rows of larger elliptical or spherical cells known as the *prickle-cell layer* or *stratum spinosum*. This term arises from the appearance of the cells when prepared for histologic examination, since they frequently shrink away from each another, remaining in contact only at points known as intercellular bridges or desmosomes (Fig. 18-9). This alignment gives the cells a spiny or pricklelike profile. It is worth noting that the Greek word for prickle, *akanthe*, is frequently used in pathologic descriptions of an increased thickness (acanthosis) or a separation of cells caused by loss of the intercellular bridges (acantholysis) in this layer.

The basal and prickle-cell layers, together, constitute from one half to two thirds the thickness of the epithelium. The next layer consists of larger flattened cells containing small granules that stain intensely with acid dyes such as hematoxylin (i.e., they are basophilic). This layer is the *granular* layer, or stratum granulosum,

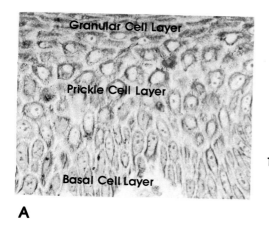

A

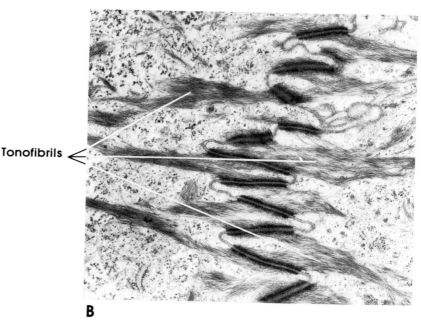

Tonofibrils

B

FIG. 18-9 Intercellular junctions. **A,** Prickle-cell layer in keratinized oral epithelium with the intercellular bridges ("prickles") between adjacent cells. Part of the basal and granular layers are also evident. **B** is an electron micrograph of similar tissue after processing for ultrastructural examination. There has been no shrinkage, so the intercellular bridges are not apparent. Tonofilament bundles (tonofibrils) insert into the attachment plaques of the desmosomes but do not pass across the intercellular space. In several of the desmosomes the specialized intercellular zone can be seen between the attachment plaque. **C,** The three types of intercellular junctions seen in oral epithelium: *A,* desmosome; *B,* tight junction; *C,* gap junction (nexus).

Tonofilaments

Attachment Plaque

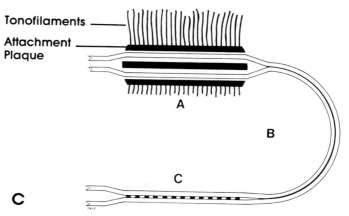

C

and the granules are called *keratohyalin granules.* In some regions of the masticatory oral epithelium, (e.g., the gingiva) it is difficult to see these granules clearly under the light microscope. The cell layers considered so far all contain nucleated living cells and are sometimes collectively termed the malpighian layer, although this term is used inconsistently and best avoided.

The surface layer is composed of very flat cells, termed *squames,* that stain bright pink with the histologic dye eosin (i.e., they appear eosinophilic) and do not contain any nuclei. This layer is the keratinized layer or stratum corneum. Other names sometimes used include cornified layer and horny layer. The pattern of maturation of these cells is often termed orthokeratinization.

It is not unusual for masticatory mucosa (e.g., parts of the hard palate and much of the gingiva) to show a variation of keratinization known as *parakeratinization.* In parakeratinized epithelium (Fig. 18-8, *B*) the surface layer stains for keratin, as described above, but shrunken (or pyknotic) nuclei are retained in many or all of the squames. Keratohyalin granules may be present in the underlying granular layer, though usually fewer than in orthokeratinized areas, so that this layer is difficult to recognize in histologic preparations. Parakeratinization is a normal event in oral tissues and does not imply disease.

Nonkeratinization

The lining mucosa of the oral cavity, which is present on the lips, cheeks, alveolar mucosa, soft palate, underside of the tongue, and floor of the mouth, has an epithelium that is usually nonkeratinized (Fig. 18-8, *C*). In many regions it is thicker than keratinized epithelium and shows a different ridge pattern at the connective tissue interface. Epithelium of the cheek, for example, may reach a thickness of more than 500 µm and has broader epithelial ridges than are seen in keratinized epithelium.

The basal and prickle-cell layers of nonkeratinized oral epithelium generally resemble those described for keratinized epithelium, although the cells of nonkeratinized epithelium are slightly larger and the intercellular bridges or prickles are less conspicuous. For this reason, some people prefer to avoid the term prickle-cell layer for nonkeratinized epithelium. There are no sudden changes in the appearance of cells above the prickle-cell layer in nonkeratinized epithelium, and the outer half of the tissue is divided rather arbitrarily into two zones: intermediate (stratum intermedium) and superficial (stratum superficiale). A granular layer is not present, and the cells of the superficial layer contain nuclei that are quite often plump. This layer does not stain intensely with eosin as does the surface of keratinized epithelium.

It is apparent from the histologic appearance of oral

| | TABLE 18-2 | Characteristics of nonkeratinocytes in oral epithelium |

Cell type	Level in epithelium	Specific staining reactions	Ultrastructural features	Function
Melanocyte	Basal	Dopa oxidase–tyrosinase; silver stains	Dendritic, no desmosomes or tonofilaments; premelanosomes and melanosomes present	Synthesis of melanin pigment granules (melanosomes) and transfer to surrounding keratinocytes
Langerhans cell	Predominantly suprabasal	ATPase; cell surface antigen markers	Dendritic, no desmosomes or tonofilaments; characteristic Langerhans granule	Unknown; proposed roles include effete melanocyte, neural element, regulatory cell, macrophage, and "antigen trap"
Merkel cell	Basal	Probably PAS positive	Nondendritic; sparse desmosomes and tonofilaments; characteristic electron-dense vesicles and associated nerve axon	Tactile sensory cell
Lymphocyte	Variable	Cell surface antigen markers (OKT-3)	Large circular nucleus; scant cytoplasm with few organelles; no desmosomes or tonofilaments	Associated with the inflammatory response in oral mucosa

epithelium that the tissue shows a well-ordered pattern of maturation and that successive layers contain cells of increasing age (i.e., progressive stages of maturation). Furthermore, the pattern of maturation differs in different regions of the oral mucosa so that two main types can be recognized: keratinization and nonkeratinization. The next section describes the fine structure of the epithelial cell and the main events that take place at the cellular level during maturation of these two types of epithelium (see in Tables 18-1 and 18-2).

Ultrastructure of the Epithelial Cell

Cells of the basal layer are the least differentiated among oral epithelial cells. They contain not only organelles (nuclei, mitochondria, ribosomes, endoplasmic reticulum, Golgi systems) commonly present in the cells of other tissues but also certain characteristic structures that identify them as epithelial cells and distinguish them from other cell types. These structures are the filamentous strands called tonofilaments and the intercellular bridges or desmosomes. Tonofilaments are fibrous proteins synthesized by the ribosomes and are seen as long filaments with a diameter of approximately 8 nm. They belong to a class of intracellular filaments called intermediate filaments and form an important structural component within the cell. Chemically the filaments represent a class of proteins known as *keratins*, which are characteristic constituents of epithelial tissues. Keratins are classified according to their size (i.e., molecular weight) and charge and the types of keratin present vary between different epithelia and even between the different cell layers of a single stratified epithelium. When they become aggregated to form the bundles of filaments called *tonofibrils*, they can often be identified with the higher magnifications of the light microscope (Fig. 18-9). One name often given to an epithelial cell because of its content of keratin filaments is *keratinocyte*. This serves to distinguish these epithelial cells from the nonkeratinocytes that are described later.

There has been a great increase recently in our understanding of the mechanisms involved in epithelial differentiation (or maturation). Information about differences between epithelia and about unusual changes such as hyperkeratinization has come about through research on the keratins and on changes that occur at the cell surface during differentiation (see Chapter 14). To recapitulate, keratins represent 30 different proteins of differing molecular weights; those with the lowest molecular weight (40 kilodaltons [kD]) are found in glandular and simple epithelia, those of intermediate molecular weight in stratified epithelia, and those with the highest molecular weight (~67 kD) in keratinized stratified epithelium. A "catalogue" of keratins has been drawn up to represent the different types. Thus, all stratified oral epithelia possess keratins 5, 14, and 15; but differences emerge between keratinized oral epithelium (which contains keratins 1, 6, 10, and 16) and nonkeratinized epithelium (keratins 4 and 13).

Stratified epithelia possess a variety of cell surface carbohydrate molecules that show differences between tissues and during differentiation. The changes are due to a sequential elongation of the cell surface carbohydrate during differentiation. This can be visualized by means of antibodies or by the use of plant-derived compounds (called lectins) that specifically bind to the carbohydrate. Much of the work on both keratins and cell surface markers has focused on identifying changes indicative of aberrant maturation to enable researchers to provide early warning of disease processes such as cancer. It has also enabled distinction of the various types of epithelia making up the dentogingival function.

An important property of any epithelium is its ability to function as a barrier, which depends to a great extent on the close contact or cohesiveness of the epithelial cells. Cohesion between cells is provided by a viscous intercellular material consisting of protein-carbohydrate complexes produced by the epithelial cells themselves. In addition, there are modifications of the adjacent membranes of cells, the most common of which is the desmosome.

Desmosomes (Fig. 18-9, *B* and *C*) are circular or oval areas of adjacent cell membranes, adhering by specialized intracellular thickenings (known as attachment plaques) into which bundles of tonofilaments insert. These filaments loop around within the plaques and pass out again; they do not cross into adjacent cells, as was once thought. If the epithelial cells shrink during histologic processing, the desmosomes usually remain intact and so appear as intercellular bridges. Adhesion between the epithelium and connective tissue is provided by hemidesmosomes, which are present on the basal membranes of cells of the basal layer (Fig. 18-22). These also possess intracellular attachment plaques with tonofilaments inserted.

The desmosomes, hemidesmosomes, and tonofilaments, together, represent a mechanical linkage that distributes and dissipates localized forces applied to the epithelial surface over a wide area. Although the term *hemidesmosome* and its morphologic appearance suggest that this structure is half a desmosome, immunocytochemical studies indicate that desmosomes and hemidesmosomes are distinct structural entities. A protein (desmoplakin) forms the attachment plaque and is found only in desmosomes. In some diseases, such as pemphigus, in which blistering of the epithelium occurs, there is a splitting of the epithelial layers to form bullous or vesicular lesions within the epithelium. This splitting is due to the breakdown of certain components of the desmosomal attachments, probably as a consequence of an immunologic reaction directed against them.

Two other types of connection are seen between cells of the oral epithelium (Fig. 18-9, *C*): gap and tight junctions. The gap junction is a region where membranes of adjacent cells run closely together, separated by only a small gap. There appear to be small interconnections between the membranes across these gaps.

Such junctions may allow electrical or chemical communication between the cells rather than have any mechanical function and are seen only occasionally in oral epithelium. Even rarer in oral epithelium is the tight junction, where adjacent cell membranes are so tightly apposed that there is no intercellular space. These junctions may serve to seal off and compartmentalize the intercellular areas.

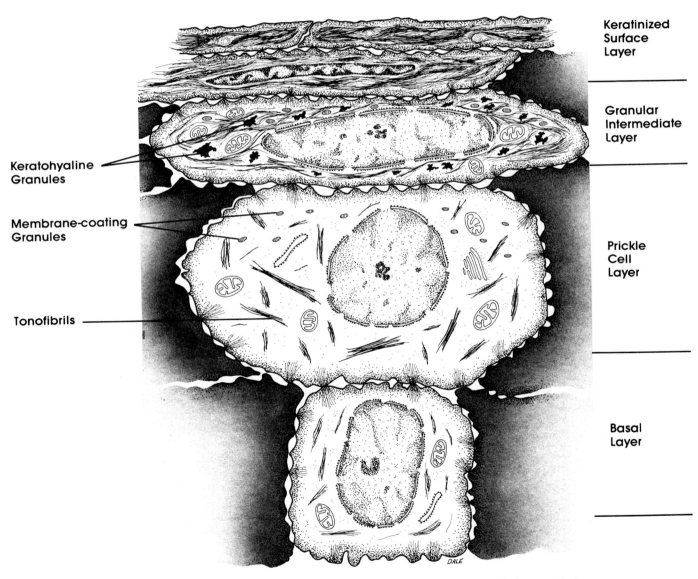

Keratinized Surface Layer

Granular Intermediate Layer

Keratohyaline Granules

Membrane-coating Granules

Prickle Cell Layer

Tonofibrils

A

Basal Layer

FIG. 18-10 Principal structural features of cells in successive layers. **A** shows orthokeratinized, and **B** nonkeratinized, oral epithelium. (Modified from Squier CA, et al: *Human oral mucosa: development, structure, and function,* Oxford UK, 1976, Blackwell Scientific Publications.)

Cellular Events in Maturation

The major changes involved in cell maturation in keratinized and nonkeratinized oral epithelium are shown in Figure 18-10 and Table 18-1. In both types of epithelia, the changes in cell size and shape are accompanied by a synthesis of more structural protein in the form of tonofilaments, the appearance of new organelles, and the production of additional intercellular material. There are, however, a number of changes that are not common in either epithelium and serve as distinguishing features. One is in the arrangement of tonofilaments. The cells of both epithelia increase in size as they migrate from the basal to the prickle-cell layer, but this increase is greater in nonkeratinized epithelium. There is also a corresponding synthesis of tonofilaments in both epithelia; but whereas the tonofilaments in keratinized epithelium are aggregated into bundles to form tonofibrils, those in nonkeratinized ep-

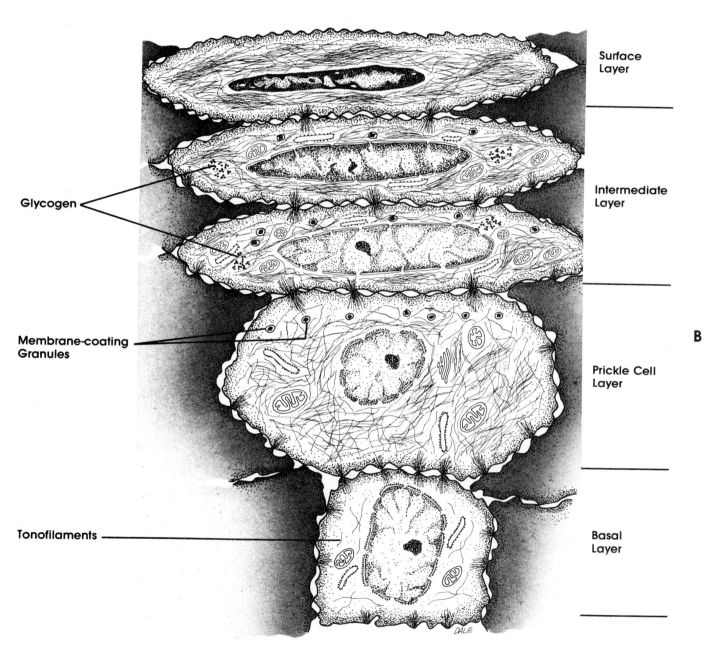

Glycogen

Membrane-coating Granules

Tonofilaments

Surface Layer

Intermediate Layer

Prickle Cell Layer

Basal Layer

B

FIG. 18-10, Continued

ithelium remain dispersed and so appear less conspicuous (Fig. 18-11). We also know that the chemical structure of keratin filaments differs between layers so that various patterns of maturation can be identified by the keratins that are present.

In the upper part of the prickle-cell layer there appears a new organelle called the *membrane-coating granule*. These granules are small membrane-bound structures, about 250 nm in size, that may originate from the Golgi system. In keratinized epithelium they are elongated and contain a series of parallel lamellae. In nonkeratinized epithelium, by contrast, they appear to be circular with an amorphous core (Fig. 18-12). As the cells move toward the surface, these granules become aligned close to the superficial cell membrane.

The next layer, called the granular layer in keratinized epithelium and the intermediate layer in nonkeratinized epithelium, contains cells that have a

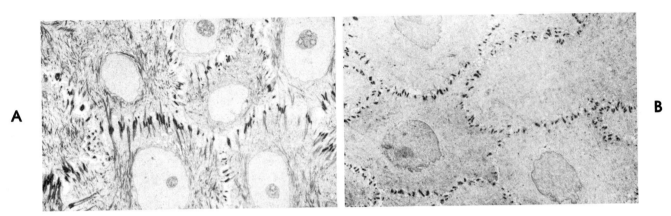

FIG. 18-11 Electron micrographs (at the same magnification) of prickle cells from, **A,** keratinized gingival epithelium, and **B,** nonkeratinized buccal epithelium. Filaments are assembled into distinct bundles (tonofibrils) in the keratinized tissue but dispersed as individual inconspicuous tonofilaments in the nonkeratinized epithelium.

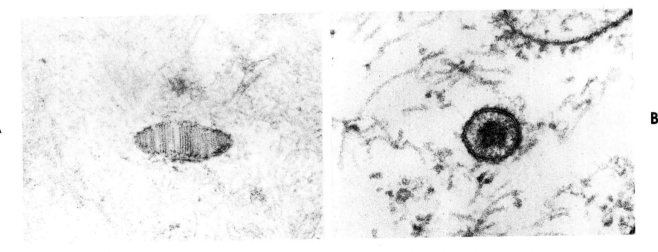

FIG. 18-12 Electron micrographs (at the same magnification) of membrane-coating granules in oral epithelium. **A** shows the elongated lamellate type seen in keratinized epithelium. **B** shows the circular type with a dense core found in nonkeratinized epithelium.

greater volume but are more flattened than those of the prickle-cell layer. In the upper part of this layer, in both keratinized and nonkeratinized epithelia, the membrane-coating granules appear to fuse with the superficial cell membrane and to discharge their contents into the intercellular space. In keratinized oral epithelium and epidermis, the discharge of granule contents may be associated with the formation of a lipid-rich permeability barrier that limits the movement of aqueous substances through the intercellular spaces of the keratinized layer. The granules seen in nonkeratinized epithelium probably have a similar function, but it is known that the contents have a different composition and do not form as effective a barrier as that in keratinized epithelia.

Cells in the superficial part of the granular layer develop a marked thickening on the inner (intracellular) aspect of their membrane that contributes to the considerable resistance of the keratinized layer to chemical solvents. One of the major constituents of this thickening is a protein known as *involucrin*. A similar, but less obvious, thickening is often seen in the surface cells of nonkeratinized epithelia. Despite their name, membrane-coating granules have nothing to do with this thickening. The remaining events during epithelial maturation are markedly different in keratinized and nonkeratinized epithelia and so will be described separately.

Keratinized epithelium

The most characteristic feature of the granular layer of keratinized epithelium is the keratohyalin granules, which appear as basophilic particles under the light microscope and as electron-dense structures in ultrathin sections (Fig. 18-13). They are irregular in shape, usually between 0.5 and 1 μm in size, and are probably synthesized by the ribosomes that can be seen surrounding them. Keratohyalin granules are also intimately associated with tonofibrils, and it is thought that they form the matrix in which filaments of the keratinized layer are embedded or aggregated. For this reason the protein making up the bulk of these granules has recently been named *filaggrin*, although there is also a sulfur-rich protein called *loricrin*. As the cells of the granular layer reach the junction with the keratinized layer, a sudden change develops in their appearance (Fig. 18-14). All the organelles, including the nuclei and keratohyalin granules, disappear. There is a dehydration, and the cells of the keratinized layer become packed with filaments surrounded by filaggrin, which facilitates their dense packing. The means by which this transformation is brought about is not well understood.

The cells of the keratinized layer become dehydrated and extremely flattened (and thus more resistant to mechanical damage and chemical solvents), and assume the form of hexagonal disks called squames (Fig. 18-

A 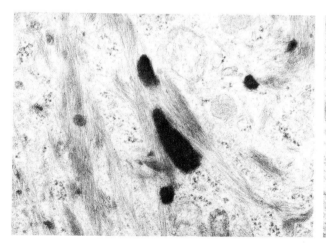 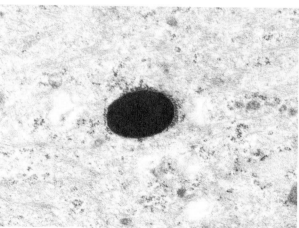 **B**

FIG. 18-13 Electron micrographs (at the same magnification) of keratohyaline granules in oral epithelium. **A,** is from the granular layer, shows irregularly shaped granules that are intimately associated with tonofilaments. **B** shows a granule of the type occasionally seen in nonkeratinized oral epithelium that is regular in shape and surrounded by ribosomes but not closely associated with tonofilaments.

14, *C*). Squames are lost (by the process of desquamation) and replaced by cells from the underlying layers. This process, which is poorly understood, may occur relatively rapidly so that a surface squame is shed in a matter of hours rather than days. Rapid clearance of the surface layer is probably important in limiting the colonization and invasion of epithelial surfaces by pathogenic microorganisms, including the common oral fungus *Candida*.

The keratinized layer in the oral cavity may be composed of up to 20 layers of squames and is thicker than that in most regions of the skin except the soles and palms.

In parakeratinization, there is incomplete removal of organelles from the cells of the granular layer, so that (although the keratinized layer contains numerous closely packed filaments) the nuclei remain as shrunken pyknotic structures and remnants of other organelles may also be present.

When gingival epithelium is prepared for histologic examination with stains such as Mallory's triple stain, a variant of keratinized or parakeratinized epithelium is sometimes seen. The outermost squames of the keratinized (or parakeratinized) layer do not look like the rest of the keratin but show a staining similar to that of deeper nucleated cells (Fig. 18-15). Such an appearance is called incomplete keratinization, or incomplete parakeratinization, and it is suggested that the cells showing this pattern have become rehydrated by taking up fluid from the oral cavity. None of these variants of keratinization, however, seems to have any pathologic significance in oral tissues.

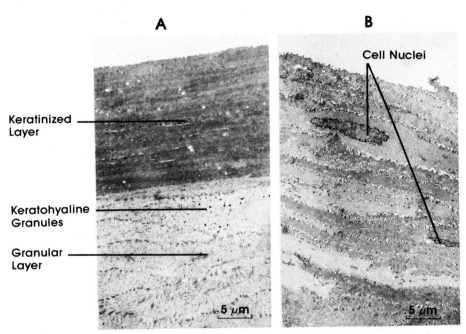

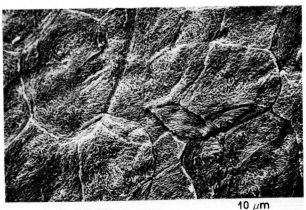

FIG. 18-14   Surface layer of keratinized and nonkeratinized oral epithelium. **A** and **B** are electron micrographs at the same magnification. **A** shows the granular and keratinized layers in gingival epithelium. Small keratohyaline granules are visible in the granular layer; the cells (squames) of the keratinized layer are flattened and appear uniformly dense. **B** shows the corresponding region of nonkeratinized buccal epithelium. Here the cells undergo only slight changes as they move to the surface. All the cells appear somewhat flattened, and organelles (including cell nuclei) can be seen even in the superficial layers. **C** is a scanning electron micrograph of the surface cells (squames) of keratinized oral epithelium. The squames are flat disks with a polygonal outline, and their surface shows a reticulate pattern of fine ridges. (**C** courtesy Dr. J. Howlett.)

Nonkeratinized epithelium

In nonkeratinized oral epithelium the events taking place in the upper cell layers are far less dramatic than those in keratinized epithelium (Fig. 18-10). There is a slight increase in cell size in the intermediate cell layer as well as an accumulation of glycogen in cells of the surface layer. On rare occasion, keratohyalin granules can be seen at this level. These differ, however, from the granules in keratinized epithelium and appear as regular spherical structures surrounded by ribosomes but not associated with tonofilaments (Fig. 18-13, *B*). Although they contain no filaggrin, loricrin is probably present. Keratohyalin granules often remain, even in the surface cells, where they are particularly obvious in surface cytologic smears.

In the superficial layer there are few further changes. The cells appear slightly more flattened than in the preceding layers and contain dispersed tonofilaments and nuclei, the number of other cell organelles having diminished (Fig. 18-14, *B*). The surface layer of non-keratinized epithelium thus consists of cells filled with loosely arranged filaments that are not dehydrated. They can thus form a surface that is flexible and tolerant of both compression and distension.

Although the distribution of keratinized and nonkeratinized epithelium in different anatomic locations is determined during embryologic development, there is often some variation of this basic pattern in adults (e.g., when the normally nonkeratinized buccal mucosa develops a thin keratin layer, the linea alba, along the occlusal line). Similarly, the normal keratin layer of the palate may become thick in smokers as a result of the tobacco smoke, but such hyperkeratotic epithelium in other ways appears normal (Fig. 18-15, *B*). Alternatively, the presence of inflammation in regions like the gingiva can reduce the degree of keratinization so that it appears parakeratinized. This change from one pattern of maturation to another or the emphasis or depression of an existing trait is usually reversible when the stimulus is removed.

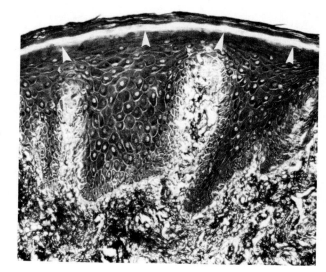

A

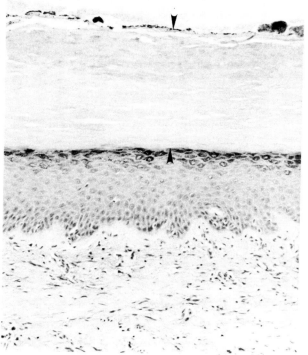

B

FIG. 18-15   Variations in keratinization. **A** is a histologic section of gingiva stained by a modified Mallory method to demonstrate incomplete orthokeratinization. Although normal keratin has formed and appears as a light band *(arrows)* beneath the surface of the epithelium, the outermost layers have become hydrated and their staining pattern reverts to that of the deeper epithelial layers. In the original preparation the light band stained orange and the dark hydrated regions blue. **B** is a histologic section through the mucosa of hard palate that has developed epithelial hyperkeratosis *(arrows)* as a result of irritation by tobacco smoke. Compare this with the normal palatal epithelium in 18-8, *A*.

Permeability and Absorption

It has already been pointed out that one function of the oral epithelium is forming an impermeable barrier; for, unlike the intestinal lining, the oral epithelium does not have an absorptive capacity. There are, however, differences in permeability between regions depending on the thickness of the epithelial barrier to be traversed and the pattern of maturation. Thus it seems that one of the thinnest epithelial regions, the floor of the mouth, may be more permeable than other areas, which is perhaps the reason why certain drugs (nitroglycerin administered to relieve angina pectoris) are successfully absorbed when held under the tongue. On the other hand, the oral mucosa is clearly able to limit the penetration of toxins and antigens produced by microorganisms present in the oral cavity except in the specialized region of the dentogingival junction.

Nonkeratinocytes in the Oral Epithelium

Many histologic sections of oral epithelium contain cells that differ in appearance from other epithelial cells in having a clear halo around their nuclei (Fig. 18-16). Such cells have been termed clear cells; but it is obvious from ultrastructural and immunochemical studies that they represent a variety of cell types, including pigment-producing cells (melanocytes), *Langerhans' cells*, *Merkel's cells*, and inflammatory cells (e.g., lymphocytes), that together can make up as much as 10% of the cell population in the oral epithelium. All of these cells, except Merkel's cells, lack desmosomal attachments to adjacent cells, so that during histologic processing the cytoplasm shrinks around the nucleus to produce the clear halo. None of these cells contains the large numbers of tonofilaments and desmosomes seen in epithelial keratinocytes, nor does any participate in the process of maturation seen in oral epithelia; therefore they are often collectively called nonkeratinocytes. Their structure and function are summarized in Table 18-2.

Melanocytes and Oral Pigmentation

It has already been mentioned that the color of the oral mucosa is the net result of a number of factors. One of these is pigmentation, which can be divided into two types: endogenous, arising in the tissues as a result of normal physiologic processes, and exogenous, caused by foreign material introduced into the body either locally or systemically. The endogenous pigments most commonly contributing to the color of the oral mucosa are *melanin* and *hemoglobin*. Melanin is produced by specialized pigment cells, called melanocytes, situated in the basal layer of the oral epithelium and the epidermis. The term melanoblast, although more accurately describing the function of these cells, is not currently applied to the pigment cells of mammals. Melanocytes arise embryologically from the neural crest ectoderm (Chapter 1) and enter the epithelium at about 11 weeks of gestation. There they divide and maintain themselves as a self-reproducing population. They lack desmosomes and tonofilaments but possess long dendritic processes that extend between the keratinocytes, often passing through several layers of cells. Melanin is synthesized within the melanocytes as small structures called melanosomes (Fig. 18-17). These are inoculated (or injected) into the cytoplasm of adjacent keratinocytes by the dendritic processes of melanocytes. Groups of melanosomes can often be identified under the light microscope in sections of heavily pigmented tissue stained with hematoxylin and eosin. These groups are referred to as melanin granules. In lightly pigmented tissues the presence of melanin can be demonstrated by specific histologic and histochemical stains. One of the most common exogenous pigments is amalgam accidentally forced into the gingiva during placement of a restoration. This circumstance gives rise to patches of bluish gray discoloration

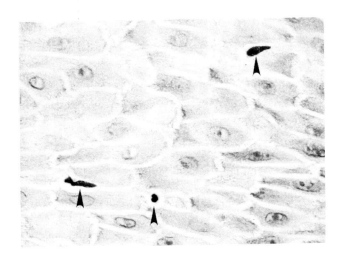

FIG. 18-16 Photomicrograph of the prickle-cell layer of gingival epithelium. The "clear cells" *(arrows)* have dark nuclei surrounded by a light halo.

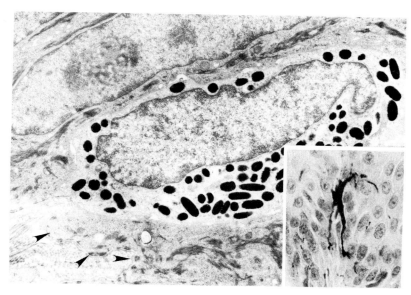

FIG. 18-17 Electron micrograph of a melanocyte in the basal layer of pigmented oral epithelium. The dense melanosomes are abundant. Arrowheads indicate the basal lamina. (Inset: Photomicrograph of a histologic secton showing a dendritic melanocyte. The cell stains darkly because it has been incubated histochemically to reveal the presence of melanin.

known as amalgam tattoo. Certain metals (e.g., lead and bismuth), when present systemically, can give rise to pigmentation of the gingival margin (sometimes called Burton's line) and may be indicative of systemic poisoning.

It is now known that both lightly and darkly pigmented individuals have the same number of melanocytes in any given region of skin or oral mucosa; color differences result from the relative activity of the melanocytes in producing melanin and from the rate at which melanosomes are broken down in the keratinocytes. In persons with very heavy melanin pigmentation, cells containing melanin may be seen in the connective tissue. These cells are probably macrophages that have taken up melanosomes produced by melanocytes in the epithelium and are sometimes termed melanophages. The regions of the oral mucosa where melanin pigmentation is most commonly seen clinically are the gingiva (Fig. 18-18), buccal mucosa, hard palate, and tongue. Although there is considerable individual variation, a direct relationship tends to be seen between the degrees of pigmentation in the skin and in the oral mucosa. Light-skinned persons rarely show any oral melanin pigmentation.

Melanocytes are involved in the development of pigmented lesions in the oral mucosa including pigmented tumors and melanoma, which is a rare but highly invasive lesion.

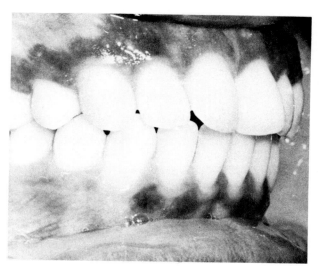

FIG. 18-18 Melanin pigmentation of the attached gingiva in a dark-skinned person.

Langerhans' Cells

Another dendritic cell sometimes seen in the suprabasal layers of epidermis and oral epithelium is Langerhans' cell. This cell lacks desmosomal attachments to surrounding cells and therefore appears clear in histologic sections. Its frequent location in the upper part of the epithelium has led to its being called a high-level clear cell, although it has now also been observed in the deeper epithelial layers. Ultrastructurally the Langerhans cell is characterized by the presence of a small rod- or flask-shaped granule, sometimes called the *Birbeck granule* (after the person who first described it under the electron microscope) (Fig. 18-19). The Langerhans cell is usually demonstrated by specific immunochemical reactions that stain cell surface antigens.

Langerhans' cells appear in the epithelium at the same time as, or just before, the melanocytes, and they may be capable of limited division within the epithelium. It is clear, however, that unlike melanocytes, they move in and out of the epithelium and their source is the bone marrow. This is in accord evidence suggesting that they have an immunologic function, recognizing and processing antigenic material that enters the epithelium from the external environment and presenting it to "helper" T lymphocytes. It is also likely that Langerhans' cells can migrate from epithelium to regional lymph nodes.

Merkel's Cells

The Merkel cell is situated in the basal layer of the oral epithelium and epidermis. Unlike the melanocyte and Langerhans' cell, however, it is not dendritic and it does possess keratin tonofilaments and occasional desmosomes linking it to adjacent cells. As a result it does not always resemble the other clear cells in histologic sections. The characteristic feature of Merkel's cells is the presence of small membrane-bound vesicles in the cytoplasm, sometimes situated adjacent to a nerve fiber associated with the cell (Fig. 18-20). These granules

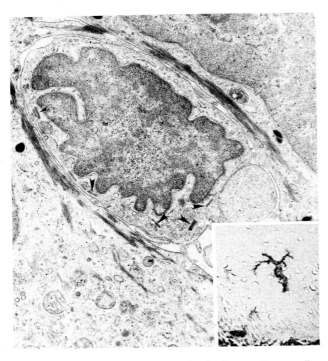

FIG. 18-19 Electron micrograph of a Langerhans cell from the oral epithelium. The cell has a convoluted nucleus, lacks tonofilaments and desmosome attachments to adjacent cells, but contains a number of characteristic rodlike granules *(arrows)*. The dark granules in the neighboring cells are melanin pigment. (Inset: Dendritic Langerhans cell in a light microscope preparation. Revealed by ATPase staining, it is seen in its characteristic suprabasal location. There is also some ATPase staining of the underlying connective tissue.) (ATPase preparation courtesy Dr. I.C. Mackenzie.)

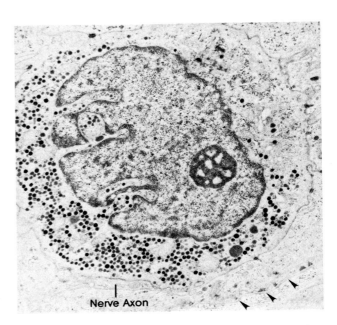

Nerve Axon

FIG. 18-20 Electron micrograph of a Merkel cell in the basal layer of oral epithelium. The cytoplasm of this cell is filled with small dense vesicles situated close to an adjacent unmyelinated nerve axon. Arrows point to the site of the basal lamina. (Courtesy Dr. S.Y. Chen.)

may liberate a transmitter substance across the synapselike junction between the Merkel cell and the nerve fiber and thus trigger an impulse. This arrangement is in accord with neurophysiologic evidence suggesting that Merkel's cells are sensory and respond to touch. The Merkel cells may arise from division of an epithelial cell (keratinocyte).

Inflammatory Cells

When sections of epithelium taken from clinically normal areas of mucosa are examined microscopically, a number of inflammatory cells can often be seen in the nucleated cell layers. These cells are transient and do not reproduce themselves in the epithelium as the other nonkeratinocytes do. The cell most frequently seen is the lymphocyte, although the presence of polymorphonuclear leukocytes and mast cells is not uncommon. Lymphocytes are often associated with Langerhans' cells, which are able to activate T lymphocytes. A few inflammatory cells are commonplace in the oral epithelium and can be regarded as a normal component of the nonkeratinocyte population.

JUNCTION OF THE EPITHELIUM AND LAMINA PROPRIA

The region where connective tissue of the lamina propria meets the overlying oral epithelium is an undulating interface at which papillae of the connective tissue interdigitate with the epithelial ridges. The interface is seen to consist of connective tissue ridges or conical papillae (or both) projecting into the epithelium (Fig. 18-21). This arrangement makes the surface area of the interface larger than a simple flat junction and may provide better attachment, enabling forces applied at the surface of the epithelium to be dispersed over a greater area of connective tissue. In this respect, it is interesting that masticatory mucosa has the greatest number of papillae per unit area of mucosa; in lining mucosa the papillae are fewer and shorter. The junction also represents a major interface for metabolic exchange between the epithelium and connective tissue, for there are no blood vessels in the epithelium.

In histologic sections of oral mucosa the basement membrane between the epithelium and connective tissue, which appears as a structureless band in H&E preparations, stains brightly with the periodic acid–Schiff (PAS) reaction (Fig. 18-21, *A*). Ultrastructurally this region is described as the basal lamina and is highly organized (Fig. 18-22). It consists of a layer of finely granular or filamentous material about 50 nm thick, called the *lamina densa*, that runs parallel to the basal cell membranes of the epithelial cells but is separated

from them by an apparently clear zone some 45 nm wide, called the *lamina lucida*. There are slight condensations of material in the lamina lucida opposite the hemidesmosomes on the epithelial cell membrane representing very fine filaments, termed *anchoring filaments,* that traverse the lamina lucida. Inserted into the lamina densa are small loops of finely banded fibrils called *anchoring fibrils*, not to be confused with the anchoring filaments. Collagen fibrils run through these loops and are thus interlocked with the lamina densa to form a flexible attachment.

Biochemically the lamina lucida contains glycoproteins—including the bullous pemphigoid antigen, which is probably associated with adhesion of the basal cell surface, and basement membrane glycoprotein (Fig. 18-22, *C*). The lamina densa contains laminin, nidogen (or entactin), and type IV collagen arranged in a "chicken-wire" configuration. The proteoglycan heparan sulfate coats both surfaces of the lamina densa and may bind proteins, thus restricting their penetration. Fibronectin and type V collagen may also be present and are referred to as extrinsic components because they are not found in all basal laminae. The anchoring fibrils consist of type VII collagen, and the collagen that runs through the loops formed by the anchoring fibrils is type I and type III.

This complex arrangement of laminae and fibrils is clearly not a membrane in ultrastructural terms and is therefore more accurately called a basal complex or *basal lamina*. Seen under the light microscope with special stains (e.g., PAS), the basement membrane is a much thicker structure than the lamina lucida and lamina densa seen under the electron microscope. It probably includes some of the adjacent subepithelial collagen fibers (sometimes termed *reticulin* fibers), which also react with many of the histologic basement membrane stains. It is now believed that all the basal lamina, except its anchoring fibrils, is synthesized by the epithelium.

The basal complex attaches the epithelium to connective tissue. When blistering of the mucosa occurs, as in the lesions of pemphigoid, there is separation of the epithelium from connective tissue at the lamina lucida. This separation is thought to be the result of antibodies that attack a specific component of the basal lamina.

LAMINA PROPRIA

The connective tissue supporting the oral epithelium is termed lamina propria and for descriptive purposes can be divided into two layers: the superficial papillary layer (associated with the epithelial ridges) and the

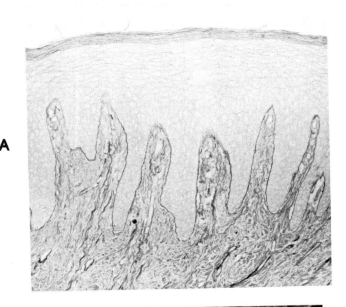

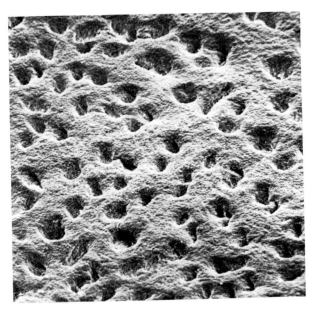

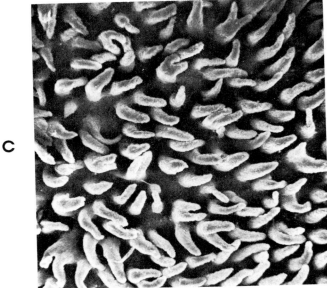

FIG. 18-21 Junction between epithelium and connective tissue. **A,** Photomicrograph of a section through gingival epithelium, stained by the PAS method, demonstrating the basement membrane and extensive interdigitations between epithelium and connective tissue. There is also staining of the intercellular substance, particularly around the keratinized epithelial squames. **B** and **C,** Scanning electron micrographs of the interface between epithelium and connective tissue in the palate. **B** shows the underside of oral epithelium and the circular orifices into which the cone-shaped papillae of connective tissue fit that are illustrated in **C.** (**B** and **C** from Klein-Szanto AJP, Schroeder HE: *J Anat* 123:93, 1977.)

FIG. 18-22 Ultrastructure of a basal lamina. **A** is a high-magnification electron micrograph of the complex in oral mucosa. Hemidesmosomes *(arrowheads)* at the plasma membrane of epithelial basal cells receive bundles of tonofilaments. Adjacent to the membrane are the lamina lucida and lamina dura. Several striated anchoring fibrils loop into the lamina densa, and some contain within their loops cross sections of collagen fibrils. **B** details the fine structure of the junction between epithelium and connective tissue. **C** presents the location of principal molecular constituents of the junction.

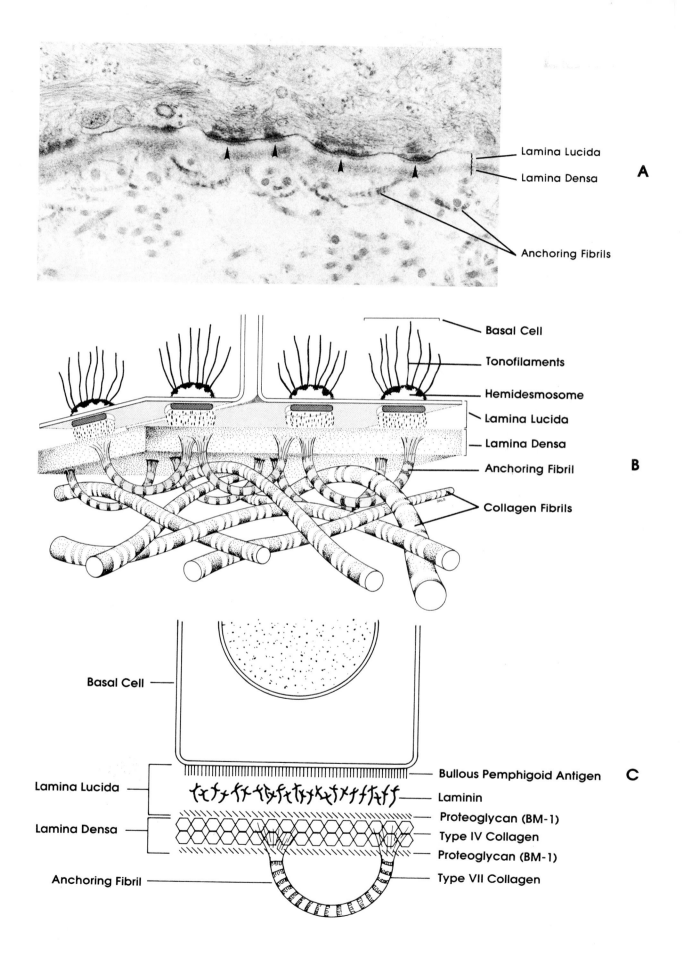

Lamina Lucida

Lamina Densa

Anchoring Fibrils

A

Basal Cell

Tonofilaments

Hemidesmosome

Lamina Lucida

Lamina Densa

Anchoring Fibril

Collagen Fibrils

B

Basal Cell

Lamina Lucida

Lamina Densa

Anchoring Fibril

Bullous Pemphigoid Antigen

Laminin

Proteoglycan (BM-1)

Type IV Collagen

Proteoglycan (BM-1)

Type VII Collagen

C

deeper reticular layer (which lies between the papillary layer and the underlying structures). The term *reticular* here means netlike and refers to the arrangement of the collagen fibers; it has nothing to do with the reticulin fibers situated beneath the basal lamina.

The difference between these two layers is poorly defined, but it essentially is based on the relative concentration and arrangement of the collagen fibers (Fig. 18-23, *A*). In the papillary layer, collagen fibers are thin and loosely arranged and many capillary loops are pres-

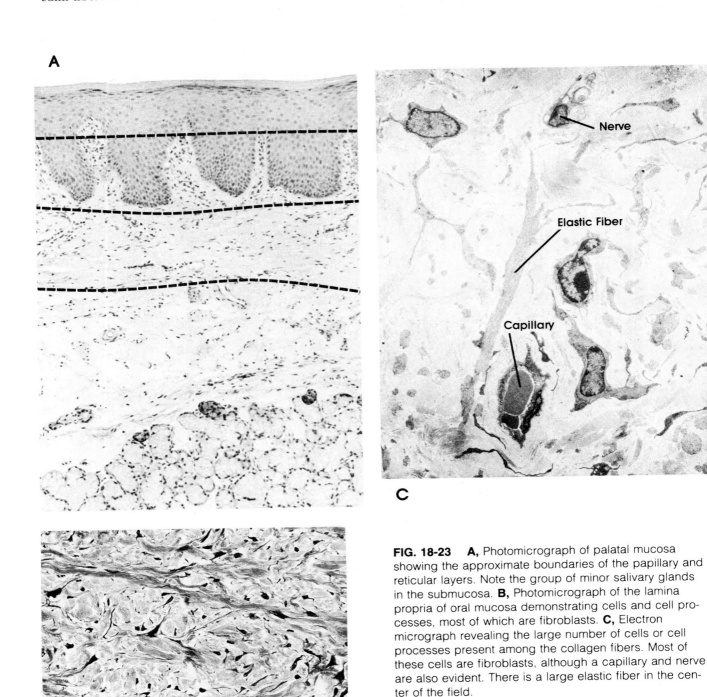

FIG. 18-23 **A,** Photomicrograph of palatal mucosa showing the approximate boundaries of the papillary and reticular layers. Note the group of minor salivary glands in the submucosa. **B,** Photomicrograph of the lamina propria of oral mucosa demonstrating cells and cell processes, most of which are fibroblasts. **C,** Electron micrograph revealing the large number of cells or cell processes present among the collagen fibers. Most of these cells are fibroblasts, although a capillary and nerve are also evident. There is a large elastic fiber in the center of the field.

ent. By contrast, the reticular layer has collagen fibers arranged in thick bundles that tend to lie parallel to the surface plane.

The lamina propria consists of cells, blood vessels, neural elements, and fibers embedded in an amorphous ground substance (Fig. 18-23, *B* and *C*). As does the overlying oral epithelium, it shows regional variation in the proportions of its constituent elements, partic-

ularly in the concentration and organization of fibers.

Cells

The lamina propria contains several different cells: fibroblasts, macrophages, mast cells, and inflammatory cells. A listing of the major cells of the lamina propria can be found in Table 18-3. At this point the structure and function of these cells will be discussed.

| **TABLE 18-3** | Main cell types found in the lamina propria of oral mucosa |

Cell type	Morphologic characteristics	Function	Distribution
Fibroblast	Stellate or elongated with abundant rough endoplasmic reticulum	Secretion of fibers and ground substance	Throughout lamina propria
Histiocyte	Spindle-shaped or stellate; often dark-staining nucleus; many lysosomal vesicles	Resident precursor of functional macrophage	Throughout lamina propria
Macrophage	Round with pale-staining nucleus; contains lysosomes and phagocytic vesicles	Phagocytosis, including antigen processing	Areas of chronic inflammation
Monocyte	Round with dark-staining kidney-shaped nucleus and moderate amount of cytoplasm	Phagocytic cell; blood-borne precursor of macrophage	Areas of inflammation
Mast cell	Round or oval with basophilic granules staining metachromatically	Secretion of certain inflammatory mediators and vasoactive agents (histamine, heparin, serotonin)	Throughout lamina propria, often subepithelial
Polymorphonuclear leukocyte (neutrophil)	Round with characteristic lobed nucleus; contains lysosomes and specific granules	Phagocytosis and cell killing	Areas of acute inflammation with lamina propria; may be present in epithelium
Lymphocyte	Round with dark-staining nucleus and scant cytoplasm with some mitochondria	Some lymphocytes participate in humoral or cell-mediated immune response	Areas of acute and chronic inflammation
Plasma cell	Cartwheel nucleus; intensely pyroninophilic cytoplasm with abundant rough endoplasmic reticulum	Synthesis of immunoglobulins	Areas of chronic inflammation, often perivascularly
Endothelial cell	Normally associated with a basal lamina; contains numerous pinocytotic vesicles	Lining of blood and lymphatic channels	Lining vascular channels throughout lamina propria

Fibroblasts

The principal cell in the lamina propria of oral mucosa is the fibroblast, which is responsible for the elaboration and turnover of both fiber and ground substance. It thus plays a key role in maintaining tissue integrity.

Under the light microscope, fibroblasts are either fusiform or stellate with long processes that tend to lie parallel to bundles of collagen fibers (Fig. 18-24). Their nuclei contain one or more prominent nucleoli. Ultrastructurally fibroblasts have the characteristics of active synthetic cells, including numerous mitochondria, an extensive granular endoplasmic reticulum (which is often distended by its contents), a prominent Golgi complex, and numerous membrane-bound vesicles. Fibroblasts have a low rate of proliferation in adult oral mucosa except during wound healing, when their number increases as a result of fibroblast division in the adjacent uninjured tissues. It is now becoming apparent that they have varied roles depending on environmental demands. Fibroblasts can become "contractile" and participate in wound contraction. In certain disease states (e.g., the gingival overgrowth sometimes seen with phenytoin, calcium channel blockers [nifedipine], and the antibiotic cyclosporine-A) fibroblasts may be "activated" and secrete more ground substance than normal. (See Chapter 6 for a more detailed description of the fibroblast and its functions.)

Macrophages

Under the light microscope the fixed macrophage (*histiocyte* is an alternate term favored by pathologists) is also a stellate or fusiform cell; and unless it is actively phagocytosing extracellular debris, it may be distinguished only with difficulty from a fibroblast. Under the electron microscope, making the distinction between the two cell types is easier: macrophages have smaller denser nuclei and less granular endoplasmic reticulum, and their cytoplasm contains membrane-bounded vesicles that, on the basis of acid hydrolytic enzyme content, can be identified as lysosomes (Fig. 18-25).

The macrophage has a number of functions, the principal one being to ingest damaged tissue or foreign material in phagocytic vacuoles that fuse, intracytoplasmically, with the lysosomes and initiate breakdown of these materials. The processing of ingested material by the macrophage may be important in increasing its antigenicity before it is presented to cells of the lymphoid series for subsequent immunologic response. Another important function is the stimulation of fibroblast proliferation necessary for repair.

In the lamina propria of the oral mucosa two types of macrophages are specifically designated: the *melanophage* and the *siderophage*. The melanophage, which is common in pigmented oral mucosa, is a cell that has ingested melanin granules extruded from melanocytes within the epithelium. The siderophage is a cell that contains hemosiderin derived from red blood cells that have been extravasated into the tissues. This material can persist within the siderophage for some time, and the resultant brownish color appears clinically as a bruise.

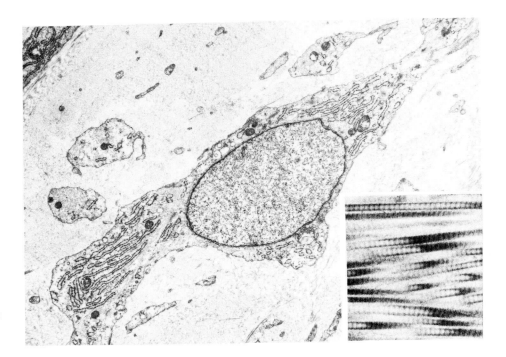

FIG. 18-24 Electron micrograph of a fibroblast in the lamina propria. (Inset: Collagen fibrils; note the typical cross-banding pattern.)

Mast cells

The mast cell is a large spherical or elliptical mononuclear cell (Fig. 18-26). Its nucleus is small relative to the size of the cell and in histologic preparations is frequently obscured by the large number of intensely staining granules that occupy its cytoplasm. These granules stain metachromatically with certain basic dyes such as methylene blue (the granules bind the dye but in so doing change its color from blue to magenta) because of the presence of heparin within the granules.

In humans the principal contents of the granules are histamine and heparin.

Because these cells are frequently found in association with small blood vessels, it has been suggested that they play a role in maintaining normal tissue stability and vascular homeostasis. Although histamine is known to be important in initiating of the vascular phase of an inflammatory process, the way it is released from the mast cells is poorly understood.

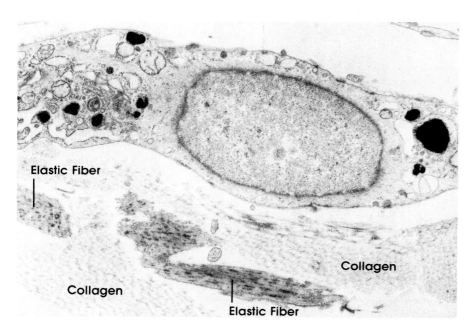

Elastic Fiber

Collagen

Collagen

Elastic Fiber

FIG. 18-25 Electron micrograph of a part of a macrophage in the lamina propria. The cell has a number of phagosomes filled with extremely dense material. Adjacent to the cell are elastic fibers composed of dark filaments embedded in a less dense matrix; they appear distinctly different from the adjacent collagen.

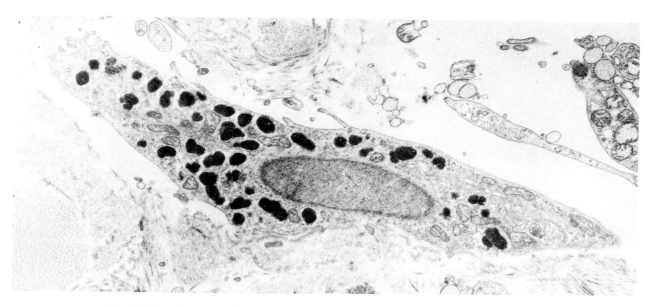

FIG. 18-26 Electron micrograph of a mast cell from the lamina propria. Note the dense granules in the cytoplasm, characteristic of this cell type in humans.

Inflammatory cells

Histologically the lymphocyte and plasma cell may be observed in small numbers scattered throughout the lamina propria; but, apart from such specialized regions as the lingual tonsil, other inflammatory cells are found in significant numbers only in connective tissue, either following an injury (e.g., a surgical incision) or as part of a disease process. When inflammatory cells are present in significant numbers, they influence the behavior of the overlying epithelium by releasing of cytokines.

As in other parts of the body, the type of inflammatory cell is dependent on the nature and duration of the injury. In acute conditions, polymorphonuclear leukocytes are the dominant cell type whereas more chronic conditions (e.g., periodontal disease) are associated with lymphocytes, plasma cells, monocytes, and macrophages. All these inflammatory cells show the same morphologic features as their circulating counterparts.

Fibers and Ground Substance

The intercellular matrix of the lamina propria consists of two major types of fibers, collagen and elastin, together with fibronectin embedded in a ground substance composed of glycosaminoglycans (GAGs) and serum-derived proteins, all of which are highly hydrated.

Collagen

Collagen in the lamina propria is primarily type I and type III, with types IV and VII occurring in the basal lamina. Type V may be present in inflamed tissue. (A full account of the biology of collagen is given in Chapter 6.)

Elastic fibers

Elastic fibers consist of two protein components that are distinctly different in both amino acid composition and morphology. The principal protein of the mature fiber is elastin, which is responsible for the elastic properties of the fiber. The second component is a glycoprotein with a microfibrillar morphology. Initially, elastic fibers consist entirely of aggregates of microfibrils, each 10 to 20 nm in diameter. As they mature, however, elastin is laid down within the microfibril matrix as a granular material until it becomes the predominant component, accounting for more than 90% of the fiber (Fig. 18-25).

Histologically, elastic fibers can be selectively stained—for example, with orcein. When stained by such methods, some elastic fibers can be seen in most regions of the oral mucosa; but they are usually found in the flexible lining mucosa, where they function to restore tissue form after stretching. Unlike collagen fi-

TABLE 18-4	Arterial blood supply to the oral mucosa

Oral region	Subterminal branches
Upper lip	Superior labial artery (anastomoses with buccal artery)
Upper gingiva	
Anterior	Anterior superior alveolar artery
Lingual	Major palatine artery
Buccal	Buccal artery
Posterior	Posterior superior alveolar artery
Hard palate	Major palatine artery
	Nasopalatine artery
	Sphenopalatine artery
Soft palate	Minor palatine artery
Cheek	Buccal artery
	Some terminal branches of facial artery
	Posterior alveolar artery
	Infraorbital artery
Lower lip	Inferior labial artery (anastomoses with buccal artery); mental artery, branch of inferior alveolar artery
Lower gingiva	
Anterior buccal	Mental artery
Anterior lingual	Incisive artery, sublingual artery
Posterior lingual	Inferior alveolar artery, sublingual artery
Posterior buccal	Inferior alveolar artery, buccal artery
Floor of mouth	Sublingual artery, branch of lingual artery
Tongue (dorsal and ventral surfaces)	
Anterior two thirds	Deep lingual artery
Posterior third	Dorsal lingual artery, to base of tongue, about posterior third

From Stablein MJ, Meyer J: In Meyer J, et al (eds): *The structure and function of oral mucosa*, New York, 1984. Pergamon Press.

bers, elastic fibers branch and anastomose and run singly rather than in bundles. Oxytalan fibers are not found in the oral mucosa.

Ground substance

Although the ground substance of the lamina propria appears by both light and electron microscopy to be amorphous at the molecular level, it consists of heterogeneous protein-carbohydrate complexes permeated by tissue fluid. Chemically these complexes can be subdivided into two distinct groups: proteoglycans and glycoproteins.

The proteoglycans consist of a polypeptide core to which GAGs (consisting of hexose and hexuronic acid residues) are attached. In the oral mucosa the proteoglycans are represented by hyaluronan, heparan sulfate, versican, decorin, biglycan and syndecan (box). Proteoglycans in the matrix are different from those associated with the cell surface, and interaction between them and with cell surface molecules (e.g., integrins) are probably important in modulating behavior and function of the cell.

The glycoproteins, by contrast, have a branched polypeptide chain to which only a few simple hexoses are attached. Uronic acids are notably absent.

The presence of these groups of substances in the lamina propria can be detected histochemically. Thus proteoglycans and glycoproteins containing a terminal sialic acid residue will bind dyes such as Alcian blue whereas all glycoproteins can be stained by the periodic acid–Schiff reaction.

BLOOD SUPPLY

The blood supply of the oral mucosa (Table 18-4) is extremely rich and derived from arteries that run parallel to the surface in the submucosa or, when the mucosa is tightly bound to underlying periosteum and a submucosa is absent, in the deep part of the reticular layer. These vessels give off progressively smaller branches that anastomose with adjacent vessels in the reticular layer before forming an extensive capillary network in the papillary layer immediately subjacent to the basal epithelial cells. From this network, capillary loops pass into the connective tissue papillae and come to lie close to the basal layer of the epithelium (Fig. 18-27). The arrangement in oral mucosa is much more profuse than in skin, where capillary loops are found only in association with hair follicles (which may explain the deeper color of oral mucosa).

Regional modifications occur in this basic pattern. For example, in the cheek a single capillary loop passes into each papilla but in the tongue each filiform papilla receives a variable number of capillaries; and in the larger fungiform and circumvallate papillae arterioles reach into them before giving off capillary loops. In

tissues such as the cheek, where the connective tissues may undergo extensive deformation, the arterioles follow a tortuous path and show more extensive branching.

Blood flow through the oral mucosa is greatest in the gingiva, but in all regions of the oral mucosa it is greater than in the skin at normal temperatures. To what extent inflammation of the gingiva (gingivitis), which is almost inevitably present, may be responsible for this greater flow is uncertain. Unlike the skin, which plays a role in temperature regulation, human oral mucosa lacks arteriovenous shunts; but it does have rich anastomoses of arterioles and capillaries, which undoubtedly contributes to its more rapid healing in response to injury as compared to skin.

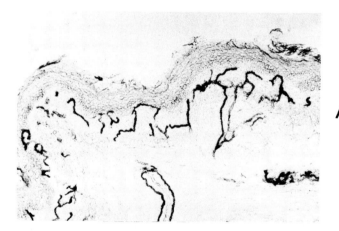

A

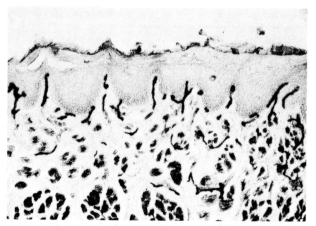

B

FIG. 18-27 Micrographs showing the relationships between capillaries in the lamina propria and overlying epithelium. Mucosal epithelium is from the floor of the mouth, **A,** and the cheek, **B.** The sections were prepared to demonstrate histochemically the distribution of alkaline phosphatase. In **B** there is also some staining of the muscle. (Courtesy Dr. G. Zoot.)

NERVE SUPPLY

Because the mouth is the gateway to the alimentary and respiratory tracts, the oral mucous membrane is densely innervated so that it can monitor all substances entering. A rich innervation also serves to initiate and maintain a wide variety of voluntary and reflexive activities involved in mastication, salivation, swallowing, gagging, and speaking. The nerve supply to the oral mucous membrane is therefore overwhelmingly sensory (Table 18-5).

The efferent supply is autonomic, supplies the blood vessels and minor salivary glands, and may also modulate the activity of some sensory receptors. The nerves arise mainly from the second and third divisions of the trigeminal nerve; but afferent fibers of the facial (VII), glossopharyngeal (IX), and vagus (X) nerves are also involved. The sensory nerves lose their myelin sheaths and form a network in the reticular layer of the lamina propria that terminates in a subepithelial plexus.

The sensory nerves terminate in both free and organized nerve endings. Free nerve endings are found in the lamina propria and within the epithelium, where they are frequently associated with Merkel's cells. Apart from the nerves associated with Merkel's cells, there are intraepithelial nerve endings that have a sensory function. Such nerves are not surrounded by Schwann cells as in connective tissue but run between the keratinocytes (which may ensheathe the nerves and so form a mesaxon). These nerves terminate as simple endings in the middle or upper layers of the epithelium (Fig. 18-28).

Within the lamina propria, organized nerve endings are usually found in the papillary region and consist of groups of coiled fibers surrounded by a connective tissue capsule. These specialized endings have been grouped according to their morphology as the Meissner or Ruffini corpuscles, the bulbs of Krause, and the mucocutaneous end organs. The density of sensory receptors is greater in the anterior part of the mouth than in the posterior region, with the greatest density occurring where the connective tissue papillae are most prominent.

The primary sensations perceived in the oral cavity are those of warmth, cold, touch, pain, and taste. Although specialized nerve endings are differentially sensitive to particular modalities (e.g., the bulbs of Krause appear to be most sensitive to cold stimuli and the Meissner corpuscles to touch), there is no evidence that any one receptor is responsible for detecting only one type of stimulus. It is possible, however, that each modality is served by specific fibers associated with each termination.

Sensory nerve networks are more developed in the oral mucosa lining the anterior than the posterior regions of the mouth, and this pattern is paralleled by the greater sensitivity of this region to a number of modalities. For example, touch sensation is most acute in the anterior part of the tongue and hard palate. By comparison, the sensitivity of the fingertips falls between those of the tongue and the palate. Touch receptors in the soft palate and oropharynx are important in the initiation of swallowing, gagging, and retching.

TABLE 18-5 Principal sensory nerve fibers supplying the oral mucosa

Oral region	Innervation
Upper lip and vestibule	Twigs from infraorbital branch of maxillary nerve
Upper gingivae	Anterior, posterior, and (when present) middle superior alveolar branches of maxillary nerve
Hard palate	Greater, lesser, and sphenopalatine branches of maxillary nerve
Soft palate	Lesser palatine branch of maxillary nerve; tonsillar branch of glossopharyngeal nerve; nerve of pterygoid canal (taste) (originating from facial nerve)
Cheek	Twigs from infraorbital branch of maxillary nerve; superior alveolar branch of maxillary nerve; buccal branch of mandibular nerve; possibly some terminal branches of facial nerve
Lower lip and vestibule	Mental branch of inferior alveolar nerve; buccal branch of mandibular nerve
Lower gingivae; buccal, lingual	Inferior alveolar branch of mandibular nerve; buccal branch of mandibular nerve; sublingual branch of lingual nerve
Anterior two thirds of tongue	Lingual branch of mandibular nerve (taste) (provided by fibers carried in lingual nerve but originating in facial nerve and passing by way of chorda tympani to lingual)
Posterior third of tongue, facial and tonsillar	Glossopharyngeal nerve (taste and general sensation)

From Holland GR: In Meyer J, et al (eds): *The structure and function of oral mucosa*, New York, 1984, Pergamon Press.

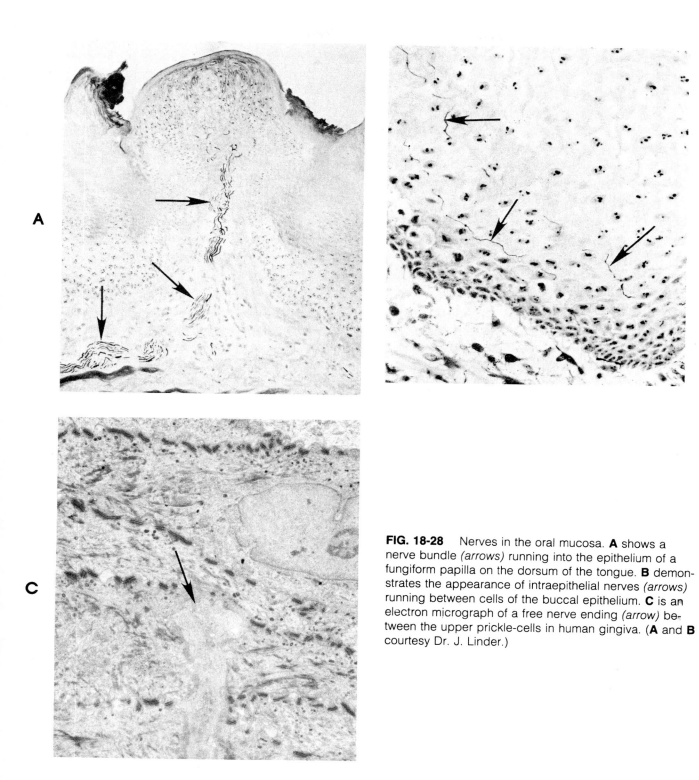

FIG. 18-28 Nerves in the oral mucosa. **A** shows a nerve bundle *(arrows)* running into the epithelium of a fungiform papilla on the dorsum of the tongue. **B** demonstrates the appearance of intraepithelial nerves *(arrows)* running between cells of the buccal epithelium. **C** is an electron micrograph of a free nerve ending *(arrow)* between the upper prickle-cells in human gingiva. (**A** and **B** courtesy Dr. J. Linder.)

Similarly, temperature reception is more acute in the vermilion border of the lip, at the tip of the tongue, and on the anterior hard palate than in more posterior regions of the oral cavity. The detection of pain is poorly understood. It appears to be initiated by noxious stimuli causing tissue damage and thereby activating polypeptides in the interstitial fluid, which in turn act on free nerve endings of slow-conducting unmyelinated and thin myelinated nerves.

A specialized receptor that occurs only in the oral cavity and pharynx is the taste bud. Although some taste buds lie within the epithelium of the soft palate and pharynx, most are found in the fungiform, foliate, and circumvallate papillae of the tongue (Figs. 18-32 and 18-33).

Histologically the taste bud is a barrel-shaped structure composed of 30 to 80 spindle-shaped cells (Fig. 18-29). At their bases the cells are separated from underlying connective tissue by the basement membrane whereas their apical ends terminate just below the epithelial surface in a taste pit that communicates with the surface through a small opening, the taste pore.

The cells of the taste bud have been divided into a number of types: light (type I), dark (type II), and intermediate (type III). Type I cells are the most common, constituting about half of all cells in the taste bud. Type II cells are morphologically similar but contain numerous vesicles and are adjacent to the intraepithelial nerves. They are continually being replaced, and their existence is dependent on the presence of a functional gustatory nerve. The apical ends of these cells

are tightly joined together by junctional complexes, somewhat similar to those occurring in intestinal mucosa, so that the initial events stimulating sensation of taste appear to involve the amorphous material within the taste pits and the microvilli of constituent cells that project into those pits.

Taste stimuli are probably generated by the adsorption of molecules onto receptors on the surface of the taste bud cells. The way in which this initial stimulation is passed to the nerves is poorly understood; but there is an extensive network of unmyelinated nerve fibers around the lower half of the taste cells, and occasional specialized synaptic connections with intermediate cells occur. These cells, together with Merkel's cells, are the only truly specialized sensory cells in the oral mucosa.

Although the sensitivity of taste buds to sweet, salty, sour, and bitter substances shows regional variation (sweet at the tip, salty and sour on the lateral aspects, and bitter and sour in the posterior region of the tongue), no distinct structural differences have been observed among taste buds in these regions. It is likely that the identification of different substances depends on the relative number and source of the associated efferent nerve fibers that are stimulated.

A special type of receptor whose function is to detect the "taste" of water has been postulated by physiologists. This function seems localized to the region of the circumvallate papillae of the tongue, but the morphologic structures responsible for it have not been described.

FIG. 18-29 Histologic section of taste buds in the epithelium of a circumvallate papilla from the dorsum of the tongue. A deep groove runs around the papilla, and the glands of von Ebner empty into it. (Inset: Enlarged view of a simple taste bud with its barrel-like appearance and the apical pore *[arrow]*. Compare this with 18-32. (From Squier CA, et al: *Human oral mucosa: development, structure, and function*, Oxford UK, 1976, Blackwell Scientific Publications.)

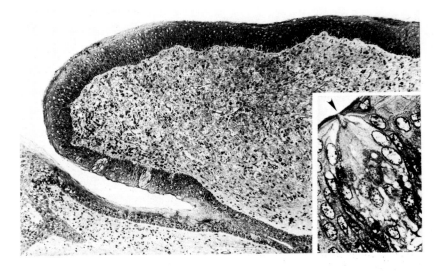

STRUCTURAL VARIATIONS

By now it should be apparent that the human oral mucosa shows considerable variation in structure, not only in the composition of the lamina propria, form of the interface between epithelium and connective tissue, and type of surface epithelium but also in the nature of the submucosa and how the mucosa is attached to underlying structures. Fortunately, the organization of component tissues shows similar patterns in many regions. It is possible to divide the oral mucosa into three main types: masticatory, lining, and specialized. The areas occupied by each type are illustrated in Figure 18-1. In the following sections, each type of mucosa will be described. A summary of the structures existing within the various anatomic regions occupied by each appears in Table 18-6. Finally, a brief account is given of several junctions between different types of mucosa that are of both morphologic interest and clinical importance.

Masticatory Mucosa

Masticatory mucosa covers those areas of the oral cavity such as the hard palate (Fig. 18-30) and gingiva (Fig. 18-35) that are exposed to compressive and shear forces and to abrasion during the mastication of food. The dorsum of the tongue has the same functional role as other masticatory mucosa but, because of its specialized structure, is considered separately.

The epithelium of masticatory mucosa is moderately thick compared to that in other regions. It is frequently orthokeratinized, although quite normally there will be parakeratinized areas of the gingiva and occasionally of the palate. Both types of epithelial surface are inextensible and well adapted to withstanding abrasion. The junction between epithelium and underlying lamina propria is convoluted, and the numerous elongated papillae probably provide good mechanical attachment and prevent the epithelium from being stripped off under shear force. The lamina propria is thick, containing a dense network of collagen fibers in the form of large closely packed bundles. These follow a direct course between anchoring points so that there is relatively little slack and the tissue does not yield on impact, enabling the mucosa to resist heavy loading.

Masticatory mucosa covers immobile structures (e.g., the palate and alveolar processes) and is firmly bound to them either directly by the attachment of lamina propria to the periosteum of underlying bone—such as in mucoperiosteum—or indirectly by a fibrous submucosa. In the lateral regions of the palate this fibrous submucosa is interspersed with areas of fat and glandular tissue that cushion the mucosa against mechanical loads and protect the underlying nerves and blood vessels of the palate.

The firmness of masticatory mucosa ensures that it does not gape after surgical incisions and rarely requires suturing. For the same reason, injections of local anesthetic into these areas are difficult and often painful, as is any swelling arising from inflammation.

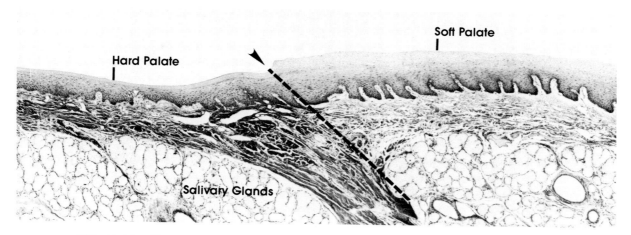

FIG. 18-30 Photomicrograph of the junction *(dashed line)* between mucosae covering the hard and the soft palate. Note the difference in thickness and the ridge pattern between keratinized epithelium of the hard palate and nonkeratinized epithelium of the soft palate. The section has been stained by the van Gieson method to demonstrate collagen; the thick dense bundles in the lamina propria of the hard palate appear different from the thinner fibers in the soft palate. There are extensive minor salivary glands beneath the mucosa.

TABLE 18-6 Structure of the mucosa in different regions of the oral cavity

REGION	MUCOSA		SUBMUCOSA
	Covering epithelium	Lamina propria	
LINING MUCOSA			
Soft palate	Thin (150 μm) nonkeratinized stratified squamous epithelium; taste buds present	Thick with numerous short papillae; elastic fibers forming an elastic lamina; highly vascular with well-developed capillary network	Diffuse tissue containing numerous minor salivary glands
Ventral surface of tongue	Thin, nonkeratinized, stratified squamous epithelium	Thin with numerous short papillae and some elastic fibers; a few minor salivary glands; capillary network in subpapillary layer, reticular layer relatively avascular	Thin and irregular, may contain fat and small vessels; where absent, mucosa is bound to connective tissue surrounding tongue musculature
Floor of mouth	Very thin (100 μm) nonkeratinized, stratified squamous epithelium	Short papillae; some elastic fibers; extensive vascular supply with short anastomosing capillary loops	Loose fibrous connective tissue containing fat and minor salivary glands
Alveolar mucosa	Thin, nonkeratinized, stratified squamous epithelium	Short papillae, connective tissue containing many elastic fibers; capillary loops close to the surface supplied by vessels running superficially to the periosteum	Loose connective tissue, containing thick elastic fibers attaching it to periosteum of alveolar process; minor salivary glands
Labial and buccal mucosa	Very thick (500 μm) nonkeratinized, stratified squamous epithelium	Long, slender papillae; dense fibrous connective tissue containing collagen and some elastic fibers; rich vascular supply giving off anastomosing capillary loops into papillae	Mucosa firmly attached to underlying muscle by collagen and elastin; dense collagenous connective tissue with fat, minor salivary glands, sometimes sebaceous glands
Lips: vermilion zone	Thin, orthokeratinized, stratified squamous epithelium	Numerous narrow papillae; capillary loops close to surface in papillary layer	Mucosa firmly attached to underlying muscle; some sebaceous glands in vermilion border, minor salivary gland and fat in intermediate zone
Lips: intermediate zone	Thin parakeratinized, stratified squamous epithelium	Long irregular papillae; elastic and collagen fibers in connective tissue	
MASTICATORY MUCOSA			
Gingiva	Thick (250 μm), orthokeratinized or parakeratinized, stratified squamous epithelium often showing stippled surface	Long, narrow papillae, dense collagenous connective tissue; not highly vascular but long capillary loops with numerous anastomoses	No distinct layer, mucosa firmly attached by collagen fibers to cementum and periosteum of alveolar process ("mucoperiosteum")
Hard palate	Thick, orthokeratinized (often parakeratinized in parts), stratified squamous epithelium thrown into transverse palatine ridges (rugae)	Long papillae; thick dense collagenous tissue, especially under rugae; moderate vascular supply with short capillary loops	Dense collagenous connective tissue attaching mucosa to periosteum ("mucoperiosteum"), fat and minor salivary glands are packed into connective tissue in regions where mucosa overlies lateral palatine neurovascular bundles
SPECIALIZED MUCOSA			
Dorsal surface of tongue	Thick, keratinized and nonkeratinized, stratified squamous epithelium forming three types of lingual papillae, some bearing taste buds	Long papillae; minor salivary glands in posterior portion; rich innervation especially near taste buds; capillary plexus in papillary layer, large vessels lying deeper	No distinct layer; mucosa is bound to connective tissue surrounding musculature of tongue

Lining Mucosa

The oral mucosa covering the underside of the tongue (Fig. 18-31), inside of the lips (Fig. 18-34), cheeks, floor of the mouth, and alveolar processes as far as the gingiva (Fig. 18-35) is subject to movement. These regions, together with the soft palate, are classified as lining mucosa.

The epithelium of lining mucosa is thicker than that of masticatory mucosa, sometimes exceeding 500 μm in the cheek, and is nonkeratinized. The surface is thus flexible and able to withstand stretching. The interface with connective tissue is relatively smooth, although slender connective tissue papillae often penetrate the epithelium.

The lamina propria is generally thicker than in masticatory mucosa and contains fewer collagen fibers, which follow a more irregular course between anchoring points. Thus the mucosa can be stretched to a certain extent before these fibers become taut and limit further distension. Associated with the collagen fibers are elastic fibers that tend to control the extensibility of the mucosa. Where lining mucosa covers muscle, it is attached by a mixture of collagen and elastic fibers. As the mucosa becomes slack during masticatory movements, the elastic fibers retract the mucosa toward the muscle and so prevent it from bulging between the teeth and being bitten.

The alveolar mucosa and mucosa covering the floor of the mouth are loosely attached to the underlying structures by a thick submucosa. Elastic fibers in the lamina propria of these regions tend to restore the mucosa to its resting position after distension. By contrast, mucosa of the underside of the tongue is firmly bound to the underlying muscle. The soft palate is flexible but not highly mobile, and its mucosa is separated from the loose and highly glandular submucosa by a layer of elastic fibers.

The tendency for lining mucosa to be flexible, with a loose and often elastic submucosa, means that surgical incisions frequently require sutures for closure. Injections into such regions are easy because there is ready dispersion of fluid in the loose connective tissue; however, infections also spread rapidly.

Specialized Mucosa

The mucosa of the dorsal surface of the tongue is unlike that anywhere else in the oral cavity because, although covered by what is functionally a masticatory mucosa, it is also a highly extensible lining and, in addition, has different types of lingual papillae. Some of these possess a mechanical function whereas others bear taste buds and therefore have a sensory function.

The mucous membrane of the tongue (Fig. 18-32) is composed of two parts, each having different embryologic origins (Chapter 2), and is divided by the V-shaped groove known as the sulcus terminalis (terminal groove). The anterior two thirds of the tongue is often called the body, and the posterior third the base. The mucosa covering the base of the tongue contains extensive nodules of lymphoid tissue, the lingual tonsils.

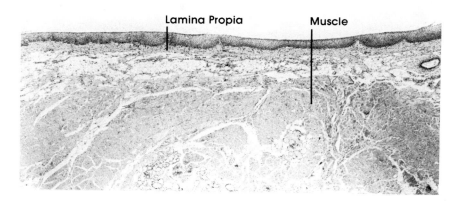

FIG. 18-31 Photomicrograph of lining mucosa from the underside of the tongue. The nonkeratinized epithelium is thin, with only a slight ridge pattern, and is bound to the underlying muscle by a narrow lamina propria. Between this lamina and the muscle is a layer of fat, appearing as light areas.

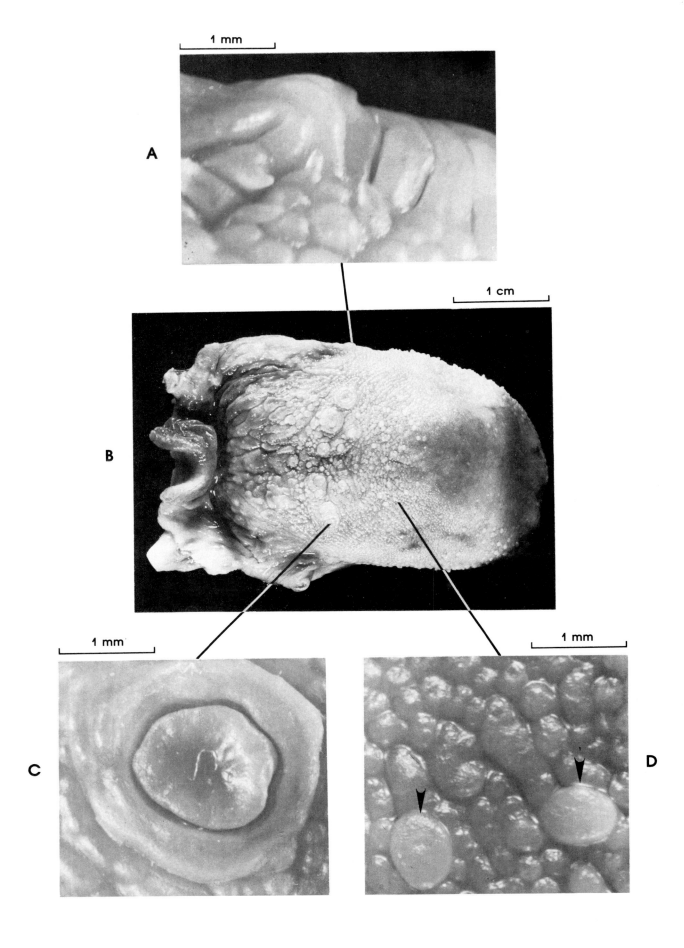

A

B

C

D

1 mm

1 cm

1 mm

1 mm

Fungiform Papillae

The anterior portion of the tongue bears the *fungiform* ("funguslike") and *filiform* ("hairlike") papillae (Fig. 18-33, *A*). Single fungiform papillae are scattered between the numerous filiform papillae at the tip of the tongue. They are smooth round structures that appear red because of their highly vascular connective tissue core, visible through a thin nonkeratinized covering epithelium. Taste buds are normally present in the epithelium on the superior surface.

Filiform Papillae

Filiform papillae cover the entire anterior part of the tongue and consist of cone-shaped structures, each with a core of connective tissue, covered by keratinized epithelium (Fig. 18-33, *A*). Together, they form a tough abrasive surface that is involved in compressing and breaking food when the tongue is apposed to the hard palate. Thus the dorsal mucosa of the tongue functions as a masticatory mucosa.

The tongue is highly extensible, with changes in its shape accommodated by the regions of nonkeratinized flexible epithelium between the filiform papillae.

Foliate Papillae

Foliate ("leaflike") papillae are sometimes present on the lateral margins of the posterior part of the tongue, although they are more frequently seen in mammals other than humans. These papillae consist of 4 to 11 parallel ridges that alternate with deep grooves in the mucosa, and a few taste buds are present in the epithelium of the lateral walls of the ridges (Fig. 18-33, *B*).

Circumvalate Papillae

Adjacent and anterior to the sulcus terminalis are 8 to 12 *circumvallate* ("walled") papillae, large structures each surrounded by a deep circular groove into which open the ducts of minor salivary glands (the glands of von Ebner) (Fig. 18-32, *C*). These papillae have a connective tissue core that is covered on the superior surface by a keratinized epithelium. The epithelium covering the lateral walls is nonkeratinized and contains taste buds.

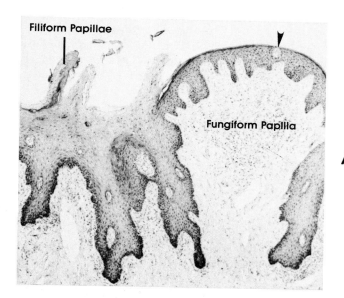

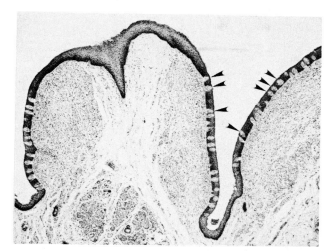

FIG. 18-32 The ridge-shaped foliate papillae, **A,** are located laterally and the circumvallate papillae, **C,** are situated in a row in front of the sulcus terminalis. **B,** Dorsal surface of a child's tongue showing the distribution and types of lingual papillae. Fungiform papillae, **D,** are interspersed among numerous filiform papillae on the anterior of the tongue, two of which are evident *(arrows).* (From Squier CA, et al: *Human oral mucosa: development, structure, and function,* Oxford UK, 1976, Blackwell Scientific Publications.)

FIG. 18-33 Histologic sections of three types of lingual papillae. **A,** Several filiform papillae and a fungiform papilla from the anterior part of the tongue. The epithelium of the filiform papillae is keratinized; that of the fungiform papilla thinly keratinized or nonkeratinized. The arrowhead points to a taste bud in the epithelium. **B,** Section through the foliate papilla. The nonkeratinized epithelium covering the papilla contains numerous taste buds *(arrowheads)* situated laterally.

JUNCTIONS IN THE ORAL MUCOSA

Within the oral mucosa are two junctions that merit further discussion: the mucocutaneous (between the skin and mucosa) and the mucogingival (between the gingiva and alveolar mucosa). The interface between the gingiva and the tooth (the dentogingival junction) is of considerable anatomic and clinical importance and is discussed in detail in Chapter 13.

Mucocutaneous Junction

The skin, which contains hair follicles and sebaceous and sweat glands, is continuous with the oral mucosa at the lips (Fig. 18-34). Here, at the mucocutaneous junction, a transitional region exists where appendages are absent except for a few sebaceous glands (situated mainly at the angles of the mouth). The epithelium of this region is keratinized but thin, with long connective tissue papillae containing capillary loops. This arrangement brings the blood close to the surface and accounts for the strong red coloration in this region, called the red (or vermilion) zone of the lip.

Because the vermilion zone lacks salivary glands and contains but a few sebaceous glands, it tends to dry out, often becoming cracked and sore in cold weather. Between it and the thicker nonkeratinized labial mucosa is an intermediate zone covered by parakeratinized oral epithelium. In infants this region is thickened and appears more opalescent, which represents an adaptation to suckling (called the suckling pad).

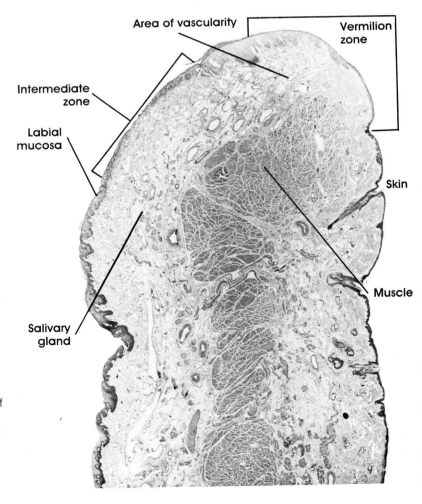

FIG. 18-34 Sagittal section through the lip. The skin covering the external aspect has an extremely thin epidermis and contains hair follicles. Continuous with this is the vermilion zone, which has a thin epithelium overlying an area of extensive vascularity. Between the vermilion zone and the labial mucosa of the oral cavity is the intermediate zone. There are minor salivary glands beneath the labial mucosa, and the extensive muscular tissue represents part of the orbicularis oris.

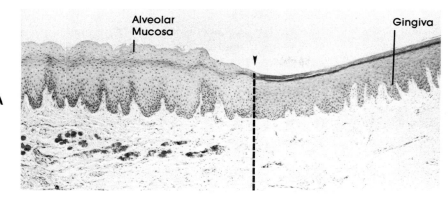

A

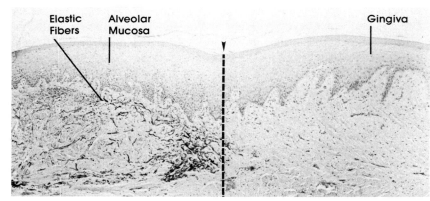

B

FIG. 18-35 Sections through the mucogingival junction *(dashed line)*. In **A** the differences in thickness, ridge pattern, and keratinization between epithelium of the gingiva and alveolar mucosa are seen. The preparation was stained by Papanicolaou's method, which reveals variations in keratinization. The junction in **B** was stained by Hart's method to demonstrate elastic fibers in the connective tissue. Although there is very little change in the epithelium in this specimen, a striking difference appears in the concentration of elastic fibers in the lamina propria between masticatory mucosa of the gingiva and lining mucosa of the alveoli. (From Squier CA, et al: *Human oral mucosa: development, structure, and function,* Oxford UK, 1976, Blackwell Scientific Publications.)

Mucogingival Junction

Although masticatory mucosa meets lining mucosa at several sites, none is more abrupt than the junction between attached gingiva and alveolar mucosa. This junction is identified clinically by a slight indentation called the mucogingival groove and by the change from bright pink of the alveolar mucosa to paler pink of the gingiva (Fig. 18-2, *B*).

Histologically there is a change at this junction, not only in the type of epithelium but also in the composition of the lamina propria (Fig. 18-35). The epithelium of the attached gingiva is keratinized or parakeratinized, and the lamina propria contains numerous coarse collagen bundles attaching the tissue to periosteum. The stippling seen clinically at the surface of healthy attached gingiva probably reflects the presence of this collagen attachment; the surface of free gingiva is smooth. The structure of mucosa changes at the mucogingival junction, where the alveolar mucosa has a thicker nonkeratinized epithelium overlying a loose lamina propria with numerous elastic fibers extending into the thick submucosa. These elastic fibers return the alveolar mucosa to its original position after it is distended by the labial muscles during mastication and speech.

Coronal to the mucogingival junction is another clinically visible depression in the gingiva, the free gingival groove, whose level corresponds approximately to that of the bottom of the gingival sulcus (Chapter 13). This demarcates the free and attached gingivae, although, unlike the mucogingival junction, there is no significant change in the structure of the mucosa at the free gingival groove.

DEVELOPMENT OF THE ORAL MUCOSA

The primitive oral cavity develops by fusion of the embryonic stomatodeum with the foregut after rupture of the buccopharyngeal membrane, at about 26 days of gestation, and thus comes to be lined by epithelium derived from both ectoderm and endoderm. The precise boundary between these two embryonic tissues is poorly defined, but structures that develop in the branchial arches (e.g., tongue, epiglottis, pharynx) are covered by epithelium derived from endoderm whereas the epithelium covering the palate, cheeks, and gingivae is of ectodermal origin. (see Chapter 2).

By 5 to 6 weeks of gestation the single layer of cells lining the primitive oral cavity has formed two cell layers, and by 8 weeks there is marked thickening in the region of the vestibular dental lamina complex. In the central region of this thickening, cellular degeneration occurs at 10 to 14 weeks, resulting in separation of the cells covering the cheek area and the alveolar mucosa and thus forming the oral vestibule. At about this time (8 to 11 weeks) the palatal shelves elevate and close, so that the future morphology of the adult oral cavity is apparent.

The lingual epithelium shows specialization at about 7 weeks when the circumvallate and foliate papillae first appear, followed by the fungiform papillae. Within these papillae taste buds soon develop. The filiform papillae that cover most of the anterior two thirds of the tongue become apparent at about 10 weeks. By 10 to 12 weeks the future lining and masticatory mucosa show some stratification, and although the superficial cells are still represented by the primitive hexagonal cells, these two areas already show different structures.

Those areas destined to become keratinized (e.g., hard palate and alveolar ridge of gingiva) have darkly staining columnar basal cells that are separated from the underlying connective tissue by a prominent basement membrane. Low connective tissue papillae are also evident. By contrast, the epithelium that will form areas of lining mucosa retains cuboidal basal cells, and the epithelium–connective tissue interface remains relatively flat. Between 13 and 20 weeks of gestation all the oral epithelia thicken (Fig. 18-36), and with the appearance of sparse keratohyalin granules a distinction between the prickle-cell and granular layer can be made. Differences are evident between the cytokeratins of epithelia of the developing masticatory and lining regions. During this period both melanocytes and Langerhans' cells appear in the epithelium. The surface layers of the epithelium show parakeratosis; orthokeratinization of the masticatory mucosa does not occur until after the eruption of teeth during the postnatal period.

While these changes are occurring in the oral epithelium, the underlying ectomesenchyme shows progressive changes. Initially the ectomesenchyme consists of widely spaced stellate cells in an amorphous matrix, but by 6 to 8 weeks extracellular reticular fibers begin to accumulate. As in the epithelium, regional differences can be seen in the ectomesenchyme. The connective tissue of lining mucosa contains fewer cells and fibers than that of the future masticatory mucosa. Between 8 and 12 weeks, capillary buds and collagen fibers can be detected; and although the collagen initially shows no particular orientation, as the fibers increase in number they tend to form bundles. Immediately subjacent to the epithelium these bundles are arranged perpendicular to the basement membrane. Elastic fibers become prominent only in the connective tissue of lining mucosa between 17 and 20 weeks.

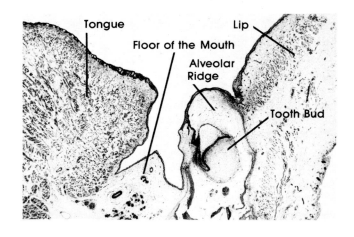

FIG. 18-36   Part of a sagittal section through the oral cavity of a 15-week human embryo showing the tongue, floor of the mouth, alveolar ridge with a tooth bud in situ, and lip. Differences in thickness are already apparent between the epithelia of the labial mucosa, alveolar ridge, floor of the mouth, and tongue; however, keratinization has not yet begun.

AGE CHANGES

Clinically, the oral mucosa in an elderly person often has a smoother and dryer surface than that in a youngster and may be described as atrophic or friable, but it is likely that these changes represent the cumulative effects of extrinsic insults over the lifetime of the individual (masticatory wear, disease processes, drug therapy) rather than an intrinsic biologic aging process.

Histologically the epithelium appears thinner, and a smoothing of the epithelium–connective tissue interface results from the flattening of epithelial ridges. The dorsum of the tongue may show a reduction in the number of filiform papillae, such changes being exacerbated by any nutritional deficiency of iron or B complex vitamins. The reduced number of filiform papillae may make the foliate papillae more prominent, and patients may erroneously consider this to be a disease state.

Aging is associated with decreased rates of metabolic activity, but studies on epithelial proliferation and rate of tissue turnover are inconclusive. Langerhans' cells become fewer with age, and this may contribute to a decline in cell-mediated immunity. Vascular changes may be quite prominent, with the development of vascular nodules and nevi. A striking and relatively common feature seen in elderly persons is the development of nodular varicose veins on the undersurface of the tongue ("caviar tongue"). Although such changes appear to be unrelated to the cardiovascular status of the patient, they are more frequent in patients with varicose veins of the legs.

In the lamina propria there is decreased cellularity with an increased amount of collagen, which is reported to become more highly cross linked. Sebaceous glands (Fordyce's spots) of the lips and cheeks also increase with age, and the minor salivary glands show marked atrophy with fibrous replacement.

Elderly patients, particularly postmenopausal women, may present with symptoms such as dryness of the mouth, burning sensations, and abnormal taste. Whether such symptoms reflect systemic disturbances or are a manifestation of local tissue changes is not clear.

BIBLIOGRAPHY

Dabelsteen E, Mandel U, Clausen H: Cell surface carbohydrates are markers of differentiation in human oral epithelium, *CRC Crit Rev Oral Biol Med* 2:493, 1991.

Dale BA, Salonen J, Jones AH: New approaches and concepts in the study of differentiation of oral epithelia, *CRC Crit Rev Oral Biol Med* 1:167, 1990.

Hill MW: The influence of aging on skin and oral mucosa, *J Gerontol* 3:35, 1984.

Meyer J, Squier CA, Gerson SJ (eds): *The structure and function of oral mucosa,* New York, 1984, Pergamon Press.

Milam SB, Haskin C, Zardeneta G, et al: Cell adhesion proteins in oral biology, *CRC Crit Rev Oral Biol Med* 21:451, 1991.

Rahemtulla F: Proteoglycans of oral tissues, *CRC Crit Rev Oral Biol Med* 3:135, 1992.

Squier CA: The permeability of oral mucosa, *CRC Crit Rev Oral Biol Med* 2:13, 1991.

Uitto VJ, Larjava H: Extracellular matrix molecules and their receptors: an overview with special emphasis on periodontal tissues, *CRC Crit Rev Oral Biol Med* 2:323, 1991.

CHAPTER 19

Temporomandibular Joint

THE articulation of the lower jaw with the cranium and upper facial skeleton involves two separate joints and the teeth when in occlusion. It is important to recognize that the joints, through anatomically distinct, function in unison and independent movements are not possible.

The bones involved are the mandible and the os temporale, and the joint is therefore designated the temporomandibular joint (TMJ). It is unique to mammals. In other vertebrates the lower jaw is compound—consisting of several bones, including the dentary (bearing teeth) and the articular bone (formed from the posterior part of Meckel's cartilage)—and articulates with the quadrate bone of the skull (Fig. 19-1). As mammals evolved, the compound lower jaw was reduced to a single bone (the mandible) bearing teeth that articulated with the newly developed articulating surface on the temporal bone. Thus, in phylogenetic terms, the TMJ is a secondary joint. The primary vertebrate jaw joint is still present in human anatomy (as the incudomalleolar articulation), with the bones involved (incus and malleus) now positioned in the middle ear (Fig. 19-2).

CLASSIFICATION OF JOINTS

Joints are classified in a number of ways. A common and simplistic classification is given here (Fig. 19-3).

Fibrous Joints

In a fibrous joint 2 bones are connected by fibrous tissue. 3 types are described: The first is the *suture* (Chapter 8), a joint that permits little or no movement. Its histology clearly indicates that its function is to permit growth, since its articulating surfaces are covered by an osteogenic layer responsible for new bone formation to maintain the suture as the skull bones are separated by the expanding brain. The second type of fibrous joint is the *gomphosis*, the socketed attachment of tooth to bone by the fibrous periodontal ligament (PDL). Here functional movement is restricted to intrusion and recovery in response to biting forces. (Long-term movement of teeth in response to environmental pressures or orthodontic treatment represents remodeling of the joint rather than functional movement.) The third type of fibrous joint is the *syndesmosis*, examples of which are the joints between the fibula and tibia and the radius and ulna. Here the two bony components are some distance apart but are joined by an interosseous ligament that permits limited movement.

Cartilaginous Joints

In a primary cartilaginous joint bone and cartilage are in direct apposition. An example is the costochondral junction. In a secondary cartilaginous joint the tissues of the articulation occur in the sequence bone–cartilage–fibrous tissue–cartilage–bone. An example is the pubic symphysis. Cartilaginous joints and fibrous joints permit little if any movement between the bones involved.

Synovial Joints

In a synovial joint, which generally permits significant movement, two bones (each with an articular surface covered by hyaline cartilage) are united and surrounded by a capsule that, thereby, creates a joint cavity. This cavity is filled with synovial fluid formed by a synovial membrane that lines the nonarticular surfaces. The cavity may, in some joints, be divided by an articular disk. Various ligaments are associated with synovial joints to strengthen the articulation and check excess movement. Synovial joints are further classified by the number of axes in which the bones involved can move (uniaxial, biaxial, or multiaxial) and by the shapes of the articulating surfaces (planar, ginglymoid [hinged], pivot, condyloid, saddle, ball-and-socket). Movements of a synovial joint are initiated and effected by muscles working together in a highly coordinated manner. This coordination is achieved, in part, through the joint's sensory innervation—which establishes Hilton's law, that the muscles acting on a joint have the same nerve supply as the joint.

A good way to describe any joint is with the following headings:

Type of joint
Development of the joint

Bones and cartilage involved in the joint
Capsule, synovial membrane, and disk of the joint
Ligaments associated with the joint
Muscles bringing about movement
Biomechanics of the joint
Innervation of the joint
Blood supply to the joint

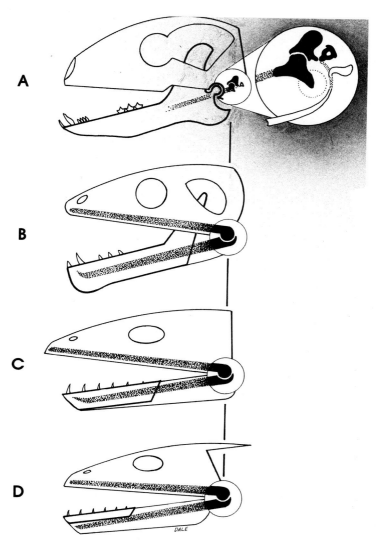

FIG. 19-1 Evolution of the mammalian jaw joint. **A** depicts an amphibian skull. The teeth are confined to the dentary bone. The articulation is between the terminal portion of Meckel's cartilage (the articular) and the palatoquadrate bar. **B** depicts a reptile skull. The jaw joint is still between the articular and the palatoquadrate, but the dentary is of increased size. **C** shows the skull of a fossil mammallike reptile. The dentary is greatly enlarged and has a coronoid process. The jaw articulation, however, is still between the articular and palatoquadrate. In mammals, **D,** the dentary has formed an articulation with the temporal bone. The original joint now constitutes part of the inner ear. (Based on a diagram from DeBrul EL: In Sarnat BG, Laskin DM, [eds]: *The temporomandibular joint,* ed 3, Springfield Ill, 1979, Charles C Thomas.)

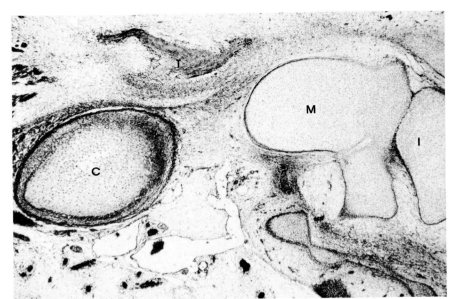

FIG. 19-2 Sagittal section through a 67 mm fetus showing both the primary and the secondary jaw joints. The developing temporal bone *(T)* and condylar blastema *(C)* together form the secondary joint. The malleus *(M)* and incus *(L)* represent the primary joint. (From Perry HT, et al: *J Craniomandib Pract* 3:125, 1985.)

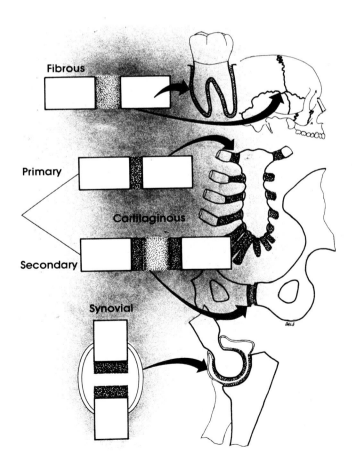

FIG. 19-3 Classification of joints.

TYPE OF JOINT

The temporomandibular articulation is a synovial joint. Its anatomy varies considerably among mammals, depending on masticatory requirements, so that a single all-embracing descriptive classification is not possible. For example, in carnivores movement is restricted to a simple hinge motion by the presence of well-developed anterior and posterior bony flanges that clasp the mandibular condyle. The badger provides an extreme example of this: the flanges clasp and envelop the condyle to such an extent that it is not possible to dislocate the mandible from the skull. In humans a different situation exists: the masticatory process demands that the mandible be capable of not only opening and closing movements but also protrusive, retrusive, and lateral movements and combinations thereof. To achieve these, the condyle undertakes translatory as well as rotary movements; and therefore the human TMJ is described as a *synovial sliding-ginglymoid joint* (Fig. 19-4).

DEVELOPMENT OF THE JOINT

Meckel's cartilage (Chapter 2) provides the skeletal support for development of the lower jaw and extends from the midline backward and dorsally, where it terminates as the malleus (or, in cephalometric terminology, the *articulare*). It articulates with the incal cartilage (the quadrate in nonmammals); and if there is any movement of the early jaw, it occurs between these two cartilages. This primary jaw joint exists for about 4 months until the cartilages ossify and become incorporated in the middle ear. At 3 months of gestation the secondary jaw joint, the TMJ, begins to form. The first evidence of its development is the appearance of two distinct regions of mesenchymal condensation, the temporal and condylar blastemas. The temporal blastema appears before the condylar, and initially both are positioned some distance from each other. The condylar blastema grows rapidly in a dorsolateral direction to close the gap. Ossification begins first in the temporal blastema (Fig. 19-5, *A*). While the condylar blastema

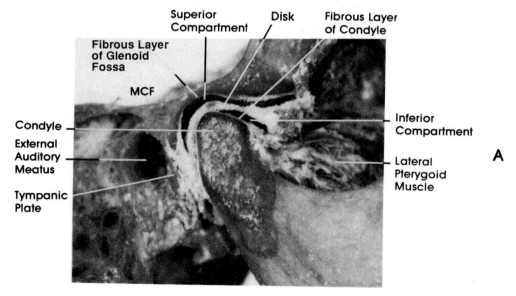

FIG. 19-4 The temporomandibular joint. In **A** the macroscopic appearance of the joint is depicted. (**A** from Liebgott WB: *The anatomical basis of dentistry*, St. Louis, 1986, Mosby.)

Continued.

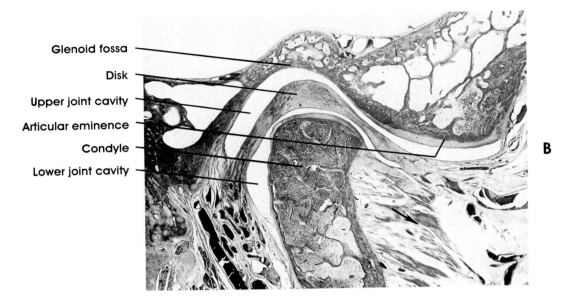

Glenoid fossa

Disk

Upper joint cavity

Articular eminence

Condyle

Lower joint cavity

B

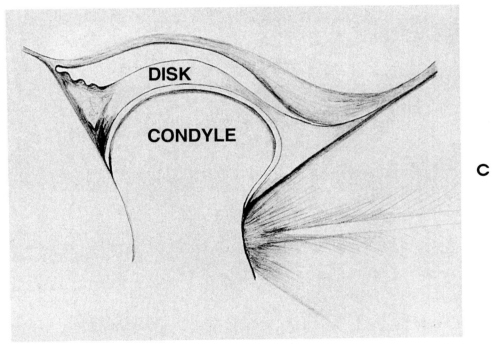

DISK

CONDYLE

C

FIG. 19-4, cont'd. **B** is a histologic section through the joint. **C** diagrams the joint. (**B** from Griffin CJ, et al: *Monogr Oral Sci* 4:1, 1975.)

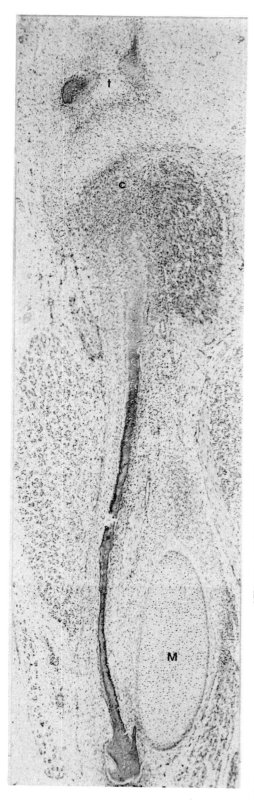

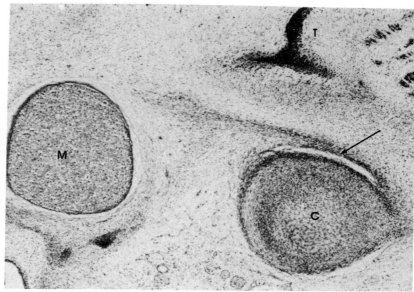

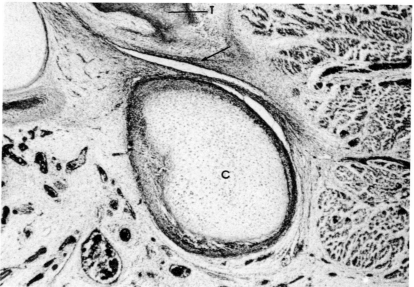

FIG. 19-5   Developing temporomandibular articulation.
A, Coronal section through a 12 week (61 cm CR) fetus. Bone formation has begun in the temporal blastema *(T)*. The condylar blastema *(G)* is still undifferentiated. Note the membranous bone forming the body of the mandible on the lateral aspect of Meckel's cartilage *(M)*. **B,** Sagittal section of the TMJ in a fetus (67 mm CR) showing the developing inferior joint cavity *(arrow)*. Bone formation has begun in the temporal blastema, but the condylar blastema still consists of undifferentiated cells. Meckel's cartilage is to the left of the developing joint. **C,** Sagittal section of the temporomandibular joint of a fetus (70 mm CR) showing the developing superior joint cavity *(arrow)*. Cartilage has formed in the condylar blastema, and the developing temporal bone is indicated. (**A** from Chi JG, et al: *Sequential atlas of human development,* Seoul Korea, 1992, Medical Publishing Co; **B** and **C** from Perry HT, et al: *J Craniomandib Pract* 3:125, 1985.)

is still condensed mesenchyme, a cleft appears immediately above it that becomes the inferior joint cavity (Fig. 19-5, *B*). The condylar blastema differentiates into cartilage (condylar cartilage), and then a second cleft appears in relation to the temporal ossification that becomes the upper joint cavity (Fig. 19-5, *C*). With the appearance of this cleft the primitive articular disk is formed.

BONES OF THE JOINT

The bones of the temporomandibular articulation are the *glenoid fossa* (on the undersurface of the squamous part of the temporal bone) and the *condyle* (supported by the condylar process of the mandible). The glenoid fossa is limited posteriorly by the squamotympanic and petrotympanic fissures. Medially it is limited by the spine of the sphenoid, and laterally by the root of the zygomatic process of the temporal bone. Anteriorly it is bounded by a ridge of bone described as the articular eminence, which is also involved in the articulation (Fig. 19-6). The middle part is a fairly thin plate of bone whose upper surface forms the middle cranial fossa (housing the temporal lobe of the brain). The condyle is the articulating surface of the mandible. Viewed sagittally, it is some 15 to 20 mm long (from medial to lateral extreme) and 8 to 120 mm thick, superficially

resembling a date stone perched atop a column. Its articular surface is strongly convex in the anteroposterior direction and slightly convex mediolaterally. Its medial and lateral ends are termed *poles*. The medial pole extends farther beyond the condylar neck than the lateral pole does and is positioned more posteriorly so that the long axis of the condyle deviates posteriorly and meets a similar axis drawn from the opposite condyle at the anterior border of the foramen magnum. Variations in the shape of the condyle are frequent, and often the condylar surface is divided by a sagittal crest into medial and lateral slopes.

Unlike most synovial joints, whose articular surfaces are covered hyaline cartilage, the temporomandibular articulation is covered by a layer of fibrous tissue. This histologic distinction has been used to argue that the TMJ is not a weight-bearing joint but the reality for this distinction can be found in the developmental history of the joint. The only other synovial joints with articular surfaces covered by fibrous tissue are the acromioclavicular and sternoclavicular, linking the clavicle to the appendicular skeleton. Both the mandible and the clavicle are bones formed directly from an intramembranous ossification center and are not preformed in cartilage—cartilage that persists in the long bones to cover articular surfaces following the appearance of ossification centers.

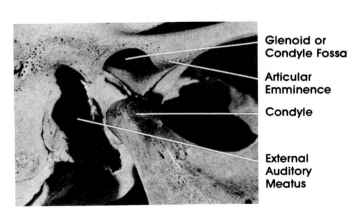

FIG. 19-6 Bones involved in the temporomandibular articulation.

Labels: Glenoid or Condyle Fossa; Articular Emminence; Condyle; External Auditory Meatus

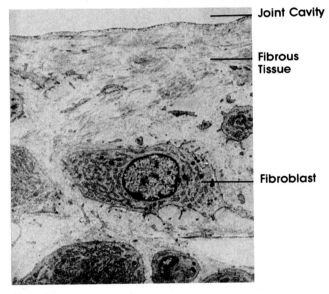

FIG. 19-7 Transmission electron micrograph showing the fibrous articular tissue covering the mandibular condyle. (From Goose DH, Appleton J: *Human dentofacial growth*, New York, 1982, Pergamon Press.)

Labels: Joint Cavity; Fibrous Tissue; Fibroblast

The fibrous layer covering the condyle consists of fibroblasts scattered through a dense, largely avascular, layer of type I collagen limited by an electron-dense membrane (the lamina splendens) (Fig. 19-7). The fibrous layer sits on a proliferative zone of cells associated with the formation of condylar cartilage. Whether this proliferative zone also contributes to the cellular content and renewal of the fibrous zone is undecided (and indeed unlikely). Studies in rats indicate that cell division occurs within fibroblasts occupying the deeper part of the fibrous layer; and since there is no convincing demonstration that cells from the proliferative layer contribute to the fibrous layer, it must be assumed that the fibrous articular layer is a self-contained and self-replicating structure.

The glenoid fossa is always covered by a thin fibrous layer that directly overlies the bone, much as periosteum does (Fig. 19-8), but this layer becomes appreciably thicker where it covers the slope of the articular emminence (Fig. 19-9).

CARTILAGE ASSOCIATED WITH THE JOINT

Some accounts of TMJ histology indicate that the surface coverings of the joint consist of fibrocartilage rather than fibrous tissue. Although it is possible that with age the fibrous covering layer might contain some

cartilage cells, there is no evidence that this is the norm. There is firm evidence, however, that fibrocartilage is associated with the articulation deep to the fibrous layer both in the condyle and on the articular eminence. The occurrence of such cartilage has a developmental explanation: A secondary growth cartilage associated with the developing TMJ forms within the blastema the *condylar cartilage*—and is in some ways akin to the epiphyseal cartilage of a developing long bone. It consists essentially of a proliferative layer of replicating cells that function as progenitor cells for the growth cartilage. These cells become chondroblasts and elaborate an extracellular matrix consisting of proteoglycans and type II collagen to form the extracellular matrix of cartilage. At the same time there is an increase in size of the chondroblasts (hypertrophy). Following the production of this cartilage, endochondral ossification occurs involving mineralization of the cartilage, vascular invasion, loss of chondrocytes and differentiation of osteoblasts to produce bone on the mineralized cartilaginous framework (Fig. 19-10). The only difference in this process between condylar and epiphyseal cartilages in long bones is the absence of ordered columns of cartilaginous cells (which characterize the epiphyseal growth cartilage and are the result of chondroblast cell division). The absence of elongated columns of chondroblast daughter cells in condylar carti-

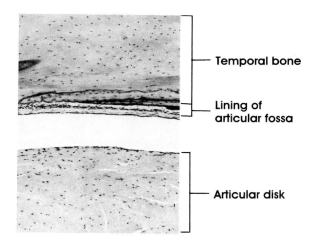

FIG. 19-8 Section through the temporal bone showing the very thin lining of the articular surface of the glenoid fossa. (From Blackwood HJJ. In Cohen B, Kramer IRH [eds]: *Scientific foundations of dentistry,* London, 1976, William Heinemann Medical Books.)

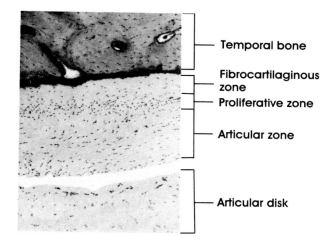

FIG. 19-9 Section through the articular eminence in the adult mandibular joint showing the relatively thick articular covering of this area of the joint. (From Blackwood HJJ. In Cohen B, Kramer IRH [eds]: *Scientific foundations of dentistry,* London, 1976, William Heinemann Medical Books.)

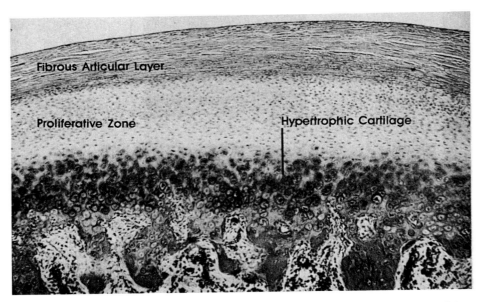

FIG. 19-10   Section through the growing condylar cartilage of a 13-year-old child. (From Goose DH, Appleton J: *Human dentofacial growth,* New York, 1982, Pergamon Press.)

lage has key significance. A typical long bone epiphyseal plate characterized by well-defined columns, is committed to an essentially unidirectional mode of growth; that is, the proliferation of cells by mitotic division is such that the whole bone necessarily elongates in a manner determined by the columns of dividing cells. The mandibular condyle, by contrast, has a multidirectional growth capacity and its cartilage can proliferate in any combination of superior and posterior directions as needed to provide for the best anatomic placement of the mandibular arch. It has also been established that in rat condylar cartilages cell proliferation and enlargement and extracellular matrix production all contribute to the growth of cartilage (in a ratio of 1:1.6:4).

A transient growth cartilage has also been found in association with development of the articular eminence. At birth there is no eminence; its development starts with a slender strip of growth cartilage (involving the same layers as already described for the condyle) situated along the slope of the eminence. Whereas the life span of these cartilages differs—the condylar cartilage existing until the end of the second decade, the eminence cartilage lasting a much shorter time— the subsequent history is the same for both. The

proliferative activity of cells in the proliferative layer ceases, but the cells persist (Figs. 19-9 and 19-11). The cartilage immediately below converts to fibrocartilage and, in the mandible, eventually mineralizes to a degree even greater than that of the mineralized bone (Fig. 19-12). Thus fibrocartilage is found both in the mandible and on the slope of the articular eminence. It seems certain that in both instances cells of the proliferative layer can, if the occasion demands, resume their proliferative activity. Thus remodeling of the articular surfaces can occur in response to functional changes throughout life and in response to orthodontic treatment. There can be additions to the joint surfaces, increasing the vertical dimension of the face: Regressive remodeling creates a loss of the vertical dimension, and peripheral remodeling adds tissue to the margins of the articulation (often an arthritic change). Remodeling also compensates for the changing relationships of the jaws brought about by tooth wear and loss.

In summary: Although fibrocartilage is associated with the temporomandibular articulation, it does not form part of the articulation and has no formal functional role to play in the everyday movements occurring between the two bones of the joint.

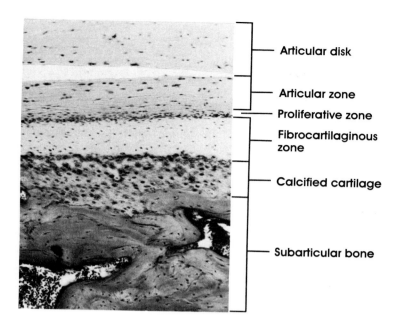

- Articular disk
- Articular zone
- Proliferative zone
- Fibrocartilaginous zone
- Calcified cartilage
- Subarticular bone

FIG. 19-11 Section through the articular covering of the adult mandibular condyle. (From Blackwood HJJ. In Cohen B, Kramer IRH, [eds]: *Scientific foundations of dentistry,* London, 1976, William Heinemann Medical Books.)

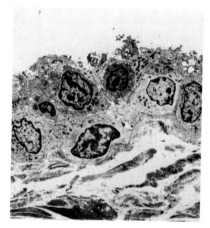

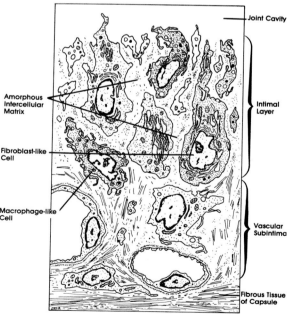

- Joint Cavity
- Amorphous Intercellular Matrix
- Intimal Layer
- Fibroblast-like Cell
- Macrophage-like Cell
- Vascular Subintima
- Fibrous Tissue of Capsule

FIG. 19-13 Synovial membrane. (Inset: Diagram of the electron micrograph.) (Micrograph courtesy Dr. W. Feagens).

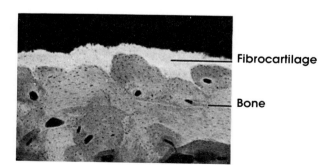

- Fibrocartilage
- Bone

FIG. 19-12 Microradiograph showing the subarticular bone and mineralization of the adjacent fibrocartilagenous layer. (From Blackwood HJJ: *J Dent Res* 45(Suppl 3): 480, 1966.)

CAPSULE, SYNOVIAL MEMBRANE, AND DISK OF THE JOINT

The TMJ is divided into two compartments by a disk and surrounded by a capsule lined with synovial membrane.

Capsule

The capsule, as it surrounds the joint, includes the articular eminence and consists of dense collagenous tissue, with its upper half (above the articular disk) forming a loose envelope that is attached to the squamotympanic fissure behind, the articular eminence in front, and the margins of the glenoid fossa elsewhere. It is also attached at its medial and lateral margins to the articular disk. Below the disk it attaches tightly to the neck of the condyle.

Synovial Membrane

The capsule is lined on its inner surface by a synovial membrane. An exact description of this delicate membrane in the human TMJ is not easy to give; several locations and structures have been described, which probably reflects the difficulty of obtaining adequately fixed specimens of the structure. Generally, the synovial membrane is considered to line the entire capsule, with folds or villi of the membrane protruding into the joint cavity, especially in its fornices and its upper posterior aspect. These folds increase in number with age and are also more prominent in joints affected by a pathologic process. Synovial membrane does not cover the articular surfaces of the joint or the disk, except for its bilaminar posterior region. The histology of the synovial membrane is also difficult to describe, since different regions of the joint capsule vary. Essentially, any synovial membrane consists of two layers, a cellular intima resting on a vascular subintima (Fig. 19-13), which in turn blends with the fibrous tissue of the capsule. The subintima is a loose connective tissue containing vascular elements together with scattered fibroblasts, macrophages, mast cells, and fat cells. The intima varies in structure, having one to four layers of synovial cells embedded in an amorphous fiber-free intercellular matrix. Often there are cellular deficiencies, so that the subintimal connective tissue directly borders the joint cavity. These cells are not connected by junctional complexes and do not rest on a basement membrane. The joint cavity is therefore not lined by epithelium. The cells forming this discontinuous layer are of two types, a predominant type A (macrophage-like) cell and a type B (fibroblast-like) cell. Type A cells have surface filopodia, many plasma membrane invaginations, and associated pinocytotic vesicles. Their cytoplasm contains numerous mitochondria and lysosomal elements and a prominent Golgi apparatus. Profiles of rough endoplasmic reticulum are few. Type B cells, on the other hand, contain many profiles of rough endoplasmic reticulum. Type A cells exhibit marked phagocytotic properties and are known to synthesize the hyaluronate found in synovial fluid. The Type B cells are thought to add protein to the fluid.

The synovial membrane is responsible for the production of synovial fluid, which is characterized by well-defined physical properties of viscosity, elasticity, and plasticity. Synovial fluid contains a small population of varying cell types such as monocytes, lymphocytes, free synovial cells, and occasionally polymorphonuclear leukocytes. The chemical composition of synovial fluid indicates that it is a dialysate of plasma with some added protein and mucin. Its function is to provide (1) a liquid environment for the joint surfaces and (2) lubrication to increase efficiency and reduce erosion. Whether it also provides nutrition for the disk and articular surfaces of the joint is debatable.

The synovial membrane is responsible for the removal of extraneous material shed into the joint cavity; the intimal cells have been demonstrated to possess marked phagocytic properties.

Disk

A fibrous disk divides the joint cavity into two compartments and is a structure with an important functional role: it provides, in effect, a largely passive movable articular surface accommodating the translatory movement made by the head of the condyle. It consists of dense fibrous tissue (Fig. 19-4) and its shape conforms to that of the apposed articular surfaces. Thus its lower surface is concave and generally matches the convex contour of the condyle. Its upper surface also presents a concave surface since its posterior and anterior components are considerably thickened, delimiting a central thinner component. At rest this central thinner component of the disk separates the anterior slope of the condyle from the slope of the articular eminence. The thickened posterior portion occupies the gap between the condyle and the floor of the glenoid fossa, and the anterior portion lies slightly anterior to the condyle. The type I collagen bundles that constitute the disk are generally loosely arranged and randomly oriented, except in the central region, where they are more tightly bound in organized bundles. Coronal sections of the disk show it to be thicker medially, its lateral and medial margins blending with the capsule. Anteriorly the disk divides into two lamellae—an upper one running forward to fuse with the capsule and periosteum on the anterior slope of the eminence, and a lower one running down to attach to the front of the neck of the condyle. In between is the "foot," which merges either with the capsule or with the upper fibers constituting the superior head of the lateral pterygoid muscle. There is some controversy as to whether fibers of the lateral pterygoid are attached to the anterior margin of the disk at its most medial aspect, and this will be discussed later with the anatomic description of this muscle. Posteriorly the disk also divides into two lamellae—an upper one, consisting of fibrous and elastic tissues, that fuses with the capsule and inserts into the squamotympanic fissure, and a lower one (nonelastic), consisting of collagen only, that turns down to blend with the periosteum of the condylar neck. Between these two lamellae a "space" is created that is filled with a loose highly vascular connective tissue (Fig 19-4, *C*). The disk is well supplied with vascular elements at its periphery but is avascular in its central region. During function it makes only relatively short movements in a passive manner to fit best with the changing relationships of the condylar head and the glenoid fossa and articular eminence. Such adaptation is permitted by the shape of the disk and the slippery environment of the joint cavity, although some influence is also exerted by superior fibers of the lateral pterygoid and the tight relationship created by taught capsular fibers running from the margins of the disk to the condyle.

LIGAMENTS ASSOCIATED WITH THE JOINT

It has been mentioned that the TM capsule is reinforced by ligamentous thickenings. Ligaments are defined as nonelastic collagenous structures that restrict and limit the movements a joint can make in that they limit the distance that the bones forming the articulation can be separated from each other without causing tissue damage. Classically, one functional ligament is described in association with the TMJ: the *lateral (or temporomandibular) ligament*, which is a fan-shaped reinforcement of the lateral wall of the capsule running obliquely backward and downward from the lateral aspect of the articular eminence to the posterior aspect of the condylar neck (Fig. 19-14). It functions in a similar way to collateral ligaments of other joints because of the bilateral nature of the articulation. Thus by preventing lateral dislocation it also prevents medial dislocation of the opposite joint. The ligament consists of two parts—an outer oblique portion arising from the outer surface of the articular eminence and extending backward and downward to insert into the outer surface of the condylar neck, and in inner horizontal portion with the same origin but inserting into the lateral pole of the condyle and the lateral margin of the disk. The position of the ligament is such that its oblique portion limits the amount of inferior displacement that can occur whereas its horizontal portion prevents, or at least limits, posterior displacement of the condyle and disk.

If the definition of a ligament is accepted, the capsule should also be considered a ligament, as should the inferior lamellae of the posterior diskal attachment, since this restricts forward extension of the disk. The capsular wall is thickened medially and laterally where

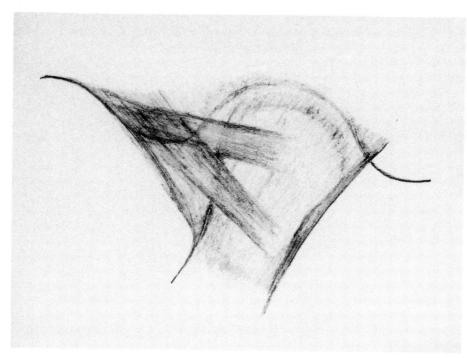

FIG. 19-14 The lateral (or temporomandibular) ligament. This diagram emphasizes two functional components of the capsular ligament preventing posterior and inferior displacement. The total ligament also prevents lateral and medial displacement (of the opposite joint).

it connects the disk to the poles of the condyle in the form of two straps, which thus firmly attach the disk to the condyle (Fig. 19-15). The lateral strap in particular, fusing as it does with the horizontal component of the lateral ligament, provides an especially firm attachment. These two thickenings have been considered to be collateral ligaments of the joint; but because they involve only the disk and head of the condyle, this can be disputed. Two other ligaments are included in conventional anatomic descriptions of the joint, although it is doubtful whether either has a functional role. The first is the *sphenomandibular ligament*, running from the lingula and shielding the opening of the inferior alveolar canal to the spine of the sphenoid. It represents the residual perichondrium of Meckel's cartilage. The second is the *stylomandibular ligament*, running from the spine of the sphenoid to the angle of the mandible. It represents the free border of the deep cervical fascia.

MUSCLES BRINGING ABOUT MOVEMENT

Before describing the muscles of mastication in detail, it is worth recalling some general features of muscle architecture and structure. Muscles may be described in a number of ways. One is by the arrangement of their fiber bundles, or fasciculi. In strap muscles the fasciculi all run parallel from origin to insertion. In fusiform muscles there is essentially the same arrangement except that the parallel-running fiber bundles converge at both the site of origin and the site of insertion of the muscle. Finally (in this grouping) there is the fan-shaped muscle, which has fasciculi that extend from a broad linear origin to a narrow insertion. Another way of describing muscles involves those that have a central tendon extending into a fleshy belly to which bundles of muscle fibers attach in an oblique direction. If all the muscle fiber bundles attach on one side; of such a tendon, the muscle is described as unipennate; if attachment occurs on both sides, bipennate and if multiple central tendons exist, multipennate.

Muscle Contraction

Muscle cells (fibers) that make up the bundles (fasciculi) are long and narrow. A fiber can be several centimeters long and up to 0.1 mm in diameter. In any given muscle the fibers tend to be of uniform length. The cell membrane of the fiber is called the *sarcolemma*, immediately beneath which the nucleus of the cell is found. Within each cell the sarcoplasm is packed with myofibrils, arranged in such a way that their close packing creates the pattern of striations seen under the

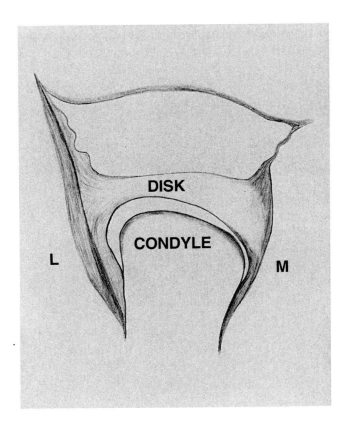

FIG. 19-15 Lateral and medial attachments of the disk to the condyle. Note how the lateral attachment is reinforced by the temporomandibular ligament.

light microscope. For a detailed account of the molecular basis of muscle contraction, standard histology textbooks should be consulted. Another feature of the muscle fiber is its sarcoplasmic reticulum, a branching endoplasmic network that surrounds each myofibril. Muscle contraction depends on the availability of calcium ions, which are transferred back and forth from the sarcoplasmic reticulum. Finally, the sarcoplasm contains variable numbers of mitochondria, glycogen, and myoglobin (the last acts as an oxygen-storing pigment).

You are all familiar with the distinction between red meat and white meat. This distinction reflects the greater amounts of myoglobin (a pigment similar to hemoglobin) found in red meat, which is characterized as muscle and is capable of slow but sustained contraction, as opposed to the more rapidly contracting fast muscle of white meat.

This distinction is mirrored in the histology and histochemistry of the individual muscle fiber, so that the slow-twitch fiber (type I) is generally narrower than the fast-twitch (type II) fiber, has poorly defined myofibrils, contains slow myosin, possesses many mitochondria, and exhibits high oxidative enzyme and low phosphorylase activity. This last trait reflects the fact that slow fibers also have a well-developed aerobic metabolism. As a result they are resistant to fatigue. By contrast, the type II or fast-twitch fibers have fewer mitochondria, possess an extensive sarcoplasmic reticulum, contain fast myosin, and show a lower oxidative enzyme activity (which is balanced by increased phosphorylase activity). Fast-twitch fibers thus rely more on anaerobic (glycolytic) activity and fatigue more easily.

This distinction understood, it is important to recognize that most if not all muscles contain a mixture of fast and slow fibers in varying proportions reflecting the function of that muscle (Fig. 19-16). It is also important to recognize that individual muscle fibers can be transformed (e.g., as a result of training) and that the innervation of the fibril determines its characteristics. In experiments in which nerves to red and white muscle fibers are cut, crossed, and reconnected, the fibers change their morphology and physiology accordingly.

Histochemical analyses of muscle fibers involving the demonstration of activity of the enzyme adenosine triphosphatase easily show the distinction between type I and type II fibers and also indicate that some fibers fall into an intermediate (IM) category. Furthermore, by varying the pH of the substrate during the histochemical reaction it is possible to differentiate subtypes of type II fibers (i.e., types IIA, IIB, and IIC). Types IIA and IIB contain fast myosin exclusively but can be distinguished on the basis of an inhibition of enzyme activity that occurs at pH 4.6 in the type IIA fiber. The IIA fiber is more fatigue resistant. Type IIC differs from A and B in that it contains a mixture of slow and fast myosins, with fast myosin predominating. Intermediate fibers also contain a mixture of fast and slow myosins, but in this case the slow myosins predominate. Although it is generally thought that IM fibers are those undergoing transformation, there is evidence from studies involving the muscles of mastication that at least some IM fibers are part of a stable population of fibers in muscle.

Motor Unit

Voluntary skeletal muscle, obviously, requires innervation for contraction to take place. A single nerve may innervate a single muscle fiber (fine control) or, by branching, supply as many as 160 fibers. No matter the pattern, the complex is known as a *motor unit* (Fig. 19-17) and innervation is achieved through a structure known as the *motor end plate*. At the site of innervation the nerve loses its myelin sheath, but not the covering of Schwann cells, and forms a terminal dilation that comes to occupy a corresponding dimple in the muscle cell surface. Between the nerve termination and the sarcolemma is a gap known as the synaptic cleft where the sarcolemmal surface is thrown into a series of junctional folds. A motor unit supplies fibers of a single type.

Two other neuronal structures need to be described in relation to muscle contraction: the muscle spindle and the Golgi tendon organ.

Muscle spindle

The muscle spindle is an encapsulated proprioceptor (Fig. 19-18) that detects changes in length. It consists of a connective tissue sac some 5 mm long and 0.2 mm in diameter containing 2 to 12 specially adapted muscle fibers, designated as intrafusal fibers. Intrafusal fibers are narrower than extrafusal fibers and assume two forms: the first is described as a nuclear bag fiber, because of the concentration of many nuclei in its centrally expanded portion, and the second as a nuclear chain fiber, because its nuclei are aligned in a single row. The nuclear bag fiber receives innervation from a nerve that spirals around the bag, the primary afferent. The nuclear chain fiber receives innervation from a primary terminal supplying the central region of the chain and a secondary terminal on either side of the primary (Fig. 19-19). The primary terminal is thought to be involved with responses to the degree and rate of stretch, the secondary terminal only with the degree of stretch. Muscle spindle intrafusal fibers retain their efferent supply.

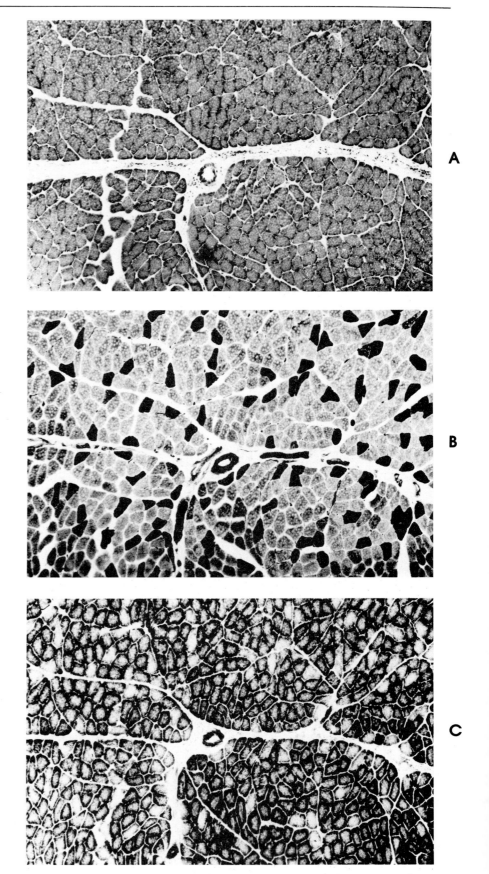

FIG. 19-16 Three successive sections of the lateral pterygoid muscle. In **A** the muscle has been stained with H&E, and all the fibers appear the same. In **B** the muscle has been stained to demonstrate adenosine triphosphatase (ATPase) activity, and this treatment clearly distinguishes two types of fiber, the slow-oxidative (unstained) and the fast glycolytic. The same muscle is stained in **C** to demonstrate reduced nicotinamide adenine dinucleotide (NADH). The majority of fibers that stained strongly with ATPase are now not stained, but some indicate a fast oxidative fiber. (Courtesy Dr. G. Altuna.)

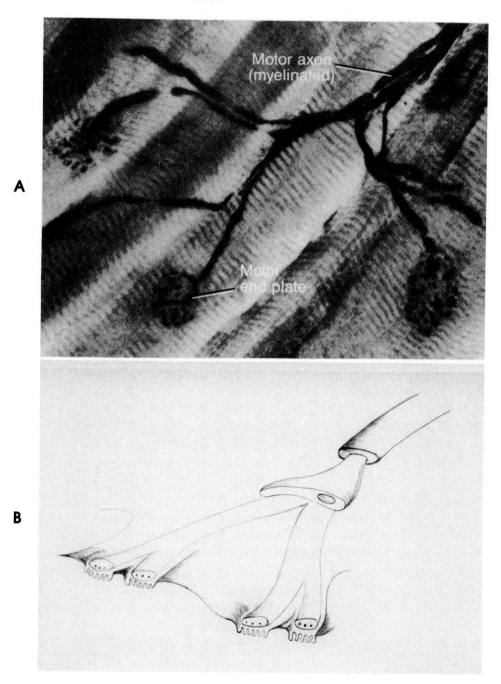

FIG. 19-17 **A,** Motor end plates on skeletal muscle fibers (stained with gold chloride). **B,** Functional relationship between the nerve and muscle fiber. (**A** from Cormack D [ed]: *Ham's Histology,* ed 9, Philadelphia, 1987, JB Lippincott.)

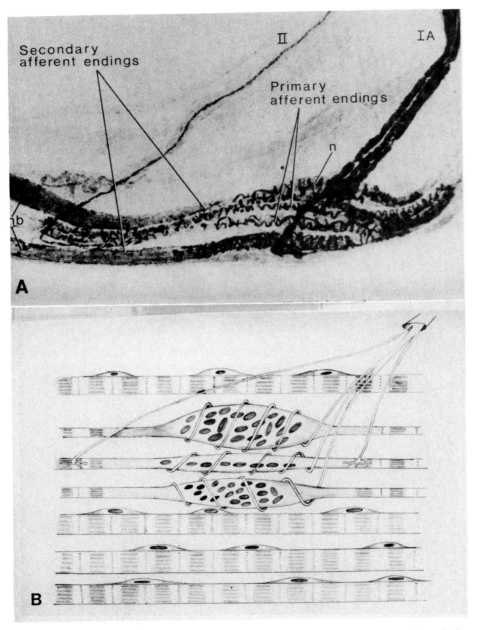

FIG. 19-18 **A,** Photomicrograph of the structure and innervation of a muscle spindle (cat) (stained with gold chloride) showing primary annulospiral afferent endings at the *right* and secondary flower spray endings at the *left.* **B,** The spindle. (For clarity the capsule has been omitted.) Primary annulospiral fibers envelop both the nuclear bag and the nuclear chain intrafusal fibers. Note the flower spray secondary endings associated with the nuclear chain fiber. (**A** from Boyd IA: *Philos Trans R Soc Lond [Biol]* 245:81, 1962.)

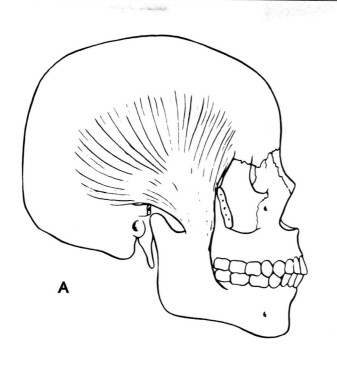

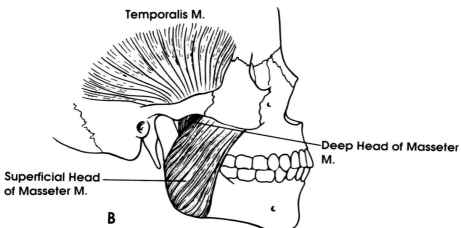

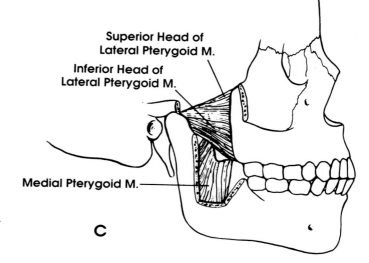

FIG. 19-19 Muscles of mastication: **A,** temporalis; **B,** masseter; **C,** lateral and medial pterygoids. (From Liebgott B [ed]: *The anatomical basis of dentistry,* Philadelphia, 1982, WB Saunders.)

Golgi tendon organ

Golgi tendon organs are found at the junction between muscles and the tendons or aponeuroses on which they pull. They are about half the size of a muscle spindle and consist of a capsule surrounding a group of collagen fibrils. The afferent nerve breaks up within the capsule and the terminal fibers ramify between the collagen bundles. The nerves are stimulated by compression between the bundles when the tendon is under compression.

From this abbreviated account of muscle, its heterogenity can be appreciated as providing the tremendous adaption of structure necessary to function, which is especially evident in the muscles of mastication.

Muscles of Mastication

Classically the muscles of mastication are the masseter, the medial (inferior) pterygoid, the lateral (superior) pterygoid, and the temporalis (Fig. 19-20). In functional terms other muscle groups are involved in mastication, such as the postcervical group (which stabilizes the cranial base) and the infrahyoid groups (which stabilizes the hyoid bone and permits the mylohyoid muscle and anterior belly of the digastric muscle to influence mandibular position). The anatomic configurations of all these muscles are well described, except for the insertion of the lateral pterygoid (which is still problematic).

The masseter and medial pterygoid muscles, together, have a slinglike configuration clasping the angle of the mandible and are the principal elevators of the jaw. Both muscles are multipennate and quadrate, and each has two heads.

The masseter consists of a superficial and a deep portion (or head), which, though originating separately, have a common insertion and blend together at the anterior border of the muscle. The superficial head has both a tendinous portion, originating from the zygomatic process of the maxilla, and a fleshy portion, arising from the inferior border of the anterior two thirds of the zygomatic arch. Its fibers run inferoposteriorly to insert into the angle and lower border of the mandibular ramus. They cover the fibers of the deep portion of the muscle, which arise from the inner aspect and inferior border of the posterior third of the zygomatic arch and run almost vertically downward to insert into the upper border and lateral aspect of the ramus. Although anatomically there are two components of this muscle, they can be readily distinguished and seen in functional terms to consist of four components: deep anterior, deep posterior, superficial anterior, and superficial posterior.

The medial pterygoid also has two portions or heads. The bulk of the muscle originates from the medial aspect of the lateral pterygoid plate, with a slip of fibers originating from the maxillary tuberosity. Little functional significance can be attributed to the latter origin.

Analysis of fiber composition of these two powerful elevator muscles confirms regional differences. Both exhibit a preponderance of type I fibers, indicating a muscle that (in conjunction with the multipennate structure) is adapted to resisting fatigue at low force levels. The posterior portions of both muscles, however, are characterized by possessing a relatively high concentration of type IIB fibers. Thus these fibers belong to fast-twitch rapidly contracting motor units and are sensitive to fatigue; they are able to generate large forces intermittently in the molar region of the mandible.

The temporalis is a fan-shaped muscle arising from the side of the skull that inserts into the coronoid process and the anteromedial border of the mandibular ramus. It is covered by a strong sheet of fascia attached (above) to the superior temporal line and (below) to the medial and lateral aspects of the zygomatic arch, whose undersurface also provides origin for fleshy muscle fibers. It is a bipennate muscle. An inner layer of fibers converges vertically down the lateral wall of the cranium to form a central tendon that inserts into the coronoid process and the anterior edge of the ascending ramus. The outer layer fibers (arising from the temporal fascia) descend in a more medial direction.

Functionally the temporalis acts as two muscles, its anterior fibers as an elevator and its posterior horizontally disposed fibers as a retractor or of the mandible. The muscle also shows variation in its fiber composition. The bipennate superfical portion has 50% type IIB fibers, indicating a capacity for acceleration coupled with an ability to develop tension. The posterior portion, however, contains a preponderance of type I fibers and many muscle spindles (indicating adaptation to a postural function).

In general, then, the masseter and the medial pterygoid are power producers and the temporalis is concerned more with moving and stabilizing the mandible.

There is still some controversy about the lateral pterygoid concerning not only its anatomy but also its exact functional role. The muscle has two heads, superior and inferior, arising from the roof of the infratemporal fossa and the lateral pterygoid plate respectively. No debate exists over the insertion of fibers of the lower head: they run posteriorly, inferiorly, and slightly laterally to insert into the pterygoid fovea (on the anterior surface of the condylar neck) and, upon contraction, bring about downward-forward and medial movement of the condyle. It is the insertion of the fibers of the superior head that is debatable; and the debate ranges around whether some of the superior fibers insert into

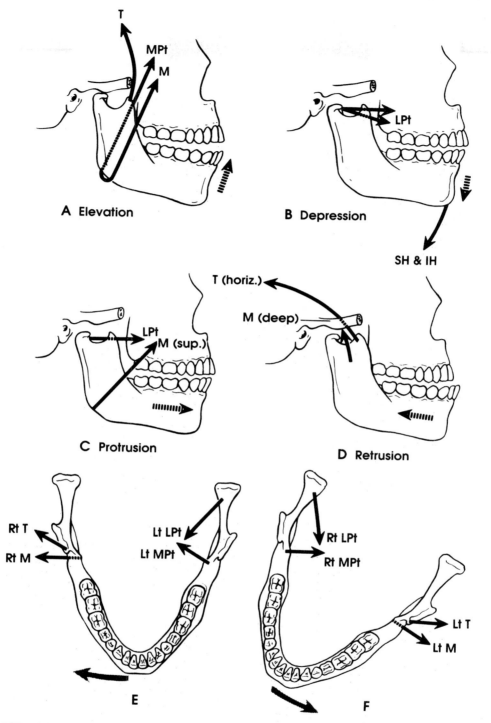

FIG. 19-20   Actions of the muscles of mastication. **A,** Elevation. *T,* Temporalis; *M,* masseter; *MPt,* medial pterygoid. **B,** Depression. *LPt,* Lateral pterygoid; *IH,* infrahyoid; *SH,* suprahyoid. **C,** Protrusion. *M(sup),* Masseter, superficial fibers; *LPt,* lateral pterygoid. **D,** Retrusion. *T(horiz),* temporalis, horizontal fibers; *M(deep),* masseter, deep fibers. **E,** Right lateral excursion of the mandible. *Rt T,* Right temporalis; *Rt M,* right masseter; *Lt Mpt,* left medial pterygoid; *Lt LPt,* left lateral pterygoid. **F,** Left lateral excursion of the mandible. *Rt LPt,* Right lateral pterygoid; *Rt Mpt,* right medial pterygoid; *Lt T,* left temporalis; *Lt M,* left masseter. (From Liebgott B: *The anatomical basis of dentistry,* Philadelphia, 1982, WB Saunders.)

the disk. There is no doubt that most of the fibers in the lower part of the muscle insert into the pterygoid fovea on the condyle. It is the upper fibers of the muscle that shows some variation. These may (1) gain insertion into the condyle by merging with the central tendon of the muscle, (2) insert directly into the pterygoid fovea, (3) blend with the collagenous fibers of the anterior joint capsule and thereby gain attachment to the condyle indirectly via the capsule,* or (4) insert directly into the disk at its most medial aspect. In dissected cadavers, if the upper fibers are pulled manually, the condyle and disk will move in unison, suggesting that the muscle either directly or indirectly exerts some effect on the disk. Because the bulk of the muscle inserts into the condyle, however, its main activity (obviously) is to move the condyle. Electromyographic studies indicate a reciprocal activation of the two heads of the muscle, with the inferior head involved in opening the jaw and the superior head involved in closure (by seating the condylar head against the posterior slope of the articular eminence). The attachment of the upper fibers to the disk either directly or indirectly is thought to stabilize the disk at closure. Again, these functional differences are reflected in fiber composition, with the type I fiber predominating (indicating a capacity for endurance during continuous work at relatively low force levels).

It has been argued that that the relatively high proportion of type IIC and IM fibers in the muscles of mastication indicates such fibers to be permanent residents in masticatory muscle, suggesting special functional characteristics for them.

Finally, the intrafusal fibers of muscle spindles in the masseter not only have a different enzyme profile from that in the extrafusal fibers but also are different from the intrafusal fibers in the limbs and trunk; and, again, this suggests special functional characteristics for this masticatory muscle.

---

*Since the foot of the disk merges with the inner surface of the anterior portion off the joint capsule, the functional effect here is as if the muscle inserted into the disk.

BIOMECHANICS OF THE JOINT

The muscles act on the TMJ to achieve opening and closure of the jaw, protrusion and retrusion, and alternate lateral movements and to provide stability. Since these movements rarely occur in isolation, most involve complex combinations of muscle activity. The role of the muscles in providing stability is one that should not be overlooked, for during mastication the forces applied to the joint not only are great but also are constantly changing; and when this is considered with the destabilizing effects of translatory movement, the functional role of muscle becomes more obvious. An example would be the situation found in biting, which demands that the disk be stabilized in a slightly forward position. This stabilization is achieved by the upper fibers of the lateral pterygoid muscle.

Based on the anatomic configuration of the muscles, and remembering that most movements of the joint involve both rotatory and translatory movement, we can now group muscle function as follows (Fig. 19-21):

The masseter, medial pterygoid, anterior part of the temporalis, and upper head of the lateral pterygoid combine to close the jaw.

The inferior head of the lateral pterygoid plus the anterior belly of the digastric and the mylohyoid (the latter two not strictly muscles of mastication as defined) are responsible for opening movements.

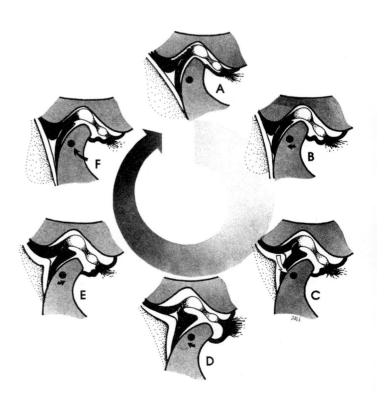

FIG. 19-21 Changing position of the mandible during the opening and closing. **A** to **D**, During opening. **E** and **F**, During closing. (Based on the original work of Rees LA: *Br Dent J* 96:126, 1954.)

The inferior head of the lateral pterygoid plus the elevator group bring about protrusive movement, and the posterior fibers of the temporalis plus the elevator group retrude the mandible.

Lateral movement is achieved by combined action of the elevator muscles, the posterior part of the temporalis (retrusion on the working side), and the lateral pterygoid (protrusion on the nonworking side).

Because movements at the joint involve both rotation and translation, the functional significance of the disk becomes more apparent (Figs. 3-13 and 19-21). The disk is not comparable to the meniscus in some other joints but is a unique feature of the TM articulation in that it enables a complexity of movement to be performed that are not found in any other joint. As has already been pointed out, the disk moves passively according to and dictated by its shape and the changing relationships of the bones involved in the TM articulation. This is somewhat simplistic, however, since the direct and indirect relationships of the superior head of the lateral pterygoid to the disk clearly play a part in its function. At present the cumulative evidence is that at rest a few slips of the upper head function to maintain the position of the disk, opposing the retractive forces created by elastic fibers in the upper lamella that connect the posterior aspect of the disk to the capsule of the joint. It may also be that this muscle attachment compensates for the weaker attachment of the medial surface of the disk to the condyle than exists laterally, or (vice versa) that the lateral attachment is stronger because of the medial muscle attachment.

INNERVATION OF THE JOINT

The innervation of any joint (the TMJ included) involves four types of nerve endings: the first (type I) are *Ruffini corpuscles*, the second (type II) *Pacinian corpuscles*, the third (type III) *Golgi tendon organs*, and the fourth (type IV) *free nerve endings*. The first three types are encapsulated, with the first two (Ruffini and Pacini) limited to the capsule of a joint and the third (Golgi) confined to the ligaments associated with the joint. Free nerve endings have a wider distribution. Ruffini corpuscles show a striking resemblance to Golgi tendon organs (already described) so that it is difficult to justify making a distinction between them other than to point out that Golgi tendon organs are specfically located in tendons or ligaments. The Pacini corpuscle has a characteristic microanatomy. It is an ovoid encapsulated structure, some 1 to 2 mm long and 0.5 to 1 mm in diameter. Within the capsule concentric layers of modified elongated Schwann cells wrap around a central axon much as the successive layers of an onion,

with the inner layers being compacted and the outer ones having wider connective tissue spaces between the cells. The corpuscle is adapted to register changes in pressure and vibration.

The TMJ is no different from other joints with respect to its innervation. Free nerve endings are the most abundant, with Ruffini, Golgi, and Pacini following in descending order. Generally the anatomic and functional designations for each type of nerve ending, together with their reflex role, can be listed as in the box.

Ruffini	Posture (proprioception)	Dynamic and static balance
Pacini	Dynamic mechanoreception	Movement accelerator
Golgi	Static mechanoreception	Protection (ligament)
Free	Pain (nociception)	Protection (joint)

It has been pointed out, however, that neurophysiologic studies are limited in their ability to attribute single nerve discharges to specific endings. In particular, the role of free nerve endings is confusing since elsewhere in the body such endings are sensitive to thermal and mechanical as well as noxious stimuli.

Regardless, there seems to be a common pattern for innervation of the TMJ that can be summarized as follows: *Ruffini endings* exist in clusters in the superficial layers of the joint capsule and are thought always to be active in every position of the joint (even when the joint is immobile) so that they signal static joint position, changes in intraarticular pressure, and the direction, amplitude, and velocity of joint movements. *Pacini corpuscles* are rapidly acting mechanoreceptors with a low threshold found mainly in the deeper layers of the capsule that signal joint acceleration and deceleration. *Golgi tendon organs*, limited as they are to the ligaments and sparsely distributed in the superficial layers of the lateral ligament, remain completely inactive in immobile joints, becoming active only when the joint is at the extremes of its range of movement. The distribution and significance of *free nerve endings* in joints are usually considered secondary to the roles of the other specialized receptors. Yet they are the most frequently occurring terminal in a joint, are generally thought to be associated with nociception, and are widely distributed. There has been some debate as to whether free nerve endings occur in the disk of the TMJ and the synovial membrane. Recent studies have supported the theory that they do indeed occupy the anterior and posterior bands of the disk and the synovial membrane, where (it is speculated) they may function to control the activity of macrophagelike cells.

As previously mentioned, Hilton's law states that the trigeminal nerve (V) provide the afferent innervation to a joint, and this is also the case with branches supplying the joint. Branches of the mandibular division of the fifth cranial nerve (i.e., the auriculotemporal, deep temporal, and masseteric) supply the joint.

BLOOD SUPPLY TO THE JOINT

The vascular supply to the TMJ comes from branches of the superficial temporal, deep auricular, anterior tympanic, and ascending pharyngeal arteries, all branches of the external carotid.

BIBLIOGRAPHY

Anderson DJ, Matthews BJ (eds): *Mastication*, Bristol UK, 1976, John Wright & Sons.

Appleton J: The ultrastructure of the articular tissue of the mandibular condyle in the rat, *Arch Oral Biol* 20:823, 1975.

Appleton J: The fine structure of a surface layer over the fibrous articular tissue of the rat mandibular condyle, *Arch Oral Biol* 23:719, 1978.

Barnett CH, Davies D, MacConaill MA: Synovial joints: their structure and mechanics, London, 1961, Longmans.

Baume LJ, Holz J: Ontogenesis of the human temporomandibular joint: development of the temporal components, *J Dent Res* 49:864, 1970.

Blackwood HJJ: The mandibular joint: development, structure, and function. In Cohen B, Kramer IRH (eds): *Scientific foundations of dentistry*, London, 1976, Heinemann.

Carpentier P, Yung JOP, Marguelles-Bonnet R, Meunissier M: Insertions of the lateral pterygoid muscle: an anatomic study of the human temporomandibular joint, *J Oral Maxillofac Surg* 46:477, 1988.

Dixon AD: Structure and functional significance of the intra-articular disk of the human temporomandibular joint, *Oral Surg* 15:48, 1962.

Durkin JF, Heeley JD, Irving JT: The cartilage of the mandibular condyle, *Oral Sci Rev* 2:29, 1973.

Eriksson PO, Eriksson A, Ringqvist M, Thornell LE: Special histochemical muscle-fiber characteristics of the human lateral pterygoid muscle, *Arch Oral Biol* 26:495, 1981.

Eriksson PO, Thornell LE: Histochemical and morphological muscle-fiber characteristics of the human masseter, the medial pterygoid and the temporal muscles, *Arch Oral Biol* 28:781, 1983.

Eriksson PO, Thornell LE: Variation in histochemical enzyme profile and diameter along human masseter intrafusal fibers, *Anat Rec* 226:168, 1990.

Furstman L: The early development of the human temporomandibular joint, *Am J Orthod* 49:672, 1963.

Gage JP: Mechanisms of disc displacement in the temporomandibular joint, *Aust Dent J* 34:427, 1989.

Goose DH, Appleton J: *Human dentofacial growth*, New York, 1982, Pergamon Press.

Griffin CJ, Hawthorn R, Harris R: Anatomy and histology of the human temporomandibular joint. In Sarnat BG (ed): *The temporomandibular joint*, ed 2, Springfield Ill, 1964, Charles C Thomas.

Griffin CJ, Sharpe CJ: Distribution of elastic tissues in the human temporomandibular meniscus, especially in respect to compression areas, *Aust Dent J* 7:72, 1962.

Ichikawa H, Matsuo S, Wakisaka S, Akai M: Fine structure of calcitonin gene-related peptide–immunoreactive nerve fibers in the rat temporomandibular joint, *Arch Oral Biol* 35:727, 1990.

Kido MA, Kondo T, Ayasaka N, et al: The peripheral distribution of trigeminal nerve fibres in the rat temporomandibular joint studied by an anterograde axonal transport method with wheat germ agglutinin–horseradish peroxidase, *Arch Oral Biol* 36:397, 1991.

Luder HU, Leblond CP, von der Mark K: Cellular stages in cartilage formation as revealed by morphometry, radioautography and Type II collagen immunostaining of the mandibular condyle from weanling rats, *Am J Anat* 182:197, 1988.

Marguelles-Bonnet R, Yung JP, Carpentier P, Meunissier M: Temporomandibular joint serial sections made with mandible in intercuspal position, *J Craniomandib Pract* 7:97, 1989.

Matthews B: Mastication. In Lavelle CLB (ed): *Applied physiology of the mouth*, Bristol UK, 1975, John Wright & Sons.

Miles AFW, Dawson JA: Elastic fibers in the elastic fibrous tissues in the human temporomandibular meniscus especially in respect to compression areas, *Aust Dent J* 7:72, 1962.

Mizuno I, Saburi N, Taguchi N, et al: Mitotic activity of cells in the fibrous zone of the rat mandibular condyle, *Arch Oral Biol* 37:29, 1992.

Moffett BC: The morphogenesis of the temporomandibular joint, *Am J Orthod* 52:401, 1957.

Moffett BC: The prenatal development of the human temporomandibular joint, *Contrib Embryol* 36(243):21, 1957.

Muntener M: A rapid and reversible muscle fiber transformation in the rat, *Exp Neurol* 77:668, 1982.

Noble HW: Comparative functional anatomy of the temporomandibular joint, *Oral Sci Rev* 2:3, 1973.

Perry HT, Xu Y, Forbes DP: The embryology of the temporomandibular joint, *J Craniomandib Pract* 3:125, 1985.

Rees LA: The structure and function of the mandibular joint, *Br Dent J* 96:126, 1954.

Ringqvist M: Histochemical fiber types and fiber sizes in human masticatory muscles, *Scand J Dent Res* 79:336, 1971.

Ringqvist M: Fibre sizes of human masseter muscle in relation to bite force, *J Neurol Sci* 19:297, 1973.

Ringqvist M: Histochemical enzyme profiles of fibres in human masseter muscles, with special regard to fibres with intermediate myofibrillar ATPase reaction, *J Neurol Sci* 18:133, 1973.

Ringqvist M: A histochemical study of temporal muscle fibers in denture wearers and subjects with natural dentition, *Scand J Dent Res* 82:28, 1974.

Ringqvist M: Size and distribution of histochemical fiber types in masseter muscle of adults with different states of occlusion, *J Neurol Sci* 22:429, 1974.

Symons NBB: The development of the human mandibular joint, *J Anat* 86:326, 1952.

Thilander B: Innervation of the temporo-mandibular joint capsule in man, *Trans R Sch Dent Stockholm Umea* 7:7, 1961.

Thilander B: Innervation of the temporomandibular joint, *Acta Odontol Scand* 22:51, 1964.

Thornell LE, Billeter R, Eriksson PO, et al: Heterogeneous distribution of myosin in human masticatory muscle fibers as shown by immunocytochemistry, *Arch Oral Biol* 29:1, 1984.

Wilkinson T, Chan KK: The antomic relationship of the insertion of the superior lateral ptrygoid muscle to the artic-

ular disc in the temporomandbular joint of human cadavers, *Aust Dent J* 34:315, 1989.

Wilkinson TM: The relationship between the disk and the lateral pterygoid muscle in the human temporomandibular joint, *J Prosthet Dent* 60:715, 1988.

Wright W, Dowson D, Kerr J: The structure of joints, *Rev Connect Tissue Res* 6:105, 1973.

Yuodelis RA: The morphogenesis of the human temporo-mandibular joint and its associated structures, *J Dent Res* 45:182, 1966.

Yuodelis RA: Ossification of the human temporomandibular joint, *J Dent Res* 45:192, 1966.

Yung JP, Carpentier P, Marguelles-Bonnet R, Meunissier M: Anatomy of the temporomandibular joint and related structures in the frontal plane, *J Craniomandib Pract* 8:101, 1990.

Zimny ML: Mechanoreceptors in articular tissues, *Am J Anat* 182:16, 1988.

CHAPTER 20

Repair and Regeneration of Dental Tissue

ONE purpose in studying the structure and development of dental tissues is to understand how they respond to insult caused by function or dental disease and how this response can and should determine subsequent clinical practice.

Tissue response is always a question of degree. Thus there are responses (e.g., hyperkeratinization of epithelium or tubular occlusion in dentin following attrition) that do not necessarily involve inflammation. If, however, an insult is sufficient to elicit an inflammatory response, the healing process is evoked. The outcome of healing is either (1) complete restoration of tissue architecture tissue (regeneration) or (2) restoration of tissue continuity with scarring and distortion of the normal architecture (repair).

REPAIR OF THE SKIN

The repair process follows a predictable series of orderly biologic events, differs little from one kind of tissue to another, and is independent of the type of injury. To explain the repair process in dental tissues, it is best to give first a simplified account of repair in skin after it has been incised and where healing is uncomplicated by infection. Repair of skin wounds involves both an epithelial and a connective tissue response.

Epithelial Response

The response of epithelium is straightforward, and the desired outcome is a reestablishment of epithelial continuity and the covering of exposed connective tissue. This is achieved by the mobilization and migration of epithelial cells at the wound margin. The cells lose their firm attachment to each other and to the underlying connective tissue, seen histologically as a widening of the intercellular spaces (Fig. 20-1). There is

also an increase in the amount of cytoplasm, permitting the development of profiles of rough endoplasmic reticulum, and the metabolism of the cells switches from the Krebs cycle to the pentose phosphate shunt. Basal epithelial cells adjacent to the immediate margin of the wound show increased mitotic activity. All these changes are characteristic of epithelium supported by a disturbed connective tissue and have been discussed with development of the dentogingival junction (Chapter 13). As a result of this mobilization, epithelial cells migrate across and eventually cover the exposed wound surface. In the instance of a clean incised wound, epithelialization can occur in about 24 hours.

Connective Tissue Response

The response of connective tissues involves hemostatic, inflammatory, proliferative, and secretory stages.

Hemostasis

Immediately following an injury, hemorrhage occurs into the tissue defect, with an aggregation of platelets and coagulation to form a clot. This clot not only serves as a hemostatic barrier, it also unites the wound margins and eventually provides a scaffold for the subsequent migration of reparative cells.

Inflammation

Neutrophils are the first inflammatory cells to invade the wound. They appear within a few hours of injury, reaching a maximum at 24 hours, and they have a short life span at the wound site before they degenerate. Although their degeneration releases enzymes that help destroy damaged tissues, their prime function is to control bacterial invasion and hence infection. If a wound is not infected, the absence of neutrophils does not hinder the repair process. Macrophages (Fig. 20-2) en-

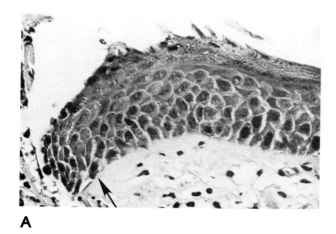

A

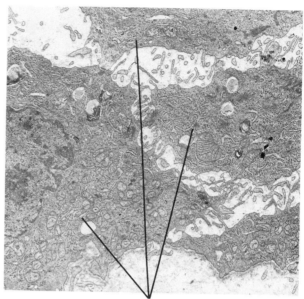

Rough Endoplasmic Reticulum

B

FIG. 20-1 Light and electron microscopic views of the eptithelial response to a wound of lip epithelium in the rat. **A,** The epithelial cells bordering the wound margin (arrow) are beginning to separate from each other before migrating across the defect. **B,** The migrating cells show, in addition to widened intercellular spaces, the amount of cytoplasm which contains added profiles of rough endoplasmic reticulum.

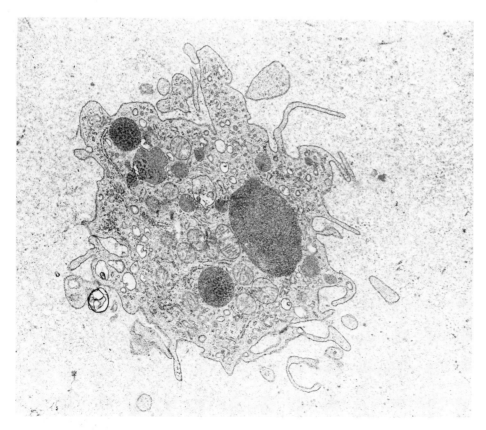

FIG. 20-2 Electron micrograph of a macrophage in the wound defect 24 hours after wounding.

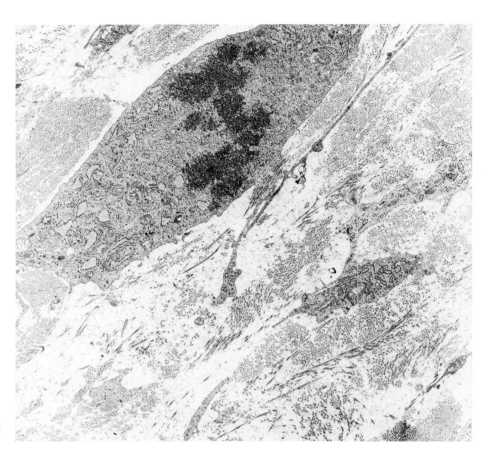

FIG. 20-3 Cell division within a fibroblast peripheral to the wound margin.

ter the wound after about 48 hours and are the predominant inflammatory cell at 5 days. Their function is to "mop up" foreign and damaged materials, but they also secrete a variety of biologically active peptides (including a mitogen specific for fibroblasts). In the absence of macrophages, fewer fibroblasts are stimulated during healing, so that the rate of repair is slowed and the amount of repair tissue diminished. Thus macrophages have a direct bearing on the repair process.

Proliferation and synthesis

This stage involves the proliferation of fibroblasts and the synthesis of collagen to form scar tissue. The fibroblasts for wound repair are derived from two sources: (1) the division of undamaged fibroblasts at the wound periphery (Fig. 20-3) and (2) the differentiation and proliferation of undifferentiated perivascular cells (Fig. 20-4). The resulting daughter cells from both sources

migrate into the wound defect to form the collagen of scar tissue (Figs. 20-5 and 20-6). Figure 20-7 is a summary of this simple account of repair.

REPAIR OF ENAMEL

It has already been pointed out that enamel cannot repair itself in the conventional sense, since the cells that formed it no longer exist. Enamel is capable of repair in a limited way, however, by physicochemical means. If the carious process is arrested while confined to enamel and there has been no breakdown of the surface layer, remineralization can occur in the subsurface enamel. This depends on an added supply of calcium and phosphate ions from the saliva, and if fluoride is present the remineralized enamel may be more resistant than normal enamel to further demineralization.

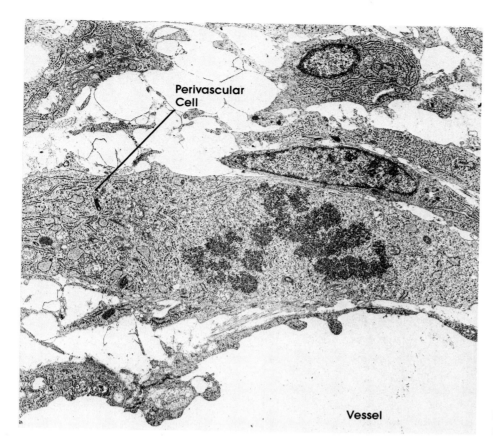

FIG. 20-4 Cell division in an undifferentiated perivascular cell.

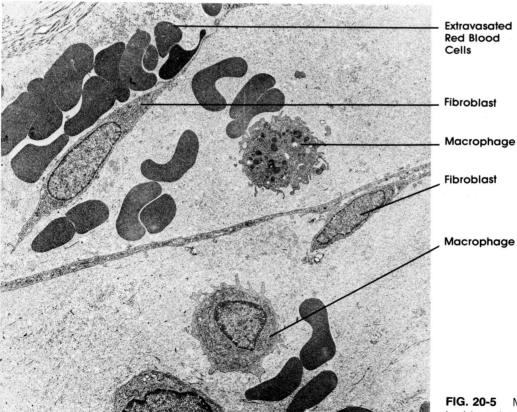

FIG. 20-5 Migration of pioneer fibroblasts into the wound defect.

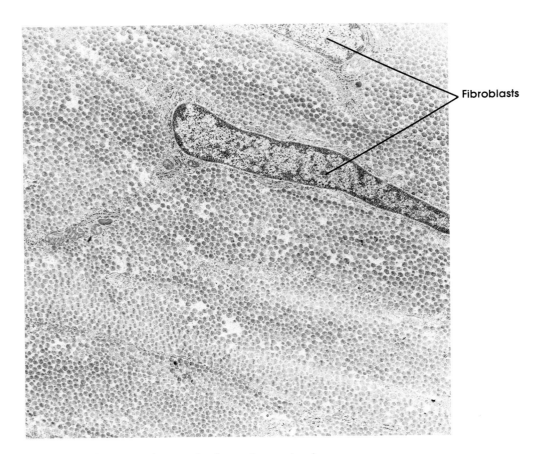

FIG. 20-6 Electron micrograph of scar tissue showing a dense mass of collagen fibrils (cut in cross section) and two quiescent fibroblasts.

REPAIR OF THE DENTIN-PULP COMPLEX

Dentin is a vital tissue whose response to damage is both varied and complex; some of these responses have already been discussed (Chapter 10). Essentially they can be divided into two categories: (1) changes within the dentin and (2) deposition of reparative dentin. Changes within dentin are represented by occlusion of the dentinal tubules. Occlusion is achieved in a number of ways. First, there can be occlusion by the deposition of collagen, which remains unmineralized, to simply plug the tubule (Fig. 20-8). Second, there can be mineral deposition within the tubule, which, if collagen is present, will occur around the collagen fibrils (Fig. 10-11).

Reparative dentin formation is confused by the fact that this form of dentin may be the product of either (1) pre-existing odontoblasts stimulated to deposit additional dentin or (2) new cells differentiated from the pulp following odontoblast death that are odontoblast-

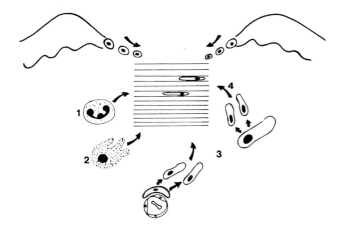

FIG. 20-7 Summary of tissue repair. The epithelial response is achieved by proliferation and migration of cells to cover the defect. The connective tissue response involves successively *(1)* a polymorph response (12 to 24 hours), *(2)* a macrophage response (2 to 5 days), and *(3)* a fibroblast response (2 days and on) from undifferentiated perivascular cells and undamaged fibroblasts. The new fibroblasts *(4)* form the collagen of scar tissue. (See Fig. 20-6.)

like and produce a substance not strictly identical to normal dentin.

Once death of the odontoblast has occurred, for whatever reason (which may include caries and the outcome of cavity preparation), the reaction of the pulp can be compared to that of connective tissue in the skin. There is inflammation, leading to a proliferative and secretory response. New cells differentiate from undamaged pulpal cells and lay down collagen (scar tissue), which becomes mineralized to form tertiary or reparative dentin.

This basic reparative response of the dentin-pulp complex can be impaired by a number of local factors: First is the fact that restorative materials do not precisely mimic the epithelium's ability to cover and seal. It is now recognized that microleakage can occur around some restorative materials, so that a low-grade persistent infection modifies and delays the pulpal response.

Second is the age of the tooth. Formation of dentin continues throughout life, so that the pulp chamber grows progressively smaller. At the same time there is a relative increase in the pulp's collagen content, a decrease in its cellularity, and a loss of water from the ground substance. The blood supply to the pulp is diminished, and there is a loss with degeneration of both myelinated and unmyelinated axons as well as demyelination and a decrease in neuropeptide content (all of which affect hemoregulation).

Third is the fact that it was assumed, on the basis of normal embryologic development, that an epithelial factor was needed for the differentiation of odontoblasts. This fact, combined with the recognition that mature odontoblasts cannot divide, led to the conclusion that cells able to form hard tissue were generally unavailable in the dental pulp.

We now understand much more about the reparative potential of the pulp. As has been clearly shown, in the absence of bacteria (i.e., germ-free animals) or when steps are taken to prevent microleakage around the epithelial substitute restorative material, cells can differentiate and deposit a calcific tissue as early as 5 days in germ-free experimental animals and certainly by 10 days—a time-frame that shows the healing potential of the pulp to be similar to that of other soft connective tissue.

The cells constituting this hard tissue originate from cell divisions in deeper layers of the pulp. Which populations of cells divide has not been established. They might be undifferentiated perivascular cells, pulpal fibroblasts, or cells formed from the odontoblast lineage but not exposed to the final epithelial influence. Regardless, they form a hard tissue without the usual requirement for epithelial contact. What does seem to be required is a surface. Thus in various experimental sit-

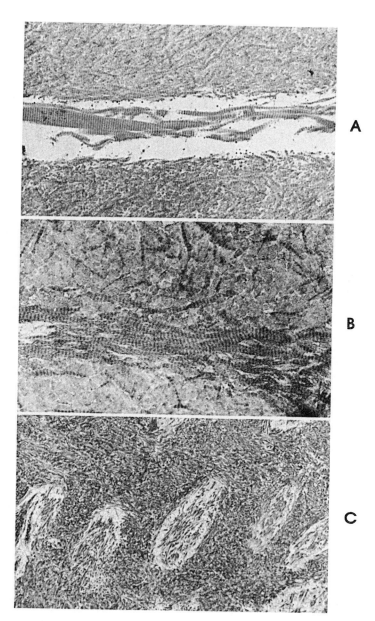

FIG. 20-8 Occlusion of a dentinal tubule with collagen (all sections demineralized). In **A** collagen fibrils occupy the patent tubule. In **B** they have occluded the tubule. **C** shows a number of collagen-containing tubules in cross section.

uations dentinlike tissue can form as long as a surface of predentin is present. When no surface is available (e.g., after pulpal exposure), these newly differentiated cells first express a mixture of collagens (including types I, II, III, and IV), which form a matrix surface. The deposition of fibronectin on this surface, or on predentin, provides the mechanism for positioning the cells, which then produce a matrix consisting of type I and type III collagen, which accepts mineral in the absence of phosphophoryn. Although it may be only a question of semantics, there is much discussion as to whether the mineralized tissue so formed is truly dentin since the odontoblasts proper express type I collagen and phosphophoryn.

Thus the dentin pulp complex has the same repair mechanism as any other connective tissue. It is not unique, as has been claimed; but the repair potential can be, and is, affected by a number of local factors.

It is now worth analyzing these responses of enamel and dentin in terms of the carious process and the dental procedures undertaken to restore the structural damage caused by that process.

DENTAL CARIES

Under the light microscope three zones can be distinguished in the early carious lesion. At the inner advancing edge is a translucent zone, which is followed by a dark zone. The third zone is the body of the lesion,

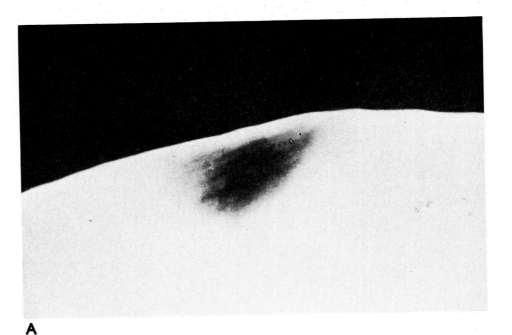

A

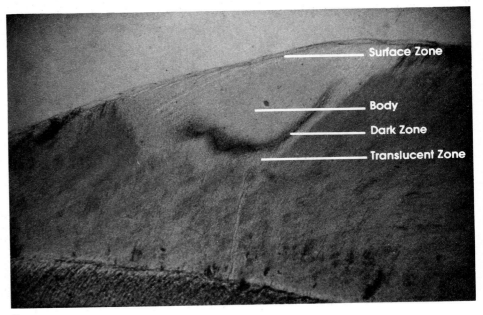

B

FIG. 20-9 Enamel caries. **A,** Microradiograph showing the subsurface location of the lesion. **B,** Same lesion viewed with polarized light. The translucent zone, dark zone, body of the lesion, and surface zone are all visible. (From Silverstone L: In Cohen B, Kramer RH [eds]: *The scientific foundation of dentistry,* London, 1976, William Heinemann Medical Books.)

which occupies the space between the dark zone and the apparently intact enamel surface (Fig. 20-9). The inner translucent zone represents the first area of change in enamel observable by light microscopy, and it has been well established that removal of mineral occurs in this region. The dark zone represents an area that was previously demineralized but is now undergoing remineralization. Thus the carious process is a dynamic one, with alternating phases of demineralization and remineralization, rather than a static simple continuing dissolution of material. The body of a lesion is where the bulk of mineral is being lost and where the most destructive morphologic changes are occurring.

An important characteristic of the early carious lesion is that most of the demineralization occurs at a subsurface level, so that a well-mineralized surface layer remains in place for some time. It is suggested that this surface zone remains intact because that is where calcium and phosphate ions are reprecipitated (from either subsurface dissolution or the saliva). Since the action of dental caries involves acid demineralization of enamel crystals, one might expect that the improved resolution of electron microscopy would reveal the structural basis of enamel dissolution in caries. Little ultrastructural change can be identified in the translucent and dark zones. It is primarily in the body of the lesion that damage to the crystals can be observed (Fig. 20-10). The electron microscope has revealed, however, that the crystals along both sides of the rod sheath in carious lesions are larger and more electron dense than elsewhere. These are reprecipitated crys-

tals, and their localization suggests that the rod sheaths have some role to play in the development of caries.

In summary: The carious process in enamel consists of a diffuse demineralization within the bulk of the lesion that affects crystals in all regions of enamel; however, varying patterns of differential dissolution are often observed.

When the carious process reaches dentin, the response is sequential. Frequently at this stage the enamel is still intact and bacterial invasion has not occurred. The lesion has increased the permeability of enamel to acid and various other chemical stimuli, however, and this stimulates a response from the dentinpulp complex. The nature of the initial response reflects the increased activity of odontoblasts, with a possible retraction of processes and an increase in collagen deposition in the periodontoblastic space plus the formation of sclerotic dentin by the mechanisms described in Chapter 10. (See Figs. 10-11 and 20-11.) This can then lead to the deposition of reparative dentin by the still vital odontoblasts. When the enamel cavitates, bacteria reach the dentin surface and destruction of dentin begins. Superimposed on this process are the death of odontoblasts, a mild inflammatory reaction in the pulp, and the bacterial invasion of dentin enclosed by the translucent zone. Because bacteria infecting dentin are acidogenic, acid diffuses ahead of them and demineralizes the dentin; consequently an additional mechanism comes into play, involving reprecipitation to enhance the zone of sclerotic dentin within dentinal tubules (Fig. 20-12). Bacteria are at first confined to the tubules (Fig. 20-13) but later escape this confinement and destroy the dentin matrix (Fig. 20-14). At

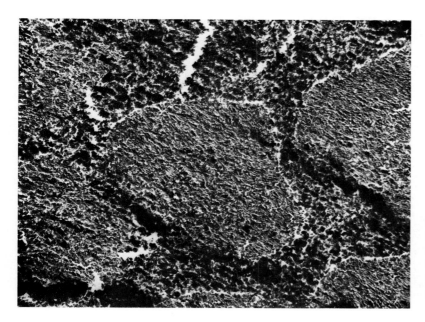

FIG. 20-10 Electron micrograph through the body of a carious lesion. Narrow channels are present at the rod junctions. (From Silverstone L: In Cohen B, Kramer RH [eds]: *The scientific foundations of dentistry,* London, 1976, William Heinemann Medical Books.)

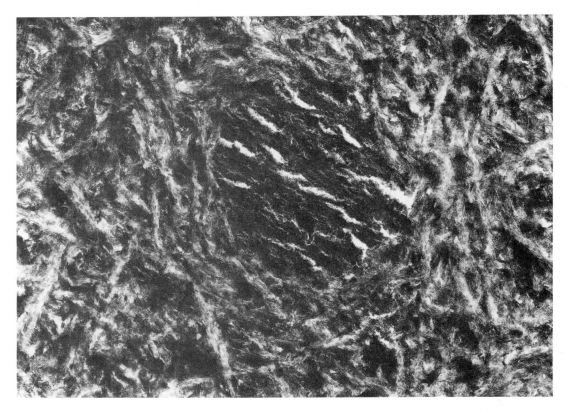

FIG. 20-11 Translucent zone in dentinal caries (undemineralized section). The tubule is filled with crystals. (Courtesy Dr. N.W. Johnson.)

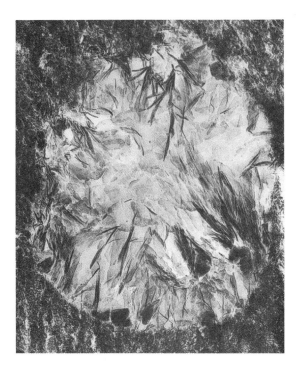

FIG. 20-12 Remineralization in a dentinal tubule. (Courtesy Dr. N.W. Johnson.)

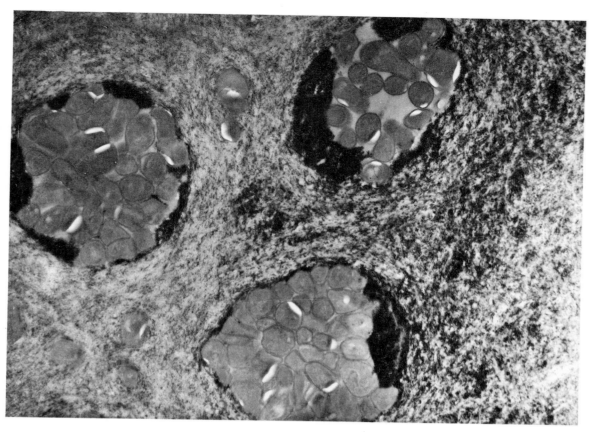

FIG. 20-13 Dentinal caries. Although microorganisms are confined to the tubules, there is demineralization of the dentin. (Courtesy Dr. N.W. Johnson.)

this stage there has been recruitment of pulpal cells, which lay down reparative dentin as previously described.

If the carious process within dentin is to be arrested (either naturally or by surgical intervention to remove infected dentin), the translucent zone and reparative dentin must provide an effective mineralized barrier. Surgical intervention is, of course, achieved by cavity preparation and the restoration of lost tooth tissue by substitute materials.

CAVITY PREPARATION

Cavity preparation in a tooth involves the removal of both enamel and dentin. Enamel is, in reality, an epithelium and the dentin-pulp complex is the connective tissue it covers, so it is not surprising that the repair response in these dental tissues is similar to that in skin (Fig. 20-15).

Epithelial response

The major difference between teeth and skin is the absence of any epithelial response, since the cells that form enamel (ameloblasts) are lost at the time of tooth eruption. To overcome this deficiency, dentistry has formulated substitute materials that not only mimic the hardness of enamel but also serve as an effective sealant against the external environment to protect the underlying dentin-pulp complex.

Connective tissue response

The basic nature of the dentin-pulp response is harnessed and involves occlusion of the dentinal tubules and, if odontoblasts are undamaged, the further deposition of dentin. Here the extent of the odontoblast processes and their response to severance become an issue. If cavity preparation involves odontoblast death or pulpal exposure, recruitment of papillary cells ensues to form a dentine like layer as already described.

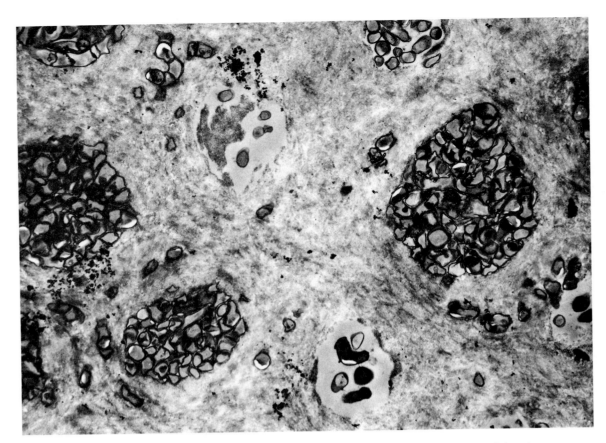

FIG. 20-14 Dentinal caries. Microorganisms have escaped the boundaries of the dentinal tubules. (Courtesy Dr. N.W. Johnson.)

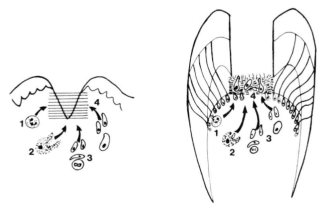

FIG. 20-15 Comparison of the repair responses in skin and teeth. There is no epithelial response in teeth; but the connective tissue response is similar in both instances and involves *(1)* polymorphs, *(2)* macrophage, *(3)* fibroblasts (by division of undamaged pulpal and perivascular cells), and *(4)* the production of scar tissue (collagen), which mineralizes in the tooth to form dentin.

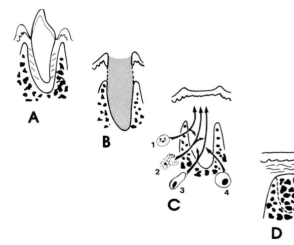

FIG. 20-16 Repair response after tooth extraction. **A** shows the tooth in situ. After extraction the socket, **B,** is filled with clot. The clot resolves, **C,** by *(1)* the polymorph response, *(2)* the macrophage response, and *(3)* the fibroblast response. In addition, the bony defect becomes colonized by new osteoblasts *(4)* that remodel the collagen scar and form bone, **D.**

REPAIR FOLLOWING TOOTH EXTRACTION

The wound created by extracting a tooth differs from an incisional skin wound in that there is substantially greater soft tissue loss and bone is involved. Even so, the repair process uses the same basic mechanisms already described. After the tooth has been extracted, the defect is immediately filled by a blood clot (the hemostatic response). Sometimes the clot can be dislodged; when this happens, infection may intervene and lead to what is known as dry socket, a painful infection of the bone lining the socket. The epithelial cells bordering the socket begin to proliferate and migrate across the clot, so that after about 10 days the socket is epithelialized. Within the clot the inflammatory reponse takes place involving first neutrophils and then macrophages. The proliferative and synthesizing phase is a little different from that in skin since the cells invading the clot are not fibroblasts but cells from the adjacent marrow that have osteogenic potential. Once in the clot they begin to form bone. Bone formation begins about 10 days after tooth extraction; and by 10 to 12 weeks the extraction site can no longer be distinguished (Fig. 20-16).

REPAIR OF THE PERIODONTIUM

Repair of the periodontium depends very much on the severity and nature of the damage inflicted. For example, when complete loss of tooth support occurs (e.g., with an avulsion), certain facts should be borne in mind. Recall (from Chapters 4 and 13) that the supporting tissues of the tooth have a specific origin, the dental follicle. Thus cells from this source are required if there is to be any reattachment of the tooth. Standard clinical practice now is to save as much of the soft tissue attached to the root of an avulsed tooth as possible before it is repositioned in its socket. If this is done, there is the chance that enough cells, programmed as they are to form the tissues for tooth support, will survive to regenerate a new attachment.

If trauma is less severe and only part of the PDL is damaged, the repair process is even more dependent on the degree of trauma. For example, when the amount of damage is such that the proliferative response derives from the cells of the bone marrow adjacent to the PDL, the synthetic response will be osteogenic and bone will form, fusing the tooth to the jawbone, a condition termed *ankylosis.* If, however, damage is slight so that the proliferative response derives from cells of the PDL (which have the potential to form all the tissues involved in tooth support), complete regeneration will be possible. In other words, the repair process in the periodontium is determined by the type of cells that repopulate the defect after injury.

Repair of the PDL may also use another, previously described, important biologic phenomenon, the ability of fibroblasts to remodel collagen. Skin repair involves formation of scar tissue. Repair of the PDL after, say, tooth movement involves the same mechanism as found in skin without scar formation. The reason is that, although the repair mechanism is identical to that in skin (and indeed collagen [scar] is the reparative tissue), this scar tissue is almost immediately remodeled by the ligament fibroblasts to restore normal architecture.

It is also appropriate here to discuss, in histologic terms, the general problem of reattachment of tooth support after its destruction by periodontal disease. The aim of periodontal therapy is, first, to eliminate the disease and, then, to restore lost tooth supportive structures. One clinical modality is to try to replace the bone around teeth by marshaling the osteogenic potential of adjacent bone marrow or of undifferentiated mesenchymal cells. This is done by implanting various materials with osteogenic potential, such as frozen dried bone, around the teeth. Such procedures certainly produce new bone around teeth, but there is no evidence that it is in any way involved in tooth attachment. Another approach is to attempt to "persuade" connective tissue other than the PDL to serve in tooth support. This approach utilizes treatment of the root surface with a mild acid (e.g., citric) to partially demineralize the cementum and dentin, thereby exposing the collagen fibers of the hard tissue matrix. It is then hoped that the exposed fibers will be remodeled by or spliced with the collagen of soft gingival connective tissue to reestablish an attachment; but there has been little evidence that such splicing occurs. More realistic approaches currently being explored clinically are to exclude gingival connective tissue from the repair process, so that repair is achieved entirely by cells from the PDL (which have the potential to differentiate into tooth supporting tissue given the correct circumstance). A further problem has arisen, however, with the recognition of a possible functional role of the root sheath in producing the hyaline layer and initiating its role in attachment. In the absence of a root sheath, it can be questioned whether true regeneration is possible.

Finally, this difficulty in regenerating tooth support has very much influenced the clinical field of implantology. For a number of years it was thought desirable to develop a fibrous connection between the implant and bone, because this mimicked the attachment of tooth to bone. When fibrous encapsulation of an implant is achieved, however, it is by cells derived from gingiva and these do not have the ability to perform in the same way as PDL fibroblasts. The consequence is eventual destruction of the connective tissue and loss of the implant—hence, the success of osseointegration (direct contact of implant with bone), which avoids the need to duplicate the PDL.

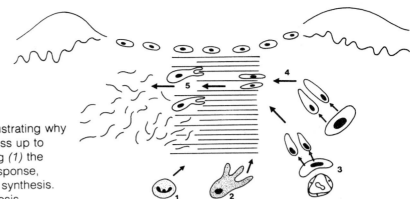

FIG. 20-17 Repair in gingival epithelium illustrating why scars are rare in the mouth. The repair process up to step *4* is as depicted in Figure 20-7, involving *(1)* the polymorph response, *(2)* the macrophage response, *(3)* fibroblast differentiation, and *(4)* collagen synthesis. The scar remodels *(5)* by collagen phagocytosis.

REPAIR OF THE ORAL MUCOSA

Although the oral mucosa has many similarities to skin and utilizes the same principle of repair, it does not form scar tissue nearly as readily. Because of this, surgery within the mouth can be undertaken without fear of producing disabling scar tissue. The reason is that, whereas the repair process does produce scarring, the scar tissue produced remodels rapidly to restore normal architecture, just as in the PDL, and using the same mechanism (Fig. 20-17).

Finally, there are a number of surgical procedures that involve detachment of the gingiva from the tooth surface with later reformation of this junction. In Chapter 13, in which the development of the dentogingival junction was described, the point was made that junctional epithelium develops from the reduced dental epithelium. After surgery a new junction with the same histologic characteristics as before develops from the phenotypically different oral epithelium. In this respect it is thought that the underlying connective tissue is significant here. Junctional epithelium has the characteristics of immature epithelium, and it is thought that when basal gingival epithelial cells reestablish contact with the tooth surface they become associated with a deep connective tissue that lacks the permissive instructions for epithelial maturation.

In summary: The dental tissues use a basic mechanism for repair, but there are local factors that both benefit and hinder this process. The absence of ameloblasts prevents the repair of enamel (although physicochemical mechanisms permit a limited form of repair). This means that substitutes for an epithelial response, in the form of dental restorative materials, are used in restorative dentistry. Dentin is capable of repair using basic mechanisms, but the scar tissue that

forms becomes mineralized. This basic response has, in the past, been obscured by the occurrence of microleakage and by age changes (which are particularly evident in the pulp). The repair of dental supportive tissues depends very much on the degree of damage. If the damage is minimal and programmed follicular cells are available, repair occurs involving scar tissue formation but this scar is rapidly remodeled to restore normal architecture. If damage is more extensive, the defect is repopulated by bone-forming cells, as in socket repair, leading to fusion of the tooth to the jaw. Finally, wounds of the oral mucosa, and especially of the gingiva, often heal without the formation of scar tissue. Scar tissue does form but is quickly remodeled to restore normal architecture.

BIBLIOGRAPHY

Boyne PJ: Osseous repair of the post-extraction alveolus in man, *Oral Surg* 21:805, 1966.

Gillman T: On some aspects of collagen formation in localized repair and in diffuse fibrotic reactions to injury. In Gould B (ed): *Treatise on collagen,* New York, 1968, Academic Press.

Krawczyk WS: A pattern of epidermal cell migration during wound healing, *J Cell Biol* 49:247, 1971.

McGaw WT, Ten Cate AR: A role for collagen phagocytosis by fibroblasts in scar remodeling: an ultrastructural stereologic study, *J Invest Dermatol* 81:375, 1983.

Ross R: The fibroblast and wound repair, *Biol Rev* 43:51, 1968.

Ross R, Odland G: Human wound repair. II. Inflammatory cell, epithelial mesenchymal interrelations, and fibrogenesis, *J Cell Biol* 39:152, 1968.

Ten Cate AR, Freeman E: Collagen remodelling by fibroblasts in wound repair: preliminary observations, *Anat Rec* 179(4):543, 1974.

CHAPTER 21

Childhood Facial Growth and Development

THE infant face is not simply a miniature of the adult face. Growth is a differential process, in which some parts develop more or less rapidly than others and in a multitude of regional directions. Growth of the face is a gradual maturational process taking many years and requiring a succession of changes in regional proportions and the relationships of various parts (Figs. 21-1 and 21-2). Many localized alterations occur that are associated with a continuous process of soft and hard tissue remodeling. An understanding of the mechanisms of growth and development of the face is essential for the practice of dentistry. To achieve this understanding, it is necessary to have some knowledge of faces.

BASIS FOR HUMAN FACIAL FORM

The human face is unusual compared to the faces of most other mammals. It lacks an elongated graceful snout and muzzle flowing back onto a streamlined neurocranium. Instead, humans possess a large rounded head with a rather bizarre combination of facial features. Extraordinarily wide, flat, and vertical, the human face has a forehead above a small, razor-thin, and fleshy proboscis. Owllike orbits point nearly straight forward, and there is a tiny mouth between muzzleless jaws with a chin. Although this description may seem exaggerated, it is given to emphasize how different the human face is; even so, the phylogenetic and functional reasons underlying our unique facial design conform to the same rules of morphology and morphogenesis that govern all mammals.

No one knows for certain what factors initiated the evolutionary events leading to the face and body of modern humans, although there are a number of hypotheses. Brachiation and/or the development of a huge brain have been suggested as possible factors leading to the subsequent evolutionary changes and adaptations; but despite the fact that precise evolutionary sequences of our facial heritage are speculative, the anatomic consequences and the functional and developmental relationships involved are fairly well understood. This knowledge is important, because it helps to explain inherent tendencies toward malocclusion and provides an insight into the causes of developmental abnormalities.

The human body has made many adaptations to its upright stance, some reflected in the skull and face. Together with the awesome enlargement of the human cerebral hemispheres, a marked flexure of the cranial floor has occurred, in contrast to the flat basicranium of other mammals (Fig. 21-3). Rather than projecting horizontally, the spinal cord has become vertically disposed; and the foramen magnum is positioned at the ventral rather than the posterior aspect of the skull. The orbits, however, still point in the horizontal direction of body movement because of the flexure in the cranial base. With a bipedal posture, the arms have been freed and the developed hands have dexterous fingers. With stereoscopic vision, the lack of an elongated muzzle allows us to see and manipulate close objects. The defensive, offensive, and vocational functions of the jaws have been taken over largely by the hands; and the decreased relative size of the jaws occasioned thereby has not presented a threat to survival. The typical mammalian snout, with its thermoregulatory function, has been replaced by a nearly hairless integument containing sweat glands and an elaborate vasomotor control system for heat loss and retention.

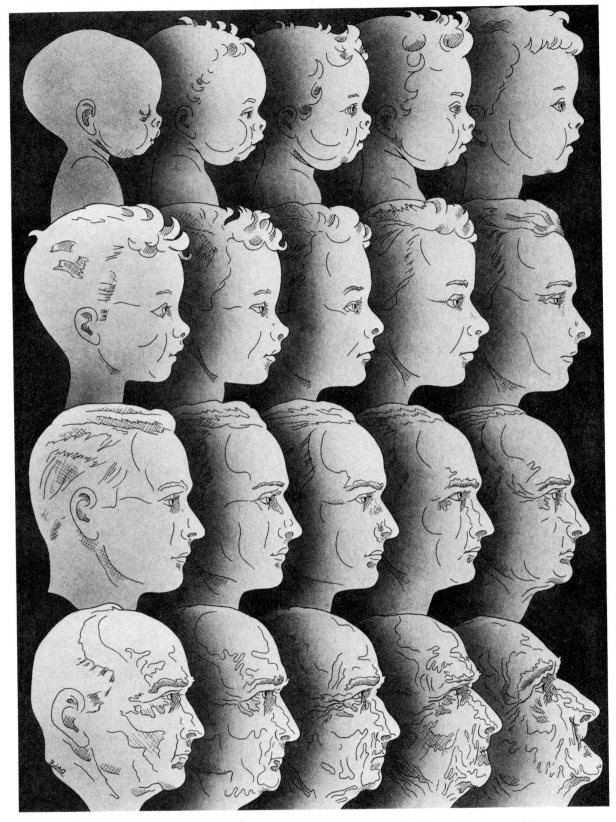

FIG. 21-1 Growth and development of the face from birth to old age. *Top row*, birth to 4 years; *second row*, 6 to 20 years; *third row*, 25 to 50 years; *bottom row*, 60 to 80 years.

Several interrelated factors have contributed to the vertical disposition of the human face, involving increases or reductions in the relative sizes of various facial regions and also a series of anatomic rotations of the facial and cranial parts. The sizable enlargement of the frontal lobes of the cerebrum has resulted in the addition of a bulging vertical forehead above the face (Fig. 21-4). The supraorbital rims have rotated to an upright position overlying the inferior orbital rims. At the same time a forward rotation of the lateral orbital rims has occurred ahead of the greatly enlarged frontal and temporal lobes of the cerebrum. The composite result is a vertically aligned set of orbits pointing nearly straight ahead that permits stereoscopic vision (Fig. 21-5).

The massive enlargement of the cerebrum also relates to another key rotation. The olfactory bulbs (and the floor of the anterior cranial fossa) have been displaced from their typical obliquely upright position to a distinctly horizontal one (Fig. 21-6). This change has a major rotational effect on the whole nasomaxillary complex because it is directly contiguous with the anterior cranial fossa and is articulated to it by sutures. As a functional generalization, the snout of a mammal

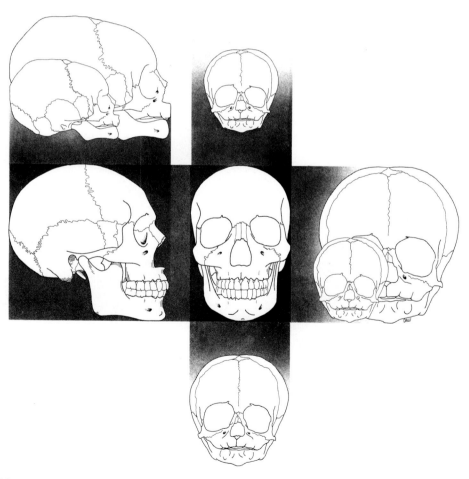

FIG. 21-2 Changes in facial proportions. The newborn skull has been enlarged to the same size as the adult skull to show the regional differences in height, depth, and breadth.

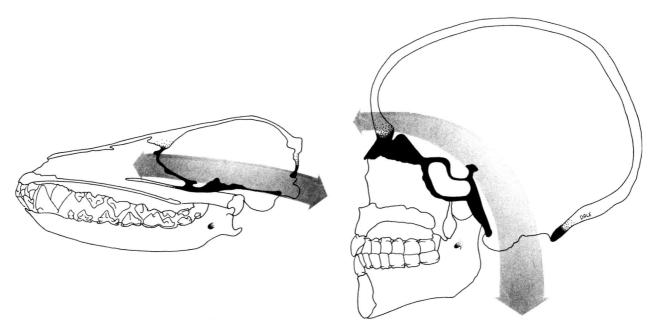

FIG. 21-3 Differences in mammalian and human crania. The flat cranial floor of mammals contrasts with the precipitous drop of the human basicranium.

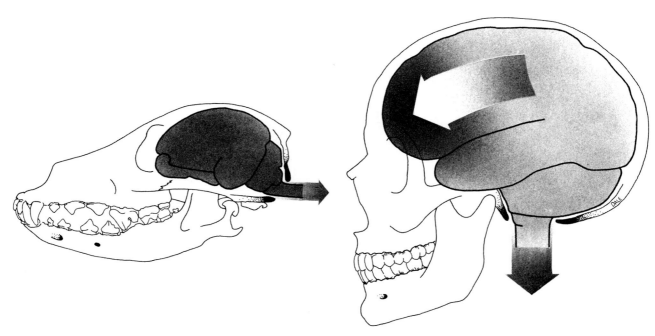

FIG. 21-4 Differences in mammalian and human crania. Concomitant with massive enlargement of the cerebrum, the human forehead and supraorbital rims rotated vertically to a position overlying the mouth and dentition.

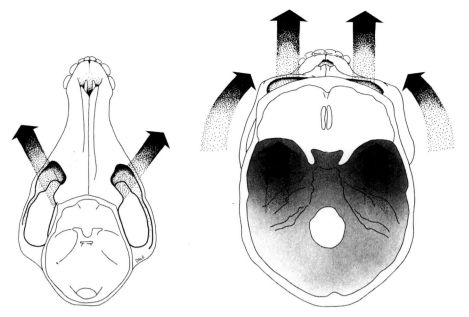

FIG. 21-5   Rotation of the orbits horizontally to a forward-pointing binocular position. Because of cerebral expansion also, the human face as a whole has become considerably widened.

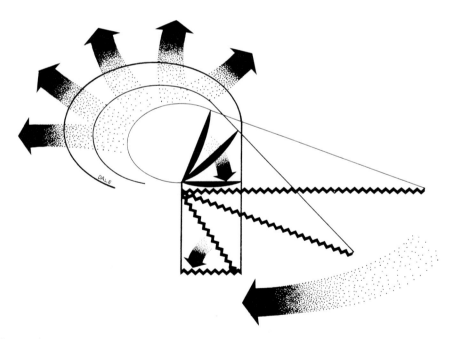

FIG. 21-6   Progression from the mammalian to the human cranium. As the cerebral hemispheres enlarged *(outwardly directed arrows)*, the olfactory bulbs *(black edgewise saucers)* rotated from an obliquely vertical position typical of mammals to the horizontal position of humans. In almost all mammals (including humans) the nasomaxillary complex *(triangle of solid and zig-zag lines)* projects in a perpendicular direction from the olfactory bulbs. Thus, as the bulbs became displaced horizontally, the human face correspondingly assumed an upright alignment. To provide a horizontal occlusal plane, a new compartment (the suborbital region, occupied by the maxillary sinus) was added to the human maxilla, thus lowering the occlusion to a functional position.

points in a direction essentially parallel to the neutral axis of olfactory nerve spread, which in turn is perpendicular to the olfactory bulbs. With the downward rotational displacement of the olfactory bulbs from a nearly vertical to a horizontal plane, and of the olfactory nerves from horizontal to vertical, the fleshy proboscis of the human face with its downward-directed nares guides inflowing air toward the ceiling of the nasal chambers. Because of the rotation of the olfactory bulbs and sensory nerves, the nerve endings are located in the roof of the nasal chambers rather than the posterior walls, as in other mammals. The nasomaxillary complex also has correspondingly become rotated downward and backward into an upright rather than a horizontally prominent position.

Because of the orbital rotation toward midline (biorbital convergence), the anatomic region between the eyes has undergone a reduction in size (Fig. 21-7). This region houses the root of the nose, and a markedly thinned nose results. A nose with a more narrow base must also necessarily be less protuberant. As the snout underwent reduction, a corresponding reduction in jaw prominence and maxillary arch length occurred, because the nasal and oral regions share a common bony palate. The swing of the orbits forward and toward midline placed the cheekbones in wide bilateral positions.

All these various rotations, brain enlargements, facial reductions, and realignment adaptations have produced a wide, flat, and vertically disposed face and contributed to the anatomic basis for the various malocclusions that can occur in the human face.*

*For a more detailed account, see Enlow DH: *Handbook of facial growth*, Philadelphia, 1990, WB Saunders.

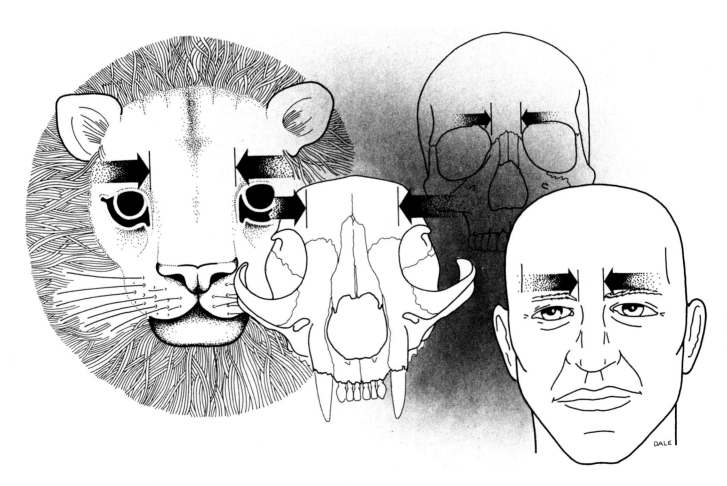

FIG. 21-7   Decreasing relative dimensions of the interorbital region. The result is a thinner, less protrusive, snout between close-set eyes.

FACIAL TYPES

There are two general facial types—long and narrow (leptoprosopic) and round and broad (euryprosopic)—each associated with a type of head. The dolichocephalic head is relatively narrow and long, and the brachycephalic head wider and rounder. Because the floor of the neurocranium (basicranium, cranial base) is the platform to which the facial bones articulate, the head form provides the template that establishes either a correspondingly narrow or a correspondingly broad facial skeleton. Although many intermediate types of head forms and facial patterns exist in any general population, these two skull configurations (Fig. 21-8) tend to be associated with the characteristic facial features.

The narrow facial type tends to have a convex profile with a prognathic maxilla and a retrognathic mandible. The forehead slopes because the forward growth of the upper part of the face carries the outer table of the frontal bone with it. A larger frontal sinus than is characteristic of the broad facial type exists because of the greater separation of inner and outer bony tables of the forehead, whereas the inner table remains fixed to the dura of the frontal lobe of the cerebrum. The glabella and supraorbital rims are prominent, and the nasal bridge is high. There is a tendency toward an aquiline or Roman nose, because the more prominent upper part of the nasal region induces a bending or curving of the nasal profile. Because the face is relatively narrow, the eyes appear close set and the nose is correspondingly thin. The nose also is typically prominent and quite long, and its point has a tendency to tip downward. The lower lip and mandible are often set in a somewhat recessive position, because the long dimension of the nasal chambers leads to a downward and backward rotational placement of the lower jaw. (The dolichocephalic head form also has a more open cranial base flexure, which adds to the downward mandibular rotation.) These factors contribute to a downward inclination of the occlusal plane and a marked curve of occlusion. The anterior mandibular teeth drift upward to compensate for the downward mandibular rotation (Fig. 21-49); however, an anterior open bite is often the result of inadequate drift (Fig. 21-48). Because individuals with a dolichocephalic head form tend to have a more open cranial base angle, a stooped posture of the body with anterior inclination of the neck and head may result (Fig. 21-9).

The round broad facial type is characterized by a more upright and bulbous forehead, with the upper nasal part of the face less prominent than in the dolichocephalic face. The nasal chambers are horizontally shorter but wider, in contrast to the narrow but more

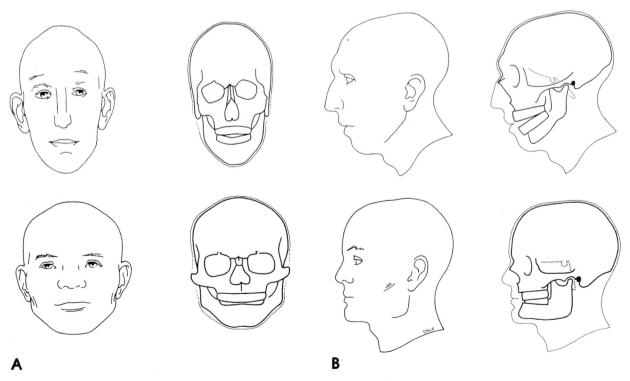

A   **B**

FIG. 21-8   **A,** Dolichocephalic head form. **B,** Brachycephalic head form.

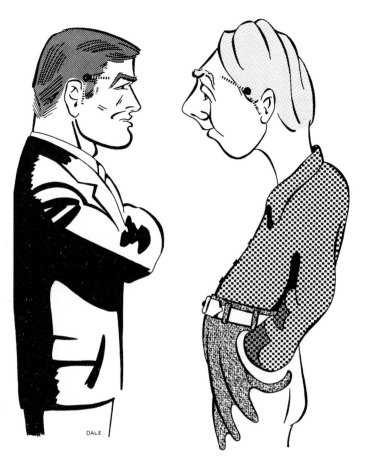

FIG. 21-9 Influence of head form on posture. Persons with a dolichocephalic head form tend toward a more stooped posture whereas a more erect posture characterizes brachycephalic individuals.

prominent nasal region characterizing the dolichocephalic head form. The net capacity of the airway in both instances is thus equivalent. There is less protrusion by the supraorbital ridges, the glabella is less prominent, and the frontal sinus is smaller. The nose is shorter vertically as well as horizontally and tends to be more puglike. The nasal bridge is lower, the nasal alae are broader, and the end of the nose often tips upward. The eyes appear widely set and the cheekbones seem prominent because the nose and forehead are less prominent. The face appears quite flat and broad, in contrast to the more angular, narrow, deep, and topographically bold appearance of the dolichocephalic face. Because the cranial base angle of the brachycephalic skull tends to be more closed, the body and head posture tend to be more erect. There is also a greater tendency toward an orthognathic (straight-jawed) profile.

The Negroid (Black) head form tends to be dolicho-cephalic, although (as in any population group) a range of variations exists. The narrow facial form is characterized by relatively close-set eyes, as in many dolichocephalic Caucasians (Whites). The interorbital compartment is correspondingly narrow. Rather than providing for airway volume by a marked degree of forward nasal prominence, as in a typical Caucasian dolichocephalic, the nose of Blacks is characterized by a lateral enlargement of its lower part. This produces a less prominent nose having a narrow upper bridge but with bilateral flaring of the alae and the lower part of the nasal chambers. Maxillary and mandibular alveolodental protrusion is also a frequent characteristic feature among many Blacks. This characteristic results because the mandibular ramus tends to be quite broad and the resultant protrusion of the mandibular dental arch produces a labial inclination of the maxillary incisors and greatly reduces the incidence of protruding upper teeth in the Black population (Fig. 21-10).

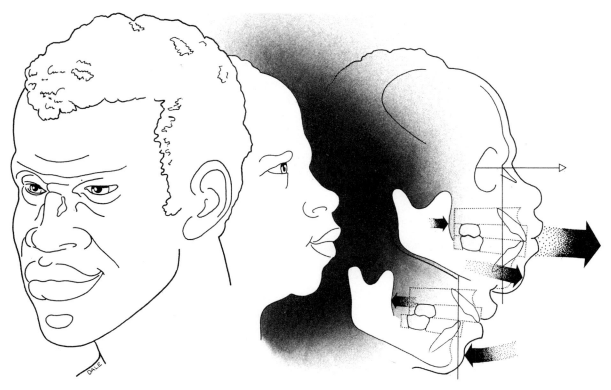

FIG. 21-10   Dolichocephalic Negroid (Black) head form. In the Black mandible the ramus has a particularly broad dimension that compensates for a downward and backward position of the mandible. The anatomic result is a more forward placement of the mandibular arch and a dentoalveolar protrusion. Because of this compensatory mechanism during facial development, severe Class II malocclusions are not nearly as frequent in the Black face as in the Caucasian face.

FACIAL PROFILES

There are three basic types of facial profiles (Fig. 21-11): The straight-jawed, or orthognathic, type is often regarded as the esthetic ideal in Western society. The retrognathic profile has a retruding chin and is the most commonly occurring profile among Western Caucasian populations. The prognathic profile is characterized by a bold lower jaw and chin; although it is generally regarded as "masculine," many men have a greater or lesser degree of mandibular retrognathism.

To identify a person's profile type, imagine a line projecting horizontally from the orbit; drop a perpendicular from this just brushing the surface of the upper lip. If the chin touches this vertical line, the profile is orthognathic; if it falls behind or ahead, the profile is retrognathic or prognathic. For a female face the vertical line will generally pass through the nose at a point about halfway along its upper slope. In male faces that are long and narrow, however, the more marked extent of the upper nasal prominence is such that more of the nose sometimes lies forward of the vertical line.

People with a dolichocephalic head form (a characteristic feature of some Caucasian populations in northernmost and southernmost Europe, North Africa, and the Middle East) tend to have a retrognathic face. Those with a brachycephalic head form (a characteristic feature of Middle Europe and East Asia) have a greater tendency toward prognathism. Also, Asians commonly have a maxillary and mandibular alveolodental protrusion characterized by labial tipping of the maxillary incisors resulting from a protrusive mandibular dentition. Thus there are more malocclusions involving protruding maxillary teeth in some Caucasian populations and more malocclusions involving protruding mandibular teeth with alveolodental protrusion in Asian populations.

An important intrinsic developmental process of compensation functions to offset and reduce the anatomic effects of built-in tendencies toward malocclusions. A genetically determined retrognathic mandibular placement caused, for example, by some rotational factor in the cranial base can be compensated by the development of a broader mandibular ramus. Thus the whole mandible becomes longer and reduces the amount of retrognathism. Because latitude exists for compensatory adjustments, only a relatively slight degree of retrognathism, or some other anatomic imbalance, occurs in most persons (Fig. 21-12). For narrow-faced individuals, 3 to 4 mm of mandibular retrognathism (a mild malocclusion with some crowding of the incisors) is typical. A perfect occlusion is hardly to be considered normal since relatively minor dental arch or facial skeleton irregularities are almost universal. Only when the compensatory process fails do severe malocclusions occur.

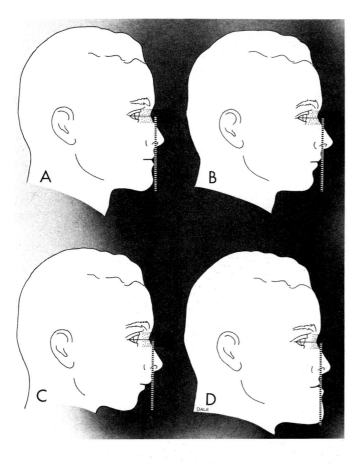

FIG. 21-11 In **A**, an orthognathic profile, the chin touches a vertical line along the upper lip perpendicular to the neutral orbital axis. In **B**, a slightly retrognathic profile, the chin tip falls several millimeters behind this line. In **C**, a severely retrognathic face, the chin is well behind the vertical line. The lower lip also is much less prominent. In **D**, a prognathic profile, the chin tip lies well forward of this vertical line.

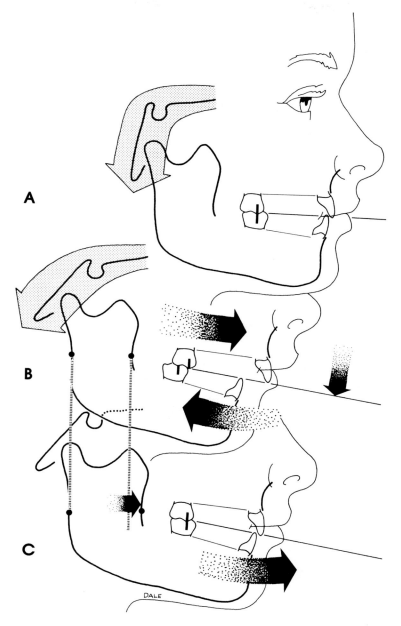

FIG. 21-12 Mandibular compensation. **A** represents the normal mandible. A more open-angled cranial base, **B,** has the anatomic effect of placing the mandible in a retrognathic position. Because the whole mandible is in a backward and downward position, the occlusal plane has a slight downward inclination. The retruding tendency of the mandible is often compensated during facial growth by the development of a wider ramus, **C,** thus placing the mandibular arch in a more forward position.

MALE AND FEMALE FACES

Until about 12 years of age boys' and girls' faces are essentially comparable. Shortly after puberty, the female face has attained most of its size and structural maturity and growth ceases. Growth and development of the male facial complex, however, continue into the early 20s, bringing about noticeable differences between male and female faces (Fig. 21-13).

Male and female faces, whether of the narrow or broad type, have a composite of key topographic characteristics. On a scale from extreme masculine to extreme feminine, most individuals usually have some features that are intermediate between the two extremes. In general, however, the male face tends to be noticeably more protuberant and more knobby, bulky, or coarse. Female faces tend to be flatter, more delicate, and less bumpy.

The characteristically larger nose of the male face creates several related facial differences. The whole nasal region is larger because of the requirement for a greater airway capacity. Thus the relatively wide and long male nose contrasts with the thinner and less prominent female nose. The hard palate forms the floor of the nasal cavity and the roof of the oral cavity. When the upper skeletal part of the nasal region becomes markedly prominent, a constraint is imposed on the lower part of the nasal skeleton by the palate and maxillary arch. This means that the upper part of the nose can become so prominent that the nasal profile necessarily bends to give a resultant aquiline or Roman nose configuration. Alternatively, upper nasal prominence can produce a rotation of the whole nasal profile into a distinctively more vertical alignment. This is the classic male Greek nasal configuration, in which the nasal profile drops nearly straight down from the prominent forehead (Fig. 21-14). It should always be remembered that there is a great deal of ethnic variation in nasal shapes; in some population groups an aquiline configuration, for example, is as common among females as males (e.g., the Dinaric type of head form). Generally, however, the smaller thinner female nose tends to have a concave-to-straight profile whereas the male nose has a tendency toward a straight-to-convex profile.

A major difference exists between the sexes in the forehead. In females the supraorbital ridges lie on or very near to the same vertical plane as the inferior orbital rims and cheekbones. There are usually no more than a few millimeters of supraorbital overhang in the female face. The female cheekbones therefore tend to appear more prominent, which is especially noticeable in a 45-degree view of the face (Fig. 21-13). The entire midfacial region, including the upper jaw, also seems more prominent in female faces, and for the same reason. The outer bony plate of the forehead in males, because of the greater nasal prominence, is carried forward. The result is a sloping forehead with large frontal sinuses and a supraorbital and glabellar overhang. Because of the more massive extent of both nasal and

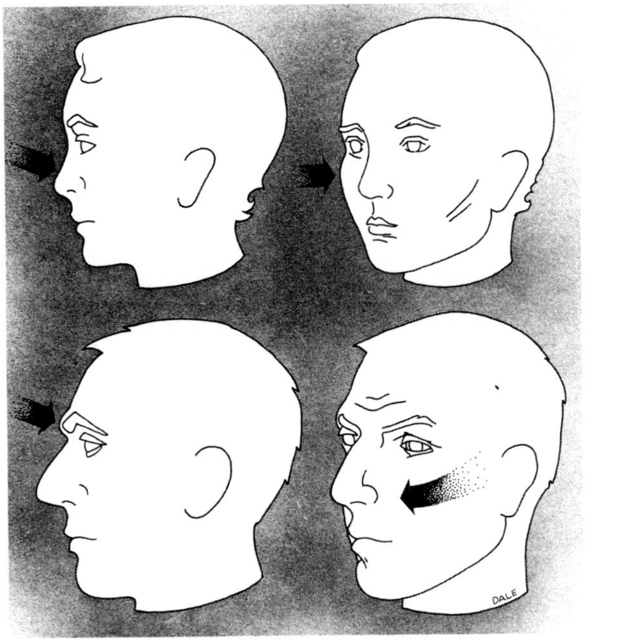

FIG. 21-13 Comparison of male and female facial features in profile and at a 45-degree angle.

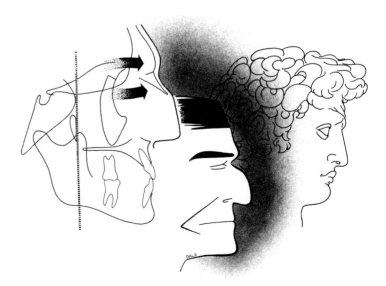

FIG. 21-14 Male nasal profiles.

supraorbital skeleton in males, the cheekbones appear less prominent, as does the whole upper jaw. Although such basic sex differences in the face exist, recall that there are also similar facial differences between long and broad head form types as well. Among the differences between male and female faces and between narrow and broad faces, many permutations exist. A female dolichocephalic, for example, may present greater forehead slope and a more prominent but thinner nose than a male brachycephalic.

AGE CHANGES

An infant's face is round and wide, because lateral facial growth occurs earlier and to a greater extent than vertical growth (Figs. 21-1 and 21-15). With increasing age and body size, however, vertical facial enlargement exceeds lateral facial growth as the nasal chambers progressively expand inferiorly to provide an increased airway for the enlarging lungs. A baby's face also appears rather flat because the nose is small relative to the broad but short face. Since forward growth of the face has not yet occurred, the forehead is upright and bulbous. Buccal and labial fat pads give a full appearance to the cheeks. Brachycephalic adults usually have a rather juvenile facial character compared to the relatively angular and topographically bolder adult dolichocephalic face. If an adult "round face" also tends toward obesity, thus presenting a fat-padded face, the youthful parallel is augmented. Subcutaneous adipose tissue also tends to smooth out any age wrinkles, which further adds to the illusion of youth. Any marked loss of facial adiposity exaggerates an aged appearance because of consequent skin wrinkling. The effect is also seen in children who have undergone significant weight loss for any reason, as evidenced by the aged, sagging, wrinkled face of a child suffering from severe malnutrition.

The firm, turgid, velvety skin of youth becomes progressively more open pored, leathery, spotted, crinkled, and flabby with advancing age. Overexposure to the sun greatly hastens some of these changes. In middle age the skin begins to sag and droop noticeably because the hypodermis becomes less firmly anchored to the underlying facial muscles and bone. This may be the result of weight loss, but biochemical and physical alterations in the connective tissue of the dermis and hypodermis also exert an effect. There is a diminished flexibility of component fibers with a marked decrease in the content of water-bound proteoglycans. The latter results in a widespread subcutaneous dehydration, contributing significantly to a shrunken facial volume and consequent skin surplus. These factors, in turn, lead to the onset of facial lines and wrinkles, sunken eyes, drooping bags, and suborbital creases.

Facial lines and furrows appear in characteristic locations (Fig. 21-15). One of the first to appear, and the one associated with middle age, is the nasolabial furrow (extending down along the sides of the nasal alae lateral to the corners of the mouth). This "smile line" is seen at any age when a face grins, but it becomes a permanent integumental mark during the late 30s or early 40s. In the happy individual who looks younger than his or her years, the onset of these and other telltale lines may be delayed or are at least less noticeable. Other permanent lines that appear with advancing age include forehead furrows, suborbital creases, crow's-feet at the lateral corners of the eyes, vertical corrugations over the glabella and on the upper lip, lines extending down from the corners of the mouth on both sides of the chin, bags below the cheekbones, and jowls along the sides of the mandible. In advanced old age the face can become an expansive carpet of "noble ripples" and may also be characterized by a decrease in the vertical dimension resulting from the loss of teeth.

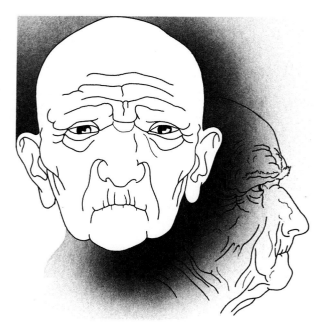

FIG. 21-15 Facial characteristics of old age. Note the development of lines and furrows in specific locations.

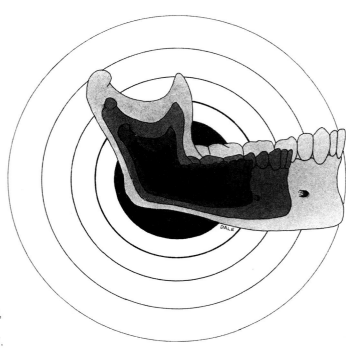

FIG. 21-16 Erroneous schema of bone growth. Bone does not simply "grow" by symmetric expansion. Rather, it undergoes a complex remodeling process throughout all its regions and parts. Compare this with Figure 21-17.

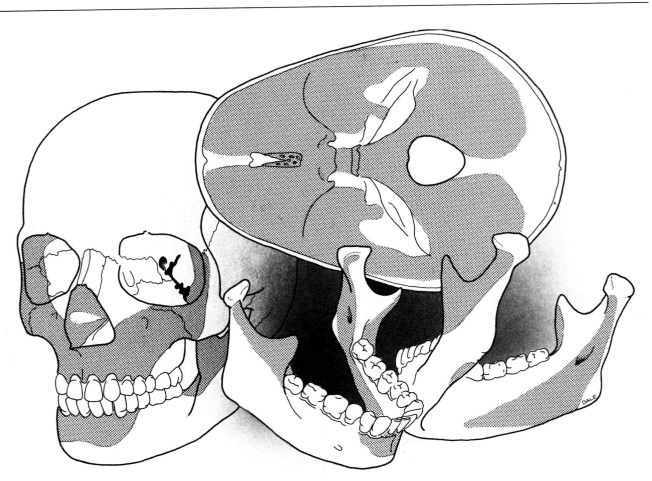

FIG. 21-17 Growth and remodeling fields. The entire facial and neurocranial skeleton is covered, inside and out, by a characteristic spread of regional growth and remodeling fields. Resorptive fields are shaded. Depository fields are free of shading.

BASIC CONCEPTS OF FACIAL GROWTH

There are two common but incorrect assumptions that must be discarded before an understanding of facial growth is possible. The first is that various individual bones (e.g., mandible, maxilla, ethmoid, and sphenoid) enlarge simply by a symmetric expansion of the outer contours (Fig. 21-16). The second is that a bone grows by a combination of periosteal deposition on its outer surface and endosteal resorption on its inner surface. Beginning students often assume (incorrectly) that the bone of growing cortex must necessarily be produced by the periosteum. Actually about half or more of the compact bone tissue of the face and cranium is laid down by endosteum, the inner membrane lining the medullary cavity, and about half the periosteal surfaces of most bones in the face and neurocranium are resorptive (with about half depository) (Fig. 21-17). The reason for this is that remodeling is required to increase the size of any given bone.

Three essential processes bring about the growth and development of various cranial and facial bones: size increase, remodeling, and displacement. The first two are closely related and are produced simultaneously by a combination of bony resorption and deposition. The third (displacement) is a movement of all the bones away from each other at their articular junctions as each undergoes size increases (Fig. 21-18). To control properly and thereby make use of the complex processes of growth in clinical procedures, it is essential that the various concepts described below be fully and thoroughly understood.

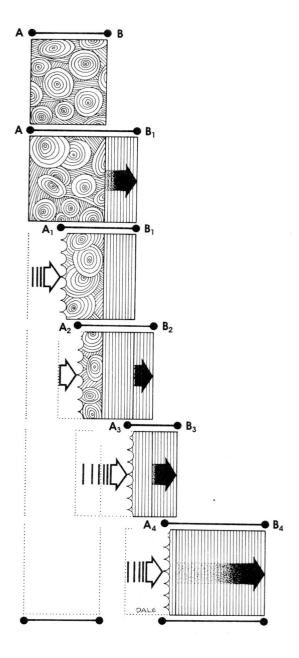

FIG. 21-18 Remodeling and relocation of bone. *A-B* represents a cortical plate of bone. Apposition on one surface increases its dimension to *A-B₁*. Resorption on the opposite surface decreases its dimension: from *A-B₁* to *A₁-B₁*. When apposition on one surface equals resorption on the opposite surface, the dimension is maintained: *A₁-B₂* to *A₂-B₂*. When apposition is less than resorption, the dimension is decreased: *A₂-B₂* to *A₃-B₃*. When apposition is greater than resorption, the dimension is increased: *A₃-B₃* to *A₄-B₄*. Note that the cortical plate has completely relocated to the right, from *A-B* to *A₄-B₄*, by the process of remodeling.

Size Increases and Remodeling

A bone enlarges and remodels by the addition of new bone on one side of a cortical plate and the removal of old bone from the opposite side of the same cortex. This process produces one of the two basic kinds of growth movements, termed *relocation;* the other is *displacement*. The cortex actually moves, and it is the composite of all such changes throughout the bone that brings about its overall enlargement. Simultaneously, internal regional remodeling adjustments are also made.

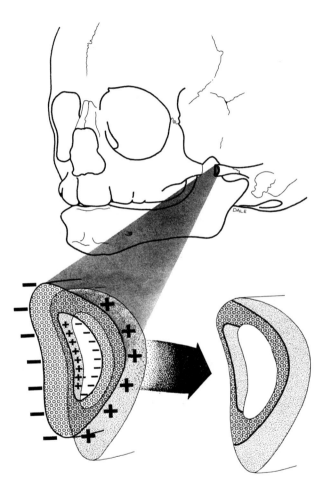

FIG. 21-19 Process of relocation. This is the basis for the developmental process of remodeling. Deposition is indicated with a *positive sign*, resorption with a *negative sign*. As the face, brain, basicranium, muscles of mastication, etc. progressively enlarge, the right and left zygomatic arches become relocated to the right and left, respectively, thus enlarging the distance between them to accommodate the growth of the remainder of the head. This relocation movement is produced by remodeling that involves combinations of resorption and deposition, as shown.

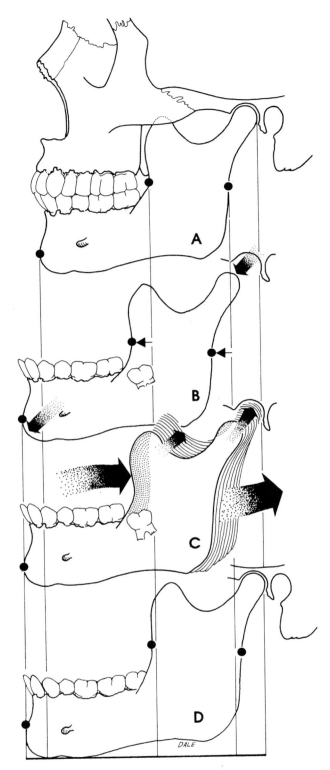

FIG. 21-20 Two basic types of growth movements. From the original position, **A,** as all of the facial soft tissues enlarge, the whole mandible is displaced, **B,** in a forward and downward direction away from its articulation with the basicranium. The condyle and ramus are then stimulated simultaneously to enlarge by remodeling, **C,** posteriorly and superiorly by an amount that equals the displacement movement, with the result shown in **D.**

As examples, consider the zygomatic arches, the mandible, and the palate. The right and left zygomatic arches grow bilaterally to the right and left, which increases the space between them and allows for the bilateral enlargement of brain tissue and the remainder of the face and cranium. This relocation of the zygomatic arches is achieved through the combination of resorption and deposition (Fig. 21-19). About half the surfaces, inside as well as outside, are resorptive; the others are depository. About half the compact bone is produced by endosteum, and half is laid down by periosteum. Because the extent of depository activity on one side of each bony cortex slightly exceeds the amount of resorption on the other side, the arch continuously increases in thickness as it moves (relocates) laterally.

The assumption that the mandible grows downward and forward not only is an oversimplification but is inaccurate. As the human mandible enlarges, it remodels primarily in posterior and superior directions (Fig. 21-20); a displacement movement carries it downward and forward. The mandibular ramus relocates in a backward direction; because the progressive amounts of bone addition on its backward-facing surfaces slightly exceed resorptive removal from its forward-facing surfaces, the ramus simultaneously enlarges as it moves slowly posteriorly over a period of years. Because of the posterior manner of ramus relocation, the body (corpus) of the mandible has space within which to elongate. It does this by remodeling; that is, what was formerly part of the ramus becomes converted by bony remodeling into an addition onto the corpus, which thereby lengthens the mandibular arch to house the enlarging tooth buds and erupting teeth (Fig. 21-21). This is a continuous, ongoing, and sequential process that proceeds from the early fetal period through the attainment of adult form and size.

In a young child the level of the palate is only slightly inferior to the orbital floor (Fig. 21-22). The nasal chambers progressively enlarge by a growth process in which the palate descends for a considerable distance. One of the mechanisms that achieve this positional change involves palatal relocation by remodeling. The bony palate has two cortical plates, one on the nasal side and one on the oral side, with a medullary space and cancellous bone between. On the nasal side, the mucosal (periosteal) surface is resorptive, and the medullary (endosteal) surface is depository (Fig. 21-23). On the oral side, the periosteal surface is depository and the endosteal surface is resorptive. This combination produces a growth movement of the bony palate in a downward direction, and the whole bony palate thereby relocates inferiorly to provide for a vertical expansion of the overlying nasal region. The various inner and outer

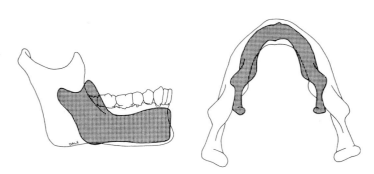

FIG. 21-21 Posterior and superior condylar and ramal remodeling. This produces a backward relocation of the whole ramus. In turn, the mandibular corpus becomes lengthened by remodeling conversions from former parts of the backward-moving ramus.

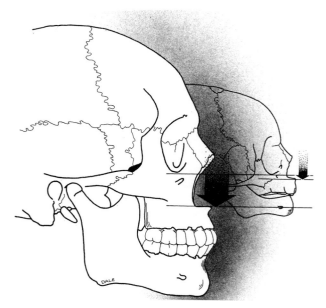

FIG. 21-22 Growth of the hard palate, illustrating the processes of relocation and remodeling. In the newborn skull *(right)*, note that the level of the palate is just slightly inferior to the level of the inferior orbital rim. As the nasal chambers progressively expand, the bony palate becomes relocated downward. What used to be hard palate is remodeled into additions for the nasal chambers.

surfaces are thus about half resorptive and half depository; about half the compact bone is of endosteal origin and half periosteal. In young children the facial level occupied by the maxillary arch is later occupied, in adulthood, by the expanded nasal region. As the palate relocates downward by remodeling, what was formerly the palate and the bony maxillary arch becomes part of the nasal chambers.

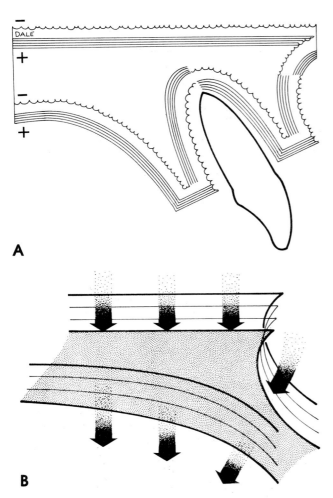

FIG. 21-23 Downward remodeling of the palate. This is produced by deposition on the inferior-facing (oral) side and resorption from the superior-facing (nasal) side, thus bringing about a progressive and continuous inferior relocation of the whole palate and maxillary arch, **A.** The maxillary teeth are moved downward at the same time by a process of vertical drift associated with remodeling (resorption and deposition) of alveolar bone **B.**

The term *growth site* is often used to designate some area or part that plays a noteworthy role in the growth process (e.g., the mandibular condyle). All parts and areas of a bone and their covering membranes, however, participate directly in the growth sequence, whether they are specially designated or not. A mosaic of remodeling fields totally blankets all outside and inside surfaces of all the individual bones (Fig. 21-17), and these growth fields produce the enlargement of each bone. Although some changes in a given bone's shape may be involved, the essential function of remodeling is to move the various parts of a bone to successively new locations (relocation) so that the whole bone can then enlarge. Remodeling fields represent the morphogenetic activity of the enclosing periosteum, endosteum, and other soft tissues. Thus the entire bone is involved in the growth process, not just certain restricted growth sites or growth centers.

Displacement Process

As all the various muscles, epithelia, connective tissues, and other soft tissues of the head grow and expand, a separation effect occurs at the articular joints among the different bones, which are physically carried away from each other by masses of enlarging soft tissue. This process is termed displacement, and the bone's osteogenic membranes and cartilages are immediately triggered to respond by producing overall bone enlargement and remodeling. The bones grow by an amount proportional to the increases in soft tissue mass. As the bones become separated at their various contacts with each other (e.g., sutures, condyles, and synchondroses), their osteogenic membranes and cartilages are stimulated to enlarge them by amounts equal to the extent of their separation, thereby sustaining constant articulations. The displacement movements of the bones, in effect, create the space into which bones grow. Spaces as such never develop, of course, because displacement and subsequent bone growth are virtually simultaneous. When a functional and biomechanical equilibrium is attained between the soft tissues and the bones, the stimulus for skeletal growth ceases.

Thus, as already stated, the mandible is continuously displaced in an anteroinferior direction but enlarges by equal amounts posteriorly and superiorly (Fig. 21-24). All the various bones of the nasomaxillary complex also become separated from each other at their various sutural junctions by displacement, and the sutural membranes (comparable to periosteal membranes) deposit bone in an amount equal to that lost by the displacement separation (Fig. 21-25).

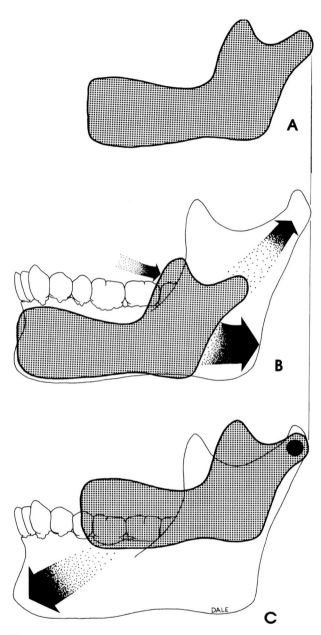

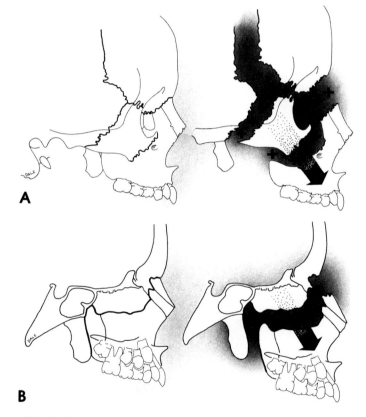

FIG. 21-24 Superimposed growth stages of the mandible. From the original position, **A,** remodeling occurs by regional combinations of resorption and deposition, **B.** This relocates the ramus in posterior and superior directions and provides for a lengthening of the corpus. **C** demonstrates the anterior and inferior displacement of the whole mandible.

FIG. 21-25 Displacement of the nasomaxillary complex. As a result of enlargement of the facial soft tissues, the bones of the nasomaxillary complex are displaced away from each other at their various sutural articulations. New bone is added, virtually simultaneously, at the sutural edges of each bone, thus enlarging the perimeter of each bone by amounts that equal the extents of regional displacement. All other bony surfaces also enlarge by the remodeling activity of periosteum and endosteum. **A** is a lateral view; **B,** a sagittal view.

BONE AND CARTILAGE

Because cartilage can exist without a surface vascular membrane and its matrix is nonvascular, and also because it is noncalcified, turgid, and able to grow interstitially, it has the special capacity to function and grow while withstanding direct pressure. By contrast, bone cannot withstand any undue amount of direct pressure on its outer surface because compression closure of the vascular bed in the periosteum results from such pressure. The matrix of bone is mineralized and requires vascularization. A mineralized matrix also precludes interstitial growth, so that growth can occur only by appositional activity of its surface membranes. The periosteum is, in fact, structurally adapted to tension by virtue of its dense connective tissue design, and the traction anchorage of muscles, tendons, ligaments, and other soft tissues represents one of its principal functional roles.

For each region the two basic components of the growth process, displacement and remodeling, will be shown separately. Vertical and horizontal reference lines are included so that the directions and amounts of displacement and remodeling can be visualized.

During postnatal growth and development there are two modes of bone growth, endochondral and intramembranous (Chapter 8). In direct surface pressure areas, cartilage permits a bone's elongation by the endochondral replacement process. In noncompression or surface tension sites intramembranous growth process takes place. Thus, in the growing face and cranium, there is an appropriate distribution of intramembranous and endochondral systems for growth. Endochondral growth sites in a child's face and cranium involve principally the mandibular condyles and various synchondroses of the cranial base (although some other localized endochondral growth sites also exist). All other areas in these same bones, as well as all remaining parts of the craniofacial skeleton, grow and remodel intramembranously by means of the periosteum, endosteum, periodontal membrane, and sutures.

Biomechanical pressures and tensions are believed to contribute to the stimuli that cause the membranes and cartilages to activate bone growth. Body mass and muscle actions cause bones or parts of bones to undergo minute "bending" actions, which creates very small bioelectric potentials (the piezo effect; Fig. 21-26). When a bone undergoes such slight distortions, pressures and tensions are produced within the fibrous matrix of the bone. The resultant negative and positive bioelectric effects are, in turn, believed to generate corresponding osteoblastic and osteoclastic responses.

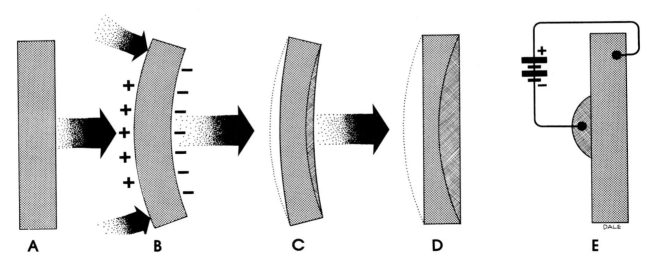

FIG. 21-26 Piezo response. When the matrix of bone tissue undergoes minute distortions, caused by mechanical stress, negative and positive polarity is established on the bony surfaces. (The *positive* and *negative signs* used here represent polarity rather than the conventional symbols for deposition and resorption.) A negative charge triggers osteoblasts to function, and positive charges stimulate osteoclasts to respond. Compressive stress (as on a concave surface) produces a negative charge, and tensile stress (as on a convex surface) a positive charge. Thus, starting at **A,** the charges produced in **B** by deforming the bone lead to bone deposition and resorption, as shown in **C** and **D.** The end effect, **E,** is a remodeling of bone to accommodate the mechanical forces placed on it.

GROWTH SEQUENCE

To illustrate the process of facial and cranial growth as a whole, the key events involved are outlined below, largely pictorially, as a series of separate regional changes in each of the major parts and areas of the growing head. Understand that all these various growth processes occur more or less simultaneously. The changes are presented in a manner that demonstrates perfectly balanced growth, with everything in constant dimensional proportion relative to everything else. Since the growth process is differential in nature, however, the face and cranium never actually grow in such a balanced way. Normal growth is indeed imbalanced and therefore progressive, and quite noticeable alterations in facial form and pattern take place. These differential growth processes not only produce a wide range of topographic facial variations, they also constitute the developmental basis for malocclusions and congenital facial abnormalities. Nevertheless, the presentation of growth changes as a perfectly balanced sequence promotes a better understanding of the developmental basis for all variations and also allows a recognition of where and how much the growth pattern has departed from the normal in different individuals (Fig. 21-27).

We begin arbitrarily with the horizontal growth of the maxillary arch. The whole maxilla is continuously displaced anteriorly throughout the growth period (Fig. 21-28). This displacement occurs because expansion of all the facial soft tissues causes a "carrying" effect, moving the bony maxillary complex with them. An older, but controversial, theory holds that the growth expan-

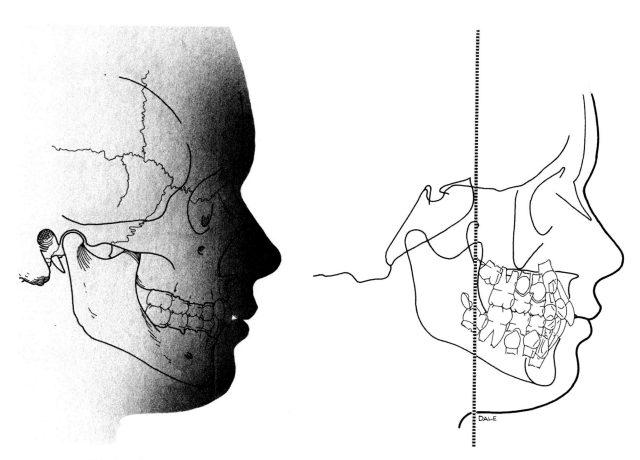

FIG. 21-27 Facial and neurocranial growth. This skull and cephalometric tracing of a 9-year-old child will be used in the subsequent figures to illustrate the composite of facial and neurocranial growth changes. In the cephalometric tracing the *vertical line* demonstrates the directions and amounts of regional growth. Note that it passes along the maxillary tuberosity to a point exactly dividing the anterior from the middle endocranial fossae. For each region in the face and basicranium displacement and remodeling will be shown separately.

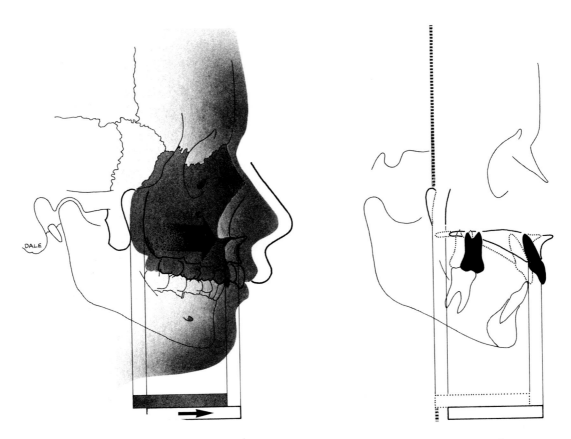

FIG. 21-28 Displacement of the whole palate and maxillary arch in an anterior direction.

sion of the cartilaginous nasal septum causes the maxilla to move forward. Whichever model is more accurate, as the maxillary arch moves anteriorly by displacement a "space" is continuously being created in the region behind the maxilla. In Figure 21-28 the pterygomaxillary fissure is shown moving forward. This fissure, which appears as an inverted teardrop structure on lateral radiographs of the head, is used to locate and represent the maxillary tuberosity—the posterior end of the bony maxillary arch. A real space, of course, never develops behind the tuberosity, because simultaneous maxillary growth fills it in as soon as it forms.

The bony maxillary arch grows and elongates posteriorly by bone deposition on the posterior-facing surface of the maxillary tuberosity (Fig. 21-29). Resorption occurs on the inner surface of the tuberosity, which is the posterior wall of the maxillary sinus. The sinus thereby progressively enlarges. The amount of posterior growth of the maxillary arch equals the amount of its anterior displacement (Fig. 21-28). The displacement of the whole nasomaxillary complex also causes a

progressive separation at all the various facial sutures, which triggers the growth of new bone at the sutural edges by activity of the sutural membranes (Fig. 21-25). This sustains constant skeletal articulation at the sutural junctions. All other inside and outside surfaces of the maxillary complex are also involved in regional resorption and deposition, and the result is a progressive enlargement and reshaping of the entire region (Fig. 21-53).

Although the maxilla is being displaced anteriorly, it has an anterior surface that is actually surface resorptive. The maxillary arch, therefore, does not "grow" forward through bone deposition on its front surface. Only in the human face is the anterior surface of the upper and lower jaws resorptive, which is one factor relating to the extreme gnathic reduction in humans and explains why this region grows essentially straight downward rather than downward *and* forward as in other mammals.

As the maxillary complex becomes displaced anteriorly, the mandible is also similarly displaced by an

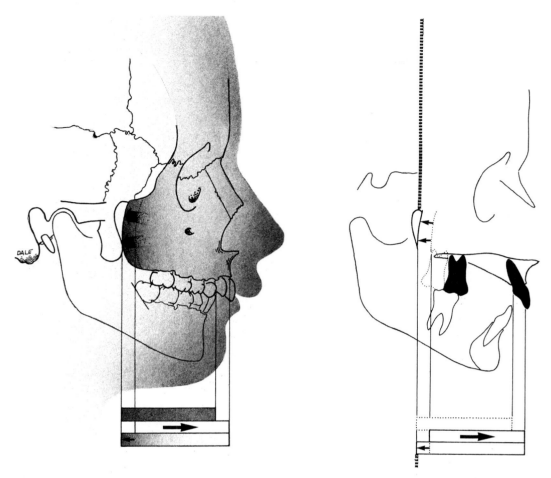

FIG. 21-29   Posterior lengthening by remodeling of the palate and maxillary arch. New bone is deposited on the posterior-facing surface of the maxillary tuberosity. Resorption occurs on the inner surface of the tuberosity (which is the inside wall of the maxillary sinus).

equivalent amount in a corresponding forward direction (Fig. 21-30), given there is perfectly balanced growth in both amount and timing. Anterior mandibular displacement continuously causes a "space" to occur at the condylar articulation, as well as in the whole region just behind the mandible (Fig. 21-31). Mandibular remodeling, however, is virtually simultaneous. The displacement of the whole mandible in a forward direction caused by expansion of the enclosing soft tissue mass triggers the condyle and ramus to grow backward (and also upward) by an amount that equals the continuous displacement movement.

The anterior-facing surface of the ramus undergoes progressive resorption by an amount that equals new bone deposition on the posterior-facing surface (Fig. 21-32). The result is that (1) a relocation of the whole

ramus occurs posteriorly and (2) the anterior part of the old ramus becomes remodeled into an addition for the mandibular corpus. Consequently the bony mandibular arch is lengthened. To this point, lengthening of the maxillary arch has been matched by an elongation of the mandibular arch and both structures have been displaced anteriorly by an equivalent amount.

As all the above changes proceed continuously and more or less simultaneously, the right and left middle cranial fossae are also enlarging in conjunction with growth expansion of the temporal lobes of the cerebrum (Fig. 21-33). The endocranial surface is mostly resorptive, and the ectocranial side depository. In the midline part of the cranial base, endochondral bone growth also occurs in conjunction with the cartilaginous synchondroses.

Text continued on p. 496.

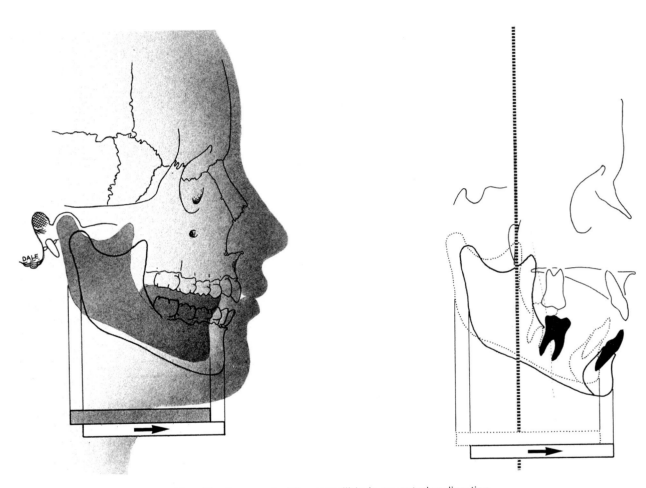

FIG. 21-30 Displacement of the mandible in an anterior direction.

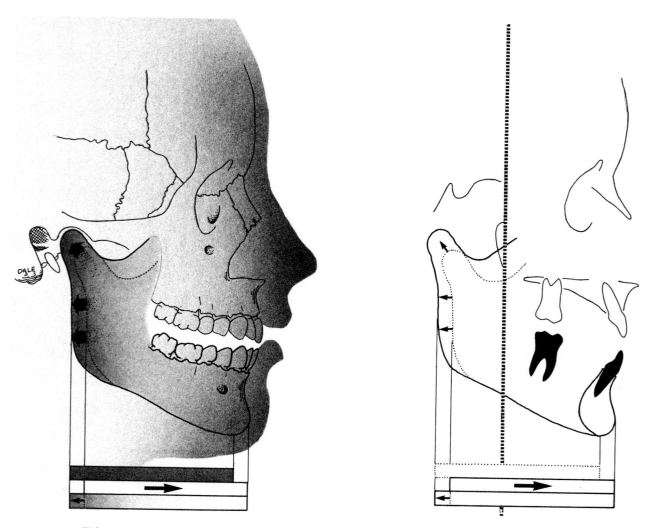

FIG. 21-31 Mandibular condylar and ramal growth. The mandibular condyle and posterior border of the ramus grow posteriorly (and superiorly) by an amount equal to the extent of the whole mandibular anterior displacement.

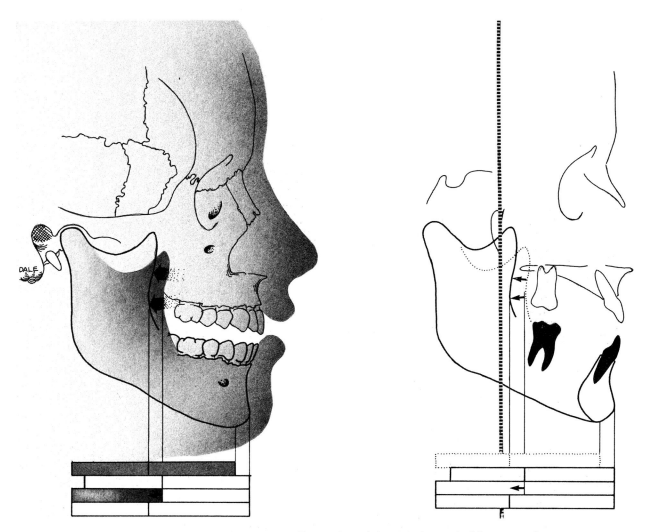

FIG. 21-32 Relocation of the ramus. Resorption of the anterior part of the ramus by an amount that equals deposition along the posterior part results in a posterior relocation of the whole ramus. The corpus is thereby lengthened by an equivalent amount.

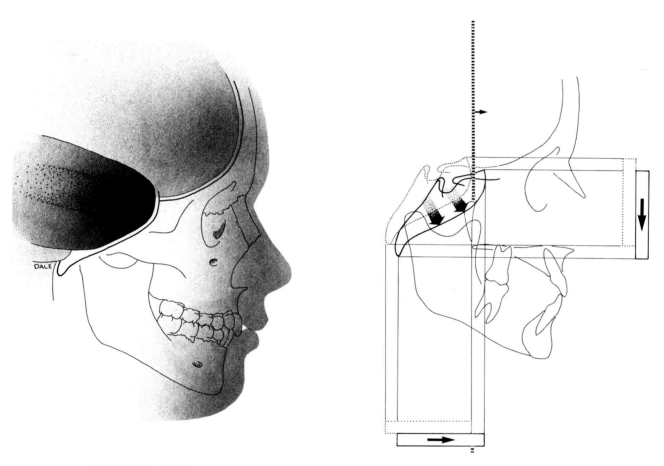

FIG. 21-33   Middle cranial fossa enlarging to accommodate the growing temporal lobe of the cerebrum.

The enlargement of the brain and middle cranial fossa causes displacement of the entire nasomaxillary complex and the anterior cranial fossa anteriorly (Fig. 21-34). The mandible responds by a horizontal enlargement of the whole ramus. The condyle and posterior part of the ramus continue to grow posteriorly, so that the ramus now increases in breadth by an amount that equals the size increase of the overlying middle cranial fossa (Fig. 21-35). As this occurs, the whole mandible is being displaced anteriorly (Fig. 21-36) to keep pace with the anterior displacement of the maxilla caused by brain and middle cranial fossa growth.

Thus far, two phases of displacement have occurred for the maxillae. The first (Fig. 21-28) involved growth of the facial soft tissue mass, and the second (Fig. 21-34) growth of the brain and middle cranial fossa. Two remodeling changes have also occurred for the mandibular ramus. The first (Figs. 21-30 and 21-32) involved its posterior relocation to allow for mandibular arch lengthening, and the second (Fig. 21-35) its increasing breadth to match the enlargement of the middle cranial fossa.

In the meantime, the frontal lobes of the cerebrum have also continued to grow and the anterior cranial

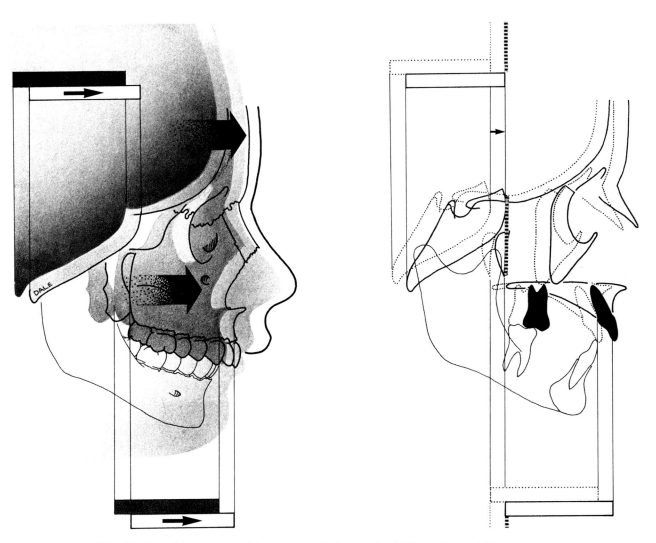

FIG. 21-34 Enlargement of the temporal lobes and middle endocranial fossae, causing anterior displacement of the nasomaxillary complex and the anterior endocranial fossae.

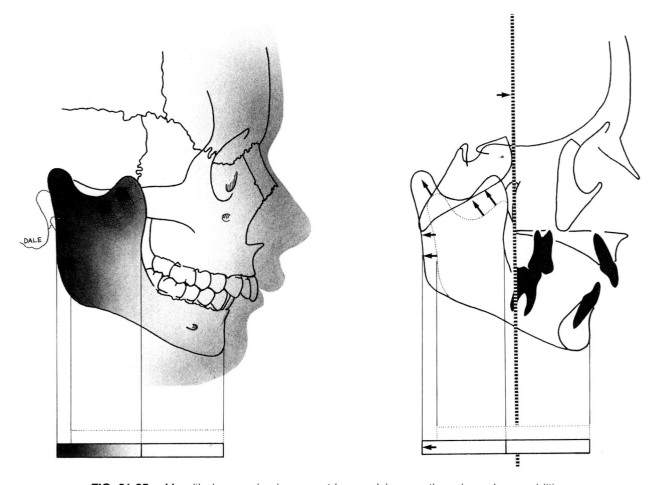

FIG. 21-35 Mandibular ramal enlargement by condylar growth and new bone addition along the posterior part of the ramus. The amount equals the extent of middle cranial fossa enlargement. (See Fig. 21-32.)

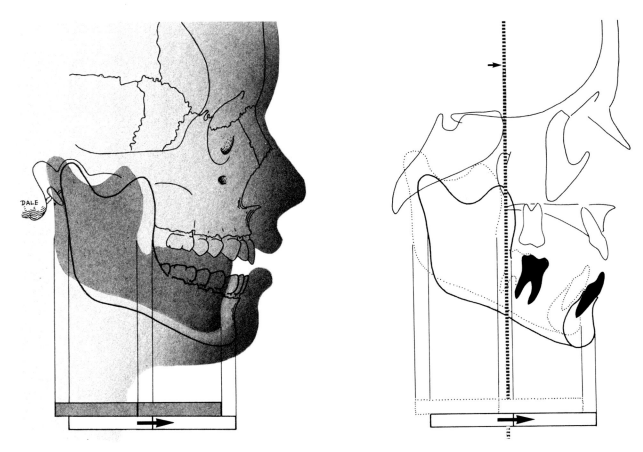

FIG. 21-36 Mandibular displacement. This matches the displacement of the maxilla caused by middle cranial fossa enlargement (Fig. 21-34) and ramal widening (Fig. 21-35).

fossae enlarge to accommodate them (Fig. 21-37). The endocranial surfaces of the fossae are largely resorptive, and the outer surfaces are depository. These particular growth activities essentially cease by 5 or 6 years of age, whereas most other parts of the face and cranium continue to grow and develop for many more years.

The nasomaxillary complex also becomes displaced inferiorly (as well as anteriorly, outlined above) by the expansion of soft tissues of the face (Fig. 21-38). As shown in Figure 21-25, all the various sutures receive bone deposits by amounts that equal the extent of ongoing displacement. The entire dental arch is carried downward by this displacement process, and all the teeth are thereby moved inferiorly from level 1 to level 2.

In addition to the downward displacement movement and sutural growth process just seen, the palate and maxillary arch grow directly downward by remodeling (Fig. 21-23). The combination of these growth processes provides for the total progressive vertical enlargement of the overlying nasal chambers to keep pace with lung growth. In general, upward-facing surfaces are resorptive and downward-facing surfaces are depository, thus producing a downward direction of progressive growth. The nasal side of the hard palate thereby has a resorptive surface, and the oral side a depository surface. Other similar combinations of resorption and deposition occur in other parts of the nasomaxillary complex to produce an inferiorly directed composite of remodeling changes. In Figure 21-23, for example, the alveolar bone of the incisor region is remodeling downward along with other parts of the whole maxilla.

The maxillary teeth are moving inferiorly by the same two growth processes just mentioned, displacement and remodeling. Although shown separately, they occur simultaneously. In Figure 21-38 the entire dental arch is being displaced as a unit (from level 1 to level

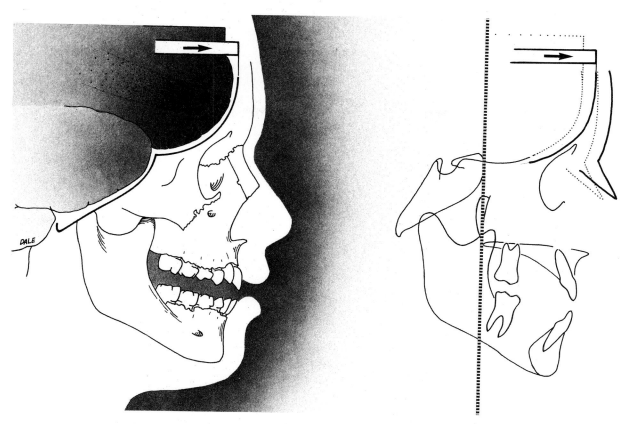

FIG. 21-37 Anterior endocranial fossa enlargement to accommodate growth of the frontal lobes.

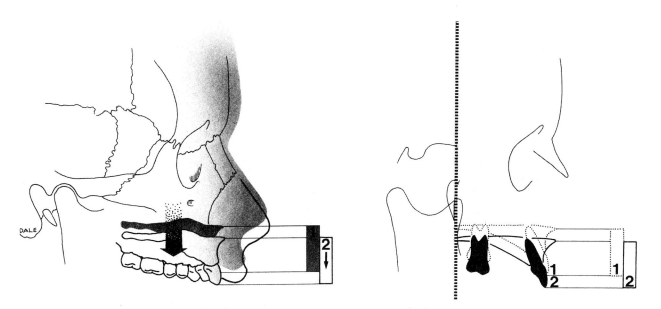

FIG. 21-38 Vertical displacement of the nasomaxillary complex. Just as the expansion of all facial soft tissues causes a forward displacement of the whole nasomaxillary complex (Fig. 21-28), a concomitant inferior displacement from level *1* to level *2* is produced. (Compare this with Figure 21-25, in which the forward and downward movements are combined in a single illustration.) These movements "separate" the bones at their various sutural junctions, and sutural bone deposition simultaneously enlarges the circumference of each bone by an amount that equals its displacement.

2), and in Figure 21-39 each tooth is moving downward (from level *2* to level *3*) in conjunction with the remodeling of its bony alveolar socket. The latter process is termed *vertical drift*, and the PDL produces it. The same deposition and resorption of bone that are involved in medial drift also provide for the vertical drifting of each tooth at the same time (Fig. 21-40). This vertical growth process is often, but incorrectly, called eruption or extrusion, which is a separate movement of the teeth. Eruption is the movement of a tooth out of its socket whereas vertical drift is a combined movement of the tooth and its socket and constitutes a posteruptive event. (See Chapter 15.)

"Working with growth" is a fundamental principle of clinical dentistry. From the foregoing account, it can be recognized that an understanding of the details of the growth process is quite necessary to harness them for various clinical treatment procedures. One must know just which component of the growth process is to be involved in different clinical objectives. For example, in the movement of the dentition from level 2 to level 3 the periodontal ligament (membrane) is the target for certain orthodontic procedures intended to provide positional adjustments of individual teeth and their alveolar sockets. The displacement movement from level 1 to level 2, however, has the sutural membranes as targets for adjustment and repositioning of the whole maxilla and dental arch.

Most of the downward displacement of the mandibular dentition is provided by vertical enlargement of the ramus (Figs. 21-30 and 21-35). As the maxillary arch descends and the nasal region correspondingly expands, the obliquely upward and backward lengthening of the mandibular ramus produces an equivalent extent of inferior and anterior placement for the lower arch (Fig. 21-41). Much less vertical upward drift occurs for the mandibular teeth than vertical downward drift for the maxillary teeth. There is thus less growth (alveolar remodeling) for the lower teeth to work with (which is one reason why orthodontists often use maxillary rather than mandibular dentition for certain clinical procedures, even though it is usually the size or placement of the mandible, or both, that actually underlies many severe malocclusions). The displacement process of the mandible, however, offers considerable growth movement that can be used in selected clinical procedures, through efforts to increase or decrease the rate or direction of condylar growth and ramus remodeling activity.

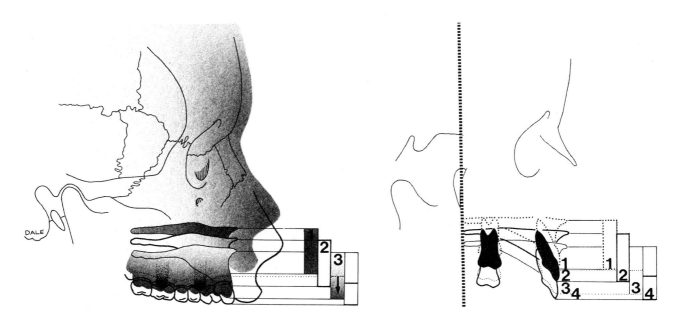

FIG. 21-39 Downward remodeling of the palate and maxillary arch. This takes place in addition to the displacement movement shown in Figure 21-38. Displacement moves the palate and arch from level *1* to level *2*. Remodeling (deposition on the oral side and resorption on the nasal side) moves the palate and arch from level *2* to level *3*. The anterior teeth tend to drift inferiorly more than the posterior teeth, which relates to a frequently occurring clockwise rotation of the occlusal plane.

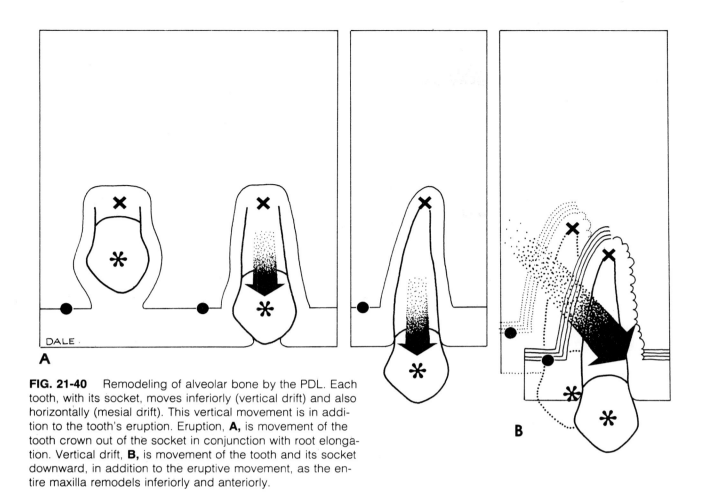

FIG. 21-40 Remodeling of alveolar bone by the PDL. Each tooth, with its socket, moves inferiorly (vertical drift) and also horizontally (mesial drift). This vertical movement is in addition to the tooth's eruption. Eruption, **A,** is movement of the tooth crown out of the socket in conjunction with root elongation. Vertical drift, **B,** is movement of the tooth and its socket downward, in addition to the eruptive movement, as the entire maxilla remodels inferiorly and anteriorly.

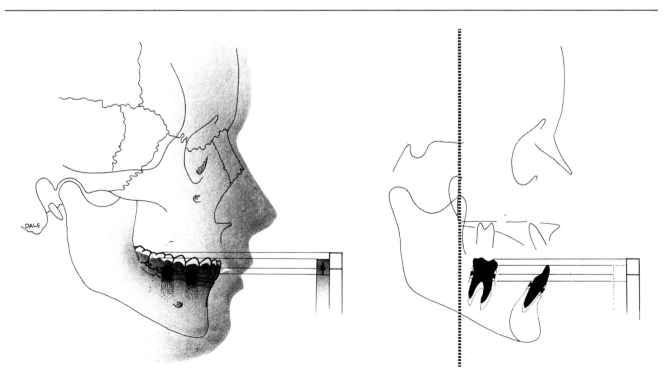

FIG. 21-41 Mandibular teeth drift vertically in a superior direction.

Mandibular incisors, as they erupt and drift upward into occlusion along with the other mandibular teeth, come into a normal overbite and overjet relationship with the maxillary incisors (Fig. 21-42). In other words, the upper teeth overlap the lower, involving a backward tipping of the mandibular incisors as they drift superiorly. The labial side of the alveolar bone is resorptive; and, together with bone remodeling by the periodontal membrane within the alveolar socket, the tooth drifts lingually as well as upward. Bone deposition on the mental protuberance, with retroclination of the incisors, produces a gradually enlarging chin.

As the maxillary complex becomes displaced anteriorly, the malar region and the contiguous orbital part of the zygoma are likewise displaced in a forward direction (Figs. 21-43 and 21-44). The whole region simultaneously remodels posteriorly to keep pace with the posteriorly lengthening maxillary arch. By this growth process, remodeling and displacement changes of the cheekbone region match those of the maxillary arch.

Whereas almost all components (nasal region, maxillary arches, cheekbones) are displaced anteriorly, divergent directions of remodeling occur among the nasal, frontal, and cheekbone areas. The nasal bones, supraorbital rims, and lateral walls of the nasal chambers remodel and expand anteriorly. The malar protuberance and lateral orbital rim remodel posteriorly. The topography of the face becomes bolder and deeper as a result. In Figure 21-45, note that a line drawn

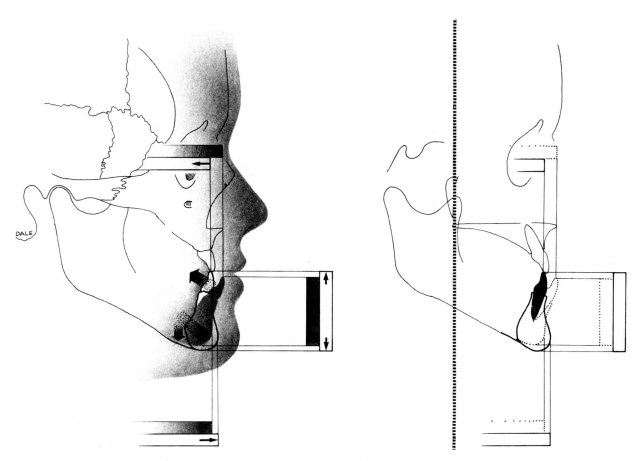

FIG. 21-42 Two-way remodeling movements in the anterior part of the mandibular arch. The mental protuberance receives new bone deposits slowly and over a long period. The incisors, however, undergo an uprighting (lingual tipping) into their overlap position behind the upper centrals. The labial side of the alveolar bone is resorptive, the lingual side depository, and the composite effect is a progressive enlargement of the chin.

through the upper and lower orbital rims is angled slightly posteriorly in the young child but inclines more anteriorly in the adult because of the divergent directions of remodeling between the forehead–nasal region and the cheekbone–lateral orbital rim.

If the first and last stages of the preceding series (Figs. 21-27 and 21-44) are superimposed with the sella turcica as a registration point, the forward and downward growth of the face relative to the cranial base is apparent (Fig. 21-46). At one time it was believed that this overlay represented the picture of how the face

actually grew. It is now realized that the growth process itself is a complex of many regional displacement and remodeling changes. The overlay in Figure 21-46 shows the composite results of all these regional growth changes and the locations of various facial parts at the two ages involved relative to an arbitrary point in the cranial base (the sella). Although this method of superimposing cephalograms does not demonstrate the actual process of growth itself, it is nonetheless useful to clinicians and researchers in measuring and quantifying the anatomic products of growth.

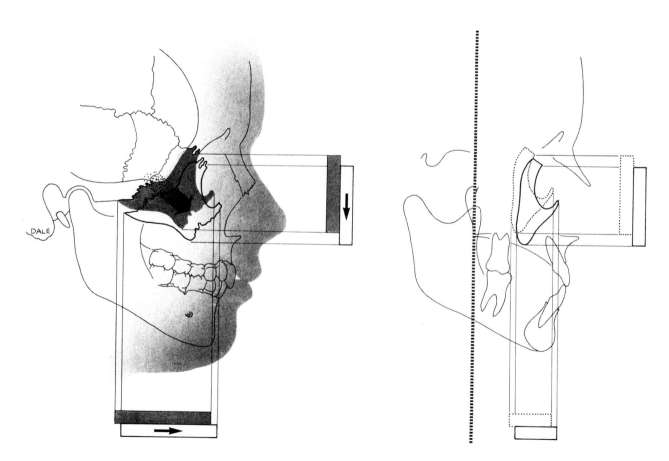

FIG. 21-43 Anterior and inferior displacement of the zygoma.

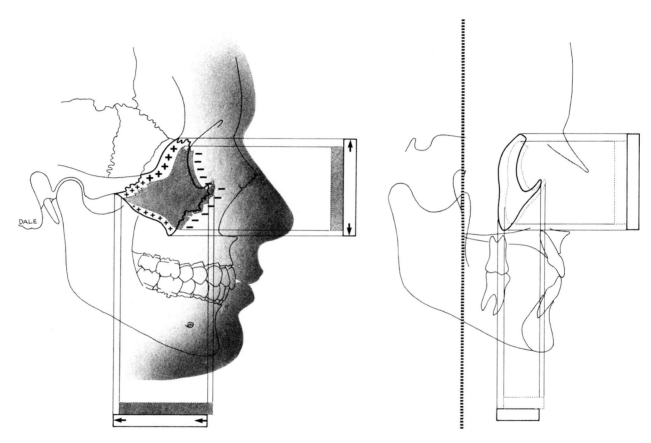

FIG. 21-44 Remodeling process of the zygoma comparable to that of the maxilla. Note that the anterior part of the malar protuberance is resorptive (as is also the anterior part of the maxilla).

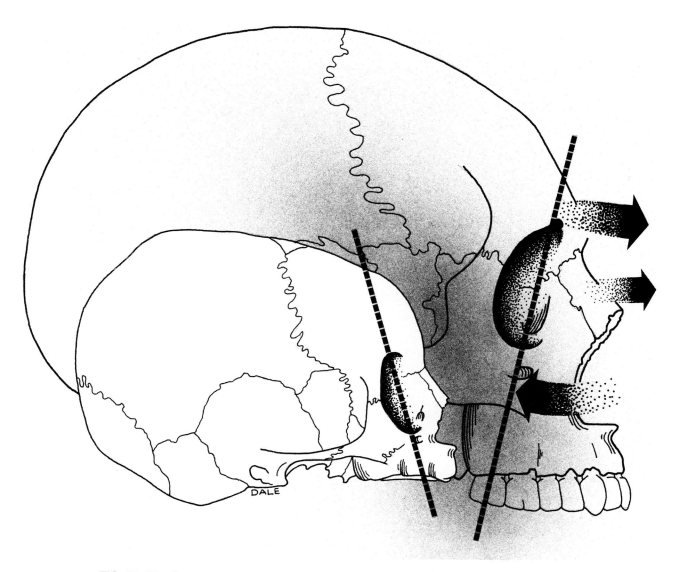

FIG. 21-45 Two-way remodeling movements between the upper and lower regions of the nasomaxillary complex. The upper nasal region, forehead, and superior orbital rim remodel and enlarge anteriorly whereas the inferior orbital rim and cheekbone remodel posteriorly. Note that the facial plane (shown here by a vertical line passing through the upper and lower orbital rims) rotates into an anteriorly inclined alignment. The topographic depth of the face is increased considerably. Although the cheekbone region is remodeling backward along with the maxillary tuberosity, it is also displaced forward together with the tuberosity, maxillary arch, nasal region, palate, and all other parts of the face. Thus some facial parts remodel posteriorly and some remodel anteriorly, but everything is displaced anteriorly.

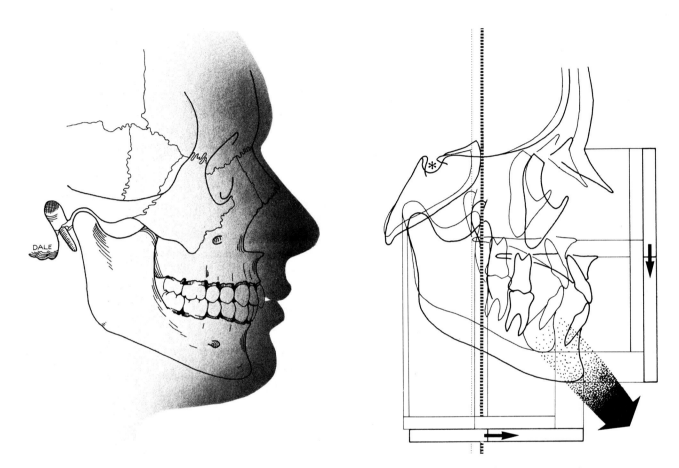

FIG. 21-46 First and last stages of the craniofacial growth sequence (Figs. 21-27 and 21-44) superimposed on the cranial base. In this method of superimposing serial cephalometric tracings, the center of the sella turcica is the point for registration (asterisk) of the tracings. Note that this method does not show how the face actually grows. Rather, it shows the aggregate result of all the regional changes described in Figures 21-27 through 21-44 when visualized relative to the cranial base. It illustrates the locations of the growing mandible, maxilla, and other parts relative to the sella turcica at the two ages represented, not the biologic processes of remodeling and displacement that actually bring about the growth changes involved.

CURVE OF OCCLUSION

Because of the notably long vertical human face, there is a tendency for the mandible and occlusal plane to have a downward and backward rotated position. This rotational alignment would produce an anterior open bite but for a compensatory action on the part of the dentition (Figs. 21-47 to 21-49). The mandibular incisors and their alveolar sockets undergo additional upward drift, which closes the occlusion in the incisor region. The occlusal plane has a characteristic curve as a result that tends to be more or less marked according to the downward rotation of the mandible produced by vertical growth of the nasomaxillary region. As the mandibular anterior teeth undergo this vertical drifting process, their axial inclinations shift to a more upright alignment, which continues until they come into occlusion with the upright-oriented maxillary teeth. Incisor alignment contrasts with alignment of the mandibular posterior teeth, which tend to be inclined slightly anteriorly because of the downward mandibular rotation.

A long-faced (dolichocephalic) head form with a hyperdivergent facial pattern, a short-faced (brachycephalic) head form with a hypodivergent facial pattern, the degree of vertical overbite of the incisor teeth, and the maxillary and mandibular curves of occlusion all have a bearing on whether certain procedures will be beneficial or detrimental to the orthodontic correction of a malocclusion (Figs. 21-50 and 21-51).

Text continued on p. 512.

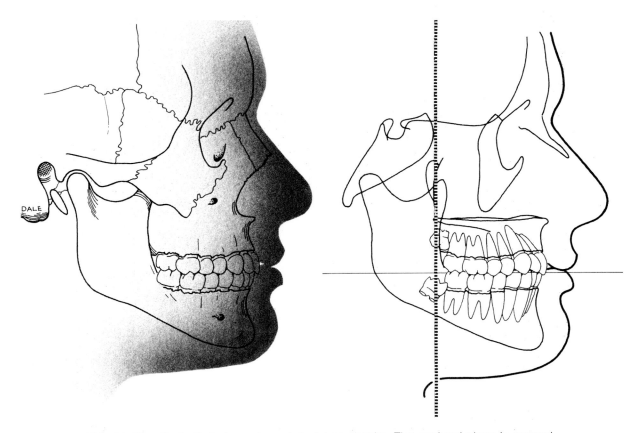

FIG. 21-47 Perfectly balanced craniofacial composite. The occlusal plane is approximately perpendicular to the maxillary tuberosity (the vertical reference line shown in Fig. 21-27). It is rotated neither upward nor downward to any marked extent and is approximately parallel to the neutral orbital axis. In most faces some degree of occlusal plane rotation occurs.

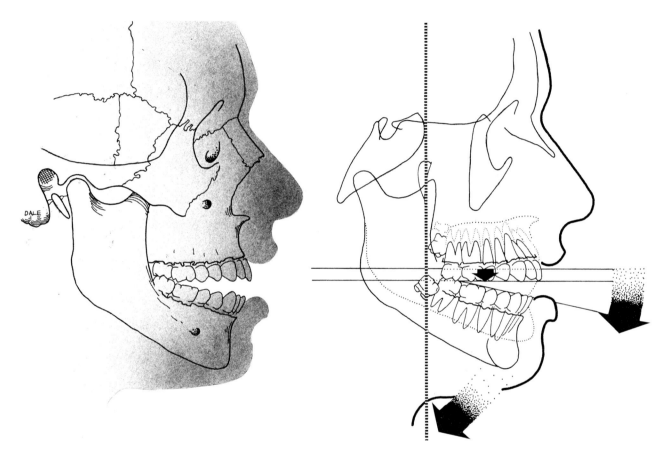

FIG. 21-48 Lowered maxillary arch, resulting in a downward and backward alignment of the mandible. Note also the retrusion of the chin and lower incisors. This, in part, is the anatomic basis for a Class II malocclusion among persons having a long narrow head form. (An open cranial base angle has the same effect and adds to the extent of the mandibular retrognathism, as seen in Figure 21-12.)

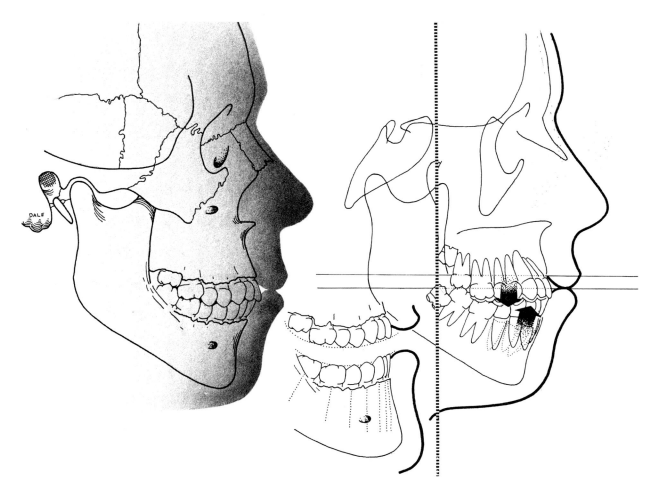

FIG. 21-49 Dental compensations precluding an anterior open bite as a consequence of the mandibular rotation seen in Figure 21-50. The anterior mandibular teeth drift vertically in a superior direction, the anterior maxillary teeth drift inferiorly, and the result (frequently encountered) is the curve of occlusion.

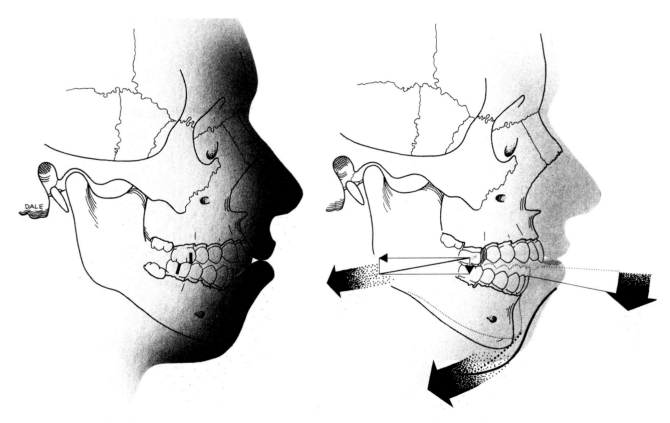

FIG. 21-50   How posterior cervical-pull headgear has a tendency to produce a vertical drift of the maxillary first molars during the correction of a Class II malocclusion. As may vertical development of the nasomaxillary region, this therapy can produce a downward and backward rotation of the mandible. If the patient has a hyperdivergent leptoprosopic facial pattern, such a response could increase the length of an already long face and accentuate the tendency toward an open bite.

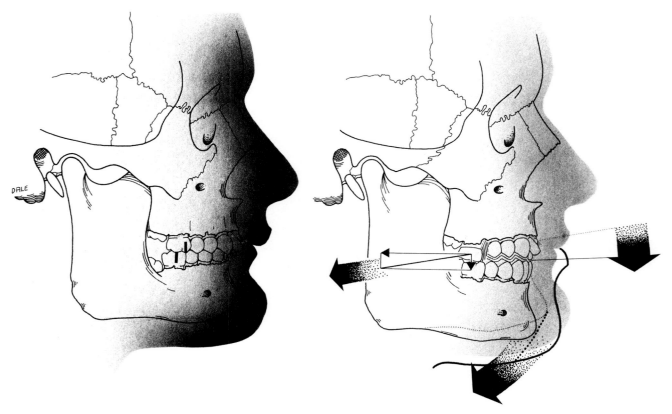

FIG. 21-51 How a posterior cervical-pull headgear tends to produce a favorable response in patients with a hypodivergent euryprosopic facial pattern. The vertical force in this instance increases a short lower face height, reduces prominence of the chin, provides space to upright the mandibular incisors labially, and opens a deep overbite while the Class II molar malocclusion is being corrected.

MANDIBULAR CONDYLE AND GROWTH

Historically the condyle has been thought to have special significance with regard to the mandibular growth process. Although this belief is true, its conceptual basis has changed considerably. Formerly the condyle and its condylar cartilage were presumed to contain the genetic programming that provided the primary pacemaker role for overall mandibular growth and development. In light of experimental research, this presumption is no longer fully acceptable. Significantly, however, the role of the condyle is becoming better understood and now gives a far more noteworthy developmental function to this structure.

In Chapter 19 the condylar cartilage was described as having, along with the remainder of the ramus, a special developmental role to accomplish—an adaptive function involved in the continued placement of the mandibular arch in juxtaposition with the maxillary arch and basicranium as all grow to become an interrelated whole. Because the mandible articulates with the cranial base at one end (at the TMJs) and also with the maxilla through tooth contact in the occlusal plane, its growth must be adaptable to the wide range of dimensional, anatomic, rotational, and developmental variations that occur in the nasomaxillary complex, dentition, and neurocranium. The ramus and its condyle have the capacity to provide for this developmental adaptability, within a normal latitude, by varying the amount and direction of their growth to accommodate whatever nasomaxillary and dental height, length, and width exist during the changing course of growth. Similar variations occurring in the cranium are also accommodated.

The mandibular growth process involves a feedback mechanism. Continuously changing growth circumstances (e.g., physiologic changes, soft tissue increases, biomechanical forces, bioelectric alterations, neurologic changes, hormones, and possibly other factors) trigger the ramus and condyle to grow or stop growing, in more or less upward and backward directions. This

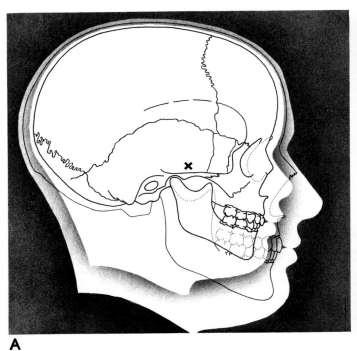

A

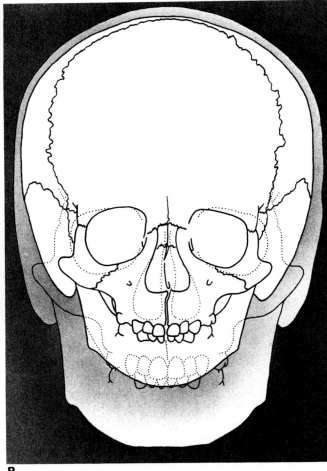

B

FIG. 21-52 Summary of postnatal growth and development from 3 to 18 years of age. **A** is a lateral view, and **B** a frontal view. The location of the sella turcica is denoted by *x*.

is an exceedingly important and fundamental growth function, carried out by the condyle and the ramus as a whole.

A summary of the growth changes that have been discussed in this chapter appears in Figure 21-52, which depicts the face and skull from 3 to 18 years of age.

BIBLIOGRAPHY

Babula WJ, Smiley GR, Dixon AD: The role of the cartilaginous nasal septum in midfacial growth, *Am J Orthod* 58:250, 1970.

Bjork A: The face in profile, *Svensk Tandlak Tidskr* 40(Suppl):180, 1947.

Bjork A, Skieller V: Facial development and tooth eruption: an implant study at the age of puberty, *Am J Orthod* 62:339, 1972.

Brodie AG: On the growth pattern of the human head from the third month to the eighth year of life, *Am J Anat* 68:209, 1938.

Coben SE: The integration of facial skeletal variants, *Am J Orthod* 41:407, 1955.

Droschl H: The effect of heavy orthopedic forces on the maxilla in the growing *Saimiri sciueus* (squirrel monkey), *Am J Orthod* 63:449, 1973.

Durkin JF, Heeley JD, Irving JT: The cartilage of the mandibular condyle, *Oral Sci Rev* 2:29, 1973.

Enlow DH: *The human face,* New York, 1968, Harper & Row.

Enlow DH: Growth of the problem of the local control mechanism, *Am J Anat* 136:403, 1973.

Enlow DH: *Handbook of facial growth,* ed 3, Philadelphia, 1990, WB Saunders.

Enlow DH, Harris DB: A study of the postnatal growth of the human mandible, *Am J Orthod* 50:25, 1964.

Enlow DH, Harvold EP, Latham RA, et al: Research on control of craniofacial morphogenesis: an NIDR state-of-the-art workshop, *Am J Orthod* 71:509, 1977.

Ford EHR: Growth of the human cranial base, *Am J Orthod* 44:498, 1958.

Gianelly AA, Moorrees CFA: Condylectomy in the rat, *Arch Oral Biol* 10:101, 1965.

Johnston LE: A statistical evaluation of cephalometric prediction, *Angle Orthod* 38:284, 1968.

Koski K: Cranial growth centers: facts or fallacies? *Am J Orthod* 54:250, 1968.

Koski K: Some characteristics of cranio-facial growth cartilages. In Meyers RE, Krogman WM (eds): *Cranio-facial growth in man,* New York, 1971, Pergamon Press.

Koski K, Ronning O: Growth potential of intracerebrally transplanted cranial base synchondroses in the rat, *Arch Oral Biol* 15:1107, 1970.

Latham RA: The septopremaxillary ligament and maxillary development, *J Anat* 104:584, 1969.

Latham RA: Maxillary development and growth: the septopremaxillary ligament, *J Anat* 107:471, 1970.

Latham RA, Burston WR: The postnatal pattern of growth at the sutures of the human skull, *Dent Pract* 17:61, 1966.

Luder HU, Leblond CP, von der Mark K: Cellular stages in cartilage formation as revealed by morphometry, radioautography and Type 11 collagen immunostaining of the mandibular condyle from weanling rats, *Am J Anat* 182:197, 1988.

Martone VD, Enlow DH, Hans MG, et al: Class I and Class II malocclusion subgroupings related to headform type, *Angle Orthod* 62:35, 1992.

McNamara JA Jr: Neuromuscular and skeletal adaptation to altered function in the orofacial region, *Am J Orthod* 64:578, 1973.

Meikle MC: The role of the condyle in the postnatal growth of the mandible, *Am J Orthod* 64:50, 1973.

Moss ML: The primary role of functional matrices in facial growth, *Am J Orthod* 55:566, 1969.

Moss ML, Bromberg BE: The passive role of nasal septal cartilage in midfacial growth, *Plast Reconstruct Surg* 41:536, 1968.

Nanda RS: The rates of growth of several facial components measured from serial cephalometric roentgenograms, *Am J Orthod* 41:658, 1955.

Sarnat BG: Clinical and experimental considerations in facial bone biology: growth, remodeling and repair, *J Am Dent Assoc* 82:876, 1971.

Sarnat BG: Surgical experimentation and gross postnatal growth of the face and jaws, *J Dent Res* 50:1462, 1971.

Scott JH: The cartilage of the nasal septum, *Am J Orthod* 42:381, 1956.

Scott JH: The cranial base, *Am J Phys Anthropol* 16:319, 1958.

Sicher H: Growth of the mandible, *Am J Orthod* 33:30, 1947.

Washburn SL: The relation of the temporal muscle to the form of the skull, *Anat Rec* 99:239, 1947.

Index

A

Acellular cementum, 52, 279
  formation of, 264
Acellular zone in dental papilla, 67
Acetylcholine, 382-383
Achondroplasia, 2
Acid etching, 254-255
Acinus in salivary glands, 361, 362, 363
Actin, 373
Adenosine monophosphate, 383
Adenosine triphosphate, 445
African American, facial form in, 476, 477
Age changes; see Aging
Aggregation in plaque formation, 345
Aging
  in dentin-pulp complex, 210-212
  in dentogingival junction, 272, 307
  in enamel, 254
  in face, 481
  fibroblasts and, 86-87
  in oral mucosa, 431
  in salivary gland, 383
Alanine, 221
Alkaline phosphatase
  in early tooth germ, 63, 64
  in hard tissue formation, 115
  in osteoblasts, 125
Alveolar bone, 47, 50, 55
  orthodontic tooth movement and, 334
  remodeling of, 500, 501
Alveolar cleft, 42
Alveolar crest fiber, 262, 267
Alveolar mucosa
  structure of, 424
  surface areas of, 45
Alveolar nerve, 34, 35
Alveolar plates, maxillary, 38
Alveolar process, 55
  in periodontal ligament, 298-299, 300
Amalgam in oral mucosa, 408-409
Ameloblast
  in amelogenesis, 218-219
  in crown stage, 71, 72
  in enamel
    maturation of, 227, 231, 232
    rods of, 244
  life-cycle of, 233, 234

Ameloblast—cont'd
  micrograph of functioning, 72
Amelogenesis, 71, 72, 218-238
  ameloblast in, 269
    differentiation of, 218-219
  defects of, 236-237
  electron microscopy of, 226-233, 234
    maturation stage in, 227-231, 232, 233
    morphogenetic stage in, 226
    protective stage in, 233, 234
    secretory stage in, 227, 228, 229, 230
  enamel in, 269
    matrix formation of, 219-223
  light microscopy of, 223-226
  mineral pathway in, 235-236
Amelogenesis imperfecta, 2
Amelogenin, 111, 219, 220
Amino acid
  in collagens, 88
  in enamel, 221
AMP; see Adenosine monophosphate
Amplifying cells, 395
Amylase in saliva, 53, 357
Anchoring fibril, 411, 413
  of collagens, 88
Anchoring filaments, 411
Androgen in salivary gland regulation, 383
Ankylosis
  avulsed tooth and, 267
  in periodontium repair, 467
Antibodies in saliva, 357
Antigen, bullous pemphigoid, 411
Antimicrobial action in saliva, 357
Apatite crystallite
  in enamel mineralization and maturation, 222-223
  in hard tissue formation, 115
  in intertubular dentin, 178
  in mineralized tissue, 111-113
Apoptosis of periodontal ligament, 327, 328
Approximal drift of tooth, 322
Arch
  branchial, 15-20
  dental, displacement of, 498-500
  mandibular, 502
  maxillary
    alignment of mandible and, 507, 508
    displacement of, 489, 490, 491

Arch—cont'd
  maxillary—cont'd
    downward remodeling of, 500
  zygomatic
    in mastication, 450
    relocation of, 485
Arginine, 221
Arteriovenous shunt in dental pulp, 201, 202
Articular bone, 432
Articular disc, 56, 57
Articular eminence, 56
Articulare, 435
Aspartic acid, 221
Attachment plaque, 401
Autocrine regulation, 101
Autoradiography in proliferating cell identification, 396
Autosomal dominant inheritance, 2
Autosomal recessive inheritance, 2
Avulsion of tooth, 267
Axon in dental pulp, 204-205

B

Bacterial plaque, 342, 344-345, 347
Band
  epithelial, 58-60, 61
  Hunter-Schreger, 249, 250
Basal bone, 55
Basal lamina, 66
  epithelial–lamina propria junction and, 411, 413
  epithelial-mesenchymal relationship and, 102
Basement lamina, 66
Basement membrane
  of oral mucosa, 392, 411
  of seromucous cell, 365, 367
  of terminal secretory end piece, 362
Basicranium, 469, 472, 473
BdU; *see* Bromodeoxyuridine
Bell stage of tooth development, 62-64, 65, 69
  crown pattern determination in, 67
  dental papilla in, 67
  fragmentation of dental lamina in, 67
Bicarbonate in saliva, 357
Biglycan in oral mucosa, 419
Bilaminar embryonic disk, 7
Biorbital convergence, 474
Bipartite secretory granule, 368
Birbeck granule, 410
Black persons, facial form in, 476, 477
Blastema in temporomandibular joint, 435-438
Blastocyst, 3, 4, 5
Blood clot
  saliva and, 358
  in tissue repair, 456
  in tooth extraction repair, 466, 467
Blood supply
  of dentogingival junction, 306-307
  of oral mucosa, 418, 419
  of periodontal ligament, 294
  of salivary gland, 383
  of temporomandibular joint, 454
BMP; *see* Bone morphogenetic protein
Bone, 120-146
  alveolar, 47, 50, 55
    orthodontic tooth movement and, 334
    remodeling of, 500, 501

Bone—cont'd
  alveolar—cont'd
    cancellous, 144, 145
    cells in, 124-129, 130
    in childhood facial growth and development, 488
    compact, 120, 121, 122
    composition of, 120
    displacement of, 486, 487
    evolution of terminology of, 124
    flat, 120
    formation of
      endochondral, 130, 131-134
      intramembranous, 134-137
      in mandible formation, 35
      in periodontium, 267-268
      in tooth extraction repair, 466, 467
    frozen dried, 467
    gross histology of, 120-121, 122, 123
    growth of
      endochondral, 488
      erroneous schema of, 482, 483
      intramembranous, 488
      sutural, 137, 138, 139, 140
    immature, 136, 137
    incremental lines in, 117
    lamellar, 136, 137
    long, 120
    in mandible formation, 35
    relocation of, 483, 484
    remodeling of, 320-321, 483, 484-486, 488
      in childhood facial growth and development, 484-486
      in neurocranial skeleton, 482
    tooth movement and, 317, 320-321, 334
    trabecular, 120, 121, 122
    turnover of, 137-145
    woven coarse-fibered, 135, 136
Bone morphogenetic protein
  in cell communication, 101
  osteoblasts and, 125
Brachiation, 469
Brachycephalic head, 475
  facial profile of, 478
  in orthodontic malocclusion correction, 507, 508, 509
Brain enlargements in evolution, 469
Branchial arches in embryology, 15-20
Branchial grooves, 15
Bromodeoxyuridine in proliferating cell identification, 396
Buccal mucosa
  linea alba of, 392, 407
  nonkeratinized, 398, 404
  structure of, 424
  surface areas of, 45
Buccal salivary gland, 384
Buccopharyngeal membrane in embryology, 15, 16, 17
Bud stage in tooth development, 60, 61
Bulbs of Krause, 420
Bullous pemphigoid antigen, 411

C

Calcitonin in bone metabolism, 126
Calcium
  in forming enamel, 235, 236
  free cytosolic, 235, 236
  in mineral transport to hard tissue, 116
  in saliva, 357, 358

Calcium-adenosine triphosphatase, 235, 236
Calcium hydroxyapatite, 111-113
Calcium phosphate, fluoride and, 254
Calculus, 342
Cambium of skull suture, 137, 140
Canal
    gubernacular, 318, 319
    root, 210
Canaliculus in seromucous cells, 367
Cancellous bone, 144, 145
Canine
    epithelial-mesenchymal relationship in, 105
    formation of, 105, 107
    impacted, 332
    resorption of, 325
Cap stage of tooth development, 65
Capillary in oral mucosa, 419
Capsule of temporomandibular joint, 442
Cardiac plate, 7
    embryology of, 15, 16
Caries
    dentin and, 175
    development of, 462-465, 466
    fluoridation and, 254
Cartilage
    in childhood facial growth and development, 488
    in endochondral bone formation, 130, 131-134
    Meckel's, 18
    Reichert's, 18
    remodeling of, 488
    symphysial, 37
    in temporomandibular joint, 432
Caucasian person, facial forms in, 476, 477
Caudocephalic folding of embryo, 8-9, 11
Cavity preparation, 465, 466
CD44 in fibroblast, 93
Cell cycle
    deoxyribonucleic acid replication during, 1
    phases of, 395
Cell surface marker, 401
Cell surface receptor
    in cell communication, 100-102
    in tooth morphogenesis, 104, 105
Cells; *see also* specific cell type
    communication between, 100-102
    in hard tissue formation, 111
    matrix interaction of, 98
Cellular cementum, 52, 279
    formation of, 262, 265
Cellular intima, of temporomandibular joint, 441, 442
Cement line of osteoblasts, 144
Cementoblast
    in cementum, 279, 281
        primary, 257, 258, 262, 264
    progenitor cells of, 268
Cementocyte, 279, 281
Cementoenamel junction, 277, 278
Cementogenesis, 77, 257-262, 263, 264, 265
Cementum, 47, 52
    acellular, 52, 264, 279
    cells of, 279, 281
    cellular, 52, 262, 265
    classification of, 279, 280
    coronal, 342
    extrinsic fiber, 279

Cementum—cont'd
    formation of, 77, 257-262, 263, 264, 265
    incremental lines in, 117
    intrinsic fiber, 279
    mixed fiber, 279
    organic matrix in, 279
    orthodontic tooth movement and, 334, 336
    in periodontal ligament, 287
Cephalometric tracing, 503, 506
Cerebrum
    evolution of, 471, 472
    growing temporal lobe of, 491, 495
Cervical loop of dental organ, 64, 66
Cervical margin of tooth, 48
Cervical-pull headgear, 510, 511
Chairside microscopy in examination, 353, 354
Cheek
    arterial blood supply to, 418
    innervation of, 420
    mucosa of; *see* Buccal mucosa
    surface areas of, 45
Cheekbone
    male verus female, 480, 481
    remodeling of, 502-503, 505
Child, facial growth and development of, 469-513
    age changes in, 481
    basis for human facial form in, 469-474
    bone and cartilage in, 488
    bone remodeling and increases in, 484-486
    curve of occlusion in, 507, 508, 509, 510, 511
    displacement process in, 486, 487
    facial profiles in, 478, 479
    facial types in, 475-476, 477
    growth sequence in, 489-503, 504, 505, 506
    male and female faces in, 480
    mandibular condyle in, 512-513
Chondroclast in endochondral bone formation, 131, 133
Chromosome in germ cell formation, 1
Circumferential lamellae of bone, 121, 122, 123
Circumvalate papillae in oral cavity, 426, 427
Citric acid, 467
Class II malocclusion, 507, 508
    cervical-pull headgear and, 510, 511
Clear cell, 408
    Langerhans' cell as, 410
    of salivary ducts, 376, 379
Cleft
    alveolar, 42
    gill, 15
    orofacial, 40-43
    synaptic, 445
Cleft lip, 40, 41, 42
Cleft palate, 40, 42
Cleidocranial dysostosis, 2
Clinical crown, 48
Clot, blood; *see* Blood clot
Coarse-fibered woven bone, 135, 136
Cocci
    in periodontal disease diagnosis, 353, 354
    in plaque
        gingival sulc:, 351
        occlusal fissure, 349
        smooth-surface, 346, 347, 348
Col in dentogingival junction, 306-307
Colchicine in cell identification, 396

Collagen
  aggregation of, 92
  aging and, 210
  banded, 92, 94, 95
  in cementum, 52, 276
    primary, 257-262
    secondary, 262
  degradation of, 92-93, 94, 95
  in dental pulp, 199
  in dentin, 50
    intertubular, 178
  in dentin-pulp complex repair, 461-462
  in dentinal tubule, 195, 196, 197, 460, 461
  in developing salivary gland, 359
  in enamel mineralization and maturation, 222
  fibrillogenesis and, 92
  in fibroblasts, 81, 82, 88-93, 94, 95
  lamina densa, 411
  in lamina propria, 418
  mineral location in bones and, 117
  in odontoblast formation, 153-157
  in oral mucosa repair, 468
  osteoblasts and, 125
  in periodontal ligament, 50, 285
  remodeling of, 285, 287
  synthesis and assembly of, 88, 91, 458, 459, 460
  in tissue mineralization, 114, 115
  in tissue repair, 458, 459, 460
  types of, 88, 90
3,4-Collagen endopeptidase, 93, 95
Collagenase, 93, 95
Compact bone, 120, 121, 122
Competence as embryologic concept, 2-3
Concentric lamellae of bone, 121, 122, 123
Condensation of ectomesenchyme, 62
Condylar blastemas in temporomandibular joint, 435-438
Condyle
  cartilage of, 37, 439-440
  mandibular
    childhood growth of, 512
    displacement of, 491, 493
    remodeling of, 485
    in temporomandibular joint, 56, 435, 438-439
    in temporomandibular ligament, 444
Congenital defect, 2
  in embryology of head, face, and oral cavity, 40-43
  germ cell formation and, 1
Connective tissue
  in cavity preparation, 465
  in dentogingival junction, 304-306, 307
  in oral mucosa, 389
  papillae of, 392, 412
  in salivary gland, 380
  in tissue repair, 456-458, 459, 460
Contour lines of Owen, 181
Cord
  enamel, 64, 65
  gubernacular, 319
Corium, 392, 393
Corncob formation in plaque, 346, 347, 348
Cornification, 399
Coronal cementum, 342
Coronoid cartilage, 37
Corpuscle, Meissner, 420
Costochondral junction in temporomandibular joint, 432

Cranial base, 31
Cranial fossa, 491, 495, 496, 497
Cranial vault, 31
Craniofacial composite, 507
Craniofacial growth sequence, 503, 506
Cranium
  mammalian to human progression, 471, 473
  versus other mammals, 469, 472, 473
Crease, suborbital, 481
Cribriform plate, 294
Cross striations in enamel, 248, 249
Crown, 47
  clinical, 48
  determination of pattern in, 67-68
  in erupting tooth, 77
  intratubular nerves distribution in, 206, 207
Crown-rump length, 2
Crown stage in tooth formation, 71-73
Crow's feet, 481
Crystal in dental caries, 463
Cuboidal cell, 375
Curve of occlusion, 507, 508, 509, 510, 511
Cuticle, dental, 342, 343
Cutting cone in bone turnover, 139, 140, 141, 142, 143, 144
Cyst, 68, 262
Cystine, 221
Cytokine
  in cell division, 396, 397
  osteoblasts and, 125
Cytoplasm
  in active odontoblast, 151, 152
  in epithelium tissue repair, 456, 457
  in fibroblasts, 81, 82, 83
  in fine structures of tooth germ, 67
  in salivary glands, 364
  of seromucous cells, 365
Cytosolic free calcium, 116

D
Dead tracts in dentin, 211, 212
Deciduous dentition, 48
  chronology of, 337
  formation of, 68
Deciduous molar, 313-317, 326
Decorin
  in fibroblasts, 93
  in oral mucosa, 419
Dehydration, subcutaneous, 481
Dendritic cell, 199
Dental cuticle, 342, 343
Dental follicle, 257
  development of, 62, 63
  eruptive tooth movement and, 320, 321
Dental lamina
  formation of, 60
  fragmentation of, 67-68
    formation of permanent dentin and, 68, 89
Dental organ
  in amelogenesis, 217
  in crown stage, 71-73
  development of, 62
  replaced by dental papillae, 105
Dental papilla
  in bell stage tooth development, 67
  in crown stage tooth development, 71

Dental papilla—cont'd
in dentin formation, 147, 148, 149, 150
development of, 62, 63
at epithelium and lamina propria junction, 411
formation of, 62, 63
in oral cavity, 426, 427
replaced by dental organ, 105
Dental pulp; *see* Pulp
Dentary bone of temporomandibular joint, 432
Dentin, 47, 49, 50
aging in, 210-212
basic anatomy of, 169-170
caries of, 175, 463
in cavity preparation, 465
cementum and, 257
dentinocementum junction in, 184
dentinoenamel junction in, 183, 184
deposition rate of, 147
formation of, 71, 72, 73, 147-168
incremental nature of, 160
mineralization in, 157, 158, 159
odontoblast differentiation in, 147-149, 150
odontoblast movement in, 163-165
pattern of, 147, 148
primary physiologic, 157, 158
resting odontoblast in, 153
secretory odontoblast in, 151-152, 153
successive stages of, 161
transitional odontoblast in, 152
von Korff fibers in, 165
granular layer of Tomes in, 182
incremental growth lines in, 117, 180, 181
innervation of, 204-207, 208
interglobular, 157, 178, 179
intratubular, 161, 162, 176, 177, 178
mantle, 153-157
peritubular, 161, 162
physical properties of, 169
physiologic, 157, 158
primary, 170
dentinal tubules in, 173-175
repair of, 460-463
root, 147, 162, 163, 164
sclerotic, 176, 177, 178
secondary, 165-166, 170-171
sensitivity in, 208-209, 210
terminology and distribution of, 170
tertiary, 165-166, 171-172, 173
Dentin-pulp complex; *see also* Dentin; Pulp
aging and, 210-212, 213
anatomy of, 169-170
environmental stimuli and, 213
innervation of, 204-207, 208
repair of, 460-463
sensitivity in, 208-209
Dentinal tubule
carious process in, 463, 464, 465, 466
contents of, 189, 195, 196, 197
in dental pulp innervation, 207
in dentin-pulp complex repair, 460, 461
in dentin sensitivity, 209
in intratubular and sclerotic dentin, 176, 177, 178
odontoblast process in, 189-194
in primary dentin, 173-175
remineralization of, 463, 464

Dentinocementum junction, 184
Dentinoenamel junction, 183, 184, 251
Dentinogenesis, 71, 72, 73, 147-168
incremental nature of, 160
intratubular, 161, 162
mantle, 153-157
mineralization in, 157, 159
odontoblast in
differentiation of, 147-149, 150
movement of, 163-165
resting, 153
secretory, 151-152, 153
transitional, 152
pattern of, 147, 148
primary physiologic, 157, 158
root, 162, 164
secondary, 165-166, 170-171
successive stages of, 161
tertiary, 165-166
von Korff fibers in, 165
Dentinogenesis imperfecta, 2
Dentition
downward displacement of, 500
primary, 48, 68, 337
secondary, 68, 69, 70, 338
Dentogingival junction, 268-274, 299-307
aging and, 307
blood supply of, 306-307
connective tissue in, 304-306, 307
epithelium in
col, 306-307
gingival, 299, 301
junctional, 301-303
sulcular, 299-301, 302
formation of, 77
innervation of, 307
Deoxyribonucleic acid in germ cell formation, 1
Deposition
in bone relocation, 484, 485
in neurocranial skeleton, 482
Desmoplakin, 401
Desmosome, 399, 401
in fibroblast junctions, 86
in salivary myoepithelial cells, 370, 372
Dichophase, 395
Differentiation in embryology, 2-3
Digestion, saliva in, 357
1,25-Dihydroxyvitamin D in bone metabolism, 126
Disk of temporomandibular joint, 442-443, 444
Displacement of bone, 484, 486, 487, 488
Displacement of cartilage, 488
Dolichocephalic head, 475
facial profile of, 478
in orthodontic malocclusion correction, 507, 508, 509
posture and, 476
Down's syndrome, 1
Drugs in congenital defects, 40
Dry socket, 467
Ductal system, of salivary glands, 361-362, 375-379, 380
obstruction of, 383-384
Dysostosis, cleidocranial, 2
Dysplasia, frontonasal, 41

E

Ectoderm, 6, 7

Ectoderm—cont'd
　of branchial arch, 18
Ectomesenchyme, 13, 58, 59, 430
　condensation of, 62
　in developing salivary gland, 359
　in epithelial-mesenchymal reactions, 102-103
　in formation of head, 16, 18ʹ
　in odontoblast differentiation, 149, 150
　recombined with epithelium, 105
EGF; *see* Epidermal growth factor
Elastic fiber in lamina propria, 418-419
Elastin
　in fibroblasts, 95
　in lamina propria, 418
　in periodontal ligament, 292-293
Electron microscopy
　in amelogenesis, 226-233, 234
　in dental plaque studies, 344
　in odontoblast process, 190, 193
Eluanin
　in fibroblasts, 95
　in periodontal ligament, 292-293
Embryo
　bilaminar, 5, 6
　cells of, 2, 3
　environmental factors affecting, 40-42
　folding of, 8-14
　oral mucosa development and, 430
　stages in, 2, 3
　three-layered, 3-7
　trilaminar, 6
Embryoblast, 4
Embryology, 1-14
　concepts of, 2, 3
　embryo in
　　folding of, 8-14
　　three-layered, 3-7
　germ cell formation and fertilization in, 1-2
　head, face, and oral cavity in, 15-44
　　branchial arches and primitive mouth in, 15-20
　　congenital defects in, 40-43
　　face formation in, 21-22, 23, 24
　　mandible and maxilla development in, 34-39
　　palate formation in, 22-24, 25-27
　　skull development in, 31-32, 33
　　temporomandibular joint development in, 40
　　tongue formation in, 25-28, 39-30
　induction, competence and differentiation in, 2-3
　neural crest and germ layers in, 7-8, 9, 10
Eminence cartilage, 440
Enamel, 47, 48
　acid etching and, 254-255
　aging and, 254
　amino acids and; *see* Enamel protein
　in cavity preparation, 465
　fluoridation and, 254
　formation of
　　ameloblast in, 218-219, 269
　　defects of, 236-237
　　electron microscopy of, 226-233, 234
　　light microscopy of, 223-226
　　matrix in, 219-223
　　maturation stage in, 227-231, 232, 233
　　mineral pathway in, 235-236
　　morphogenetic stage in, 226

Enamel—cont'd
　formation of—cont'd
　　protective stage in, 233, 234
　　secretory stage in, 227, 228, 229, 230
　gnarled, 250
　incremental lines in, 117
　mineralization and maturation in, 115, 222-223
　physical characteristics of, 240
　repair of, 458
　rod sheath in, 242, 244
　structure of, 240-253
　　cross striations in, 248, 249
　　dentinoenamel junction and spindles in, 251
　　Hunter-Schreger bands in, 249, 250
　　rods in, 241, 242-244, 245
　　striae of Retzius in, 246, 247
　　surface in, 252-253
　　tufts and lamellae in, 250-251
　synthesis of, 227, 228, 229, 230
Enamel cord, 64, 65
Enamel knot, 64, 65
Enamel niche, 64, 65
Enamel organ, 62
Enamel prism, 240
Enamel protein, 250, 257
　in amelogenesis, 227, 230
　in matrix formation, 219, 220, 221
Enamel rod, 240
Enamel septum, 64, 65
Enamel spindle, 184
Enamelin, 219
Enameloid, 257
Endochondral bone growth, 488
Endocranial fossae, 496-497, 498
Endocrine in cell communication, 100-101
Endoderm, 6, 7
　of branchial arch, 18
Endoplasmic reticulum
　in active odontoblast, 151, 152
　in epithelium tissue repair, 456, 457
Endosteum of compact bone, 121, 122
Endothelial cell, 415
Environment, dentin-pulp complex and, 213
Epidermal growth factor in cell communication, 101
Epilemmal innervation of salivary gland, 381
Epiphyseal growth plate in endochondral bone formation, 131
Epithelial band in developing tooth, 58-60, 61
Epithelial cell
　fibroblast junctions and, 86
　fragmentation of dental lamina and, 68, 69
　fusion of processes and, 24
　in periodontal ligament, 285-286
　rests of Malassez in, 73, 286
　　Hertwig's root sheath and, 262
Epithelial cement, 276
Epithelial cuff, 270
Epithelium
　aging and, 431
　in amelogenesis, 223, 224
　in cavity preparation, 465
　cell function in, 233
　in crown stage, 71, 72
　in dentin formation, 147, 148, 149
　in developing salivary gland, 359
　in erupting tooth, 76, 77

Epithelium—cont'd
external, 64, 66, 67
gingival
in dentogingival junction, 299, 301
repair of, 468
internal, 63, 64, 66, 67
junctional, 270-271, 273
in dentogingival junction, 301-303
keratinized versus nonkeratinized, 397
mesenchymal relationship to, 100-110
basal lamina in, 102
cell communication in, 100-102
neural crest cells in, 102-103
tooth formation in, 105-110
tooth morphogenesis in, 104, 105
in mucosa
lining, 425
masticatory, 423
in odontoblast differentiation, 147, 149
odontogenic, 23
oral, 52, 389, 392, 393, 395-419
cellular events in maturation of, 402, 403-407
inflammatory cells of, 411
junctions of, 411, 412, 413
keratinization of, 398, 399-400, 405-406, 407
lamina propria of, 411-419
Langerhans' cells of, 410
maturation of, 397-401
melanocytes and pigmentation of, 408-409
Merkel's cells of, 410-411
nonkeratinization of, 400-401, 402, 405, 406, 407
nonkeratinocytes in, 408
permeability and absorption of, 408
proliferation of, 395-397
ultrastructure of cell of, 401-402, 413
recombined with ectomesenchyme, 105
reduced, 342
in dentogingival junction formation, 268, 270, 271
in skin repair, 456, 457
sulcular, 272, 299-301, 302
turnover time of, 396
Eruption cysts of tooth, 68
Eruptive tooth movement, 318-322
Esthetics, 45
Estrogen
in bone metabolism, 126
in salivary gland regulation, 383
Euryprosopic face, 475
cervical-pull headgear and, 511
Evolution
of face, 469-474
of teeth, 50
Excretory duct, 53
Extraction of tooth, 466, 467
Extrinsic fiber cementum, 279

F

Face
bones of, 16
clefts of, 40, 41
embryology of, 21-22, 23, 24
congenital defects in, 40-43
embryonic formation of, 19
euryprosopic, 475
cervical-pull headgear and, 511

Face—cont'd
growth and development of, 469-513
aging and, 481
basis for human facial form in, 469-474
bone and cartilage in, 488
bone remodeling and increases in, 484-486
curve of occlusion in, 507, 508, 509, 510, 511
displacement process in, 486, 487
facial profiles in, 478, 479
facial types in, 475-476, 477
growth sequence in, 489-503, 504, 505, 506
male and female faces in, 480
mandibular condyle in, 512-513
leptoprosopic, 475
cervical-pull headgear and, 510, 511
postnatal growth summary of, 512
proportions in, 471
Facial lines, 481
Facial nerve, 420
Facial processes, fusion of, 24
Fasciculi, 444
Fast-twitch fiber muscle, 445, 446
Febrile disease in forming enamel, 236
Female face, 480-481
Fertilization of germ cell, 1-2
Fetal alcohol syndrome, 40
Fetus; *see* Embryo
FGF; *see* Fibroblast growth factor
Fibril of collagens, 88
Fibrillogenesis, 92
Fibroblast, 81-99
active, 82
aging and, 86-87
collagens in, 88-93, 94, 95
contraction and motility of, 86
cytoskeleton of, 81-85
in dental pulp, 198
elastin, oxytalin, eluanin, and reticulin in, 95-97
in eruptive tooth movement, 318-319, 321-322
glycoproteins in, 97
ground substance in, 97
heterogeneity in, 86
inactive, 82
integrins in, 97-98
junctions in, 86, 87
in lamina propria of oral mucosa, 414, 415, 416
of mandibular condyle, 438, 439
in oral mucosa repair, 468
in periodontal ligament, 266, 267, 284, 285, 286, 287
progenitor cells of, 268
proteoglycans in, 96, 97
in tissue repair, 458, 459, 460
in tooth extraction repair, 466
Fibroblast growth factor
beta, 126
in cell communication, 101
Fibrocartilage in temporomandibular joint, 439-440, 441
Fibrocellular follicle, 319
Fibronectin
in fibroblasts, 93
in lamina densa, 411
in lamina propria, 418
Fibronexus, 285
in fibroblast junctions, 86, 87, 91
Fibrous joint in temporomandibular joint, 432

Filaggrin, 405
Filaments of fibroblast, 85
Filiform papillae in oral cavity, 427
Filling cone of osteon, 144
Fissure plaque, 349
Floor of mouth
   arterial blood supply to, 418
   mucosal structure of, 424
Fluoride, 48
   in amelogenesis defects, 236
   in enamel, 233, 254
Foliate papillae in oral cavity, 427
Follicle, dental, 62, 63, 320, 321
Fordyce's spots, 391
   aging and, 431
Foregut in branchial arches, 15
Forehead
   evolution of, 471, 472
   furrows in, 481
   male verus female, 480
   remodeling of, 502-503, 505
Forensic science, 50
   secondary cementum formation and, 262
Fossa
   cranial, 491, 495, 496, 497
   glenoid, 56, 438-439
   tonsillar, 15
Free cytosolic calcium, 235, 236
Free gingival groove, 429
Free nerve ending in temporomandibular joint, 453-454
Frontal lobe, 496-497, 498
Frontal process of maxilla, 39
Frontal prominence, 21
Frontonasal dysplasia, 41
Frontonasal process, 21
Frozen dried bone, 467
Fungiform papillae in oral cavity, 426, 427
Furrow, forehead or nasolabial, 481

G

Gamete in germ cell formation, 1
Gap junction, 399, 402
Gelatinase in collagen degradation, 93, 95
Genetic defects, 2
Germ cell, 1-2
Germ layers, 7-8, 9, 10
German measles, 40
Germinative layer of oral epithelium, 399
Gill cleft, 15
Gingiva, 53
   amalgam in, 408-409
   arterial blood supply to, 418
   blood flow in, 419
   in dentogingival junction, 299, 301
   innervation of, 420
   keratinized, 404
   mucosa in, 45
      masticatory, 423
      structure of, 424
   orthokeratinization and parakeratinization in, 398
   prickle-cell layer of, 408
   repair of, 468
   surface of, 391-392
Gingival groove, free, 429
Gingival sulcus, 270
Gingival sulcus microbiota plaque, 350-351, 352
Gingivectomy, 272
Glenoid fossa in temporomandibular joint, 56, 438-439
Glossopharyngeal nerve, 420
Glucocorticoid
   in bone metabolism, 126
   in salivary gland regulation, 383
Glutamic acid, 221
Glycine, 221
Glycogen
   in amelogenesis, 217
   in internal dental epithelium, 63, 64, 65
Glycoprotein
   basement membrane and, 411
   in fibroblasts, 97
   in lamina propria, 419
   in saliva, 357
Glycosaminoglycan
   in dental organ, 62-64
   in palate formation, 22
   in proteoglycans, 93
Golgi complex in secretory odontoblast, 151, 152
Golgi tendon organ, 450, 453-454
Gomphosis joint, 432
Granular layer
   in oral epithelium, 399-400, 405
   of Tomes, 182
Granule
   Birbeck, 410
   keratohyalin, 400, 405
   membrane-coating, 404-405
   secretory, 368-370
      bipartite, 368
Greek nose, 480
Grooves
   branchial, 15
   embryology of, 15-18
Ground substance
   in cementum, 276, 283, 285
   in dental pulp, 199
   in fibroblasts, 97, 416
   in lamina propria, 419
Growth factor
   in cell communication, 101
   in tooth morphogenesis, 104, 105
Growth plate, 131
Growth sequence in childhood facial development, 489-503, 504, 505, 506
Growth site, 486
Gubernacular canal, 318, 319
Gubernacular cord, 319
Gustin, 357

H

Haploid number, 1
Hard palate
   arterial blood supply of, 418
   innervation of, 420
   mucosa in
      masticatory, 423
      structure of, 424
   relocation of, 485
   remodeling of, 485, 486
   surface of, 391
Hard tissue, formation and destruction of, 111-119

Hard tissue—cont'd
  alkaline phosphatase in, 115
  cells in, 111
  degradation in, 117-119
  incremental lines in, 117
  minerals in, 111-115
  organic matrix in, 111
Head
  African American, 476, 477
  brachycephalic, 475
    facial profile of, 478
    in orthodontic malocclusion correction, 507, 508, 509
  Caucasian, 476, 477
  dolichocephalic, 475
    facial profile of, 478
    in orthodontic malocclusion correction, 507, 508, 509
    posture and, 476
  embryology of, 15-44
    branchial arches and primitive mouth in, 15-20
    congenital defects in, 40-43
    face formation in, 21-22, 23, 24
    mandible and maxilla development in, 34-39
    palate formation in, 22-24, 25-27
    skull development in, 31, 32, 33
    temporomandibular joint development in, 40
    tongue formation in, 25-28, 29-30
Head fold of embryo, 8-9, 10
Headgear, 510, 511
Helix in collagen, 88, 89, 91
Hemidesmosome, 401, 413
  in enamel maturation, 233
  in fibroblast junctions, 86
Hemoglobin in oral mucosa, 408
Hemostasis in tissue repair, 456
Heparan sulfate
  lamina densa and, 411
  in oral mucosa, 419
Heparin in mast cell, 416
Hertwig's epithelial root sheath, 73, 74, 75
  fragmentation of, 77
  in periodontium development, 262
Heterogeneity of fibroblast, 86
Heterogenous mineralization, 113
Heterogenous nucleation, 113, 115
Hilton's law, 433, 454
Histamine in mast cell, 416
Histidine, 221
Histiocyte in oral mucosa, 415
Histodifferentiation
  of dental organ, 67
  of tooth germ, 62, 64
Homogenous nucleation, 113
Hopewell-Smith hyaline layer, 257
Hormone
  in congenital defects, 40
  parathyroid, 126
  peptide, 383
Howship lacunae, 126
Hunter-Schreger bands, 249, 250
Hyaline layer of Hopewell-Smith, 257
Hyalinization, 334
Hyaluronan in oral mucosa, 419
Hybridization, 100
Hydration shell of crystallite, 113
Hydrostatic pressure in eruptive tooth movement, 320

Hydroxyapatite, 276
Hydroxyapatite crystals
  in cementum, 52
  in dentin, 50
  in enamel, 48, 239, 240, 242-243
  in mantle dentin formation, 156, 157
Hyperkeratosis, 407
Hypobranchial eminence, 25, 28
Hypolemmal innervation of salivary gland, 381

I

IGF; *see* Insulinlike growth factor
Immature bone, 136, 137
Immunocytochemistry in cell identification, 396
Immunoglobulin A in saliva, 357
Implantology, 467
Incisor
  formation of
    epithelial-mesenchymal relationship in, 105
    morphogenetic fields in, 107
  mesial inclination of, 322, 323
  remodeling of, 502
Incremental lines
  in dentinogenesis, 180, 181
  in hard tissue formation, 117
Incudomalleolar articulation, 432
Incus bone, 432
Induction in embryology, 2-3
Infant
  abnormal tooth movement in, 332
  face of, 481
Infectious agent in congenital defects, 40
Inflammation
  in dentogingival junction formation, 270
  in lamina propria, 418
  mitotic activity and, 397
  in oral epithelium, 411
  in tissue repair, 456-458
Infrahyoid muscle, 450
Infraorbital nerve, 38
Inhibins in cell communication, 101
Injury to pulp-dentin complex, 213
Innervation
  of dentin-pulp complex, 204-207, 208
  of dentogingival junction, 307
  of developing tooth, 68
  of oral mucosa, 420-422, 426, 427
  of periodontal ligament, 294-296, 297
  of periodontium, 268, 307
  of salivary gland, 381-383
  of temporomandibular joint, 453-454
Insulinlike growth factor
  in cell communication, 101
  osteoblasts and, 126
Integrins in fibroblast, 97-98
Intercalated duct, 53
  in parotid gland, 384
  in salivary gland, 373, 376
Interglobular dentin, 157, 178, 179
Interorbital region, 476
Interproximal wear in tooth movement, 322
Interstitial lamellae of bone, 121, 122, 123
Intertubular dentin, 178
Intestinal mucosa, 394
Intima of temporomandibular joint, 441, 442

Intrafusal fiber in muscle spindle, 445
Intramembranous bone growth, 488
Intratubular dentin, 176, 177, 178
    formation of, 161, 162
Intrinsic fiber cementum, 279
Involucrin, 405
Ion
    alkaline phosphatase and, 115
    in mineralized tissue, 111-113, 116
Isoleucine, 221

J

Jaw; *see also* Mandible; Maxilla
    bone of, evolution in, 433
    bones of, 55
    tooth movement and
        posteruptive, 322
        preeruptive, 313-317
Joint
    classification of, 432-433, 434
    temporomandibular; *see* Temporomandibular joint
Junctional epithelium, 270-271, 273
    in dentogingival junction, 301-303

K

Keratin, 401
Keratinization of oral epithelium, 398, 399-400, 405-406, 407
Keratinocyte, 401
Keratohyalin granule, 400, 405

L

Labial mucosa, 424
Labial sulcus, 52
Lactoferrin in saliva, 357
Lacunae
    in cementum, 279, 281
    Howship, 126
    osteocytic, 126
Lamellae
    of bone, 121, 122, 123
    enamel, 250-251
Lamina
    dental, 60, 67-68
    in dentogingival junction formation, 268, 270
    vestibular, 60
Lamina densa, 411, 413
Lamina limitans, 195, 197
Lamina lucida, 411, 413
Lamina propria, 52
    aging and, 431
    nerve endings in, 420
    in oral epithelium, 411-419
    in oral mucosa, 392, 393, 425, 431
    sebaceous glands in, 395
Lamina splendens, 439
Laminin in salivary gland, 359
Langerhans' cell
    characteristics of, 400
    in oral epithelium, 410
Lectin, 401
Leptoprosopic face, 475
    cervical-pull headgear and, 510, 511
Leucine, 221
Ligament
    periodontal; *see* Periodontal ligament

Ligament—cont'd
    sphenomandibular, 444
    stylomandibular, 444
    temporomandibular, 443-444
    transseptal, 322-323
Ligament fibroblast, 285
Light microscopy
    in amelogenesis, 223-226
    in odontoblast process, 190, 191, 192
Linea alba of buccal mucosa, 392, 407
Lingual salivary gland, 384
Lingual swelling, 25, 28
Lingula, 35
Lining cell, 125
Lining mucosa, 425, 428, 429
Lip, 21
    arterial blood supply to, 418
    clefts of, 40, 41, 42
    innervation of, 420
    mucosal structure of, 424
Lipids in tissue mineralization, 115
Loricrin, 405
Lumina in salivary gland, 359, 360, 361
Lymphatic supply in dental pulp, 201, 202, 203
Lymphocyte
    characteristics of, 400
    in lamina propria, 415
    in oral mucosa, 411
    in pulp, 199
Lymphoid tissue of oral cavity, 395
Lysine, 221
Lysozyme in saliva, 357

M

Macrophage
    in lamina propria, 415, 416-417
    in oral mucosa, 415
        repair of, 468
    in pulp, 199
    in skin repair, 456-458
    in tooth extraction repair, 466
Macula adherens in fibroblast junction, 86
Malassez rest, 73, 286
    Hertwig's root sheath and, 262
Male face, 480-481
Malleus bone, 432
    in temporomandibular joint, 435
Mallory method, 407
Malocclusion
    class II, 507, 508
        cervical-pull headgear and, 510, 511
    facial profile in, 478
    orthodontic correction of, 507, 508, 509
Malpighian layer, 400
Mandible; *see also* Jaw
    alignment of, 507, 508
    development of, 34-38, 39
    displacement of, 491, 492, 498
    facial profile and, 478, 479
    malocclusion and, 478, 479
    maxilla and, 39
    osteogenesis of, 35
    remodeling of, 486, 487
Mandibular arch, 502
Mandibular cleft, 41

Mandibular condyle
  displacement of, 491, 493
  growth of, 496, 497, 512
  remodeling of, 485
  in temporomandibular joint, 435, 438-439
  in temporomandibular ligament, 444
Mandibular dentition, 500
Mandibular nerve, 34
Mandibular process, 20, 21, 23
Mandibular ramus, 485, 491, 493, 494, 496, 497
Mandibular third molar, 332
Mandibulofacial dysostosis, 8, 10
Mantle dentin, 153-157
Masseter muscle, 449, 450, 451, 452-453
Mast cell
  in lamina propria, 415, 417
  in oral mucosa, 411
Mastication
  muscles of, 449, 450-452
  teeth and, 45
Masticatory mucosa, 52-53, 423, 429
  keratinization of, 400
  papillae in, 411
Matrix
  in dental pulp, 199
  in dentin formation, 156, 157, 160
  in hard tissue formation, 111
  mineralization of, 157, 158
  in tooth morphogenesis, 104, 105
Matrix metalloendoproteinase, 93
Matrix vesicle
  in primary cementum formation, 257, 261
  in tissue mineralization, 112, 113-115
Maxilla; *see also* Jaw
  development of, 38-39
  displacement of, 490
  mandible and, 39
  remodeling of, 504
Maxillary arch
  alignment of mandible and, 507, 508
  displacement of, 489, 490, 491
  downward remodeling of, 500
Maxillary canine, 332
Maxillary process, 22, 23
Maxillary tuberosity, 316
Measles, German, 40
Meckel's cartilage, 18, 35, 36
  in mandible formation, 34
  in temporomandibular joint, 435, 437
Meiosis, 1
Meissner corpuscle, 420
Melanin in oral mucosa, 408-409
Melanoblast, 408
Melanocyte
  characteristics of, 400
  in oral epithelium, 408-409
Melanophage, 409, 416
Melanosome, 408, 409
Membrane-coating granule, 404-405
Merkel's cell
  characteristics of, 400
  in oral epithelium, 410-411
Mesenchymal cell
  in dental pulp, 198
  in endochondral bone formation, 131, 132

Mesenchymal cell—cont'd
  in periodontal ligament, 286
Mesenchyme, 13
  epithelial relationship to, 100-110
    basal lamina in, 102
    cell communication in, 100-102
    neural crest cells in, 102-103
    tooth formation in, 105-110
    tooth morphogenesis in, 104, 105
  in head development, 16
Mesial drift, 322
Mesoderm, 6, 7, 9-12
Mesodermal mesenchyme, 16
Methionine, 221
Microfilament
  in fibroblasts, 81, 84, 85
  in salivary myoepithelial cells, 370, 372
Microscopy
  chairside, 353, 354
  electron; *see* Electron microscopy
  light; *see* Light microscopy
  in plaque
    studies of, 344
    subgingival, 353, 354
Microtubule of fibroblast, 81, 84
Mineral pathway, 235-236
Mineralization
  in deep fissure plaque
  in dentinogenesis, 157, 159
  in enamel matrix formation, 222-223
  in hard tissue formation, 111-117
  heterogenous, 113
Mitochondrion in calcium transport, 116-117
Mitosis, 395
  in embryology, 1
Mixed fiber cementum, 279
Mixed saliva, 53
Molar
  deciduous
    exfoliated, 326
    preeruptive tooth movement and, 313-317
  development of, 68, 69
  epithelial-mesenchymal relationship in, 105
  horizontally impacted, 332
  permanent, 313-317
  resorption and, 326
  third, 332
  vertical drift of, 510, 511
Monocyte, 415
Monopartite secretory granule, 368
Monosomy, 1-2
Morphodifferentiation of tooth germ, 62-64
Morula, 4
Motor unit in muscle, 445, 447
Mouth; *see also* entries under Oral
  embryology of, 15-20
  floor of, 45
    arterial blood supply to, 418
    mucosal structure of, 424
  structures of, 45
  surface areas of, 45
Mucocutaneous junction, 428
Mucogingival junction, 429
Mucoperiosteum, 394, 395

Mucosa
  alveolar
    structure of, 424
    surface areas of, 45
  buccal
    linea alba of, 392, 407
    nonkeratinized, 398, 404
    structure of, 424
    surface areas of, 45
  gingival
    masticatory, 423
    structure of, 424
    surface areas of, 45
  intestinal, 394
  labial, 424
  masticatory, 52-53, 423, 429
    keratinization of, 400
    papillae in, 411
  oral; *see* Oral mucosa
Mucous cell
  in salivary glands, 368-370
  versus seromucous cell, 370
Mucous membrane, 389; *see also* Mucosa
Muscle in temporomandibular joint, 444-450
Myoepithelial cell in salivary gland, 370-372, 373, 374
Myoglobin in muscle contraction, 445

N

Nasal pit, 21, 23, 29
Nasal placode, 23
Nasal process, 21, 22, 23
Nasal septum, 25, 26, 60
Nasolabial furrow, 481
Nasomaxillary complex
  displacement of, 486, 487, 496
    vertical, 498, 499
  of mammals, 473
  remodeling of, 502-503, 505
Nerve; *see* specific nerve
Nerve growth factor, 101
Nerve growth factor receptor, 204, 205
Nerve supply; *see* Innervation
Neural crest cell
  derivatives of, 13
  formation of, 7-8, 9, 10
  migration of, 9
    epithelial-mesenchymal relationship and, 102-103
  in neural tube development, 16
  origin and development of, 8
Neural fold, 7
Neural plate, 7, 8
Neural tube, 16
Neurocranium, 31, 32
Neutrophil
  in oral mucosa lamina propria, 415
  in skin repair, 456
Newborn
  abnormal tooth movement in, 332
  skull of, 471
NGF; *see* Nerve growth factor
NGFR; *see* Nerve growth factor receptor
Noble ripples, 481
Node, primitive, 6, 7
Nonkeratinization of oral epithelium, 400-401, 402, 405, 406, 407,
    408

Nonmyelinated axon in dental pulp, 204, 205
Norepinephrine, 382-383
Nose
  evolution of, 474
  Greek, 480
  male versus female, 480, 481
  remodeling of, 502-503, 505
  Roman, 480
Notochord, 6, 7
Nuclear bag fiber in muscle, 445
Nuclear chain fiber in muscle, 445
Nucleation
  in crystallite formation, 115
  in tissue mineralization, 113, 115
Nutritional deficiency in congenital defect, 43

O

Occipital somite, 28
Occlusal fissure plaque, 349
Occlusal force in tooth movement, 322
Occlusal wear in tooth movement, 322
Occlusion
  curve of, 507, 508, 509, 510, 511
  of dentinal tubules, 460, 461
Odontoblast
  in dentin, 49, 50
    formation of, 151-152, 153
    repair of, 460-461
    sensitivity of, 209
  differentiation of
    in crown stage, 71, 72
    in dentinogenesis, 147-149, 150
    in root formation, 74
  functional stages in, 151
  in hard tissue, 118, 119
  junction between, 188-189
  life cycle of, 186
  in pulp, 184-189
  resting, 153
  secretory, 151-152, 153
  in tooth shedding, 324, 325-327, 328
  transitional, 152
Odontoblast process, 187, 188
  in dental pulp, 189-194
    innervation of, 206
  formation of, 155, 157
  in sclerotic dentin, 176, 177
Odontogenic epithelium, 23
Oncocyte of salivary gland, 383
Open bite, 507, 509
Oral cavity
  development of, 20, 29
  embryology of, 22-28, 23, 30, 34-42
    congenital defects in, 40-43
    mandible and maxilla development in, 34-39
    palate formation in, 22-24, 25-27
    temporomandibular joint development in, 40
    tongue formation in, 25-28, 29-30
  saliva and, 357
  temperature reception in, 422
Oral epithelium
  basal layer, 399
    cells of, 401
  dental lamina fragmentation and, 68
  in erupting tooth, 76, 77

Oral mucoperiosteum, 394, 395
Oral mucosa, 52-55, 389-431
  aging and, 431
  alveolar, 45
  blood supply to, 418, 419
  buccal vestibular, 45
  component tissues and glands of, 392-395, 412
  development of, 430
  epithelium in, 395-419
    cellular events in maturation of, 402, 403-407
    inflammatory cells of, 411
    junctions of, 411, 412, 413
    keratinization of, 398, 399-400, 405-406, 407
    lamina propria of, 411-419
    Langerhans' cells of, 410
    maturation of, 397-401
    melanocytes and pigmentation of, 408-409
    Merkel's cells of, 410-411
    nonkeratinization of, 400-401, 402, 405, 406, 407
    nonkeratinocytes in, 408
    permeability and absorption of, 408
    proliferation of, 395-397
    ultrastructure of cell of, 401-402, 413
  functions of, 389-390
  gingival, 45
  innervation of, 420-422, 426, 427
  junctions in, 428-429
  organization of, 390-392
  repair of, 468
  structural variations of, 423-427
    lining mucosa in, 425, 428, 429
    masticatory mucosa in, 423, 429
    papillae in, 426, 427
  surface areas of, 45
Oral tissue, structures of, 45-57
  jaw bones in, 55
  mouth in, 45
  oral mucosa in, 52-55
  temporomandibular joint in, 57
  tooth in, 45-52
Orbit, rotation of, 471, 473
Orbital rim, 502-503, 505
Organelle
  in fibroblasts, 81, 82, 83
  in salivary glands, 364
Organic material in enamel, 239, 240
Organic matrix
  in cementum, 279
  in dentin formation, 160
  in hard tissue formation, 111
Orofacial cleft, 40-43
Orthodontics
  in malocclusion correction, 507, 508, 509
  tooth movement in, 334-335, 336, 337, 338
Orthognathic profile, 478
Orthokeratinization, 400
Ossification
  mandibular, 34, 35
  in maxilla development, 38
  of premaxilla, 39
Osteoblast
  in bone, 124-126
    turnover of, 139, 141, 142, 143, 144
  progenitor cells of, 268
  in tooth extraction repair, 466

Osteoblast-osteocyte complex, 126
Osteoclast
  in bone remodeling, 320
  in bone turnover, 139, 141, 142, 143, 144
  in hard tissue degradation, 118
  hematopoietic origin of, 128, 129, 130
Osteocytic lacuna, 126
Osteodentin, 171
Osteogenesis
  endochondral, 130, 131-134
  intramembranous, 134-137
  in mandible formation, 35
  in periodontium, 267-268
  in tooth extraction repair, 466, 467
Osteogenesis imperfecta, 2
Osteoid, 124
Osteon
  in bone formation, 137
  in bone turnover, 139, 140, 141, 142, 143, 144
Ova in germ cell formation, 1
Oxytalan
  in fibroblasts, 95
  in periodontal ligament, 283, 292-293

P

Pacinian corpuscle, 453-454
Pain
  in dentin sensitivity, 208
  detection of, 422
Palatal process, fusion of, 20
Palatal salivary gland, 384
Palatal shelf, 25, 26
Palate
  cleft of, 40, 42
  downward remodeling of, 500
  formation of, 22-24, 25-27
  hard
    arterial blood supply of, 418
    innervation of, 420
    mucosa in, 423, 424
    relocation and remodeling of, 485, 486
    surface of, 391
  primary, 29, 30
  remodeling of, 489, 490, 491
  secondary, 25, 30
  soft
    arterial blood supply to, 418
    innervation of, 420
    mucosal structure of, 424
  surface areas of, 45
Palatine shelves, 22
Palatine tonsil, 15
Papillae
  in bell stage tooth development, 67
  in crown stage, 71
  in dentin formation, 147, 148, 149, 150
  development of, 62, 63
  at epithelium and lamina propria junction, 411
  formation of, 62, 63
  in oral cavity, 426, 427
  replaced by dental organ, 105
Paracrine regulation, 101
Parakeratinization, 400
  incomplete, 406
Parathyroid gland in embryology, 15

Parathyroid hormone in bone metabolism, 126
Parenchyma in salivary gland, 359, 360
Parotid duct, 384
Parotid gland, 53, 358, 384, 385
Passive eruption, 272
PDGF; *see* Platelet-derived growth factor
PDL; *see* Periodontal ligament
Peking man, 50
Pellicle, salivary, 342, 343
   in plaque formation, 344-345
Pemphigus, 401-402
Peptide hormone, 383
Perikymata, 252, 253
Periodontal disease, 353
Periodontal ligament, 45, 50, 51, 279-299, 300
   alveolar bone remodeling and, 500, 501
   alveolar process in, 298-299, 300
   apoptosis of, 327, 328
   blood supply to, 294
   cells of, 285-287
   development of, 73, 75, 78, 262-267
   in eruptive tooth movement, 321-322
   fibers of, 288-293
   fibroblasts of, 84
   ground substance of, 293
   innervation of, 294-296, 297
   repair of, 467
   vertical drift and, 500
Periodontium, 276-312
   alveolar process in, 298-299, 300
   blood supply to, 294
   cementum in, 276-279, 280, 281
   dentogingival junction in, 299-307
   development of, 257-275
      bone formation in, 267-268
      cementogenesis in, 257-262, 263, 264, 265
      dentogingival junction formation in, 268-274
      Hertwig's root sheath in, 262
      nerve and vascular supply in, 268
      periodontal ligament formation in, 262-267
   functions of, 307-309
   innervation of, 294-296, 297
   organic matrix in, 279
   periodontal ligament in, 279-299, 300
      cells of, 285-287
      fibers of, 288-293
      ground substance of, 293
      repair of, 467
   sensory function of, 308
Periodontoblastic space, 195
Periosteum of compact bone, 121, 122
Peritubular dentin, 161, 162
Perivascular cell
   in periodontal ligament formation, 268
   in skin repair, 458, 459
Perlecan in fibroblast, 93
Permanent dentition, 68, 69, 70
   chronology of, 338
   formation of, 68, 69, 70
Pharyngeal arch
   development of, 17, 18
   embryology of, 15-20
Pharyngeal pouch, 15
Pharyngeal wall, 15
Phase-contrast photomicrograph, 353, 354

Phenotype in embryology, 2
Phenylalanine, 221
Phosphate in saliva, 357, 358
Phosphatidylinositol-4,5-biphosphate, 383
Phosphophoryn, 157, 462
Phosphoric acid in etching, 254
Physiologic dentin, 157, 158
Piezo response, 488
Placode
   nasal, 23
   olfactory, 21
Plaque, 54, 55
   bacterial, 342, 344-345, 347
   in enamel surface, 253
   formation of, 344-345
   gingival sulcus microbiota, 350-351, 352
   morphology in, 346, 347-351, 352
      factors determining, 345
   occlusal fissure, 349
   smooth-surface, 346, 347, 348
   study of, 344
   subgingival, 350-351, 352
   sulcus microbiota, 350-351, 352
Plasma cell, 415
Plate
   alveolar, 38
   cardiac, 7
   cribriform, 294
   epiphyseal growth, 131
   neural, 7, 8
   prochordal, 5, 6, 7
Platelet-derived growth factor
   in cell communication, 101
   osteoblasts and, 126
Pleuripotent stem cell, 126-129
Plexus of Raschkow, 203
   in dental pulp innervation, 204, 207
Pole of mandibular condyle, 438
Polymorphonuclear leukocyte
   in lamina propria, 415
   in oral mucosa, 411
   in oral mucosa repair, 468
   in tissue repair, 460
   in tooth extraction repair, 466
Polypeptide chain in collagen synthesis, 88, 91
Polysaccharide in plaque, 346
Postcervical muscle in mastication, 450
Posteruptive tooth movement, 322-323
Posture, 476
Pouch
   embryology of, 15-18
   pharyngeal, 15
Predentin, 172
   in dentin-pulp complex repair, 461
   in odontoblast process, 188
Preeruptive tooth movement, 313-317
Premaxilla, 39
Premolar, 31
Preosteoblast, 124, 126
Pressure
   in posteruptive tooth movement, 323
   in tooth shedding, 329
Prickle-cell layer, oral epithelium, 399
   cells in, 405
Primary dentition, 48

Primary dentition—cont'd
  chronology of, 337
  formation of, 68
Primary epithelial band, 58-60, 61
Primary molar, 326
Primary spongiosa, 131, 133
Primitive mouth, 15-20
Primitive node, 6, 7
Primitive streak, 6, 7
Prochordal plate, 5, 6, 7
Profile, 478, 479
Progenitor cell, 395
Prognathic profile, 478
Proliferation of tooth, 60, 62
Proliferative layer of oral epithelium, 399
Proline, 221
Protein in enamel; *see* Enamel protein
Proteoglycan
  in collagen mineralization, 114, 115
  in dentin formation, 157
  in developing salivary gland, 359
  in fibroblasts, 97
  in lamina densa, 411
  in lamina propria, 419
Proton pump, 118
Pterygoid fovea, 450-452
Pterygoid muscle, 449, 450-452
Pubic symphysis, 432
Pulp, 49, 50, 184-203
  aging and, 210-212
  basic anatomy of, 169, 170
  dentinal tubule in, 189, 195, 196, 197
  fibers of, 199
  fibroblasts in, 198
  ground substance of, 199
  immunocompetent cells in, 199
  innervation of, 204-207, 208
  matrix in, 199
  odontoblast process in, 189-194
  odontoblasts in, 184-189
  orthodontic tooth movement and, 335
  repair of, 460-463
  stones in, 210, 211
  undifferentiated mesenchymal cells in, 198
  unmyelinated axons in, 204-205
  vasculature and lymphatic supply of, 201, 202, 203
Pulp chamber, 47, 49
Pulp horn, 206, 207
Pyrophosphate, 115

R

Ramus, mandibular
  enlargement of, 496, 497
  growth of, 491, 493
  relocation of, 485, 491, 494
  remodeling of, 485
Receptor
  in oral mucosa, 389
  taste, 422
Reduced dental epithelium, 268, 270, 271
Reichert's cartilage, 18
Relocation of bone, 483, 484
Remodeling
  of bone; *see* Bone, remodeling of
  of cartilage, 488

RER; *see* Rough endoplasmic reticulum
Resorption
  in bone relocation, 484, 485
  canine, 325
  in neurocranial skeleton, 482
  pattern of, 330-331
  root, 329
    in orthodontic tooth movement, 334, 336
Resting odontoblast, 153
Rests of Malassez, 73, 286
  Hertwig's root sheath and, 262
Rete ridges, 392, 412
Reticulin, 411
  in fibroblasts, 95-97
Reticulum
  rough endoplasmic, 456, 457
  sarcoplasmic, 445
Retrognathic profile, 478
Ribosome, 405
Rod sheath, 242, 244
Roman nose, 480
Root, 47, 169, 170
  dentin in, 73
  formation of, 73, 74, 75
    in eruptive tooth movement, 319-320
  intratubular nerves in, 206, 207
  resorption of, 329
    in orthodontic tooth movement, 334, 336
Root canal, 210
Root dentin
  branching dentinal tubules in, 174
  formation of, 147, 163, 164
Root sheath, Hertwig's epithelial, 73, 74, 75
  fragmentation of, 77
  in periodontium development, 262
Rouget's cell, 201
Rough endoplasmic reticulum
  in collagen synthesis, 88
  in epithelium tissue repair, 456, 457
Rubella virus, 40
Ruffini corpuscle, 420
  in temporomandibular joint, 453-454

S

Saliva, 53-55
  formation of, 363-364
  functions of, 357-358
  mixed, 53
  oral mucosa and, 389
Salivary duct, 53, 361-362, 375-379, 380
  obstruction of, 384
Salivary gland, 356-388
  aging and, 383
  anatomy of, 358-359
  blood supply to, 383
  connective tissue of, 380
  development of, 359-361
    defects in, 383
  disease of, 383
  ductal system in; *see* Salivary duct
  functions of saliva in, 357-358
  innervation of, 381-383
  lobular organization of, 54
  mechanism for secretion in, 364
  minor, 358-359, 384

Salivary gland—cont'd
  oral mucosa and, 389, 391, 395
  parotid, 358, 384, 385
  structure of, 361-372
    fluid component development in, 364
    macromolecular component development in, 363
    mucous cells in, 368-370
    myoepithelial cells in, 370-372, 373, 374
    serous cells in, 365-367, 368-370
  sublingual, 358, 384-385
  submandibular, 358, 384, 385
Salivary pellicle, 342, 343
  in enamel surface, 253
  in plaque formation, 344-345
Sarcolemma, 444
Sarcoplasmic reticulum, 445
Scar tissue
  in oral mucosa repair, 468
  in skin repair, 458, 459, 460
Sclerotic dentin, 176, 177, 178
Sebaceous glands in oral mucosa, 295, 391, 392
Sebum, 395
Secondary dentition
  chronology of, 338
  formation of, 68, 69, 70
Secondary nucleation in crystallite formation, 115
Secretory granule, 368-370
Secretory odontoblast, 151-152, 153
Sella turcica, 512
Sensory nerve, 18-19
Septum
  enamel, 64, 65
  nasal, 25, 26, 60
Serial cephalometric tracing, 503, 506
Serine, 221
Seromucous cell
  versus mucous cell, 370
  in salivary glands, 365-367, 368-370
Serous cell; *see* Seromucous cell
Sharpey's fibers, 291
Shedding of tooth, 324, 325-329, 330, 331
Siderophage, 416
Skin
  aging and, 481
  oral mucosa versus, 391
  repair of, 456-458, 459, 460
    versus tooth repair, 465, 466
Skull
  bones of, 16
  development of, 31, 32, 33
  newborn, 471
  postnatal growth summary of, 512
  subdivision of, 31
Slow-twitch fiber muscle, 445, 446
Smile lines, 481
Smoking, 407
Sodium in salivary duct, 379
Soft palate
  arterial blood supply to, 418
  innervation of, 420
  mucosal structure of, 424
Somite, 9, 28
  occipital, 28
Speech, teeth and, 45
Spermatozoa in germ cell formation, 1

Sphenomandibular ligament, 444
Spindle, enamel or muscle, 251
Spirochete
  in periodontal disease diagnosis, 353, 354
  in subgingival plaque, 351, 352
Spongiosa, 131, 133
Squame, 400, 405-406
Stellate reticulum of dental organ, 64, 66
Stem cell
  epithelial, 395
  pleuripotent, 126-129
Stomatodeum, 28
  development of, 20
  embryology of, 15, 16, 17
Straight-jawed profile, 478
Stratum basale, 399
Stratum corneum, 400
Stratum granulosum, 399-400
Stratum intermedium, 67
  in amelogenesis, 217
  formation of, 64
Stratum spinosum, 399
Striae of Retzius
  in enamel, 246, 247
  perikymata and, 252, 253
Striated duct, 53
  in parotid gland, 384
  in salivary gland, 377-379
  in submandibular gland, 385
Stromelysin, 93, 95
Stylomandibular ligament, 444
Subcutaneous dehydration, 481
Subintima in temporomandibular joint, 441, 442
Sublingual gland, 53, 358, 384-385
Submandibular gland, 53, 358, 384, 385
  developing, 359
Submandibular gland duct, 385
Submucosa, 392-395
Suborbital crease, 481
Suckling pad, 428
Sulcular epithelium, 272
  in dentogingival junction, 299-301, 302
Sulcus
  gingival, 270
  labial, 52
Sulcus microbiota plaque, 350-351, 352
Sulcus terminalis, 425
Supraorbital rims, 471, 472
Suture joint, 432
Symphysial cartilage, 37
Symphysis pubis, 432
Synaptic cleft, 445
Syndecan
  in fibroblasts, 93
  in oral mucosa, 419
Syndesmosis joint, 432
Syndrome
  Down's, 1
  Treacher-Collins, 8, 10
Synovial joint, 432-433, 434
Synovial membrane, 57, 441, 442

T

Taste
  oral mucosa and, 389

Taste—cont'd
  saliva in, 357
Teeth; *see* Tooth
Telopeptidase, 93, 95
Temperature reception in oral cavity, 422
Temporal blastema, 435-438
Temporal lobes, 496
Temporalis muscle, 449, 450, 452-453
Temporomandibular joint, 56, 57, 432-455
  biomechanics of, 452-453
  blood supply to, 454
  bones of, 438-439
  capsule of, 442
  cartilage and, 439-440, 441
  cartilaginous, 432
  development of, 40, 435-438
  disk of, 442-443
  evolution of, 433
  fibrous, 432
  innervation of, 453-454
  ligaments and, 443-444
  muscles of, 444-452
    mastication and, 450-452
  subintima in, 441, 442
  synovial, 432-433, 434
  synovial membrane of, 441, 442
Temporomandibular ligament, 443-444
Tenascin
  in fibroblasts, 93
  in neural crest cells, 102
Teratogen, 40
Teratology, 2
Terminal excretory duct in salivary gland, 379, 380
Terminal groove of tongue, 425
Terminal secretory end piece, 361
  developing, 359, 361
  in myoepithelial cells, 370, 371, 372, 374
  spherical, 362
  tubular, 362, 363
Tertiary dentinogenesis, 165-166, 171-172, 173
Tetracycline, 236
Tetraploid in embryology, 1
TGF beta; *see* Transforming growth factor beta
Thalidomide, 40
Thermal regulation, 389-390
Third molar, 332
Threonine, 221
Thumb-sucking, 319
Thymidine, 396
Thymus gland in embryology, 15
Tight junction, 399, 402
Tissue
  cell communication in, 100-102
  repair and regeneration of, 456-468
    cavity preparation in, 465, 466
    dental caries in, 462-465, 466
    dentin-pulp complex in, 460-462
    enamel in, 458
    oral mucosa in, 468
    periodontium in, 467
    saliva in, 358
    skin repair and, 456-458, 459, 460
    tooth extraction in, 466, 467
TMJ; *see* Temporomandibular joint

Tomes process
  enamel and
    formation of, 223, 225, 227, 228, 229
    surface of, 243-244
  striae of Retzius and, 246, 247
Tongue
  aging and, 431
  arterial blood supply to, 418
  formation of, 25-28, 29-30
  innervation of, 420
  mucosal structure of, 424
  muscles of, 25, 28
  salivary gland of, 384
  surface of, 45, 391
  swelling of, 25, 28
  taste buds and, 422
  terminal groove of, 425
Tonofibril, 399, 401
  keratohyalin granules and, 405
Tonofilament, 399, 401
  keratinized versus nonkeratinized epithelium and, 403-404
Tonsil, palatine, 15
Tonsillar fossa, 15
Tooth
  alveolar remodeling and, 500
  animal, 45
  cavity preparation in, 465
  darkening of, 254
  in dentin-pulp complex repair, 461
  development of, 58-80
    bell stage in, 62-64, 65, 67
    bud stage in, 60, 61
    cap stage in, 60, 62, 65
    crown pattern determination in, 67-68
    dental papilla in, 67
    dentogingival junction formation and, 270
    enamel knot, enamel cord, and enamel niche in, 64, 65
    epithelial-mesenchymal relationship in, 105-110
    eruption in, 73-77, 270
    fine structures of tooth germ in, 67
    fragmentation of dental lamina in, 67-68
    hard tissue formation in, 71-73
    innervation in, 68
    long-term potential for, 105
    permanent dentition in, 68, 69, 70
    primary epithelial band in, 58-60, 61
    root formation in, 73, 74, 75
    supporting tissue formation in, 77-79
    time scale for, 73
    vascular supply in, 68
  displacement and remodeling of, 498-500
  erupted, 47, 272
  extraction of, 466, 467
  functions of, 45
  ground section of, 47
  morphogenesis of, 104, 105
  neural crest and, 8
  position of, 323
  regenerating support of, 467
  repair of, 465, 466
  saliva in, 357-358
  shape of, 108-110
  structures of, 45-50
    dentin in, 49, 50
    enamel in, 48

Tooth—cont'd
  structures of—cont'd
    pulp in, 49, 50
  supporting tissues of, 50-52
  surface areas of, 45
  surface coatings of, 342-355
    calculus in, 342
    chairside microscopy in, 353, 354
    coronal cementum in, 342
    dental cuticle in, 342, 343
    dental plaque in, 342, 344-351, 352
    reduced dental epithelium in, 342
    salivary pellicle in, 342, 343, 344-345
  three-rooted, 75
  two-rooted, 75
  vertical drifting of, 500, 501, 502
Tooth germ
  development of, 60, 61
  fine structures of, 67
  mandibular, 34, 35
  maxillary, 38
  molar, 68, 69
  of permanent dentition, 70
  preeruptive tooth movement and, 317
Tooth movement
  abnormal, 332-333
  eruptive, 318-322
    bony remodeling in, 320-321
    histologic features of, 318-319
    hydrostatic pressure in, 320
    periodontal ligament in, 321-322
    root formation in, 319-320
  orthodontic, 334-335, 336, 337, 338
  posteruptive, 322-323
    growth accomodation in, 322
    interproximal wear compensation in, 322
    occlusal force in, 322, 323
    occlusal wear compensation in, 322
    soft tissue pressures in, 323
    transseptal ligament contraction in, 322-323
  preeruptive, 313-317
  shedding in, 324, 325-329, 330, 331
    odontoclasts in, 324, 325-327, 328
    pattern of, 329, 330, 331
    pressure in, 329
Trabecular bone, 120, 121, 122
Transforming growth factor beta
  in cell communication, 101
  osteoblasts and, 125
Transitional odontoblast, 152
Transseptal ligament, 322-323
TRAP; see Tyrosine-rich amelogenin protein
Treacher-Collins syndrome, 8, 10
Trigeminal nerve
  mandibular branch of, 34
  oral mucosa and, 420
Trilaminar disk, 7, 12
Tripartite secretory granules, 368
Trisomy, 1-2
Trophoblast, 4
Tryptophan, 221
Tuberculum impar, 25, 28

Tuberosity, maxillary, 316
Tubulin, 81, 84
Turnover time of epithelium, 396
Tyrosine, 221
Tyrosine-rich amelogenin protein, 219
  in enamel, 239

U
Unmyelinated axons in dental pulp, 204-205

V
Vagus nerve, 420
Valine, 221
Vascular subintima in temporomandibular joint, 441, 442
Vascular system
  in dental pulp, 201, 202, 203
  in developing tooth, 68
  in periodontium, 268
Versican
  in fibroblasts, 93
  in oral mucosa, 419
Vertical drift, 500
Vesicle of Merkel's cell, 410
Vestibular lamina, 60
Vimentin of fibroblast, 85
Virus, rubella, 40
Viscerocranium, 31, 32
Vitamin C in collagen synthesis, 88, 91
Vitamin D in bone metabolism, 126
Vitamin deficiencies, 43
von Ebner
  incremental lines of, 180, 181
  mineralization of dentin and, 160
von Korff's fibers, 165, 167

W
Waldeyer's ring, 395
Weil, zone of, 184, 185
Wound
  contraction of, 358
  healing of, 416
Woven bone, 135, 136
Wrinkling of skin, 481

X
X-irradiation in congenital defects, 40

Y
Yolk sac, 4, 5

Z
Zone of Weil, 184, 185
Zonula adherens, 86
Zonula occludens, 86
Zygoma, remodeling of, 502, 503
  versus maxilla, 504
Zygomatic arch
  in mastication, 450
  relocation of, 485
Zygomatic process, 39
Zygote, 1